Progress in

Obstetrics and Gynaecology

Progress in Obstetrics and Gynaecology
Edited by John Studd

Contents of Volume 15

First published 2003

ISBN 0 443 072221
ISSN 0261 0140

Progress in
Obstetrics and Gynaecology

VOLUME 16

Edited by

John Studd DSc MD FRCOG

Professor of Gynaecology and Consultant Gynaecologist
Academic Department of Obstetrics and Gynaecology,
Chelsea and Westminster Hospital, London, UK

ELSEVIER
CHURCHILL
LIVINGSTONE

EDINBURGH LONDON NEW YORK OXFORD PHILADELPHIA ST LOUIS SYDNEY TORONTO 2005

ELSEVIER

First published 2005

ISBN 0 443 074224
ISSN 0261 0140

British Library Cataloguing in Publication Data
A catalogue record for this book is available from the British Library

Library of Congress Cataloging in Publication Data
A catalog record for this book is available from the Library of Congress

Note
Medical knowledge is constantly changing. As new information becomes available, changes in treatment, procedures, equipment and the use of drugs become necessary. The editor, contributors and the publishers have taken care to ensure that the information given in this text is accurate and up to date. However, readers are strongly advised to confirm that the information, especially with regard to drug usage, complies with the latest legislation and standards of practice.

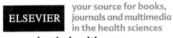

ELSEVIER your source for books,
journals and multimedia
in the health sciences
www.elsevierhealth.com

Commissioning Editor – Ellen Green
Project Manager – Frances Affleck
Designer – Sarah Russell
Editorial services and Typeset – BA & GM Haddock
Printed in UK

The
publisher's
policy is to use
**paper manufactured
from sustainable forests**

Contents

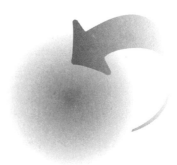

Contributors

Masoud Afnan FRCOG
Consultant Obstetrician and Gynaecologist, Assisted Conception Unit, Birmingham Women's Hospital, Birmingham, UK

Elizabeth N. Anionwu RN NV Tutor PhD CBE
Head, Mary Seacole Centre for Nursing Practice, Faculty of Health and Human Sciences, Thames Valley University, Ealing, London, UK Honorary Professor, London School of Hygiene and Tropical Medicine, London, UK

William Atiomo MBBS DM MA MRCOG
Clinical Senior Lecturer and Consultant Gynaecologist, Division of Obstetrics and Gynaecology, School of Human Development, University of Nottingham, Queen's Medical Centre, Nottingham, UK

Roksana Begum MBBS MRCOG
Staff Grade, Warwick Hospital, Warwick, UK

Debra L. Bogen MD FAAP
Assistant Professor of Pediatrics, Children's Hospital of Pittsburgh, University of Pittsburgh Medical Center, Pittsburgh, Pennsylvania, USA

Tom Bourne PhD MRCOG
Early Pregnancy, Gynaecological Ultrasound and MAS Unit, St George's Hospital Medical School, London, UK

Rianna Burrill BMedSci
Medical Student, University of Nottingham, Nottingham, UK

Linda Cardozo FRCOG
Professor of Urogynaecology, Department of Obstetrics and Gynaecology, King's College Hospital, London, UK

George Condous MRCOG
Early Pregnancy, Gynaecological Ultrasound and MAS Unit, St George's Hospital Medical School, London, UK

Diaa M. El-Mowafi MD
Professor, Obstetrics and Gynecology Department, Benha Faculty of
Medicine, Egypt; Educator and Researcher, Wayne State University, Detroit,
Michigan USA; and Fellow of Geneva University, Switzerland; Consultant
and Head of Obstetrics & Gynaecology Department, King Khalid General
Hospital, Hafr El-Batin, Saudi Arabia.

Alaa El-Ghobashy MBChB MSc MRCOG
Specialist Registrar in Obstetrics and Gynaecology, University Hospital of
North Staffordshire, West Midlands, UK

Horace M. Fletcher BSc MB BS DM(O&G) FRCOG FACOG
Senior Lecturer and Consultant, Department of Obstetrics and Gynaecology,
University of the West Indies, Kingston, Jamaica

Robert Fox MB MRCOG
Consultant Obstetrician, Division of Obstetrics, Gynaecology & Paediatrics,
Taunton & Somerset Hospital, TauntonA, UK

Joseph Frederick MB BS DM(O&G) FRCOG FACOG
Professor and Consultant, Department of Obstetrics and Gynaecology,
University of the West Indies, Kingston, Jamaica

Carole Gilling-Smith MA PhD FRCOG
Assisted Conception Unit, Chelsea & Westminster Hospital, London, UK

Joanna C. Girling MRCP MA MRCOG
Consultant Obstetrician and Gynaecologist, Department of Obstetrics and
Gynaecology, West Middlesex University Hospital, Middlesex, UK

Nahed Hammadieh MD MRCOG
Subspeciality Trainee in Reproductive Medicine, Cardiff Assisted
Reproduction Unit, University Hospital of Wales, Cardiff, UK

Joseph Hanoch MD
Gynaecological Oncology Fellow, Department of Gynaecological Oncology,
Hammersmith Hospital, Imperial College Medical School, London, UK

Simon Herrington DPhil FRCPath
Professor of Pathology, University of St Andrews, Bute Medical School, St
Andrews, Fife, UK

Jo Hockey MBBS MD MRCOG
Speciaist Registrar, Queen Charlotte's and Chelsea Hospital, London, UK

Judith Hyde MB MRCOG
Specialist Registrar, Southmead Hospital, Westbury-on-Trym, Bristol, UK

Sharif I. M. F. Ismail MSc MBA MA MMedSci(Ed) LLM MRCOG
Specialist Registrar in Obstetrics and Gynaecology, Singleton Hospital, Sketty,
Swansea, UK

Anna P. Kenyon MBChB MD
Specialist Registrar Obstetrics and Gynaecology, Department of Obstetrics and Gynaecology, West Middlesex University Hospital, Middlesex, UK

Asma Khalil MB BCh
Senior Resident in Obstetrics and Gynaecology, Ain Shams University Hospital, Cairo, Egypt

Ronald F. Lamont BSc MB ChB MD FRCOG
Consultant and Honorary Reader, Department of Obstetrics and Gynaecology, Northwick Park and St Mark's Hospital and Division of Paediatrics, Obstetrics and Gynaecology, Imperial College, London, UK

Frank Lawton MD FRCOG
Consultant Gynaecological Cancer Surgeon, Guy's, King's and St Thomas' Gynaecological Cancer Centre, King's College Hospital, London, UK

Martin Lupton MA MRCOG
Consultant Obstetrician and Gynaecologist, Chelsea and Westminster Hospital, London, UK

Tahir A. Mahmood MD FRCOG FRCPI MBA
Consultant Obstetrician and Gynaecologist/Clinical Director, Department of Obstetrics and Gynaecology, Forth Park Hospital, Kirkcaldy, Fife, UK

Angus McIndoe PhD FRCS MRCOG
Consultant Gynaecological Oncologist, Hammersmith Hospital, Imperial College Medical School, London, UK

Sharon Mensah RGN SCM
Haemoglobinopathy Specialist Nurse Counsellor, Ealing Sickle Cell and Thalassaemia Service, Southall, London, UK

Jack Moodley MBChB FCOG FRCOG(UK) MD
MRC/UKNZ Pregnancy Hypertension Research Unit and Department of Obstetrics and Gynaecology, Nelson R. Mandela School of Medicine, University of Natal, Durban, South Africa

James D. M. Nicopoullos MBBS BSc
Clinical Research Fellow, Assisted Conception Unit, Chelsea & Westminster Hospital, London, UK

Patrick O'Brien MB BCh MRCOG MFFP
Consultant in Obstetrics and Gynaecology, Obstetric Hospital, University College London Hospitals, London, UK

Emeka Okaro MRCOG
Early Pregnancy, Gynaecological Ultrasound and MAS Unit, St George's Hospital Medical School, London, UK

Reeba Oliver MBBS MRCOG
Clinical Research Fellow, Department of Obstetrics and Gynaecology, Northwick Park Hospital and St Mark's Hospital, Harrow, UK

Olufemi Olufowobi MRCOG
Clinical Research Fellow in Reproductive Medicine, Assisted Conception Unit, Birmingham Women's Hospital, Birmingham, UK

Eugene Oteng-Ntim MBBS MRCOG
Consultant Obstetrician, Guy's and St Thomas' Hospital, London, UK

Nicholas Panay BSc MRCOG MFFP
Consultant Obstetrician and Gynaecologist, Queen Charlotte's and Chelsea Hospital, London, UK

Fathima Paruk MBChB FCOG
Department of Anaesthesiology, Faculty of Health Sciences, University of Witwatersrand, Johannesburg, South Africa

Nicholas J. Raine-Fenning MBChB MRCOG PhD
Clinical Lecturer, Academic Division of Reproductive Medicine, School of Human Development, Queen's Medical Centre, Nottingham, UK

Jonathan W. A. Ramsay MS FRCS
Assisted Conception Unit, Chelsea & Westminster Hospital, London, UK

Dudley Robinson MRCOG
Sub-specialty Trainee – Urogynaecology, Department of Obstetrics and Gynaecology, King's College Hospital, London, UK

Khaldoun Sharif FRCOG MFFP MD
Consultant Obstetrician and Gynaecologist, Assisted Conception Unit, Birmingham Women's Hospital, Birmingham, UK

Aarti Sharma MBBS MRCOG
Specialist Registrar in Obstetrics and Gynaecology, City Hospital, Nottingham, UK

Kamal I. Shehata MRCOG
Senior Specialist Registrar, Department of Obstetrics and Gynaecology, University Hospital of Wales, Heath Park, Cardiff, Wales, UK

Olanrewaju O. Sorinola MBBS MRCOG MMedSci
Consultant Obstetrician and Gynaecologist and Honorary Senior Lecturer University of Warwick, Warwick Hospital, Warwick, UK

Philip Steer MD FRCOG
Professor of Obstetrics and Gynaecology, Chelsea and Westminster Hospital, London, UK

John W. W. Studd DSc MD FRCOG
Professor of Gynaecology and Consultant Gynaecologist, Academic Department of Obstetrics and Gynaecology, Chelsea and Westminster Hospital, London, UK

Keerthy R. Sunder MD MS DRCOG
Senior Resident Physician in Psychiatry, Magee Women's Hospital and
Western Psychiatric Institute and Clinic/University of Pittsburgh Medical
Center, Pittsburgh, Pennsylvania, USA

Emma Treloar MB MRCOG
Specialist Registrar, Gloucester Royal Infirmary, Gloucester, UK

Geoffrey Trew MBBS MRCOG
Consultant in Reproductive Medicine and Surgery, Hammersmith and Queen
Charlotte's Hospital and Honorary Senior Lecturer, Imperial College,
London, UK

Vineeta Verma MBBS MD MRCOG
Specialist Registrar, Queen Charlotte's and Chelsea Hospital, London, UK

Andrew D. Weeks MD MRCOG
Clinical Lecturer in Obstetrics and Gynaecology, Department of Obstetrics
and Gynaecology, Liverpool Women's Hospital, Liverpool, UK

Katherine L. Wisner MD MS
Professor of Psychiatry, Obstetrics and Gynecology and Reproductive
Sciences, and Epidemiology, Director, Women's Behavioral HealthCARE,
Western Psychiatric Institute and Clinic/University of Pittsburgh Medical
Center, Pittsburgh, Pennsylvania, USA

Mohammed Yousef MBBCh MA MRCOG
Staff Grade Doctor in Obstetrics and Gynaecology, Queen's Medical Centre,
Nottingham, UK

George Condous Emeka Okaro Tom Bourne

Complimentary role of ultrasound and serum hormone measurements in the management of early pregnancy complications

Early pregnancy units (EPUs) have revolutionised the management of early pregnancy complications both in terms of diagnostic accuracy and varied treatment options. In the latest UK triennial report into *Why Mothers Die?*, ectopic pregnancies (EP) accounted for 80% of early pregnancy deaths.[1] Access to such facilities for all women in the first trimester with vaginal bleeding and/or abdominal pain is the ideal. This is not feasible in all clinics, but a thorough understanding of the behaviour of serial hormone measurements in both normal and abnormal pregnancy as well as their ultrasonographic appearances are essential for all those managing these conditions.

In this review, we aim to assess the role of ultrasound and serum hormonal measurements in the management of early pregnancy complications. These include miscarriage, ectopic pregnancies, hydatidiform mole, pregnancies of unknown location (PUL) and ovarian cysts in early pregnancy. PUL is an ultrasonographic descriptive term and not a pathological entity *per se*. Transvaginal ultrasonography is an extension of the clinical examination and should be combined with the clinical scenario in order to make a diagnosis and formulate a management plan. The introduction of dedicated EPUs, has coincided with a shift away from a surgical approach to one based on either medical management or an expectant 'watch and wait' policy.[2]

George Condous MRCOG
Early Pregnancy, Gynaecological Ultrasound and MAS Unit, St George's Hospital Medical School, Cranmer Terrace, London SW17 0RE, UK (for correspondence, E-mail: gcondous@hotmail.com)

Emeka Okaro MRCOG
Early Pregnancy, Gynaecological Ultrasound and MAS Unit, St George's Hospital Medical School, Cranmer Terrace, London SW17 0RE, UK

Tom Bourne PhD MRCOG
Early Pregnancy, Gynaecological Ultrasound and MAS Unit, St George's Hospital Medical School, Cranmer Terrace, London SW17 0RE, UK

THE EARLY PREGNANCY ASSESSMENT UNIT

The EPU should provide an open access, ultrasound-based assessment of pregnancy duration, viability and location, which allows for informed and individualised management of the woman.

The cost benefits of the early pregnancy unit are well established[3] as admission can be avoided in about 40% of patients, with a further 20% requiring a shorter stay. Ideally, there should be a dedicated unit for the assessment and investigation of those women with suspected complications of early pregnancy. This will be centred on a scan room, run by dedicated ultrasound practitioners. There should be a private area in which the patient can change and also a separate counselling room with access to a counselling service and an outside line telephone.

Referral to the EPU may be by appointment only or a 'walk-in' self-referral system can operate. The latter will provide the patient with the means to contact a unit directly when problems arise, although this may make clinics busy. The patient's history can be collected on a proforma highlighting relevant factors predisposing to ectopic pregnancy.

A number of commercially available computer databases now exist which aid data collection and archiving. This means that the patient can leave the clinic with a detailed report and follow-up plan and a report distributed to the referring clinician immediately. This database also facilitates audit and research.

Availability of rapid serum hCG and progesterone assays will vary within units, but the judicious use and follow-up of serum hormonal levels are essential for a diagnosis where the pregnancy location is not readily identified or following treatment. This may be achieved in a number of ways but typically will be dependent upon a dedicated staff member to record and interpret results either via a computer database or log book. The patient is either contacted with further follow-up/intervention plans or the patient contacts the unit herself for these results.

Fortunately, the majority of women presenting with pain or bleeding in early pregnancy will present sub-acutely; in all cases, however, an initial assessment of haemodynamic compromise must be made. Facilities for resuscitation, obtaining venous access and commencing intravenous volume replacement should be available. All patients with a miscarriage or possible miscarriage who are booked for surgical evacuation require a full blood count and grouping as a minimum.

Anti-D immunoglobulin should be given to non-sensitised Rhesus D negative women in the following circumstances: (i) an ectopic pregnancy; (ii) a therapeutic termination of pregnancy (surgical or medical); (iii) a threatened or spontaneous miscarriage after 12 weeks' gestation; and (iv) a surgical evacuation of retained products of conception prior to 12 weeks' gestation.[4] Where there is heavy, recurrent or painful bleeding prior to 12 weeks' gestation, anti-D 500 IU prophylaxis is also recommended.

The psychological morbidity associated with early pregnancy loss is documented.[5] Women, and their partners, who are diagnosed with early pregnancy failure, should be offered support and counselling.

Transvaginal sonography (TVS) should be the primary imaging modality in the assessment of early pregnancy patients. Transvaginal probes provide high-resolution images of the pelvic organs, providing reliable and reproducible information. The use of a vaginal probe can be thought of as a natural extension of the conventional bimanual examination. The fact that a full bladder is not required improves patient acceptability.

The minimum requirements are a transvaginal probe (6–7.5 MHz), a 3.5 MHz abdominal transducer and facilities for capturing images – either as a hard copy or digitally. The facility to perform Doppler studies, although not mandatory, can be helpful in difficult cases. Appropriate cleaning of the transducer using a germicidal (e.g. 70% alcohol) cloth or spray, after first wiping off the gel, is effective in preventing cross infection.

ULTRASONOGRAPHIC MILESTONES

Knowledge of the normal milestones in early pregnancy that can be seen by ultrasonography is important. The first definitive sign of pregnancy is the gestational sac. Before the gestational sac becomes visible, the endometrium is markedly echogenic and the arcuate vessels are somewhat prominent.[6] This is known as the decidual reaction and is non-diagnostic as it can also be seen in the normal late secretory phase.

The gestational sac becomes visible during the fourth week and appears as a thick echogenic ring surrounding a sonolucent centre. This sonolucent centre is the fluid-filled chorionic sac[6] and is eccentrically placed within the endometrium. As the gestation progresses, the yolk sac is the first structure visualised inside the chorionic sac.[7] The yolk sac appears during week five. The embryonic pole will follow this (embryonic growth rate is 1 mm/day), with a detectable heartbeat first seen in the sixth week.[8] Eventually the amnion surrounding the embryo, which is distinctly different to the yolk sac, will be visualised.

The yolk sac when normal is regular and spherical, being up to 6 mm in diameter. It has a very bright echogenic rim around a sonolucent centre, appearing like a 'halo'. The normal embryo first appears as a thickening along the yolk sac and embryonic cardiac activity can be visualised as a 'flickering signal'.

It is important to distinguish the true intra-uterine gestational sac from the so-called 'pseudogestational sac'. The 'pseudosac' is a misnomer and probably represents a fluid collection or debris in the cavity.[9] This sign is largely based on historical data and relates to the use of transabdominal ultrasonography. Using high-resolution vaginal probes, misinterpretation is less likely.

MISCARRIAGE

Ultrasound and the diagnosis of miscarriage

Miscarriage is known to occur in at least 10–20% of clinical pregnancies.[10] The majority occur before the thirteenth week. The risk of miscarriage is reduced to 3% if a viable embryo has been seen by ultrasonography. EPUs have been introduced in order to improve the efficiency of dealing with women with early pregnancy loss.[11]

The gestational age of the pregnancy may be uncertain, and in these circumstances early fetal demise can be difficult to diagnose. If the gestation

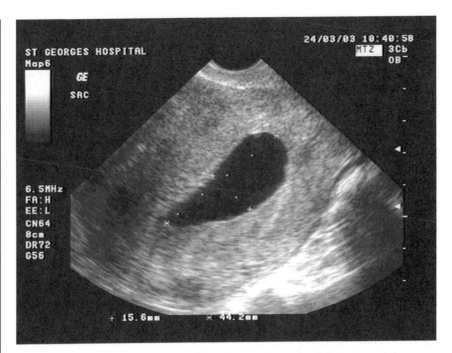

ST GEORGES HOSPITAL

24/03/03 10:40:58

Fig. 1 Anembryonic pregnancy – gestational sac > 20 mm in diameter.

sac diameter is > 20 mm without a yolk sac, this is classified as an anembryonic pregnancy or early embryonic demise (Fig. 1).[12] If the crown rump length is at least 6 mm and there is no fetal cardiac activity or if the crown rump length is < 6 mm with no change at the time of a repeat scan 7 days later, this is classified as a missed miscarriage or early fetal demise.[12] Care must be taken when making this diagnosis as approximately one-third of embryos with a crown rump length of less than 5 mm have no demonstrable cardiac activity.[13] Whenever there is uncertainty about the viability of a pregnancy, a repeat scan at an interval of 1 week is necessary before a definite diagnosis can be made. Small or irregular gestational sacs, discrepancies between the crown rump length and gestational age, or an abnormal embryonic heart-rate pattern are predictors of a poor pregnancy outcome.[14] An incomplete miscarriage is characterised by a heterogeneous appearance and the presence of irregular tissues (Fig. 2), with or without a gestational sac within the uterine cavity.[12] The endometrial midline echo will usually be distorted. According to Neilsen *et al.*,[15] if the endometrial thickness is < 15 mm and there is no evidence of retained products of conception, then the miscarriage is classified as being complete.[12] There is a wide variation in the published literature on the optimal cut-off levels to diagnose incomplete miscarriage. Cut-offs between 8 and 15 mm have been used to differentiate between incomplete and complete miscarriage.[15,16] However, these cut-offs have never been prospectively validated. In our unit, if the endometrial thickness is < 15 mm and there is no evidence of retained products of conception, then the miscarriage is classified as being complete; however, we place more emphasis on the clinical picture. Care should be taken in women thought to have a complete miscarriage. As no

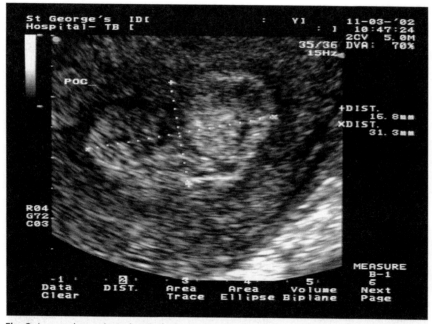

Fig. 2 Incomplete miscarriage – heterogeneous tissue within the endometrial cavity. [Reproduced from Condous G, Okara E and Bourne T[63] with permission]

pregnancy has been seen at any time, it is possible that such patients, in fact, have an ectopic pregnancy. We, therefore, manage patients with a presumed complete miscarriage in the same way as those with a pregnancy of unknown location (PUL). This will be discussed in detail below.

The management of miscarriage

More women with a miscarriage are choosing expectant management. In a recent large prospective observational trial, Luise et al.[12] demonstrated that 70% of 451 women with retained products of conception will choose expectant management after appropriate counselling. This cohort of women underwent weekly follow-up with TVS and over 80% of those with an incomplete miscarriage who were managed expectantly completed their miscarriage without surgical intervention within 2 weeks. For other types of miscarriage, expectant management was less successful. The rate of spontaneous completion of a missed miscarriage may be as high as 84%;[17] in a more recent study, 76% of missed miscarriages and 66% of anembryonic pregnancies resolved without intervention.[12] Other authors have reported a success rate for expectant management of missed miscarriage of as low as 24.7%.[18] Miscarriage in these two groups is often more painful and less likely to become complete in the same time span as in a patient presenting with an incomplete miscarriage. In the study by Luise et al.,[12] only 30% of missed miscarriages had resolved by the end of the first week and 25% of anembryonic pregnancies. By the end of week two the number had risen to 59% and 52%, respectively (Table 1).[12] In this study, some women persisted with expectant management for over a month; as a result, the total number of women achieving their miscarriage

Table 1 Types of miscarriage and outcomes in patients who chose expectant management

Group classification at diagnosis	Patients	Complete miscarriage By day 7	By day 14	Successful outcome by day 46
Incomplete miscarriage	221 (49)	117 (53)	185 (84)	201 (91)
Missed miscarriage	138 (31)	41 (30)	81 (59)	105 (76)
Anembryonic pregnancy	92 (20)	23 (25)	48 (52)	61 (66)
Total	451 (100)	181 (40)	314 (70)	367 (81)

Values are numbers (percentages).
Reproduced with permission from British Medical Journal.[12]

increased. However, in practice, most women will not choose such an approach. If they have a missed miscarriage or anembryonic pregnancy, women can be told that they have about a 50% chance of resolving their miscarriage without intervention within 2 weeks. After this time period, their chances of doing so diminish and in such circumstances we offer surgical evacuation of the uterus. Our anecdotal experience is that whilst expectant management is valid for women attending with symptoms to an EPU, the situation is different when the diagnosis is made as a chance finding at the time of a nuchal scan. Our view is that such cases are more likely to experience severe pain or heavy bleeding whether they receive expectant management or medical therapy; consequently, these women should be offered surgery.

The optimal follow-up for women undergoing expectant management of miscarriage is not standardised. Luise et al.[19] have shown that 91% of women presenting with an incomplete miscarriage resolved their miscarriage; 54% had done so by the end of 1 week and 83% by the end of week two.[19] After 2 weeks, the odds of a miscarriage becoming complete are significantly reduced. It is, therefore, a reasonable policy to advise women to give themselves 2 weeks to complete their miscarriage, and that intervention after this time may be reasonable. In this study, neither the presence of a gestational sac within the cavity nor the thickness of the endometrium was clinically useful in determining the outcome of expectant management.[19] Table 2 shows the number of days taken to complete a miscarriage related to the ultrasound

Table 2 The presence of a gestational sac (GS) or endometrial thickness (ET) on the outcome of expectant management for incomplete, first-trimester miscarriage

Women/ variable	Complete miscarriages n (% of total)	Days to completion n (% of group)	Mean (range)
Endometrial thickness (mm)			
< 11	30 (13.6)	28 (94.3)	6.8 (2–15)
11–15	54 (24.4)	50 (93.3)	8.8 (2–21)
16–21	41 (18.6)	38 (92.7)	8.9 (1–22)
> 21	26 (11.8)	22 (84.6)	10.4 (3–27)
Gestational sac (mm)			
3–28	70 (31.7)	64 (91.4)	8.7 (2–32)

Reproduced with permission from Ultrasound Obstetrics and Gynecology.[19]

Table 3 Follow-up data from patients undergoing expectant management for an incomplete, first-trimester miscarriage

Time from diagnosis (days)	Women	Completed spontaneous miscarriages n (% in group)	ERPC n (% in group)	Accumulated spontaneous miscarriages n (%)
1–7	221	120 (54.3)	8 (3.6)	
8–14	93	64 (68.8)	3 (3.2)	184 (83)
15–21	26	13 (50.0)	5* (19.2)	197 (89)
> 22	8	4 (50.0)	4 (50.0)	201 (91)

ERPC, evacuation of retained products of conception.
*4 elective, 1 emergency.
Reproduced with permission from *Ultrasound Obstetrics and Gynecology*.[19]

findings in this study and Table 3 the proportion of women completing their miscarriage in relation to time. The rate of complications is so low that one follow-up visit after 2 weeks to assess the clinical situation is reasonable. However, women should be able to contact the clinic at any time for advice or support. The emphasis for follow-up should be more orientated towards counselling rather than ultrasound-based assessment of the uterus.

The infective morbidity of any non-surgical approach, whether it is expectant or medical, has been a cause for concern.[20] However, the available data suggest a reduction in clinical pelvic infection using this approach.[21,22] In relation to long-term complications, it is re-assuring that Blohm et al.[23] showed no difference in future fertility rates between those whose miscarriage has been managed expectantly and those who have undergone surgical evacuation.

Threatened miscarriage is a very common first trimester problem occurring in up to one-third of pregnancies.[24] It is a clinical diagnosis defined as vaginal bleeding in the first trimester with or without abdominal pain. In this situation, ultrasound is essential to determine the viability of the pregnancy. If the uterus contains an empty gestational sac > 20 mm on TVS, this is almost certainly an anembryonic pregnancy; however, an interval scan in 7 days is recommended if there is any doubt. Sub-chorionic haematomas are common and seen in up to 18% of women with a threatened miscarriage.[25] They are insignificant sonographic findings and there is no association between the rate of premature delivery and haematoma size.[25] The confirmation of fetal cardiac activity in a threatened miscarriage confers an excellent prognosis.[26]

ECTOPIC PREGNANCY

During the past 25 years, the incidence of ectopic pregnancy has progressively increased (9.6/1000 pregnancies in the UK), whilst the morbidity and associated mortality have substantially decreased (0.4/100 ectopic pregnancies). Ectopic pregnancy is the fourth leading cause of direct maternal deaths in the UK, accounting for 80% of first trimester deaths,[1] with the ratio of intra-uterine to ectopic pregnancies as high as 50:1.

With the advent of EPUs, treatment options have become less radical as the number of stable ectopic pregnancies diagnosed increases. The evolution of treatment has progressed from salpingectomy at the time of laparotomy to conservation of the fallopian tube by laparoscopy and, more recently, to medical management in the form of systemic or local methotrexate therapy and in selected cases expectant management for failing ectopic pregnancies.

Unfortunately it is still possible to see ultrasound reports that read 'empty uterus, ectopic pregnancy cannot be excluded'. This is not helpful and will invariably lead to the patient undergoing an unnecessary laparoscopy. Advances in ultrasound technology, in particular transvaginal probes, has led to the diagnosis of ectopic pregnancy being frequently based on the positive visualisation of a pregnancy outside the uterus. In general, ectopic pregnancies (EPs) are now diagnosed at an earlier stage in their natural history and so the classic presentation of acute abdominal pain secondary to tubal rupture is less common.

The frequency of heterotopic pregnancy in spontaneous conceptions is estimated between 1:10,000 and 1:50,000, but as high as 1:100 in assisted conceptions.[27] If a woman has undergone IVF/GIFT, one should always thoroughly assess the adnexa even in the presence of an intrauterine sac.

Those women with a high risk of EPs should be advised to present to an EPU as soon as they know they are pregnant. Transvaginal ultrasonography together with the use of quantitative serum hCG levels should avoid unnecessary laparoscopy. If an ectopic pregnancy is present, TVS should see it in up to 93% of cases.[28] Misdiagnosis should be a rare event and the standard of care in any EPU should be determined by its false positive and negative rates for the diagnosis of ectopic pregnancy.

Ultrasound and the diagnosis of ectopic pregnancy

The appearances of an ectopic pregnancy on TVS may be highly variable. Classically, they are described as the 'bagel sign' with a hyperechoic ring around the gestation sac in the adnexal region (Fig. 3), but more often they are seen as a small inconglomerate mass next to the ovary – we have described this as the 'blob sign'.[29] By pressing the vaginal probe gently against the ectopic pregnancy, one sees that it moves separately to the ovary. The dimensions of the ectopic should be described, as should the presence of an embryo with or without a heartbeat. Haematoceles have a characteristic appearance, and the amount of bleeding that has occurred should be commented upon by looking for fluid or blood in the pouch of Douglas (Fig. 4). The appearances of blood and clot as opposed to serous fluid are quite different and should not be confused. This information is of importance to the clinician as the management options for EP are rapidly changing, and depend very much on the ultrasound appearances and the level of serum hCG.

A recent meta-analysis has shown that the most appropriate TVS criterion on which to diagnose EP is any non-cystic adnexal mass.[30] This leads to a positive predictive value of 96.3%, negative predictive value of 94.8%, specificity of 98.9% and sensitivity of 84.4%. This performed better than the visualisation of an embryo with a heartbeat in the adnexa, an adnexal cystic mass, or an adnexal mass with an echogenic or 'tubal' ring. This will not surprise experienced operators who will have seen many ectopic pregnancies that appear as an inhomogeneous small mass next to the ovary with no evidence of a sac or embryo – the 'blob sign' (Fig. 5).

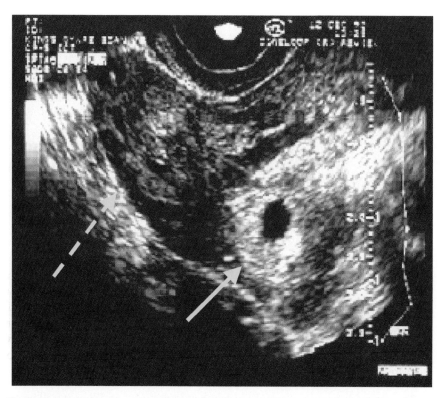

Fig. 3 Ectopic pregnancy – 'bagel' sign. Broken arrow depicts the right ovary and solid arrow shows ectopic pregnancy. [Reproduced from Condous G, Okara E and Bourne T[63] with permission]

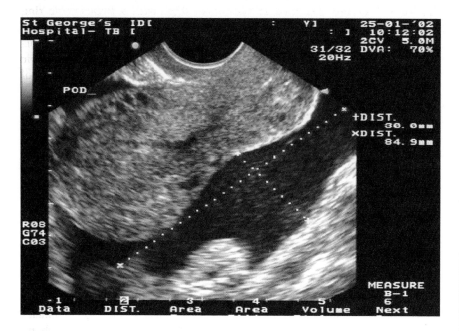

Fig. 4 Haemoperitoneum – blood in the pouch of Douglas.

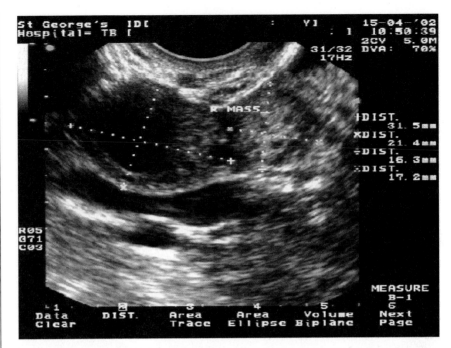

Fig. 5 Ectopic pregnancy – inhomogeneous adnexal mass. [Reproduced from Condous G, Okara E and Bourne T[63] with permission]

The corpus luteum is a useful guide when looking for an EP, as it will be on the ipsilateral side in over 85% of cases.[31]

Medical therapy with methotrexate has been reported to be successful in 71–100% of cases.[32] Successful outcome is dependent on the initial serum hCG levels (the likelihood of treatment failure is greater at higher serum hCG concentrations) and the ultrasonographic findings. The ectopic gestation should be less than 3 cm in diameter; if a crown rump is visualised in the gestational sac, there should be no cardiac activity. There should be no signs of haemoperitoneum on TVS. In the UK, 50 mg/m² methotrexate is administered intramuscularly on day 0. Up to 13% of cases require a second dose of methotrexate if the hCG levels do not fall by 15% between days 4 and 7.[33] In the US, 1 mg/kg methotrexate is given on days 1, 3 and 5 with folinic acid rescue on days 2, 4 and 6. Resolution rates between the two regimens are comparable.

In our unit, we offer medical management to 20% of women with ectopic pregnancies. These women are clinically stable, serum hCG < 10,000 IU/l, EP diameter < 30 mm, no fetal heart activity and no signs of haemoperitoneum.

Ultrasound in the management of ectopic pregnancy

TVS is not only a useful diagnostic tool, but it can also be used in the treatment of EP. Methotrexate can be administered transvaginally under sonographic guidance, but when compared to laparoscopic salpingostomy in a randomised control trial involving 100 women, it was less successful.[34]

The results of another smaller study[35] involving 36 haemodynamically stable women with a small unruptured EP showed that treatment success of

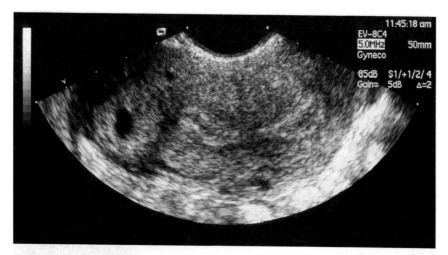

Fig. 6 Interstitial pregnancy.

methotrexate administered transvaginally under ultrasound guidance was significantly better than the 'blind' intratubal injection under laparoscopic guidance (RR, 1.6; 95% CI, 1.0–2.5).

The combined results of three studies[34,36,37] involving 95 women with a small unruptured EP showed no significant difference in the primary treatment success between methotrexate transvaginally under sonographic guidance and systemic methotrexate in a single dose intramuscular regimen (RR, 1.2; 95% CI, 0.95–1.5). The use of these transvaginal treatment techniques requires a high degree of training and skill, and one would not recommend their use especially in light of the evidence suggesting that single dose methotrexate is just as effective.

Non-tubal ectopic pregnancies

Ectopic pregnancies are classified according to their site of implantation. At least 95% of EPs will be tubal and the vast majority of these will be ampullary. Other sites account for only 5% of EPs, but they contribute a disproportionate number of serious complications. They may be difficult to diagnose, and are associated with significant haemorrhage leading to a higher morbidity and mortality than tubal EP.

Interstitial pregnancies account for about 2% of EP.[38] The sonographic image of the interstitial pregnancy is that of a bulge in the cornual area of the uterus where an extremely thin myometrial mantel surrounds the hyperechoic ring of the gestational sac (Fig. 6).[39] The gestation sac should be located more than 1 cm from the endometrial echo. Colour flow Doppler studies may help localise the pregnancy (Fig. 7). Hypo-echogenic lesions situated in the cornual region may persist for 1 year or more following treatment despite resumption of normal menstruation.[40]

Cervical ectopic pregnancies are rare (Fig. 8). The cervix is classically barrel-shaped. It is important to differentiate this from an intact gestational sac passing through the cervix, which usually causes intense pain, whereas true

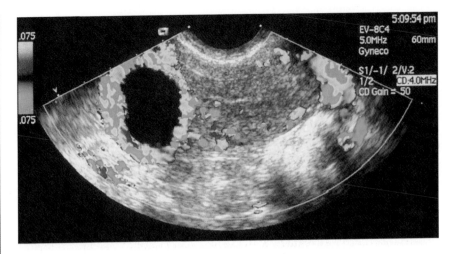

Fig. 7 Interstitial pregnancy with colour Doppler.

cervical pregnancies are often relatively asymptomatic. On TVS, a sac passing through the cervix will appear to be sliding through the cervix. Colour Doppler studies may assist in the diagnosis. The uterine artery is a useful anatomical marker and the presence of blood flow around the gestation sac is more suggestive of an implanted sac rather than one passing though the cervix. Ovarian pregnancy is also rare and has an incidence of 1:7000 deliveries and 1:34 EPs.[41] Diagnosis can be difficult, but the finding of an hyperechoic chorionic ring which moves with the ovary is suggestive.

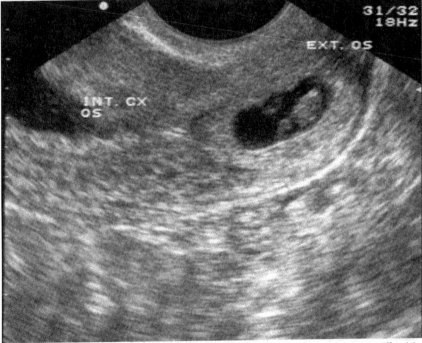

Fig. 8 Cervical pregnancy. [Reproduced from Condous G, Okara E and Bourne T[63] with permission]

Abdominal pregnancies are rare and tend to be diagnosed later in pregnancy. The ultrasound features are well described and include the finding of an empty uterus separate from the fetus, no uterine mantle around the pregnancy or fetus, placenta in an unusual location and extreme oligohydramnios resulting in crowding of the fetal structures.[42,43]

Caesarean section scar pregnancy has been described only recently. The diagnosis is based on the visualisation of trophoblast located between the bladder and the anterior uterine wall.[44] The implantation into the scar should be further confirmed by applying gentle pressure on the cervix during a TVS. A gestational sac implanted outside the uterine cavity will remain in place during such a manoeuvre, whilst a cervical miscarriage will be easily displaced.[45]

Heterotopic pregnancies are fortunately unusual; however, with the advent of reproductive technologies, their number is steadily increasing.[27] This has been mentioned above, but a high index of suspicion should be present when a patient has become pregnant with the help of an assisted conception unit.

Whilst the increased resolution obtained by transvaginal ultrasonography represents a significant advance, it creates it own problems. The earlier that patients present to the EPU the more women will have an inconclusive ultrasound scan, where no ultrasound features of either an extra- or intra-uterine pregnancy can be seen. It is the role of the early pregnancy team to follow through such patients until a diagnosis is established either on the basis of ultrasound findings or serum hCG and progesterone values.

HYDATIDIFORM MOLE

TVS has led to the early diagnosis of molar pregnancy. Classically, the 'snow-storm' effect previously described was historically seen with transabdominal sonography.[46] In modern practice, the findings seen on TVS are described as

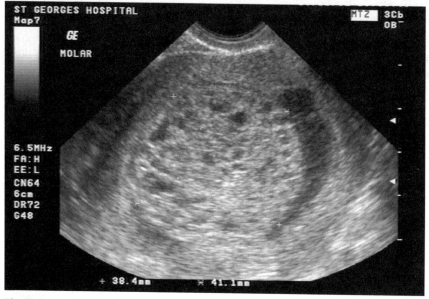

Fig. 9 Hydatidiform mole.

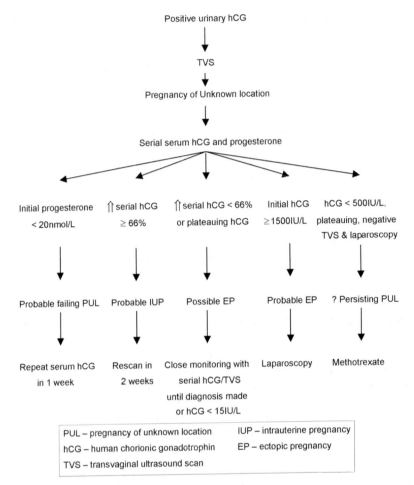

Positive urinary hCG

↓

TVS

↓

Pregnancy of Unknown location

↓

Serial serum hCG and progesterone

Initial progesterone < 20nmol/L	⇈ serial hCG ≥ 66%	⇈ serial hCG < 66% or plateauing hCG	Initial hCG ≥1500IU/L	hCG < 500IU/L, plateauing, negative TVS & laparoscopy
Probable failing PUL	Probable IUP	Possible EP	Probable EP	? Persisting PUL
Repeat serum hCG in 1 week	Rescan in 2 weeks	Close monitoring with serial hCG/TVS until diagnosis made or hCG < 15IU/L	Laparoscopy	Methotrexate

PUL – pregnancy of unknown location IUP – intrauterine pregnancy
hCG – human chorionic gonadotrophin EP – ectopic pregnancy
TVS – transvaginal ultrasound scan

Fig. 10 Flow chart for the management of pregnancies of unknown location. [Reproduced from Condous G, Okara E and Bourne T[63] with permission]

multiple small sonolucent areas (Fig. 9), which correspond to the 'grape-like' vesicles that one sees on gross pathological examination.[47]

The majority of cases of molar pregnancy (67%) seen in an EPU now present as missed or anembryonic pregnancies sonographically.[48] This highlights the importance of histological examination of products of conception to diagnose gestational trophoblastic disease. Although serum hCG levels will invariably be high, this is not specific.

PREGNANCY OF UNKNOWN LOCATION

In 8–31% of women presenting to an EPU with a positive hCG, a pregnancy will not be visualised on ultrasound and so no diagnosis can be made.[49,50] They are given the label 'pregnancy of unknown location' (PUL). The varying prevalence of PUL can be attributable to an ultrasonographer's ability to visualise intra- or extra-uterine pregnancies. An inexperienced ultrasonographer could potentially overlook early intra-uterine gestational sacs or adnexal masses which, in turn, would result in a higher prevalence of PUL for a given EPU.

In this situation there are four possible clinical outcomes: (i) a failing pregnancy; (ii) an intra-uterine pregnancy (IUP); (iii) an ectopic pregnancy; or (iv) a persisting PUL (Fig. 10).

Women with a PUL should be managed expectantly on the basis of serum hormonal measurements of hCG and progesterone. This can be on an outpatient basis. Expectant management has been shown to be safe, reduce the need for unnecessary surgical intervention and is not associated with any serious adverse outcomes. Nevertheless, 9–29%[49,51] of these women will require surgical intervention due to a worsening clinical condition or non-declining serum hCG. This management approach should also apply to women where it is thought there has been a complete miscarriage.

The discriminatory zone and serial monitoring of hormone levels

When the location of a pregnancy cannot be confirmed on the basis of an ultrasound scan, the use of hormonal markers and their interpretation are essential. An understanding of the discriminatory zone, the doubling time of serum hCG in early normal pregnancy and the correlation between low serum progesterone and spontaneous resolution of pregnancy are all important biophysiological concepts in the management of pregnancies of unknown location.

The concept of combining ultrasound with measurements of serum hCG using a discriminatory zone is well described.[52-54] By correlating the serum hCG values to the size of an intra-uterine gestational sac, a value can be chosen that corresponds to the threshold above which an intra-uterine gestation sac should be seen. If a sac cannot be seen above the threshold value, then steps must be taken to determine whether the pregnancy is abnormal or ectopic.

Barnhart et al.[52] showed that above a discriminatory level of 1500 IU/l, an intra-uterine gestation sac was seen in 91.5% of cases compared with 28.6% when levels were below 1500 IU/l. However, it should be noted that the discriminatory zone might vary among institutions due to different types of equipment, the frequency of the probe used and assay techniques. It is also dependent on operator experience. Higher serum hCG titres are seen in early multiple pregnancies and may lead to unnecessary concern about the location of the pregnancy.

In practice, a single measurement of hCG will not be diagnostic in the majority of cases. In most cases when the serum hCG is above the discriminatory zone and an ectopic pregnancy is present, it will be large enough to be visualised by ultrasonography. The problem arises at lower serum hCG levels or in the smaller number of cases when an ultrasound diagnosis cannot be made. In these cases, it is possible to distinguish between a PUL which will develop into a normal intra-uterine pregnancy and those that subsequently become ectopic pregnancies on the basis of the rate of serum hCG increase. This can be expressed as the slope of the log hCG–time curve or as the percentage increase in serum hCG over a given sampling interval. For practical purposes, the rate is most easily determined from two samples drawn 48 h apart. The differences between the two serum hCG values obtained is represented as a percentage of the initial value. In normal intra-uterine pregnancies, there should be a 66% rise over the baseline value over 48 h.[55]

Using this well-known algorithm is not without its pitfalls, as approximately 15% of normal intra-uterine pregnancies screened in this way will appear abnormal, and 13% of ectopic pregnancies will give contradictory results and delay the diagnosis beyond 48 h. It is possible to have either a 'sick' intra-uterine or a 'flourishing' ectopic pregnancy, and both can give conflicting results.

PULs should be stratified into those with either a low or high risk of ectopic pregnancy. The vast majority of these will be at low risk and, in turn, are made up of failing PUL and intra-uterine pregnancies (IUP). A failing PUL may be intra-uterine or extra-uterine and generally will resolve spontaneously. A failing PUL is not necessarily a failing intra-uterine pregnancy. These pregnancies are never seen on TVS, their baseline serum progesterone at presentation will be < 20 nmol/l and serial serum hCG levels fall. In these cases, serum hCG levels should be repeated in 1 week to confirm the diagnosis. A baseline serum progesterone level of < 20 nmol/l will identify a failing PUL with a positive predictive value of ≥ 95%.[51] This compares favourably with complex multiparameter diagnostic models.[51] In contrast, on-going IUP usually demonstrate a > 66% increase in serial serum hCG levels taken at 48-h intervals. In these cases, a repeat TVS should be repeated in 2 weeks to confirm the diagnosis.

In our series of 208 consecutive PULs, 87.3% were at low risk of ectopic pregnancy and were made up of either intra-uterine pregnancies or failing PUL.[56] Serum hormonal levels may pick out a patient who is at risk of ectopic pregnancy, but it is rarely diagnostic. Changing serum hCG and initial serum progesterone levels tell us if the pregnancy is viable, but they tell us nothing about the location of the pregnancy. If the location of pregnancy is not clear on TVS, serial ultrasound follow-up is essential to make the diagnosis. Unfortunately, this results in a very high workload for EPUs, as well as additional psychological stress for the women due to prolonged uncertainty.

One cannot overemphasise that hormonal results should not be taken in isolation and the clinical assessment and subsequent ultrasound findings are essential to the on-going management. When the diagnosis of ectopic pregnancy has been established (and this should be possible by transvaginal ultrasonography in the majority of cases), then appropriate medical or surgical management should be initiated. The overall rate of intervention for PUL managed expectantly in our series is 12.1%, which is consistent with other groups.[51]

Persisting pregnancies of unknown location

To date, there are no published data in the literature relating to persisting PUL. This small subset of women are defined as those where the serum hCG levels fail to decline, where there is no evidence of trophoblast disease, and the location of the pregnancy cannot be identified whether by ultrasound or laparoscopy. In general, the serum hCG levels are low (< 500 IU/l) and have reached a plateau. We have treated four such women successfully with methotrexate 50 mg/m² and their serum hCG levels subsequently resolved.

In our view, great care should be given before giving medical treatment for a PUL before the site of the pregnancy has been identified. A positive serum hCG does not always indicate pregnancy. Germ-cell tumours may secrete hCG and should be considered, especially if a women is adamant that she cannot be pregnant. In our unit, we have seen one posterior cranial fossa germ-cell tumour and one placental site trophoblastic tumour of the ovary present in this way.[57]

CO-EXISTENT PATHOLOGY

The incidence of adnexal pathology detected in the first trimester varies from 0.17–2.94%.[58,59] In a study of some 2245 women scanned at the end of the first trimester, 1.2% of the total persisted beyond 16 weeks and subsequently were surgically removed – there were no cases of malignancy.[58] In a study of 55,278 pregnancy terminations, there were 2 cases of malignancy.[59] Expectant management is advocated, at least until the pregnancy is beyond 14 weeks' gestation. When symptomatic, simple ovarian cysts diagnosed during pregnancy can be successfully and safely treated with sonographic-guided cyst aspiration.[60] Adnexal masses can be accurately classified according to TVS.[58,61] However, in the few cases when the nature of the cyst is in question, one must balance the risks to the pregnancy from intervention versus the risk of malignancy.

In a recent study in our unit, the majority of cysts detected in early pregnancy were physiological and resolved spontaneously.[62] Very few persisted and only 0.13% (4/3000) of all women who initially presented required acute intervention during their pregnancy.[62] The expectant management of ovarian cysts detected in the first trimester is safe and should be encouraged. We concluded that examining the ovaries in the first trimester is of limited value.

CONCLUSIONS

The wide-spread use of early pregnancy units has led to a significant improvement in the management of early pregnancy complications. This has been facilitated by the use of transvaginal sonography and access to rapid immunoassay of serum hCG and progesterone. The importance of determining viability, gestation and, most importantly, the location of the pregnancy at the first trimester ultrasound scan cannot be over emphasised.

Ideally, all women with vaginal bleeding with or without abdominal pain in the first trimester should be evaluated in a dedicated early pregnancy unit by appropriately trained staff. Once a diagnosis has been made, the clinician should individualise the management in the context of a woman's given circumstances. Her clinical and emotional state, her level of understanding and compliance, as well as her access to after-hours emergency facilities are all important factors.

The diagnosis of ectopic pregnancy is now largely based on the positive visualisation of a pregnancy outside the uterus. However, the more wide-spread use of high frequency vaginal probes and earlier presentation of women in their pregnancy has led to an increase in the number of inconclusive scans. Serum hormone levels on their own predict the viability, but not the location of PULs. Combining these results with sonographic follow-up is essential in locating the pregnancy. In the future, we hope to develop new hormonal indices that will not only predict viability, but also locate the pregnancy.

KEY POINTS FOR CLINICAL PRACTICE

- Early pregnancy complications should be assessed in dedicated early pregnancy units.

- Facilities for transvaginal sonography and same-day immunoassay of serum hCG and progesterone should be available.

- The psychological morbidity associated with early pregnancy loss is well documented and all early pregnancy units should have access to counselling services.

- Knowledge of normal sonographic milestones is essential.

- If there is any doubt as to the viability of an early pregnancy, an interval scan in 7 days is recommended.

- An understanding of various sonographic definitions of miscarriage is important.

- Anembryonic pregnancy/blighted ovum (early embryonic demise): gestational sac mean diameter of at least 20 mm with no embryonic/extra-embryonic structures present.

- Missed miscarriage (early fetal demise): CRL of at least 6 mm with no cardiac activity, or no change in size on weekly serial scanning.

- Incomplete miscarriage: disrupted endometrial echo, measuring more than 15 mm in the anteroposterior plane, with the presence of heterogeneous and irregular tissues.

- Complete miscarriage: endometrial thickness of less than 15 mm measured in the anteroposterior plane associated with the cessation of heavy bleeding and pain.

- Up to 90% of ectopic pregnancies should be visualised using TVS.

- Classically with TVS, one visualises an inhomogeneous mass adjacent to the ovary – the 'blob sign'.

- Heterotopic pregnancies occur in 1% of IVF/GIFT pregnancies.

- The majority of cases of molar pregnancy seen in an EPU are described as missed or anembryonic pregnancies sonographically; therefore, histological examination of products of conception is essential for the diagnosis of gestational trophoblastic disease.

- The rate of pregnancies of unknown location is indirectly proportional to the quality of the those scanning in an early pregnancy unit.

- Expectant management of pregnancies of unknown location is safe and the interpretation of serum hCG and progesterone levels in these cases is cornerstone to the management.

- The majority of ovarian cysts diagnosed in the first trimester are physiological.

- Expectant management of ovarian cysts diagnosed in the first trimester is advocated.

References

1 Anon. Why Mothers Die, Triennial Report Confidential Enquiry into Maternal Deaths, United Kingdom 1997–1999. London: RCOG Press, 2002

2 Hemminki E. Treatment of miscarriage: current practice and rationale. Obstet Gynecol 1998; 91: 247–253

3 Bigrigg MA, Read MD. Management of women referred to early pregnancy assessment unit: care and cost effectiveness. BMJ 1991; 302: 577–579

4 Royal College of Obstetricians and Gynaecologists. Clinical Guideline Number 22. Anti-D Immunoglobulin for Rh Prophylaxis. London: RCOG Press, 2002

5 Nielsen S, Hahlin M, Möller A et al. Bereavement, grieving and psychological morbidity after first trimester spontaneous abortion: comparing expectant management with surgical evacuation. Hum Reprod 1996; 11: 1767–1770

6 Goldstein SR. Pregnancy: embryo. In: Goldstein SR. (ed) Endovaginal Ultrasound, 2nd edn. New York: Wiley-Liss, 1991

7 Sauberbrei E, Cooperberg PL, Poland JB. Ultrasound demonstration of the normal fetal yolk sac. J Clin Ultrasound 1980; 8: 217

8 Warren WB, Timor-Tritsch IE, Peisner DB et al. Dating the early pregnancy by sequential appearance of embryonic structures. Am J Obstet Gynecol 1989; 161: 747–753

9 Goldstein SR. Early pregnancy failure. In: Timmerman D, Deprest J, Bourne T. (eds) Ultrasound and Endoscopic Surgery in Obstetrics and Gynaecology. London: Springer, 2002; 256

10 Alberman E. Spontaneous abortion: epidemiology 1992; 9–20

11 Bigrigg MA, Read MD. Management of women referred to early pregnancy assessment unit: care and cost effectiveness. BMJ 1991; 302: 577–579

12 Luise C, Jermy K, Collins WP et al. Outcome of expectant management of spontaneous first trimester miscarriage: observational study. BMJ 2002; 324: 873–875

13 Levi CS, Lyons EA, Zheng XH et al. Endovaginal ultrasound: demonstration of cardiac activity in embryos less than 5.0 mm in crown-rump length. Radiology 1990; 176: 71–74

14 Marinez JM, Comas C, Ojuel J et al. Fetal heart rate patterns in pregnancies with chromosomal disorders or subsequent fetal loss. Obstet Gynecol 1996; 87: 118–121

15 Neilsen S, Hahlin. M. Expectant management of first trimester spontaneous abortion. Lancet 1995; 345: 84–86

16 Wong SF, Lam MH, Ho LC. Transvaginal sonography in the detection of retained products of conception after first-trimester spontaneous abortion. J Clin Ultrasound 2002; 30: 428–432

17 Schwarzler P, Holden D, Nielsen S et al. The conservative management of first trimester miscarriages and the use of colour Doppler sonography for patient selection. Hum Reprod 1999; 14: 1341–1345

18 Jurkovic D, Ross JA, Nicolaides KH. Expectant management of missed miscarriage. Br J Obstet Gynaecol 1998; 105: 670–671

19 Luise C, Jermy K, Collins WP et al. Expectant management of incomplete, spontaneous first-trimester miscarriage: outcome according to initial ultrasound criteria and value of follow-up visits. Ultrasound Obstet Gynecol 2002; 19: 580–582

20 Jurkovic D. Modern management of miscarriage: is there a place for non-surgical treatment? Ultrasound Obstet Gynecol 1998; 11: 161–163

21 Hinshaw HKS. Medical management of miscarriage. Problems in early pregnancy: advances in diagnosis and management. London: RCOG Press, 1997; 284–295

22 Chipchase J, James D. Randomised trial of expectant versus surgical management of spontaneous miscarriage. Br J Obstet Gynaecol 1997; 104: 840–841

23 Blohm F, Hahlin M, Nielsen S et al. Fertility after a randomised trial of spontaneous abortion managed by surgical evacuation or expectant treatment. Lancet 1997; 349: 995

24 Sieroszewski P, Suzin J, Bernaschek G et al. Evaluation of first trimester pregnancy in cases of threatened abortion by means of Doppler sonography. Ultraschall 2001; 22: 208–212

25 Pedersen JF, Mantoni M. Prevalence and significance of subchorionic hemorrhage in threatened abortion: a sonographic study. AJR Am J Roentgenol 1990; 154: 535–537

26 Mantoni M. Ultrasound signs in threatened abortion and their prognostic significance. Obstet Gynecol 1985; 65: 471–475

27 Ludwig M, Kaisi M, Bauer O et al. Heterotopic pregnancy in a spontaneous cycle: do not forget about it! Eur J Obstet Gynecol Reprod Biol 1999; 87: 91–93

28 Cacciatore B, Stenman UH, Ylostalo P. Diagnosis of ectopic pregnancy by vaginal ultrasonography in combination with a discriminatory serum hCG level of 1000 IU/l (IRP). Br J Obstet Gynaecol 1990; 97: 904–908

29 Condous G, Okara E, Khadlid A, Timmerman D, Lu C, Zhou Y, Van Huffel S, Bourne T. The use of a new logistic regression model for predicting the outcome of pregnancies of

unknown location. Hum Reprod 2004; Jun 24 Epub 2004 Jun 17

30 Brown DL, Doubilet PM. Transvaginal sonography for diagnosing ectopic pregnancy: positivity criteria and performance characteristics. J Ultrasound Med 1994; 13: 259–266

31 Jurkovic D, Bourne TH, Campbell S et al. The diagnosis of ectopic pregnancy using transvaginal color flow imaging. Fertil Steril 1992; 57: 68–73

32 Parker J, Bisits A, Proietto AM. A systematic review of single-dose intramuscular methotrexate for the treatment of ectopic pregnancy. Aust NZ J Obstet Gynaecol 1998; 38: 145–150

33 Cobellis L. Use of methotrexate in ectopic pregnancy. Results in 55 patients treated. Minerva Ginecol 1998; 50: 513–517

34 Fernandez H, Yves Vincent SC, Pauthier S, Audibert F, Frydman R. Randomized trial of conservative laparoscopic treatment and methotrexate administration in ectopic pregnancy and subsequent fertility. Hum Reprod 1998; 13: 3239–3243

35 Tzafettas J, Anapliotis S, Boucklis A, Oxouzoglou N, Bondis J. Transvaginal intra-amniotic injection of methotrexate in early ectopic pregnancy. Advantages over the laparoscopic approach. Early Hum Dev 1994; 39: 101–107

36 Fernandez H, Bourget P, Ville Y et al. Treatment of unruptured tubal pregnancy with methotrexate: pharmacokinetic analysis of local versus intramuscular administration. Fertil Steril 1994; 62: 943–947

37 Cohen DR, Falcone T, Khalife S et al. Methotrexate: local versus intramuscular. Fertil Steril 1996; 65: 206–207

38 Kallchman GG, Meltzer RM. Interstitial pregnancy following homolateral salpingectomy: Report of 2 cases and review of the literature. Am J Obstet Gynecol 1996; 96: 1139–1141

39 Jafrie SZ, Loginsky SJ, Bouffard JA et al. Sonographic detection of interstitial pregnancy. J Clin Ultrasound 1987; 15: 253–257

40 Goldstein S, Timor-Tritsch IE. Ectopic pregnancy. In: Goldstein S, Timor-Tritsch IE. (eds) Ultrasound in Gynecology. New York: Churchill Livingstone, 1995; 169–185

41 Rimes HG, Nosal RA, Gallagher JC. Ovarian pregnancy: a series of 24 cases. Obstet Gynecol 1983; 61: 174

42 Hertz RH, Timor-Tritsch IE, Sokol RJ et al. Diagnostic studies and fetal assessment in advanced extrauterine pregnancy. Obstet Gynecol 1977; 50: 63–65

43 Stanley JH, Horger III EO, Fagan CJ et al. Sonographic findings in abdominal pregnancy. Am J Radiol 1986; 147: 1043–1046

44 Vial Y, Petignat P, Hohfeld P. Pregnancy in a Cesarean scar. Ultrasound Obstet Gynecol 2000; 16: 592–593

45 Jurkovic D, Hillaby K, Woelfer B, Lawrence A, Salim R, Elson CJ. First-trimester diagnosis and management of pregnancies implanted into the lower uterine segment Cesarean section scar. Ultrasound Obstet Gynecol 2003; 21: 220–227

46 Murphy C, Barlow R. A 'snow-storm' ultrasound pattern in the uterus. J Med Assoc Ga 1977; 66: 28–29

47 Goldstein SR. Pregnancy failure. In: Goldstein SR, Timor-Tritsch IE. (eds) Ultrasound in Gynecology. New York: Churchill-Livingstone, 1995; 155–168

48 Sebire NJ, Rees H, Paradinas F et al. The diagnostic implications of routine ultrasound examination in histologically confirmed early molar pregnancies. Ultrasound Obstet Gynecol 2001; 18: 662–665

49 Hahlin M, Thorburn J, Bryman I. The expectant management of early pregnancies of uncertain site. Hum Reprod 1995; 10: 1223–1227

50 Banerjee S, Aslam N, Zosmer N et al. The expectant management of women with pregnancies of unknown location. Br J Obstet Gynaecol 1999; 14: 231–236

51 Banerjee S, Aslam N, Woelfler B et al. Expectant management of early pregnancies of unknown location: a prospective evaluation of methods to predict spontaneous resolution of pregnancy. Br J Obstet Gynaecol 2001; 108: 158–163

52 Barnhart KT, Simhan H, Kamelle SA. Diagnostic accuracy of ultrasound above and below the beta-hCG discriminatory zone. Obstet Gynecol 1999; 94: 583–587

53 Kadar N, DeVore G, Romero R. Discriminatory hCG zone: its use in the sonographic evaluation for ectopic pregnancy. Obstet Gynecol 1981; 58: 156–161

54 Peisner DB, Timor-Tritsch IE. The discriminatory zone of beta-hCG for vaginal probes. J

Clin Ultrasound 1990; 18: 280–285

55 Kadar N, Caldwell BV, Romero R. A method of screening for ectopic pregnancy and its indications. Obstet Gynecol 1981; 58: 162–166

56 Condous G, Okaro E, Khalid A *et al.* Role of biochemical and ultrasonographic indices in the management of pregnancies of unknown location. Ultrasound Obstet Gynecol 2002; 20 Suppl 1: 36–37

57 Condous G, Thomas J, Okaro E, Bourne T. Placental site trophoblastic tumour masquerading as an ovarian ectopic pregnancy. Ultrasound Obstet Gynecol 2003; 21: 504–506

58 Czekierdowski A, Bednarek W, Rogowska W *et al.* Difficulties in differential diagnosis of adnexal masses during pregnancy: the role of greyscale and color Doppler sonography. Ginekol Pol 2001; 72: 1281–6

59 Ballard CA. Ovarian tumors associated with pregnancy termination patients. Am J Obstet Gynecol 1984; 149: 384–387

60 Caspi B, Ben-Arie A, Appelman Z *et al.* Aspiration of simple pelvic cysts during pregnancy. Gynecol Obstet Invest 2000; 49: 102–5

61 Jermy K, Luise C, Bourne T. The characterization of common ovarian cysts in premenopausal women. Ultrasound Obstet Gynecol 2001; 17: 140–144

62 Condous G, Khalid A, Okara E, Bourne T. Should we be examining the ovaries in pregnancy? Prevalence and natural history of adnexal pathology detected at first-trimester sonography. Ultrasound Obstet Gynecol 2004; 24: 62–66

63 Condous G, Okara E, Bourne T. The conservative management of early pregnancy complications: a review of the literature. Ultrasound Obstet Gynaecol 2003; 22: 420–430

Complimentary role of ultrasound and serum hormone measurements in the management of early pregnancy complications

Fathima Paruk Jack Moodley

Antihypertensive therapy for the management of mild-to-moderate hypertension?

Hypertensive disorders of pregnancy (HDP) constitute the commonest medical disorder diagnosed by obstetricians in clinical practice.[1] It is well recognised that the attendant maternal and neonatal morbidity and mortality is substantial.[1-3] The spectrum of severity of HDP, however, may range from mild to severe disease with the subset of mild-to-moderate disease being fairly substantial. Although the clinical management of severe HDP is generally standardised and acceptable to most working in this field of maternal health, there is controversy and lack of clarity on clinical issues in respect of mild-to-moderate HDP.

Despite years of research in the field of hypertensive disorders of pregnancy, there remains a lack of consensus on the classification/definition of hypertensive disorders of pregnancy, the blood pressure at which antihypertensive therapy needs to be initiated, what constitutes an appropriate antihypertensive agent in pregnancy and the materno-fetal risk-benefit ratio of treatment. These issues need urgent attention in order to minimise adverse feto–maternal outcome. This chapter addresses issues related to the definition of hypertensive disorders of pregnancy, definition of mild-to-moderate hypertension, reviews the natural history of mild-to-moderate hypertension, focuses on specific management controversies and recommends a management guideline for mild-to-moderate hypertension in pregnancy.

Fathima Paruk MBChB FCOG
Department of Anaesthesiology, Faculty of Health Sciences, University of Witwatersrand, Private Bag 3, Johannesburg, 2050, South Africa (for correspondence, E-mail: parukf@medicine.wits.ac.za)

Jack Moodley MBChB FCOG FRCOG(UK) MD
MRC Pregnancy Hypertension Research Unit and Department of Obstetrics and Gynaecology, Nelson R. Mandela School of Medicine, University of Natal, Private Bag 7, Congella 4013, South Africa (for correspondence, E-mail: gynae@nu.ac.za)

CLASSIFICATION AND DEFINITION

There exist various classifications for HDP.[4–8] In addition, there are disparities related to the diagnostic criteria in defining the different hypertensive subcategories. This lack of consensus has impacted on diagnosis, management and research and is partially responsible for the management controversies in HDP.

The most recent report from the International Society for the Study of Hypertension in Pregnancy (ISSHP) in 2001[9] has taken cognisance of other classifications, *viz* the Australian Society for the Study of Hypertension in Pregnancy (ASSHP), National High Blood Pressure Programme (NHBEP) in the US, the older ISSHP classification, World Health Organization (WHO) and the Canadian Hypertension Society.[4–8] The ISSHP classification is currently widely accepted and includes the following categories: (i) pre-eclampsia; (ii) chronic hypertension (essential or secondary); (iii) pre-eclampsia superimposed on chronic hypertension; and (iv) gestational hypertension.

The ISSHP accepts that the clinical diagnosis of pre-eclampsia may be established in the absence of proteinuria, provided the patient has hypertension with evidence of other organ affectation or fetal growth impairment. It does, however, suggest that for the purpose of research a restrictive definition be used to diagnose pre-eclampsia (*i.e.* new onset hypertension after 20 weeks' gestation with properly documented proteinuria – ≥ 300 mg/day in a timed collection or a spot urine protein/creatinine ratio ≥ 30 mg protein/mmol creatinine).[9]

It is currently accepted that a reproducible blood pressure of ≥ 140 mmHg systolic or ≥ 90 mmHg diastolic constitutes hypertension. It has been previously suggested that an increment of 30 mmHg systolic or 15 mmHg diastolic may be used to diagnose hypertension. There is a definite shift away from this opinion, which is not scientifically informed. It is, nonetheless, recommended that based on clinical opinion, the subset of patients who demonstrate this phenomenon be carefully monitored for the development of other stigmata of HDP.[5] There is currently substantial data to support the use of Korotkoff V in determining diastolic blood pressure.[10–12]

Mild-to-moderate hypertension is acceptably diagnosed in the context of a systolic blood pressure of 140–169 mmHg and a diastolic blood pressure of 90–109 mmHg.

THE COURSE OF MILD-TO-MODERATE HYPERTENSION

It is well recognised that hypertensive disorders complicate 6–8% of pregnancies.[13] The exact proportion of patients with mild-to-moderate hypertension remains unknown, but probably represents a substantial percentage of patients presenting with hypertension. Patients with uncomplicated mild-to-moderate hypertension, whose blood pressure remains so for the duration of pregnancy, generally have a maternal and fetal outcome that is comparable to their normotensive counterparts. Deaths and cardiovascular accidents are rare. Magee *et al.*[14] reported no such cases in a review of 22 trials (2552 patients). Once complications ensue or the blood pressure becomes severe, outcome is poor. Thus the natural history of progression as well as markers of poor outcome needs to be determined.

2

Antihypertensive therapy for the management of mild-to-moderate hypertension?

Literature pertaining to outcome in mild-to-moderate hypertension in pregnancy is scant. In most situations, the study populations are restricted to specific subsets of the disease, *viz* mild gestational hypertension or mild chronic hypertension. Nonetheless, they do provide important information.

Mild gestational hypertension

There is a paucity of data related to pregnancy outcome in patients with mild-to-moderate gestational hypertension. Sauden et al.,[15] in a retrospective review of 416 patients with gestational hypertension, demonstrated that 15% (62 patients) subsequently developed pre-eclampsia. An altogether separate, but prospective, arm of the study involving a cohort of 112 patients showed that 26% (29 patients) developed pre-eclampsia. Patients in whom the initial diagnosis of gestational hypertension was made beyond 36 weeks' gestation demonstrated a 10% risk (much lower than the overall risk) of developing pre-eclampsia. Multiple logistic regression analysis of the data identified previous miscarriage and early gestation at presentation as markers associated with an increased likelihood of developing pre-eclampsia.

Barton et al.[16] prospectively evaluated outcome in a cohort of 748 patients over a 3-year period. They demonstrated a 46% (343 patients) progression rate to pre-eclampsia. In addition, 9.6% (72 patients) developed severe pre-eclampsia. The development of pre-eclampsia was independent of maternal age, race (the proportion of Caucasian patients was about 60% in each group), marital status or a tobacco consumption history. Interestingly, the patients who developed pre-eclampsia were enrolled about 1 (gestational) week earlier than those who remained aproteinuric. Not unexpectedly, the pre-eclamptic patients who were more likely to develop severe pre-eclampsia and thrombocytopenia, had a longer neonatal hospitalisation period, and a higher incidence of small for gestational age babies (24.8% versus 13.8%; $P < 0.001$) compared to patients who remained aproteinuric.

Studies including mild gestational hypertension and mild pre-eclampsia patients

A prospective study assessing the effect of maternal age on outcome in mild hypertension in a cohort of 379 mature women ($\geq$ 35 years old) by Barton et al.[17] reported similar maternal outcomes but a higher still birth rate in women over 35 years of age compared with a cohort of women less than 35 years. Although this was statistically insignificant ($P = 0.63$), the sample size was too small to detect a significant difference. A *post hoc* power analysis indicated that a sample size of 1200 patients would be required to do so. A further study from Barton et al.[18] evaluated the influence of ethnicity on outcome in a prospective analysis of 1182 patients of Hispanic, African American and Caucasian ethnicity. They reported that Hispanics demonstrated a higher rate of progression to severe pre-eclampsia compared to Caucasians (<0.05). The incidence of small for gestational age (SGA) was highest among the Hispanic newborns. The rates of progression to HELLP and eclampsia were similar among all groups. African Americans when compared to White patients demonstrated a lower gestational age at delivery as well as lower birth weights

Table 1 Maternal–fetal outcome in mild chronic hypertension

Trial	Sibai et al.[22]	McCowan et al.[21]	Rey & Couturier[20]	Sibai et al.[19]
Year	1998	1996	1994	1983
Cohort	763	142	337	211
% Pre-eclampsia	25	14	21	10
% Abruptio placenta	1.5	No result	0.7	1.4
% Preterm delivery	33.3	16	34.4	12
% SGA	11.1	11	15.5	8

(< 0.05 for both parameters). In addition, African Americans had a higher stillbirth and neonatal death incidence compared to the other 2 ethnic groups.

Mild pre-eclampsia

There are no studies that focus exclusively on 'mild pre-eclamptic patients'. Hypertension may well be the *sine qua non* of pre-eclampsia; it, nevertheless, represents but one manifestation of this volatile and potentially fatal multisystem disease. Furthermore, the potential for rapid progression to severe pre-eclampsia as well as the marked lability of blood pressure measurements are well recognised issues. To label pre-eclampsia as mild, purely on the basis of a blood pressure measurement, would thus be inappropriate. Therefore, to categorise a patient into the group of mild pre-eclampsia is subject to error and not always easy to achieve. The paucity of data on mild pre-eclampsia (if it indeed does exist) is, therefore, not surprising.

Mild chronic hypertension

There are a few studies which evaluate maternal and fetal outcome in mild chronic hypertension.[19-22] Some of the results are summarised in Table 1. The rates of pre-eclampsia and abruptio placentae are evidently high and range from 10–25% and 0.7–1.5%, respectively. In a multicentre study involving 763 patients, Sibai et al.[22] reported that there was a significantly increased risk of developing superimposed pre-eclampsia in patients who had chronic hypertension for greater than 4 years (31% versus 22%) prior to the index pregnancy, a past history of pre-eclampsia (32% versus 23%) or if the baseline diastolic blood pressure ranged between 100–110 mmHg compared to a diastolic blood pressure below 100 mmHg (42% versus 24%). Maternal age and ethnic differences did not influence the incidence of pre-eclampsia. In the same series, the incidence of abruptio placentae increased once pre-eclampsia ensued. The incidence of abruptio placentae, however, was not influenced by maternal age, race or the duration of the hypertension.

The risk of preterm delivery and small for gestational age neonates in studies on mild chronic hypertension varied from 12–34% and 8–15.5%, respectively.[19-22] It is not known what proportion of the patients in these studies with mild chronic hypertension had evidence of target organ involvement at recruitment or a history of a previous perinatal loss. This is important information as it would impact on clinical management. A more

2

Antihypertensive therapy for the management of mild-to-moderate hypertension?

recent review by Sibai[23] suggests that patients with mild chronic hypertension together with target organ affectation or a previous perinatal loss should, in fact, be regarded as high-risk cases and managed accordingly.

From the above, it is clearly evident that mild-to-moderate hypertension is associated with certain adverse maternal and perinatal risks. This then raises the following pertinent issues: (i) the level of hypertension at which therapy needs to be initiated; (ii) the efficacy of antihypertensive therapy; (iii) the risk-benefit analysis of indicating antihypertensive agents including what is the ideal antihypertensive agent; and (iv) the holistic management of mild-to-moderate hypertension in pregnancy.

ISSUES IN THE MANAGEMENT OF MILD-TO-MODERATE HYPERTENSION IN PREGNANCY

The level of hypertension at which therapy needs to be initiated

The aim of antihypertensive therapy is to prevent complications associated with HDP while prolonging the course of pregnancy. It is generally agreed that severe hypertension (diastolic blood pressure ≥ 110 mmHg) requires treatment because of the risk of a cardiovascular accident or target organ damage. However, in pregnant patients with mild-to-moderate hypertension, there is no consensus regarding the blood pressure at which treatment needs to be initiated. The Canadian Hypertension Society suggests treatment initiation at a blood pressure of 140–150/90–95 mmHg, with the aim of achieving a diastolic blood pressure of 80–89 mmHg.[24] The Australian Society for the Study of Hypertension in Pregnancy, on the other hand, recommends treatment initiation at a blood pressure of ≥ 160/90 mmHg with the aim of achieving a blood pressure of 110–140/80–90 mmHg.[4] The National High Blood Pressure Education Program Working Group on High Blood Pressure in Pregnancy suggests therapy be indicated at a systolic blood pressure ≥ 160 mmHg or a diastolic blood pressure ≥ 100 mmHg, without defining the aim of treatment.[5] The agents suggested include methyldopa, nifedipine and labetalol.[4,5,24] Whilst awaiting affirmative data, it would appear to be acceptable to consider treatment initiation at a diastolic blood pressure ≥ 100 mmHg in patients with mild-to-moderate hypertension.

Efficacy of antihypertensive therapy

The issue of efficacy of antihypertensive agents in mild-to-moderate HDP has been recently addressed in a Cochrane Review by Abalos et al.[25] The primary aim of this review was to ascertain the maternal and fetal hazards of indicating antihypertensive agents for mild-to-moderate hypertension in pregnancy. A secondary aim was to compare the effects of alternative agents. The review includes 40 trials (3797 patients), of which 33 trials (3464 patients) were conducted in industrialised countries. All patients (gestational hypertension, chronic hypertension and non-specified subtypes) with mild-to-moderate hypertension were included. Twenty-four trials (2815 patients) compared an antihypertensive agent with either no drug or a placebo, whilst 17 trials (1182 patients) compared different antihypertensive agents. The vast majority of trials (14 of 17 trials) compared methyldopa to other agents(β-blockers, nifedipine and ketanserin). Overall, the largest trial (a 3-arm trial) had 300 patients. Only 5 trials had more than 100 patients per comparison arm. The authors concede that the methodological quality of the included trials range from poor to average and that concealment of allocation was adequate in only 5/40 trials.

The results of the review may be summarised as follows:

Antihypertensive agent compared to no agent

- Antihypertensive agents halve the risk of developing severe hypertension (RR, 0.52; 95% CI, 0.41–0.64) with the number needed to treat (NNT) 12 (9–17). This is independent of the class of drug, type of hypertension at trial entry or gestational age at trial entry

- No overall difference in risk of pre-eclampsia development (RR, 0.99 [0.84–1.18]), preterm birth (RR, 1.00 [0.87–1.15]) or small for gestational age (RR, 1.13 [0.91–1.42])

- No statistically significant difference in the risk of fetal/neonatal deaths (RR, 0.71 [0.46–1.09])

- With respect to other outcomes, a lesser need for additional antihypertensive agents (RR, 0.42 [0.3–0.58]), abruptio placentae (RR, 1.83 [0.77–4.37]) and a need for change in drugs due to side effects (RR, 1.88 [0.89-3.95]). A wide confidence interval is evident for the latter two outcomes

- Admission to a special care nursery was not significantly different (RR, 1.08 [0.9-1.3]).

The majority of trials evaluated β-blockers (15 trials) and methyldopa (5 trials). Subgroup analysis of different antihypertensive agents demonstrated a few differences. Calcium channel blockers (versus no drug) and β-blockers (versus no drug) yielded altered risks of pre-eclampsia (RR, 1.68 [1.17–2.41] and RR, 0.76 [0.59-0.98], respectively). β-Blockers demonstrated a statistically significant risk of SGA (RR, 1.56 [1.10–2.22]).

Comparison of different antihypertensive agents

- No clear difference in the risk of developing severe hypertension or pre-eclampsia

- A 51% reduction in the risk of fetal/neonatal deaths when any agent is compared with methyldopa (RR, 0.49 [0.24–0.99]); NNT 45 (22–1341)

- Other outcomes showed no clear differences or were reported in very few trials.

The majority of trials compared methyldopa to β-blockers (12 trials). The authors comment in their discussion that although antihypertensive agent use is associated with a halving in the risk of severe hypertension, there is insufficient data to assess for reductions in the consequences of severe hypertension (such as cardiovascular accidents). Furthermore, the expected reduction in certain clinical outcomes (Caesarean sections, preterm delivery) following a reduction in severe hypertension is not evident. There is also no clear evidence that any one agent is better than another. The wide confidence intervals for certain outcome differences

2

Antihypertensive therapy for the management of mild-to-moderate hypertension?

(pre-eclampsia, neonatal deaths) do not exclude a clinically important effect despite the lack of a statistically significant difference. The authors also agree that many outcomes were assessed on data available for a small number of studies introducing the potential to be misled by bias.

The subgroup analyses, therefore, need to be interpreted with caution. The reviewers conclude the following:

- It remains unclear whether the indication of antihypertensive agents in mild-to-moderate hypertension is worthwhile
- A treatment decision should be made by the patient in consultation with her obstetrician
- The choice of antihypertensive agent depends on the obstetrician (clinical experience) and the patient.

There are a few drawbacks that need to be mentioned, although it does need to be pointed out that, understandably, reviews of this nature are generally characterised by such problems by virtue of their retrospective nature as well as the inherent diversity of different trials. Some of the drawbacks include:

- Use of either Korotkoff IV or V was accepted to determine diastolic blood pressure
- Use of differing diastolic blood pressure measurements (in different trials) to diagnose hypertension (range from 85–100 mmHg), *i.e.* a variability in criteria to determine mild-to-moderate hypertension
- Trials which compared agents of the same class, were not included
- Many trials (14 trials) did not specify if patients with proteinuria were included or not
- A lack in clarity in 10 trials, on the issue of recruitment of patients with chronic hypertension: certain outcomes/issues of interest were documented in very few trials
- Some outcomes of interest (severe pre-eclampsia, and very low Apgar score) were not addressed in any of the trials and could not be assessed
- Variability between trials on what constituted effective therapy.

This review,[25] although adding to our knowledge on issues related to mild-to-moderate hypertension in pregnancy, highlights the point that we still do not know whether 'to treat' or 'not to treat' in the scenario of mild-to-moderate hypertension in pregnancy.

A further review of mild-to-moderate HDP by Ferrer[26] indicated that all randomised controlled trials had insufficient power to include or exclude a moderate to large benefit (20–25%) with respect to the indication of antihypertensive treatment.

It is clear that there is a paucity of information pertaining to the advantages and disadvantages of indicating antihypertensive agents for mild-to-moderate hypertension. There exists no clear evidence-based directive for obstetricians managing this common disease. There is an urgent need for well-designed, randomised, controlled trials (with structured and properly defined recruitment criteria as well a sufficient sample size) to assess prespecified maternal and fetal outcome measures (short-term and long-term) as well as the issue of cost efficiency and cost effectiveness.

The ideal antihypertensive agent including the risk-benefit analysis of indicating antihypertensive agents

Ideally, the issue of the appropriate antihypertensive agent should only be considered following clear evidence of the efficacy of such therapy. Nonetheless, it is important to focus on this subject as many obstetricians will opt to treat their patients whilst awaiting an evidence-based directive.

The Cochrane Review[25] concludes that no single class of agent is better than the other. However, this needs to be considered in light of the aforementioned drawbacks. When considering the risk-benefit analysis of indicating antihypertensive therapy, one needs to consider maternal and fetal/neonatal benefits, short- and long-term maternal– fetal/neonatal adverse effects as well as cost benefit (cost of care of antihypertensive agent use versus a system of 'intensive' maternal–fetal surveillance only).

There are many classes of drugs. In some instances, different agents within a single class of drugs may elicit a variable response. The commonly prescribed agents include methyldopa, hydrallazine, nifedipine, prazosin and β-blockers. With reference to specific agents, the Cochrane Review[25] cites the following:

- A reduced risk of pre-eclampsia development in patients administered β-blockers (compared to no agent; RR, 0.76 [0.59–0.98])
- An increased risk (statistically significant) of SGA developing in patients administered β-blockers (RR, 1.56 [1.1–2.2])
- 51% reduction in the risk of a baby dying when any drug is compared to methyldopa (RR, 0.49 [0.24–0.99]). This may, however, be a random error or reflect bias.

It is beyond the scope of this review to discuss each antihypertensive agent in detail: this has been previously addressed.[27–29] Data relating to drug teratogenicity, fetal/neonatal adverse effects and long-term outcome of infants is extremely limited and largely confined to case reports. The limited available data suggest that methyldopa, nifedipine, β-blockers and hydrallazine do not pose a major teratogenic risk.[30–32] The majority of trials have a numerically restricted cohort/sample size and lack sufficient power to detect 'lesser harmful effects'. Angiotensin converting enzyme inhibitors, although not teratogenic, are contra-indicated in pregnancy due to the associated risk of renal failure if administered in the second trimester. Atenolol, a β-blocker, is not recommended based on evidence of an increase in the risk of intra-uterine growth retardation.[33,34]

Prior to initiating therapy, one needs to individualise the drug of choice based on the obstetrician's experience, the patient's medical profile and, in some situations, patient preference.

The holistic management of mild-to-moderate hypertension in pregnancy

The aforementioned confirms that the current status of the management of mild-to-moderate hypertension is experience and opinion based rather than being scientifically informed.

2

Antihypertensive therapy for the management of mild-to-moderate hypertension?

In the absence of evidence to support or refute the use of antihypertensive agents, it is our belief that the following subset of patients should be treated until there if sufficient information to appropriately address the issue in question:

Patients from under-resourced regions

In such a situation, health care delivery is often erratic and fragmented. It is also common for the women to attend antenatal care services irregularly (due to a multitude of reasons which may include a lack of education, lack of transport, economic constraints or poor infrastructure of services). Thus appropriate maternal–fetal surveillance is not always possible and constitutes a major practical problem.[35,36] Regular blood pressure checks may not be possible and the patient may not be able to seek help timeously in the scenario of danger signs (such as persistent headaches).

Patients with proteinuria

It would be prudent to initiate an antihypertensive agent considering the potential for marked lability of blood pressure in such circumstances. Furthermore, the arteriolar vasodilatation effected by therapy may help improve organ perfusion in a disease characterised by multi-organ hypoperfusion. The management of pre-eclampsia has been reviewed elsewhere.[27]

Patients with chronic hypertension together with target organ damage or a previous perinatal loss

Sibai[23] categorised patients with mild-to-moderate chronic hypertension as low risk. He recommended that antihypertensive agents be discontinued in such cases as such treatment does not influence the rate of pre-eclampsia, abruptio placentae or preterm delivery.[19,33] However, if the patient has a history of a previous perinatal loss or has evidence of target organ damage, Sibai[23] suggested that the antihypertensive agent be continued as the patient now belongs to the high-risk category. There are short-term maternal benefits from low blood pressure in patients with target organ damage. There is evidence that in individuals with renal disease, left ventricular dysfunction or diabetes mellitus with vascular involvement the occurrence of uncontrollable mild-to-moderate hypertension may exacerbate target organ damage.[38,39] Thus, the recommendation to treat by certain authors is based on the potential of the treatment to diminish cardiovascular complications. In this context, Sibai recommended labetalol as first line therapy (initiated at 100 mg BD; maximum dose 2.4 g/day), with thiazide diuretics or nifedipine being the second line agents. Oral nifedipine is recommended for patients with diabetes mellitus and vascular disease. In addition, oral nifedipine or thiazide diuretics are recommended as the agents of choice in young Black women, as they usually manifest with a low renin type or a salt-sensitive hypertension.[40]

Informed choice made by the patient

This should follow appropriate counselling of the patient on the currently available data.

The following outlines the general principles of management of mild-to-moderate hypertension in pregnancy (Fig. 1):

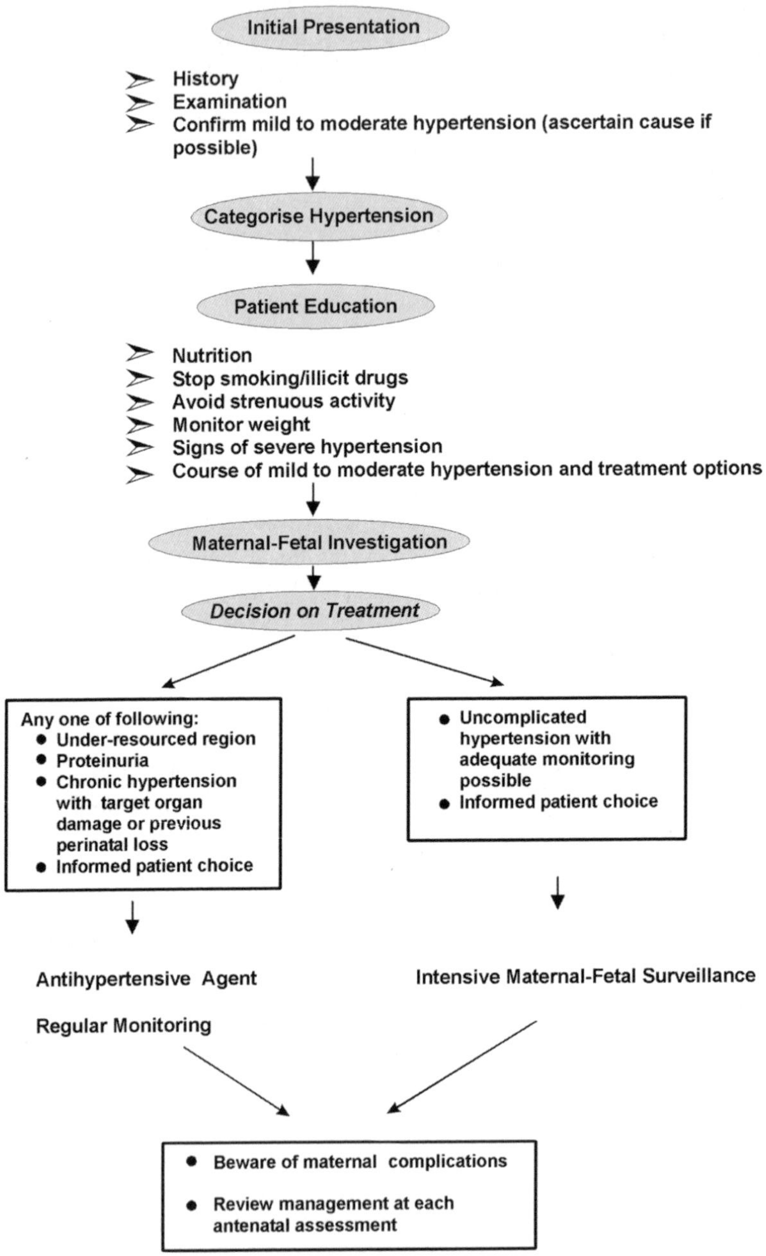

Fig. 1 Management of mild-to-moderate hypertension.

- Preconceptual counselling – this is particularly relevant to patients with chronic hypertension
- History and examination, with emphasis on important aspects pertaining to hypertension
- Confirmation of diagnosis of hypertension
- Ascertain cause of hypertension

2

Antihypertensive therapy for the management of mild-to-moderate hypertension?

Table 2 Drug regimens of commonly prescribed antihypertensive agents

Drug	Initiating dose	Maximum dose	Dosing frequency (maximum dose)
Methyldopa	250–500 mg QID	2000 mg/day	QID
Hydrallazine	20 mg QID	200 mg/day	QID
Nifedipine (long acting)	20–30 mg OD	120 mg/day	OD
Labetalol	100–200 mg BD	1200 mg/day	QID

- Categorise type of hypertension
- Patient education (balanced nutrition, stop smoking, stop illicit drugs, avoid excessive physical activity, monitor weight gain, signs of severe hypertension)
- Maternal and fetal (depending on gestational age) investigation of (i) haemoglobin, haematocrit, platelet count, urea, creatinine, uric acid, proteinuria; (ii) fetal kick count chart, ultrasound, cardiotocography, Doppler ultrasound; and (iii) additional investigations guided by results of the above tests
- Decision to initiate antihypertensive therapy (need to individualise based on aforementioned criteria – often all investigative results will not be available at initial visit). Commonly prescribed antihypertensive agent dosages are summarised in Table 2
- Patients receiving antihypertensive agents should achieve a blood pressure of 120–140/80–90 mmHg; this should prevent severe hypertension without compromising uteroplacental blood flow and fetal perfusion. These patients should be reviewed weekly in the third trimester.
- Patients who are conservatively managed (without antihypertensive drugs) require frequent antenatal visits with intensive maternal-fetal surveillance
- The detection of proteinuria or any maternal-fetal complications necessitates careful review of the patient's management plan
- Multidisciplinary management led by the obstetrician
- The timing of delivery is largely influenced by the type of hypertension and the circumstances surrounding each individual patient. The vast majority of uncomplicated cases may be allowed to await spontaneous onset of labour. Patients with proteinuria need consideration of delivery at term (37 completed weeks)
- Regional anaesthesia (if not contra-indicated)confers the dual benefit of effective analgesia and a blood pressure stabilising effect
- Meticulous intrapartum maternal–fetal surveillance (including blood pressure, pulse, neurological status and fetal heart rate) is crucial
- Post partum care should include blood pressure surveillance (treatment may need adjusting), follow-up until the blood pressure normalises, contraceptive advice and counselling with respect to future pregnancies (depending on type of hypertension and maternal–fetal outcome of the index pregnancy). Patients with hypertension (persisting beyond 6 weeks post-delivery), warrant referral to a physician.

RESEARCH AGENDA

There is a need for appropriately designed prospective multicentre randomised controlled trials (with sufficient sample size) to assess the efficacy of commonly indicated antihypertensive agents in the context of this potentially life threatening disease. The specific issues of focus should include:

- Agent efficacy
- Indication(s) for treatment (if therapy is efficacious)
- Maternal–perinatal benefits and adverse effects with treatment
- Cost benefit analysis (treatment versus non-treatment)
- Long-term follow-up of children who entered the trials as fetuses.

References

1 American College of Obstetricians and Gynaecologists. Hypertension in pregnancy. ACOG Technical Bulletin No 219, Washington, DC: The College; 1996; 1–8
2 Department of Health. Why Mothers Die. Report on confidential enquiries into maternal deaths in the United Kingdom. London: HMSO, 1998
3 Wittmann BK, Murphy KJ, King JF et al. Maternal mortality in British Columbia in 1971–86. Can Med Assoc J 1988; 139: 39–40
4 Brown MA, Hague WM, Higgins J et al. The detection, investigation and management of hypertension in pregnancy. Aust NZ J Obstet Gynaecol 2000; 40: 133–135
5 National High Blood Pressure Education Program Working Group on High Blood Pressure in Pregnancy. Report of the National High Blood Pressure Education Program Working Group on High Blood Pressure in Pregnancy. Am J Obstet Gynecol 2000; 183: S1–S22
6 World Health Organization Group. The Hypertensive Disorders of Pregnancy. Technical Report Series No. 758. Geneva: WHO, 1987
7 Davey DA, MacGillivary I. The classification and definition of hypertensive disorders of pregnancy. Am J Obstet Gynecol 1998; 158: 892–898.
8 Helewa ME, Burrows RF, Smith J et al. Report of the Canadian Hypertension Society Consensus Conference: 1: Definitions, Evaluation and Classification of Hypertensive Disorders of Pregnancy . Can Med Assoc J 1997; 157: 715–725
9 Brown MA, Lindheimer MD, de Swiet M et al. The classification and diagnosis of the hypertensive disorders of pregnancy: Statement from the International Society for the Study of Hypertension in Pregnancy. Hypertens Preg 2001; 20: ix–xiv
10 Opening AR, Barron WM. Indirect blood pressure measurements in pregnancy: Korotkoff phase 4 versus 5. Am J Obstet Gynecol 1992; 167: 577–580
11 Lopez MC, Belizan JM, Villar JL et al. The measurement of diastolic blood pressure during pregnancy: which Korotkoff phase should be used? Am J Obstet Gynecol 1194; 170: 574–578
12 Brown MA, Buddle ML, Farrell T et al. Randomised trial of management of hypertensive pregnancies by Korotkoff phase IV or phase V? Lancet 1998; 352: 777–781
13 American College of Obstetricians and Gynecologists. Hypertension in pregnancy. ACOG Technical Bulletin No. 219. Washington, DC: The College, 1996; 1–8
14 Magee LA, Ornstein MP, von Dadelszen P. Clinical review of mild-to-moderate pregnancy hypertension. BMJ 1999; 318: 1332–1338
15 Saudan P, Brown MA, Buddle ML, Jones M. Does gestational hypertension become pre-eclampsia? Br J Obstet Gynaecol 1998; 105: 1177–1184
16 Barton JR, O'Brien JM, Bergauer NK et al. Mild gestational hypertension remote from term: progression and outcome. Am J Obstet Gynecol 2001; 184: 979–983
17 Barton JR, Bergauer NK, Jaques DL et al. Does advanced maternal age affect pregnancy outcome in women with mild hypertension remote from term? Am J Obstet Gynecol 1997; 176: 1236–1243

2

Antihypertensive therapy for the management of mild-to-moderate hypertension?

18 Barton CJ, Barton JR, O'Brien JM *et al.* Mild gestational hypertension: differences in ethnicity are associated with altered outcomes in women who undergo outpatient treatment. Am J Obstet Gynecol 2002; 186: 896–898

19 Sibai BM, Abdella TN, Anderson GD. Pregnancy outcome in 211 patients with mild chronic hypertension. Obstet Gynecol 1983; 61: 571–576

20 Rey E, Couturier A. The prognosis of pregnancy for women with chronic hypertension. Am J Obstet Gynecol 1994; 171: 410–416

21 McCowan LM, Buist RG, North RA, Gamble G. Perinatal morbidity in chronic hypertension. Br J Obstet Gynaecol 1996; 103: 132–139

22 Sibai BM, Lindheimer M, Hauth J *et al.* Risk factors for pre-eclampsia, abruptio placentae and adverse neonatal outcomes among women with chronic hypertension. N Engl J Med 1998; 339: 667–671

23 Sibai BM. Chronic hypertension in pregnancy. Obstet Gynecol 2002; 100: 369–377

24 Rey E, LeLorier J, Burgess E *et al.* Report of the Canadian Hypertension Society Consensus Conference: 3. Pharmacological treatment of hypertensive disorders in pregnancy. Can Med Assoc J 1997; 157: 1245–1254

25 Abalos E, Duley L, Steyn DW, Henderson-Smart DJ. Antihypertensive drug therapy for mild-to-moderate hypertension during pregnancy (Cochrane Review). In: The Cochrane Library, Issue 3. Oxford: Update Software, 2001

26 Ferrer RL, Sibai BM, Murlow CD *et al.* Management of mild chronic hypertension during pregnancy: a review. Obstet Gynecol 2000; 96: 849–860

27 Paruk F, Moodley J. Treatment of severe pre-eclampsia/eclampsia syndrome. Prog Obstet Gynaecol 2000; 14: 103–119

28 Paruk F, Moodley J. Untoward effects of rapid acting antihypertensive agents. Clin Obstet Gynaecol 2001; 15: 491–506

29 Khedun SM, Maharaj B, Moodley J. Effects of antihypertensive drugs on the unborn child: what is known, and how should this influence prescribing? Paediatr Drugs 2000; 2: 419–436

30 Galley EDM, Hunyor SN, Gyory AZ. Plasma volume contraction: a significant factor in both pregnancy-associated hypertension (preeclampsia) and chronic hypertension in pregnancy. Q J Med 1979; 192: 593–602

31 Magee LA, Schick B, Donnenfeld AE *et al.* The safety of calcium-channel blockers in human pregnancy: a prospective, multicentre cohort study. Am J Obstet Gynecol 1996; 174: 823–828

32 Briggs GG, Freeman RK, Yaffe SJ. (eds) Drugs in Pregnancy and Lactation, 4th edn. Baltimore: Williams and Watkins, 1994

33 Magee LA. Fetal growth restriction. Lancet 2000; 355: 1366–1372

34 Butters L, Kennedy S, Rubin PC. Atenolol in essential hypertension during pregnancy. BMJ 1990; 301: 587–589

35 Paruk F, Moodley J. RHL commentary on a Cochrane Review: 'Antihypertensive drug therapy for mild-to-moderate hypertension during pregnancy'. The WHO Reproductive Health Library No. 5. Geneva: WHO, 2002

36 Paruk F, Moodley J. Practical recommendations for the management of mild-to-moderate hypertension during pregnancy. The WHO Reproductive Health Library No. 5. Geneva: WHO, 2002

37 Sibai BM, Mabie WC, Shamsa F *et al.* A comparison of no medication versus methyldopa or labetalol in chronic hypertension during pregnancy. Am J Obstet Gynecol 1990; 162: 960–966

38 Jones DC, Hayslett JP. Outcome of pregnancy in women with moderate or severe renal insufficiency. N Engl J Med 1996; 335: 226–232

39 Easterling TR, Carr DB, Brateng D *et al.* Treatment of hypertension in pregnancy: effect of atenolol on maternal disease, preterm delivery and fetal growth. Obstet Gynecol 2001; 98: 427–433

40 Umans JG, Lindheimer MD. Antihypertensive treatment. In: Lindheimer MD, Roberts JM, Cunningham JF. (eds) Chesley's Hypertensive Disorders in Pregnancy, 2nd edn. Norwalk, CT: Appleton and Lange, 1998; 581–604

Anna P. Kenyon J.C. Girling

Obstetric cholestasis

Obstetric cholestasis (also known as intrahepatic cholestasis of pregnancy or cholestasis of pregnancy) is a liver disease unique to pregnancy which presents with pruritus. It is an important condition to diagnose because of the adverse pregnancy outcome with which it is associated. While medical treatments have not been conclusively shown to be of benefit, policies of 'active management' may improve pregnancy outcome. However, itching is a common symptom amongst pregnant women, most of whom do not have obstetric cholestasis. It is important to differentiate accurately those with itching in pregnancy that is not obstetric cholestasis from those women with the disease. Thus, information regarding the risks of obstetric cholestasis, the medical treatments and the chance of recurrence in subsequent pregnancies can be given, to allow women to make informed decisions about their care and avoid unnecessary intervention. This chapter aims to review the literature to facilitate the clinician in this regard.

CLINICAL APPROACH TO PRURITUS IN PREGNANCY

Pruritus is a symptom in many dermatological conditions, some of which may present for the first time in pregnancy. However, there are a number of dermatological conditions unique to pregnancy, which result in pruritus. When a pregnant woman presents with pruritus with its onset in pregnancy, a

Anna P. Kenyon MBChB MD
Specialist Registrar, Department of Obstetrics and Gynaecology, West Middlesex University Hospital, Twickenham Road, Isleworth, Middlesex TW7 6AF, UK (for correspondence, E-mail: apkenyon@doctors.org.uk)

J.C. Girling MRCP MA MRCOG
Consultant, Department of Obstetrics and Gynaecology, West Middlesex University Hospital, Twickenham Road, Isleworth, Middlesex TW7 6AF, UK

Table 1 Causes of pruritus in pregnancy, classified according to whether it is a pregnancy-specific cause and if there is an associated rash

WITH A RASH: pregnancy specific dermatoses

Polymorphic eruption of pregnancy (PEP) *syn* pruritic urticarial papules and plaques of pregnancy (PUPP), toxaemic rash of pregnancy	Pruritus, urticarial papules and plaques, rarely vesicles. Per abdomen, along striae with umbilical sparing. May spread to thighs, buttocks and upper arms. 1 in 200–250. Onset in third trimester. Resolves on delivery
Pruritic folliculitis	Pruritus and follicular or pustular (acneiform) eruption. Trunk and thighs may be widespread. Onset after second trimester. Resolves within 2 weeks of delivery
Prurigo	Pruritus, excoriated (red-brown) nodules on trunk or limbs. Onset after second trimester. Pruritus improves on delivery. Papules may persist for several months
Pemphigoid gestationes *Syn* herpes gestationes	Pruritus. Papules and urticarial lesions, vesicles (bullous eruption). Abdomen (including umbilicus) then limbs, palms and soles. 1:60,000. Associated premature delivery, growth restriction. 10% neonates have a rash. Commonly recurs in pregnancy and COCP

WITH A RASH: inter-current dermatological disease

Eczema	Can present for first time in pregnancy: itchy flexural eruption with previous or family history of atopy. 36% of referrals to a dermatology clinic for pregnant women

WITHOUT A RASH: pregnancy specific causes

Obstetric cholestasis	Pruritus in association with increased concentrations of one or more of alanine amino-transferase, aspartate amino transferase, γ-glutamyl transpeptidase or total bile acids in the absence of other forms of liver disease that resolves on delivery. Usually onset after 30 weeks' gestation. 1:151
Pruritus gravidarum	Pruritus with its onset in pregnancy, normal liver function and bile acids. May affect up to 20% of women. May occur at any gestation

COCP, Combined oral contraceptive pill.
See references[1-7] for further details.

useful first step is to determine whether or not a rash is present. Table 1 shows possible diagnoses unique to pregnancy considered in this way. Where a rash is present, often a dermatology opinion is needed; in some cases, a skin biopsy helps to confirm the diagnosis.

All women with pruritus of onset in pregnancy in the absence of a rash should have serum testing of liver function in order to exclude obstetric cholestasis. However, severe itching can result in marked excoriations, which the patient may often interpret as a rash and so careful examination is often necessary. Where there is any doubt, liver function should be performed and a dermatology consultation requested.

LIVER FUNCTION TESTS

Laboratory tests of liver function which are widely available for clinical use are bilirubin, albumin, total protein, alanine aminotransferase (ALT), aspartate aminotransferase (AST), γ-glutamyl transpeptidase (GGT) and alkaline phosphatase (ALP). Alkaline phosphatase concentrations rise in pregnancy as the enzyme is produced and released by the placenta. Elevations in ALP are seen in cholestatic disease such as obstetric cholestasis as it is released from the damaged liver;[8] but, because the enzyme is also released from the placenta in normal pregnancies, measurements are less helpful than outside pregnancy. Upper limits of normal for pregnancy have been suggested to be 3-fold that of non-pregnant individuals and concentrations in excess of these may suggest disease. Tests are available to determine the concentration of ALP derived from the placenta (the hepatic isoform is heat stable) and can be helpful in determining the origin of elevated ALP when levels are very high.

Serum values for other tests of liver function fall in pregnancy. Possible mechanisms include a dilutional effect as a result of the expanded plasma volume of pregnancy, an increase in hepatic blood flow or reduced function of the enzymes (and, therefore, reduced release). Albumin and total protein concentrations fall and, unlike the situation outside pregnancy, albumen is not a useful marker of hepatic synthetic function. A prospective cross-sectional study on 435 pregnant women with uncomplicated pregnancies has suggested that ALT, AST, bilirubin and GGT concentrations also fall and are 20% lower than the quoted reference ranges for non-pregnant individuals.[9] These ranges were then validated in 85 women with gestational hypertension. In those developing pre-eclampsia, clinical outcome was worse where liver function was abnormal using the new ranges. These women would, using the old ranges have been identified as having 'normal liver function'. This confirms not only that results of serum tests of liver function fall in normal pregnancy but that these new ranges provide a more sensitive means of identifying liver pathology in pregnancy than had previously been available.

Bile acid concentrations can also be measured as a test of liver function. Bile acids have hydrophobic and hydrophilic portions and act as detergents to facilitate absorption of dietary fats. They are synthesised in hepatocytes from the common precursor cholesterol. Primary bile acids (cholic acid (CA) and chenodeoxycholic acid (CDCA)) enter bile after conjugation with glycine or taurine, i.e. glycocholic acid (GCA), taurocholic acid (TCA), taurochenodeoxycholic acid (TCDA) and glycochenodeoxycholic acid (GCDA). This process increases their solubility. Since bile contains significant quantities of sodium and potassium and the pH is alkaline, it is assumed that the bile acids and the associated conjugates exist in ionised form (hence the term bile salts). Once in the small intestine, primary bile acids are deconjugated via the action of intestinal microflora to form the secondary bile acids deoxycholic acid (DCA; from cholic acid) and lithocholic acid (LCA; from chenodeoxycholic acid). Primary and secondary bile acids are 98—99% re-absorbed in the ileum, returning to the liver via the portal circulation. Only trace amounts of bile acids escape absorption and are subsequently lost in the faeces. Equivalent quantities of bile acids to that lost in the faeces are synthesised from cholesterol in the liver to maintain a constant bile acid pool. As a result of efficient 'first-pass' excretion of bile acids, they are only present in small amounts in the systemic circulation in healthy individuals. Most widely available assays measure only total bile acid concentrations and are often only available at regional centres.

OBSTETRIC CHOLESTASIS

Changes in liver function

In obstetric cholestasis, the most commonly elevated liver function tests are total serum bile acids and transaminases (particularly ALT).[8,10] Despite often marked elevations in transaminases (2–10-fold) and bile acids (10–100-fold), liver failure does not occur.[8,10,11] In a prospective Scandinavian study of all pregnant women with pruritus over a 1-year period, a diagnosis of obstetric cholestasis was made if one or more of ALT, AST or bilirubin were abnormal. Serum bile acids were assessed in all women with abnormalities in these tests. Amongst cases of obstetric cholestasis, 100% (86 women) had elevated ALT, 99% elevated AST and 22% elevated bilirubin; 92% of cases had elevated serum bile acids.[10] A prospective Portuguese study of 39 women with obstetric cholestasis (elevated cholic acid, ALT, AST or bilirubin in association with pruritus) again found ALT to be elevated in 90% of cases. The reduced figure (compared to 99% in the Scandinavian population) may be explained by the slightly differing diagnostic criteria for obstetric cholestasis in the two studies. The proportion of women with elevated bilirubin was much higher than in the Scandinavian study. It has also been suggested that hyperbilirubinaemia is more common amongst Chilean obstetric cholestasis populations.[12] Despite early definitions of obstetric cholestasis suggesting the presence of hyperbilirubinaemia to be diagnostic, this is now realised not to be the case. Those with normal bilirubin concentrations but other abnormalities may be diagnosed with obstetric cholestasis. Using such criteria, bilirubin is elevated in 22–56% of cases[10,13] but clinical jaundice is rare (20%).[8] Isolated hyperbilirubinaemia in a woman with pruritus may be obstetric cholestasis, but is uncommon, and a careful consideration of other causes is necessary (see later).

More recent studies have included GGT in assessment of liver function and have reported varying levels from normal[10] to elevated in 39% (83 cases)[13] or 50% (50 cases).[14] All three studies used non-pregnant reference ranges which may have underestimated the proportion of cases with raised GGT. While GGT is not elevated as commonly as ALT in obstetric cholestasis, it may describe a sub-group of women with a different pathophysiology (see later).[15]

Serum concentrations of total bile acids and transaminases do not change in parallel with either each other or clinical symptoms in obstetric cholestasis. Indeed, there may be no correlation.[10] The Scandinavian study described earlier found no longitudinal correlation between cholic acid (the most commonly elevated individual bile acid in their series) and ALT or AST.[10]

Within the raised total pool of bile acids found in obstetric cholestasis, differential measurements of bile acids have been performed, although differential testing is not yet widely available. It may, however, provide a more sensitive marker of the disease.

Total bile acids are usually considered to be pathologically raised when concentrations exceed 14 μmol/l. However, a Scandinavian study of clinical outcome in 91 women with obstetric cholestasis described 8 μmol/l as the upper limit of normal,[16] and a Portuguese study suggested above 11 μmol/l[13] as a sensitive and specific concentration for a diagnosis of obstetric cholestasis.

Most experts would consider elevations in one or more of ALT, AST, GGT or total bile acids to be consistent with a diagnosis of obstetric cholestasis.

Presentation

While biochemical testing is clearly important in the diagnosis of obstetric cholestasis, history can also be useful. Obstetric cholestasis most commonly presents in the third trimester (80% develop symptoms after 30 weeks' gestation) and only rarely in the first trimester.[17,18] The pruritus is often severe and typically the palms of the hands and the soles of the feet but the legs, thighs, arms, back, breasts and abdomen are also reported.[8,19] On questioning, women have often had pruritus for several weeks before a diagnosis of obstetric cholestasis is made.

The disease tends to recur in every pregnancy[14,20] and so a past history of the condition is a useful clue. Women may report a positive family history, cyclical pruritus (in 35–50%), or pruritus when taking the combined oral contraceptive pill.[21,22] The disease is more common among multiple gestations (20–22% of obstetric cholestasis pregnancies are twins).[23,24]

Other signs and stigmata of liver disease are not observed in obstetric cholestasis.[8] Additional symptoms, which may be reported in common with other forms of cholestasis, are right upper quadrant pain, pale stools and dark urine.[8]

Concluding a diagnosis of obstetric cholestasis

Liver biopsy in those with obstetric cholestasis demonstrates acinar cholestasis with centrilobular bile staining and bile plugs in the canaliculi and is the only definitive diagnostic test for the disease.[25] However, taking a full history coupled with careful clinical examination, biochemical testing and methodical exclusion of alternative causes of liver disease, means that liver biopsy is rarely necessary.

Possible causes of liver pathology to consider in women with pruritus and abnormal liver function tests include acute infection with hepatitis A, hepatitis B, hepatitis C, Epstein-Barr virus (EBV) or cytomegalovirus (CMV), primary biliary cirrhosis, chronic active hepatitis or biliary obstruction. A number of drugs can also disturb liver function (Table 2).

A personal or family history of gall bladder disease is seen more commonly in obstetric cholestasis than in the general population.[26] Gall bladder volume is increased and function altered in obstetric cholestasis giving a predisposition to the formation of gallstones (and biliary sludge).[8,27,28] However, the presence

Table 2 Differential diagnosis of pruritus and abnormal liver function tests in pregnancy

Differential diagnosis	Features to note in the history	Test
Biliary obstruction	RUQ pain, jaundice, history of gallstones, steatorrhea, dark urine	USS liver, gall bladder and biliary tree
Acute cholecystitis	Severe RUQ pain, nausea, vomiting, systemic malaise, fever	
Viral hepatitides	Systemic malaise	Hepatitis A, B and C. EBV, CMV
Autoimmune liver disease (chronic active hepatitis, primary biliary cirrhosis, sclerosing cholangitis)	History of autoimmune disease	Anti-mitochondrial antibodies, anti-smooth muscle antibodies
Drug reaction	Use of antihypertensives (especially methyldopa but also atenolol and verapamil), antituberculous medication (rifampicin, isoniazid), penicillins (flucloxacillin, ampicillin, amoxacillin, co-amoxiclav), nitrofurantoin, antithyroid medication (propylthiouracil, carbimazole), phenothiazines (*e.g.* chlorpromazine) and paracetamol in high doses	
Congenital (Gilbert's, Dubin-Johnsson, Rotor)	Family history of jaundice particularly during periods of illness	Isolated hyper bilirubinaemia. Note: can also occur in dehydration

of gallstones in isolation does not in itself explain the abnormal liver function unless there is associated duct dilatation. Acute cholecystitis is often suspected clinically prior to USS when gallstones are seen in 90% of cases. However, additional USS criteria such as gallbladder wall thickening, distension, biliary sludge or pericholecystic fluid are necessary in addition to a suitable clinical scenario to confirm the diagnosis.

Hyperemesis gravidarum, the syndrome of haemolysis, elevated liver enzymes, low platelets (HELLP) and acute fatty liver of pregnancy (AFLP) must also be considered in the differential diagnosis of pruritus and abnormal liver function tests, although pruritus is not usually a dominant feature of these. It is important to note that obstetric cholestasis and AFLP may co-exist.[19,29,30]

Obstetric cholestasis has been reported to be of earlier onset in those women who are carriers of hepatitis C.[31] It is not clear if those with other forms of pre-existing liver disease are also at increased risk of developing obstetric cholestasis.

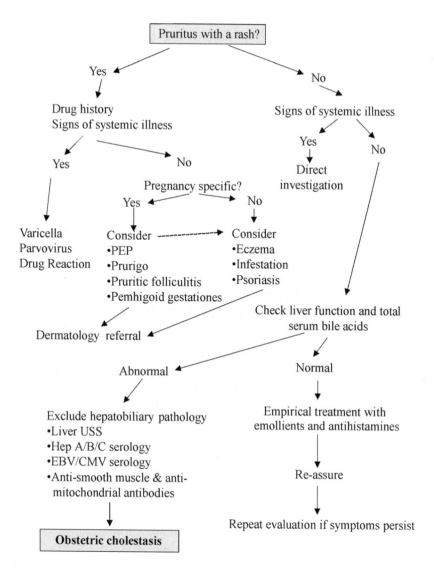

Fig. 1 A flow diagram to facilitate a systematic approach to investigation of pruritus in pregnancy. PEP, polymorphic eruption of pregnancy; EPV, Epstein-Barr virus; CMV, cytomegalovirus. Adapted from Occhipinti *et al. Prim Care Update Obstet Gynaecol* 1997; 4

It is important to note that in women who have been diagnosed with pruritus gravidarum (see Table 1), repeat testing of liver function is necessary if symptoms persist or if the history is particularly suggestive of obstetric cholestasis as pruritus may present prior to any biochemical abnormality.[32]

The diagnostic process in obstetric cholestasis is summarised in Figure 1.

Postnatal course in obstetric cholestasis

Biochemical abnormalities and pruritus in obstetric cholestasis persist until delivery following which resolution occurs. Pruritus is typically absent within

48 h[26,33] and has usually improved within 1 week.[8] A longitudinal study of 86 women demonstrated normal liver function tests (ALT, AST, and bilirubin) in 3–7 days in the majority and by 4–6 weeks post-natally in the remainder.[10] Serum bile acid levels and serum alkaline phosphatase levels may also take up to 6 weeks to return to normal levels after delivery.[8] Prolonged pruritus and biochemical abnormalities post-natally in obstetric cholestasis have been described,[34] but should prompt careful re-evaluation of the diagnosis.

On occasion, liver function tests are performed in postnatal women and, if abnormal, a retrospective search made for a possible cause. While obstetric cholestasis is one such cause it must be borne in mind that liver function tests are affected by mode of delivery. A prospective study in 91 women with normal antenatal liver function reported a rise in AST, ALT, GGT and total bilirubin following delivery. The maximum rise was at day one or two for bilirubin, day two or day five for AST and day five for ALT. Despite the observed rise when compared to pre-delivery samples, the values were only outside the pregnancy specific reference range in 15% for AST, 16% for ALT, 9% for GGT and 10% for bilirubin. Less than 2% of these remained abnormal beyond 10 days. Maternal age at delivery, use of inhalational analgesia or intramuscular injection of opioids and perineal trauma were all associated with greater or faster rises in ALT and AST. Caesarean section was strongly associated with a faster rise in AST compared to vaginal delivery. Breast-feeding was associated with a slower fall in GGT.

A suggested mechanism for the raised ALT and AST is that tissue damage releases iso-enzymes from skeletal muscle, leukocytes and erythrocytes resulting in an overall rise in total enzyme levels.[35]

Prevalence of obstetric cholestasis

The prevalence of obstetric cholestasis in the UK is unknown. One retrospective and one prospective study of UK populations (Birmingham and London, respectively) have suggested a prevalence of 0.6 and 0.7%.[7,36]

In a post-natal questionnaire, 4% (4/86) women suffering unexplained intra-uterine death (> 37 completed weeks' gestation, birth-weight over 2.5 kg, with no life-threatening congenital abnormality) reported pruritus . These women were also noted to have had abnormal liver function when tested at the time of delivery (ALT, AST, bilirubin, GGT, ALP or total bile acids). None had formally been diagnosed with obstetric cholestasis ante-natally.[37] The report does not give details about the nature of the biochemical abnormality, nor consideration of the differing normal ranges for liver function in pregnancy and puerperium or alternative causes of liver disease; none-the-less, it does suggest that obstetric cholestasis is an important cause of otherwise unexplained still-birth.

Outside the UK, the prevalence of obstetric cholestasis is 1–1.5% in Poland and Spain, and 0.2% in France.[25] In Scandinavia, however, the prevalence is higher (2%).[36] The condition is commonest in Chile, where the prevalence has fallen from 14% in 1975 to ~4% in 1995.[38] This fall is despite broadening the definition of the disease; in the earlier study, only those women with hyperbilirubinaemia were classified as having obstetric cholestasis, whereas in the latter any biochemical abnormality in liver function was considered.

Within Chile, closer analysis of the genetic mixture of the population has suggested a much higher incidence (24%) in women of Araucanian Indian descent[39] and clusters of affected women are noted amongst families. In the UK, the disease is seen more commonly among women of Asian descent with 39–41% of women with obstetric cholestasis being of Indian or Pakistani origin.[19,36]

Outcome observed in pregnancies affected by obstetric cholestasis

Historically, obstetric cholestasis and pruritus in pregnancy were thought to be benign. Adverse obstetric outcome in the disease was first quantified by Fisk et al.[40] who reported an overall peri-natal mortality amongst published studies of 70 per 1000 live births and intra-uterine deaths of 30 per 1000 pregnancies between 1966 and 1986.

On reviewing the women diagnosed with obstetric cholestasis in their own hospital between 1965 and 1975, Fisk et al.[42] noted a peri-natal mortality of 107 per 1000. When subsequent populations (1975–1984) of women with obstetric cholestasis in the same hospital were actively managed, the peri-natal mortality was lower, 35 per 1000.[40] This is the first study to suggest that a policy of active management might improve outcome in obstetric cholestasis. The term 'active management' has many different interpretations. In the study by Fisk and co-workers, a single management protocol was not applied to all 83 women. Instead, management was at the discretion of individual consultants responsible for each case. While this study may support the use of active management the fall of 66 deaths per 1000 live births (CI –9 to +139) in peri-natal mortality did not reach significance at the 5% level. The authors attribute the lack of significance to the rarity of obstetric cholestasis and thus the small numbers of women involved. Importantly, the authors did not account for the possibility of falling infant morbidity and mortality during the period of the study. A number of other studies have addressed outcome in obstetric cholestasis and most advocate policies of active management although the management varies with each study. These are shown in Table 3.

Of those studies where policies of active management were clearly described, rates of other complications remain high, e.g. meconium-stained liquor 16–58%, premature delivery 15.7–60%, fetal distress 2–33%,[14,16,23,24,26,41–46] and post-partum haemorrhage (PPH) 20–22%.[26,42] Interestingly, in two of these studies,[41,45] fetal distress, as defined by abnormal CTG (in 2% and 12%), was no more common in the obstetric cholestasis population than in the control population and in one study the premature delivery rate (14%) was not different. The Caesarean section rate was high 25.9–36%[14,16,41,46] in all studies and it is often not clear if this is as a result of active management or because of complications as a result of the disease. Only one study showed no increase in Caesarean section rates among women with obstetric cholestasis (15.1%) who were actively managed as compared to the control population (16%).[47] Most UK hospitals would adopt a policy incorporating antenatal surveillance of some form with elective delivery by 37–38 weeks; such policies must bear in mind the high rates of complications, e.g. Caesarean section, PPH. It is not clear if the latter is as a result of a high Caesarean section rate or as a result of the disease process itself. The benefit of serial ultrasound scanning (USS) has yet to be proven.

Table 3 Summary of publications giving outcome measurements in obstetric cholestasis

Country	First author	OC cases	Active management	Prematurity	C/S distress	Fetal	PPH (of OC)	Meconium (of OC)	Mortality
Chile	Rioseco[41]	320 vs controls	1	15.7% (iatrogenic) 12.1% (spontaneous)	25.9% in labour NS	NS	NE	24.8%	18/1000 NS
Scandinavia	Heinonen[16]	91 vs GP	4	14.3%	25.3% (total)	NE	NE	NE	NE
Australia	Fisk[40]	86	7	44%	NE	22%	NE	45%	35/1000
Australia	Reid[42]	56	No	36%	NE	NE	18%	27%	NE
USA	Roncaglia[43]	206 vs GP	2	27%	NE	2%	NE	16%	↓
China	Liu[44]	30 vs controls	NE	NE	NE	NE	NE	40%	NE
USA	Alsulyman[45]	79 vs controls (history of SB)	6	NS	NE	NE	NE	44%	NS
Granada	Gonzalez[46]	46 vs GP	3	22%	NE	NE	NE	NE	7% OC died
Canada	Shaw[26]	18	3	NE	NE	33%	22%	58.3%	NE
France	Bacq[14]	50	NE	60%	33%	NE	NE	NE	11% OC died
Finland	Laatikainen[24]	116 vs controls	5	NE	NE	38%	NE	28%	6.4% OC died
Sweden	Berg[33]	100 vs controls	NE	7% NS	NE	NE	NE	12% NS	2% OC died
Italy	Roncaglia[47]	206	8	27.2%	15% NS	NE	NE	15.1%	No deaths
Australia	Fisk[48]	83	No	NE	NE	NE	7%	NE	NE
UK	Kenyon[19]	70	9	17% (iatrogenic 11%) (spontaneous 6%)	36%	16% of C/S 50% of instrumentals	17%	14%	No deaths

Abbreviations: OC, obstetric cholestasis; C/S, Caesarean section; PPH, post partum hemorrhage; BWt, birthweight; Retro, retrospective study; Prosp, prospective study; NE, not examined; NS, not statistically significant; GP, general antenatal population; SB, still birth.

Active management key: (see next page)

Table 3 Summary of publications giving outcome measurements in obstetric cholestasis (*continued from previous page*)

Active management key:

1 IOL at 38 weeks. In those with hyperbilirubinaemia and fetal lungs mature delivery at 36 weeks.

2 IOL 39 weeks. > 36 weeks amnioscopy/amniocentesis delivery if meconium noted.

3 IOL when fetal lungs mature.

4 Weekly out-patient monitoring (CTG, AFI, LFTs). IOL if non-stress test non-reactive, AFI < 5, LFTs > 10 times normal. Otherwise IOL at 38–40 weeks.

5 Amnioscopy or oxytocin challenge test on alternate days. Maternal 24-h urinary oestriol excretion weekly. Weekly growth assessment.

6 Weekly non-stress tests and AFI. If normal, await spontaneous onset labour or deliver for standard obstetric indications.

7 Non-stress test or urinary oestriol and AFI with delivery at 38 weeks unless abnormal. OR amniocentesis after 29 weeks repeated weekly if clear until fetal lungs mature delivery if meconium stained.

8 Weekly transcervical amnioscopy or amniocentesis > 36 weeks. Amniocentesis > 36 weeks to assess L:S ratio if severe pruritus or ALT > 300 mg/dl. Biophysical profile if CTG non-reactive. IOL 37 weeks.

9 CTG 3 times a week, weekly USS, vitamin K, delivery at 37–38 weeks.

NO: Expectant management.

Mechanism of fetal risk in obstetric cholestasis

The underlying cause of intra-uterine death, fetal distress, meconium staining of liquor and premature delivery in obstetric cholestasis remains unclear. Prediction of those fetuses at risk of death has not been possible.

Intra-uterine deaths have been reported in those with normal CTGs in the last 5 days[41,45,49,50] and Doppler investigations of the umbilical artery have not been helpful in determining the risk of fetal compromise.[51,52] Two studies suggest an association with low birth-weight;[16,53] however, the majority do not[14,26,41,45,52] and those fetuses who are still-born, are phenotypically normal.[45] The clinical scenario would suggest that the most likely explanation for fetal demise is one of an acute anoxic event rather than chronic utero-placental insufficiency. High concentrations of bile acids have been implicated in the pathophysiology.

Bile acids can be detected not only in maternal serum but also fetal cord blood, amniotic fluid, neonatal meconium and colostrum[26,54–57] in falling concentrations, respectively. Those bile acids observed in fetal compartments are thought to be of maternal origin.[56] This source would account for the presence of secondary bile acids in the fetal bile acid pool despite the absence of intestinal microflora in the fetus.[58] It is possible that high concentrations of fetal bile acids may contribute to an acute event resulting in fetal death and possible mechanisms have been suggested. In high concentrations, CA, CDCA and DCA have a vasoconstrictive effect on placental chorionic veins which is most marked for cholic acid and is dose dependent.[59] Vasospasm such as this occurring at the placental chorionic surface may lead to fetal asphyxia. In experimental settings, meconium has been shown to cause umbilical vein constriction[60] (and fetal hypo-perfusion). The presence of meconium (a rich source of bile acids), known to be associated with a poorer outcome in obstetric cholestasis[40] would contribute to an even higher concentration of bile acids bathing the placental chorionic veins. In the clinical setting, when examining placentae and umbilical cords from pregnancies with meconium-stained liquor those with features of vascular necrosis were associated with adverse fetal outcome.[61] Alternative mechanisms by which bile acids may act as toxins are suggested by experimental work in animals. Addition of the bile acid taurocholic acid (TCA; 0.1–3.0 mmol/l) to rat cardiomyocytes has been shown to decrease their rate of spontaneous contraction and to destroy their synchronous beating.[62,63] Acute exposure to taurochenodeoxycholic acid (TCDA) in the rat induces a cell death process with apoptotic features.[64] It is important to consider, however, that experimental studies *in vitro* use much higher concentrations (*e.g.* 0.1–3 mmol/l)) of bile acids than have been measured in obstetric cholestasis cases *in vivo* (*e.g.* 0–10 µmol/l).

Other complications observed in obstetric cholestasis (*e.g.* pre-term delivery and meconium staining of liquor) might also be attributed to the effects of high concentrations of bile acids. Bile acids are known to have cellular effects that could mediate increased uterine contractility. For example CA causes dose-dependent increased contractility in rat myometrium[65] and infusion in sheep induces pre-term labour.[66] One human study has suggested that myometrium from pregnancies affected by obstetric cholestasis is more sensitive to oxytocin;[67] however, this latter study did not investigate the contribution of bile acids to the increased sensitivity. Meconium passage is commonly seen in pregnancies affected by obstetric cholestasis and again high concentrations of bile acids have been implicated following the observation in animal studies that CA increases the incidence of meconium passage. Given the observed effect of bile acids on myometrial cells, the mechanism suggested is that bile acids have an effect on colonic musculature and subsequent motility.[68]

Bile acids may be important in the pathophysiology of obstetric cholestasis both in terms of fetal demise and maternal symptoms (bile acids have been implicated as possible pruritogens in obstetric cholestasis[10,69]). One might, therefore, expect a worse obstetric outcome in those with more marked biochemical abnormalities. However, severity of symptoms or degree of abnormality in liver function has not conclusively been shown to correlate with obstetric outcome in obstetric cholestasis. Two studies have reported that intra-uterine death[10,14] is only seen in those with the most severe disease, *i.e.* highest levels of bile acids (CA > 15 µmol/l).[10] Abnormal CTG tracings have also been observed more commonly in those with high maternal and cord plasma concentrations of bile acids.[10,56,70] Other studies have reported no correlation between fetal distress (abnormal CTG) and bile acid levels in maternal serum[26,71] nor umbilical cord.[71] In addition, no correlation between maternal serum bile acid concentrations and Doppler studies on the fetal umbilical artery have been shown.[51]

Studies measuring other aspects of liver function have similar variable results. One study of 116 women reported fetal distress (abnormal CTG, meconium-stained liquor) more commonly in those with high AST and ALT (> 100 IU/l) concentrations.[24] Elsewhere, one study showed no relationship between the degree of maternal biochemical abnormality and fetal outcome.[42]

To date, few policies of active management in obstetric cholestasis pregnancies involve interventions based on degree of biochemical severity. Only one of the studies discussed earlier (see Table 3) intervened on the basis of blood results and had a high prematurity rate as a result with no clear difference in outcome compared to other studies.[47] Until the pathophysiology of obstetric cholestasis is understood more clearly, it seems appropriate to offer all women the same policy of active management regardless of the severity of the abnormal in liver function.

Treatment of obstetric cholestasis

There is, at present, no definitive treatment for obstetric cholestasis resulting in resolution of disease. Medications have been selected based on knowledge of their actions in cholestasis outside pregnancy. None have conclusively been shown to improve outcome in affected pregnancies.

Anti-histamines

Antihistamines such as chlorpheniramine (4 mg 4–6 hourly) can provide symptomatic relief in terms of pruritus. If drowsiness is proving troublesome, then limiting a single dose to evenings may be of some use.

Topical treatments

If the skin is well moisturised, pruritus may be relieved. Suitable preparations for this include Balneum plus™ bath lotion with topical Diprobase™ before and after bathing. Aqueous cream preparations with menthol (1–2%) can also provide relief.

Ursodeoxycholic acid

Ursodeoxycholic acid (UDCA) is itself a bile acid but only a minority species in the human and more hydrophilic than the other primary and secondary human bile acids. Ursodeoxycholic acid has many suggested mechanisms of action and the particular role that may be of benefit in obstetric cholestasis is not clear. Its uses outside pregnancy are in dissolution of gallstones and improving liver function in primary biliary cirrhosis.[72] Perhaps most importantly in obstetric cholestasis, it is thought to protect against the membrane damaging toxicity of other hydrophobic endogenous bile acids by displacing and replacing them in the bile acid pool (hepato-protective).[73] It improves biliary secretion both of hydrophobic bile acids and phospholipids (which are themselves hepato-protective). Additional immunomodulatory effects have been described[72] with UDCA reducing expression of major histocompatability complex (MHC) class I antigens on hepatocytes.[74] Several small studies of its use in obstetric cholestasis have reported its benefit in normalising serum bile acids and/or symptoms.[75–82] Only two of these studies involving 8[75] and 15[76] patients were randomised controlled trials. They both reported improvement in pruritus and liver function when UDCA (600 mg/day[75] and 1 g/day[76]) was given to women with obstetric cholestasis. With such small numbers involved, it is not possible to draw conclusions about effect on outcome. Although not statistically significant, treatment with UDCA in the larger study did appear to prolong pregnancy in nine treated women as compared to eight untreated women (35 ± 0.8 weeks versus 33.8 ± 0.8 weeks).[76] The recommended formulary dose is 8–15 mg/kg/day (BNF), but higher doses up to a maximum of 2 g/day[81] have been reported. The usual initial dose is 500 mg BD increasing to a maximum 1 g BD. It can often take 48 h before any improvement in symptoms is perceived. Once commenced, it should be continued until delivery. Ursodeoxycholic acid is currently not licensed for use in pregnancy; although no adverse effects have been reported in humans, appropriate counselling of women is necessary before treatment. Practice varies throughout the UK with some centres offering UDCA to all women with obstetric cholestasis on the presumption that high bile acid concentrations should be avoided and treatment should, therefore, be aimed at reducing them. Elsewhere, some feel that UDCA should be reserved for women with severe symptoms as evidence regarding its safety and effect in obstetric cholestasis with respect to outcome is lacking.

S-Adenosyl methionine

There are conflicting reports as to the benefit of S-adenosyl methionine (S-AME) in treating obstetric cholestasis. It is said to have a number of effects. When given intravenously in large doses (600–900 mg), it has variously been reported to improve symptoms and liver function when compared to controls,[83–85] or to those treated with UDCA,[84] show no effect when compared to controls[86] or treatment with UDCA[82] or to improve pruritus but not liver function when compared to UDCA.[87] One of these studies suggested a combination of UDCA and S-AME was better than either alone,[84] and another suggested a reduction in pre-term labour in those receiving treatment with S-AME.[85] Again, all of these studies were small (18–46 patients) and conclusions about outcome cannot be drawn. It must be given intravenously and is not widely used.

Dexamethasone

When given to 10 women with obstetric cholestasis, dexamethasone in high doses (12 mg orally for 7 days with a reducing dose for 3 days) resulted in resolution of pruritus in all cases and significant reduction in total bile acids and ALT. Total bile acid concentrations fell on day 4 and ALT on day 12 from the start of therapy. There was no reported recurrence of symptoms or biochemical abnormality. The drug was well tolerated and did not reveal any diabetic pregnancies.[88] The mechanism of action is suggested to be one of suppression of oestrogen production by the feto-placental unit. This remains the only clinical study of the benefits of dexamethasone in obstetric cholestasis to date. This study reported dexamethasone use in isolation but elsewhere it has been used in addition to UDCA when maximal doses of UDCA have failed to control symptoms.[19] In vitro studies with dexamethasone have suggested it may protect cultured cardiac myocytes from the arrythmogenic (and, therefore, toxic) effect of taurocholate. This effect was observed when cells were pre-incubated with dexamethasone (80 nM) for 16 h. It was not possible to reverse the effects of taurocholate by later addition of dexamethasone.[89] Further work must be done to determine if dexamethasone has any effect in improving obstetric outcome for this was not formally determined in the small Hirvioja study.

Vitamin K

The administration of oral vitamin K to reduce the risk of post-partum haemorrhage (PPH) may be beneficial. A suggested mechanism for the observed increased incidence of PPH in obstetric cholestasis is malabsorption and subsequent deficiency of vitamin K. Vitamin K is a fat-soluble vitamin and is required for the hepatic synthesis of clotting factors II, VII, IX and X. Adequate absorption of vitamin K is dependent on adequate bile secretion and formation of micelles.[14] Studies of fat excretion in women with obstetric cholestasis identified steatorrhea which may be sub-clinical (but demonstrable on faecal fat assay) but sufficient to affect maternal nutritional status and intestinal absorption of fat-soluble vitamins such as vitamin K.[90] Prothrombin time (PT) is usually normal in obstetric cholestasis but where it is not it may be corrected with vitamin K.[14] Oral vitamin K in such cases should be of the water-soluble form (menadiol sodium phosphate 10 mg orally daily). As yet, no randomised, controlled studies have been performed to establish a benefit in those with obstetric cholestasis and normal PT. A UK series of 59/70 women with obstetric cholestasis receiving vitamin K (commenced at 34 weeks' gestation) reported that in those who did not receive vitamin K, 4/11 (36%) had blood loss at delivery in excess of 500 ml compared to 10% of those who received vitamin K. However, the iatrogenic delivery rate was high (36% Caesarean sections) in the group. The post-partum haemorrhage rate may, therefore, be less than the 20–22% incidence reported in the literature without the use of vitamin K.[19]

Other treatments

Cholestyramine is a bile acid chelating agent and is reported to improve pruritus in some women. In its powder form, it is mixed with water and taken in doses of 4 g, 2–3 times daily. It is poorly tolerated and may exacerbate vitamin K deficiency; it has been associated with fetal intracranial haemorrhage in such cases.[91] Activated charcoal and guar gum act in a similar way and have been reported to be of some benefit in normalising total bile acid levels but are no longer widely used.

RESEARCH DIRECTIONS

The pathophysiology of obstetric cholestasis is not clearly understood and is the focus of much scientific work. Bile acids are thought to be important with respect to development of symptoms, liver damage (cause or effect) and fetal compromise. As described earlier, bile acids are continuously undergoing a process of hepatic synthesis, canalicular secretion and sinusoidal uptake. Transfer of bile acids into the bile canaliculus utilises multi-drug resistant gene product 3 (MDR3) which is located on the canalicular membrane. MDR3 is not involved directly in transporting bile acids but it is essential for movement of the phosphatidylcholine from the inner to the outer leaflet of the plasma membrane. This, in turn, assists in protecting the cells lining the bile ducts against the action of the free hydrophobic bile salts and is required for the formation of micelles. Defects in MDR3 (coded for on chromosome 18)[92] mean phospholipid secretion into bile is impaired, and so the bile ducts are unprotected from the damaging effects of the hydrophobic bile acids. The epithelial lining cells are thus damaged and release their membrane bound enzymes (*e.g.* GGT). This form of liver disease is known as progressive familial intrahepatic cholestasis (PFIC). When following pedigrees affected by PFIC, researchers noted that there was an increased incidence of obstetric cholestasis and that these women were heterozygous for MDR3.[93] Conversely, when investigating women with obstetric cholestasis associated with a raised GGT and no known family history of PFIC, Dixon *et al.*[15] found one case (of eight) had similar mutations in the MDR3 gene (*i.e.* were heterozygous). Defective MDR3 may be one mechanism for a particular phenotype of obstetric cholestasis in a subgroup with a raised GGT.[15] Other defective bile salt transporter proteins are known to cause familial liver disease outside pregnancy (*e.g.* benign recurrent intrahepatic cholestasis (BRIC) caused by mutations in familial intrahepatic cholestasis 1 gene (*FIC 1* gene)).[15] A family in which there were three cases of BRIC included nine members reporting pruritus and or jaundice in pregnancy (obstetric cholestasis). Two additional members reported pruritus when taking the combined oral contraceptive pill.[94]

Abnormal function of these transport proteins may explain the biochemical abnormalities seen in obstetric cholestasis. However, by definition, symptoms and biochemical abnormalities in obstetric cholestasis normalise following delivery. A genetically inherited abnormality (*e.g.* heterozygosity for MDR3) may result in a predisposition to obstetric cholestasis with subsequent development of the disease being multifactorial in origin (*e.g.* elevated oestrogen in pregnancy, environmental effects, maternal age, *etc.*). Testing for gene alterations among women with obstetric cholestasis is a research direction being undertaken at present. Other research is being conducted into identifying more subtle changes in liver metabolism in women with, or at risk of obstetric cholestasis to allow earlier identification of the disease. Indeed, it has been shown that pruritus may present before any biochemical abnormality is currently detectable.[32] One promising marker is glutathione-S-transferase, which has been shown to be abnormal as early as 24 weeks' gestation in women who developed clinical obstetric cholestasis nine weeks later.

CONCLUSIONS

Pruritus is common in pregnancy with some of these women suffering obstetric cholestasis. It is important to have a clear diagnostic protocol to follow in order to diagnose the disease, as policies of active management (elective early delivery, antenatal fetal surveillance) which may improve obstetric outcome are associated with high rates of intervention (*e.g.* Caesarean section, iatrogenic prematurity, post-partum haemorrhage). Current treatment strategies have not been shown to be of benefit in reducing perinatal morbidity but may be effective in controlling pruritus. On delivery, the condition resolves but has a high recurrence rate in subsequent pregnancies. A randomised controlled trial of elective versus anticipated delivery is needed, and we need to establish whether the severity of biochemical abnormality is related to obstetric outcome. Future research will determine if the disease has a genetic aetiology and allow earlier detection of the disease that, in turn, may allow us to better identify those fetuses at risk.

References

1 Holmes RC, Black MM. The specific dermatoses of pregnancy. J Acad Dermatol 1983; 8: 405–412

2 Vaughn Jones SA, Hern S, Nelson-Piercy C, Seed PT, Black MM. A prospective study of 200 women with dermatoses of pregnancy correlating clinical findings with hormonal and immunopathological profiles. Br J Dermatol 1999; 141: 71–81

3 Nelson-Piercy C. Skin Disease. Handbook of Obstetric Medicine. Oxford: Oxford University Press, 1997; 194–200

4 Aractingi S, Berkane N, Bertheau Ph et al. Fetal DNA in skin of polymorphic eruptions of pregnancy. Lancet 1998; 352: 1898–1901

5 Cohen LM, Capeless EL, Krusinski PA, Maloney ME. Pruritic urticarial papules and plaques of pregnancy and its relationship to maternal-fetal weight gain and twin pregnancies. Arch Dermatol 1989; 125: 1534–1536

6 Kolodney RC. Herpes gestationes; a new assessment of incidence diagnosis and fetal prognosis. Am J Obstet Gynecol 1969; 104: 39–45

7 Kenyon AP, Girling J, Nelson-Piercy C et al. Pruritus in pregnancy and the identification of obstetric cholestasis risk: a prospective prevalence study of 6531 women. J Obstet Gynaecol 2002; 22 (Suppl 1): 1–3

8 Reyes H. The spectrum of liver and gastrointestinal disease seen in cholestasis of pregnancy. Gastroenterol Clin North Am 1992; 21: 905–921

9 Girling JC, Dow E, Smith JH. Liver function tests in pre-eclampsia: importance of comparison with a reference range derived for normal pregnancy. Br J Obstet Gynaecol 1997; 104: 246–250

10 Laatikainen T, Ikonen E. Serum bile acids in cholestasis of pregnancy. Obstet Gynecol 1977; 50: 313–318

11 Heikkinen J, Maentausta O, Ylostalo P, Janne O. Changes in serum bile acid concentrations during normal pregnancy, in patients with intrahepatic cholestasis of pregnancy and in pregnant women with itching. Br J Obstet Gynaecol 1981; 88: 240–245

12 Rioseco AJ. Hyperbilirubinaemia more prevalent amongst Chilean populations. Personal communication

13 Brites D, Rodrigues CMP, van-Zeller H, Brito A, Silva R. Relevance of serum bile acid profile in the diagnosis of intrahepatic cholestasis of pregnancy in an high incidence area: Portugal. Eur J Obstet Gynecol Reprod Biol 1998; 80: 31–38

14 Bacq Y, Sapey T, Brechot MC, Pierre F, Fignon A, Dubois F. Intrahepatic cholestasis of pregnancy: a French prospective study. Hepatology 1997; 26: 358–364

15 Dixon PH, Weerasekara N, Linton KJ et al. Heterozygous MDR3 missense mutation associated with intrahepatic cholestasis of pregnancy: evidence for a defect in protein trafficking. Hum Mol Genet 2000; 9: 1209–1217

16 Heinonen S, Kirkinen P. Pregnancy outcome with intrahepatic cholestasis. Obstet Gynecol 1999; 94: 189–193

17 Kirkinen P, Ryynanen M. First-trimester manifestation of intrahepatic cholestasis of pregnancy and high fetoplacental hormone production in a triploid fetus – a case-report. J Reprod Med 1995; 40: 471–473

18 Brites D, Rodrigues CMP, Cardoso MD, Graca LM. Unusual case of severe cholestasis of pregnancy with early onset, improved by ursodeoxycholic acid administration. Eur J Obstet Gynecol Reprod Biol 1998; 76: 165–168

19 Kenyon AP, Nelson-Piercy C, Girling J, Williamson C, Tribe RM, Shennan AH. Obstetric cholestasis, outcome with active management: a series of 70 cases. Br J Obstet Gynaecol 2002; 109: 282–288

20 Reyes H. The enigma of intrahepatic cholestasis: lessons from Chile. Hepatology 1982; 2: 87–96

21 Williamson C, Hems LM, Walker I, Chambers J, Donaldson O, De Swiet DG Johnston OG. Clinical outcome in a series of cases of obstetric cholestasis identified via a patient support group. Br J Obstet Gynaecol 2004; 111: 676–681

22 Vore M. Estrogen cholestasis: membranes, metabolites or receptors? Gastroenterology 1987; 93: 643–649

23 Gonzalez CG, Reyes H, Arrese M et al. Intrahepatic cholestasis of pregnancy in twin pregnancies. J Hepatol 1989; 9: 84—90

24 Laatikainen T, Ikonen E. Fetal prognosis in obstetric hepatosis. Ann Chir Gynecol

Fenniae 1975; 64: 155–164

25 Raine Fenning N, Kilby M. Obstetric cholestasis. Fetal Maternal Med Rev 1997; 9: 1–17

26 Shaw D, Frohlich J, Wittman BAK, Willms M. A prospective study of 18 patients with cholestasis of pregnancy. Am J Obstet Gynecol 1982; 142: 621–625

27 Kirkinen P, Ylostalo P, Heikkinen J, Maentausta O. Gallbladder function and maternal bile acids in intrahepatic cholestasis of pregnancy. Eur J Obstet Gynaecol Reprod Biol 1984; 18: 29–34

28 Furhoff AK. Itching in pregnancy: a 15 year follow up study. Acta Med Scand 1974; 196: 403–410

29 Vanjak D, Moreau R, Roche-Sicot J, Soulier A, Sicot C. Intrahepatic cholestasis of pregnancy and acute fatty liver of pregnancy: an unusual but favourable association? Gastroenterology 1991; 100: 1123–1125

30 Reyes H, Sandoval L, Wainstein A et al. Acute fatty liver of pregnancy: a clinical study of 12 episodes in patients. Gut 1994; 35: 101–106

31 Locatelli A, Roncaglia N, Arreghini A, Bellini P, Vergani P, Ghidini A. Hepatitis C virus infection is associated with a higher incidence of cholestasis of pregnancy. Br J Obstet Gynaecol 1999; 106: 498–500

32 Kenyon AP, Nelson-Piercy C, Girling J, Williamson C, Tribe RM, Shennan AH. Pruritus may precede abnormal liver function tests in pregnant women with obstetric cholestasis: a longitudinal analysis. Br J Obstet Gynaecol 2001; 108: 1190–1192

33 Berg B, Helm G, Petersohn L et al. Cholestasis of pregnancy: clinical and laboratory studies. Acta Obstet Gynecol Scand 1986; 65: 107–113

34 Olsson R, Tysk C, Aldenborg F, Holm B. Prolonged postpartum course of intrahepatic cholestasis of pregnancy. Gastroenterology 1993; 105: 267–271

35 David AL, Kotecha M, Girling JC. Factors influencing postnatal liver function tests. Br J Obstet Gynaecol 2000; 107: 1421–1426

36 Abedin P, Weaver JB, Eggington E. Intrahepatic cholestasis of pregnancy: prevalence and ethnic distribution. Ethnic Health 1999; 4: 35–37

37 CESDI Consortium. Study of antepartum term stillbirths. 5th Annual Report. Maternal and Child Health Research Consortium. Confidential Enquiry into Stillbirths and Deaths in Infancy. London: HMSO, 1995; 41–50

38 Reyes H. Intrahepatic cholestasis. A puzzling disorder of pregnancy. J Gastroenterol Hepatol 1997; 12: 211–216

39 Reyes H, Gonzalez MC, Ribalta J et al. Prevalence of intrahepatic cholestasis of pregnancy in Chile. Ann Intern Med 1978; 88: 487–625

40 Fisk NM, Storey GNB. Fetal outcome in obstetric cholestasis. Br J Obstet Gynaecol 1988; 95: 1137–1143

41 Rioseco AJ, Ivankovic MB, Manzur A et al. Intrahepatic cholestasis of pregnancy — a retrospective case-control study of perinatal outcome. Am J Obstet Gynecol 1994; 170: 890–895

42 Reid R, Ivey KJ, Rencoret RH, Storey B. Fetal complications of obstetric cholestasis. BMJ 1976; 1: 870–872

43 Roncaglia N, Arreghini A, Locatelli A, Bellini P, Mariani F, Ghidini A. Intrahepatic cholestasis of pregnancy: effects of timed intervention on perinatal mortality. J Soc Gynecol Invest 1999; 6:48A

44 Liu s, Cai I, Qie M. Perinatal monitoring in intrahepatic cholestasis of pregnancy. Hua Hsi I Ko Ta Hsueh Pao 1997; 28: 98–100

45 Alsulyman OM, Ouzounian JG, Ames Castro M, Goodwin TM. Intrahepatic cholestasis of pregnancy: perinatal outcome associated with expectant management. Am J Obstet Gynecol 1996; 175: 957–960

46 Gonzalez A, Mino M, Fontes J et al. Intrahepatic cholestasis of pregnancy. Maternal and fetal implications. Revista Espanola De Enfermedades Digestivas 1996; 88: 780–784

47 Roncaglia N, Arreghini A, Locatelli A, Bellini P, Andreotti C, Ghidini A. Obstetric cholestasis: outcome with active management. Eur J Obstet Gynecol Reprod Biol 2002; 100: 167–170

48 Fisk NM, Bye WB, Bruce-Storey GN. Maternal features of obstetric cholestasis: 20 years' experience at King George V Hospital. Aust NZ J Obstet Gynaecol 1988; 28: 172–176

49 Medina Lomeli JM, Medina Castro N. Intrahepatic cholestasis of pregnancy, an unpredictable fetal risk: report of a case and review of the literature. Ginecol Obstet Mex

2000; 68: 486–488

50 Londero F, SanMarco L. Intrahepatic cholestasis of pregnancy: are we really able to predict fetal outcome? Am J Obstet Gynecol 1997; 177: 1274

51 Zimmerman P, Koskinen J, Vaalamo P, Ranta T. Doppler umbilical artery velocimetry in pregnancies complicated by intrahepatic cholestasis. J Perinat Med 1991; 19: 351–355

52 Guerra F, Guzman S, Campos G. Evaluation of maternal and fetal blood flow indices in intrahepatic cholestasis of pregnancy. Rev Chil Obstet Ginecol 1994; 59: 17–21

53 Vega J, Saez G, Smith M, Agurto M, Morris NM. Risk factors for low birth weight and intrauterine growth retardation in Santiago, Chile. Rev Med Chil 1993; 121: 1210–1219

54 Brites D, Rodrigues CMP. Elevated levels of bile acids in colostrum of patients with cholestasis of pregnancy are decreased following ursodeoxycholic acid therapy. J Hepatol 1998; 29: 743–751

55 Laatikainen T, Lehtonen PJ, Hesso AE. Fetal sulfated and nonsulfated bile acids in intrahepatic cholestasis of pregnancy. J Lab Clin Med 1978; 92: 185–193

56 Laatikainen T. Fetal bile acid levels in pregnancies complicated by maternal intrahepatic cholestasis. Am J Obstet Gynecol 1975; 122: 852–856

57 Rodrigues CMP, Marin JJG, Brites D. Bile acid patterns in meconium are influenced by cholestasis of pregnancy and not altered by ursodeoxycholic acid treatment. Gut 1999; 45: 446–452

58 Monte JM, Morales AI, Arevalo M, Alvaro I, Macias RIR, Marin JG. Reversible impairment of neonatal hepatobiliary function by maternal cholestasis. Hepatology 1996; 23: 1208–1217

59 Sepulvida WH, Gonzalez C, Cruz MA, Rudolph MI. Vasoconstrictive effect of bile acids on isolated human placental chorionic veins. Eur J Obstet Gynaecol Reprod Biol 1991; 42: 211–215

60 Altshuler G, Hyde S. Meconium-induced vasocontraction: a potential cause of cerebral and other fetal hypoperfusion and of poor pregnancy outcome. J Child Neurol 1989; 4: 137–142

61 Altshuler G, Arizawa M, Molnar-Nadasdy G. Meconium-induced umbilical cord vascular necrosis and ulceration: a potential link between the placenta and poor pregnancy outcome. Obstet Gynecol 1992; 79: 760–766

62 Williamson C, Gorelik J, Eaton BM, de Swiet M, Korchev Y. The bile acid taurocholate impairs rat cardiomyocyte function: proposed mechanism for intra-uterine fetal death in obstetric cholestasis. Clin Sci 2001; 100: 363–369

63 Gorelik J, Harding SE, Shevchuk AI et al. Taurocholate induces changes in rat cardiomyocyte contraction and calcium dynamics. Clin Sci 2002; 103: 191–200

64 Chieco P, Romagnoli E, Aicardi G, Suozzi A, Forti GC, Roda A. Apoptosis induced in rat hepatocytes by in vivo exposure to taurochenodeoxycholate. Histochem J 2001; 29: 875–883

65 Campos G, Toro F, Castillo R. Efecto de los acidos bilares sobre la contractibilidad miometral en utero gestante aislado. Chile Obstet Gynecol 1988; 53: 229–233

66 Campos G, Guerra F, Israel E. Effects of cholic acid infusions in fetal lambs. Acta Obstet Gynecol Scand 1986; 65: 23

67 Israel EJ, Guzman ML, Campos GA. Maximal response to oxytocin of the isolated myometrium from pregnant patients with intrahepatic cholestasis. Acta Obstet Gynecol Scand 1986; 65: 581–582

68 Davidson KM. Intrahepatic cholestasis of pregnancy. Semin Perinatol 1998; 22: 104–111

69 Bergasa NV, Jones EA. The pruritus of cholestasis. Semin Liver Dis 1993; 13: 319–327

70 Laatikainen T, Tulenheimo A. Maternal serum bile acid levels and fetal distress in cholestasis of pregnancy. Int J Gynecol Obstet 1984; 22: 91–94

71 Heikkinen J, Maentausta O, Tuimala R, Ylostalo P, Janne O. Amniotic fluid bile acids in normal and pathologic pregnancy. Obstet Gynecol 1980; 56: 60–64

72 Kowdley KV. Ursodeoxycholic acid therapy in hepatobiliary disease. Am J Med 2000; 108: 481–486

73 Elias E. URSO in obstetric cholestasis: not a bear market. Gut 1999; 45: 331–332

74 Hirano F, Tanaka H, Makino Y, Okamoto K, Makino I. Effects of ursodeoxycholic acid and chenodeoxycholic acid on major histocompatibility complex class I gene expression. J Gastroenterol 1996; 31: 55–60

75 Diaferia A, Nicastri PL, Tartagni M, Loizzi P, Iacovizzi C, DiLeo A. Ursodeoxycholic acid therapy in pregnant women with cholestasis. Int J Gynecol Obstet 1996; 52: 133–140

76 Palma J, Reyes H, Ribalta J et al. Ursodeoxycholic acid in the treatment of cholestasis of

pregnancy: a randomized, double-blind study controlled with placebo. J Hepatol 1997; 27: 1022–1028

77 Floreani A, Paternoster D, Grella V, Sacco S, Gangemi M. Ursodeoxycholic acid in intrahepatic cholestasis of pregnancy. Br J Obstet Gynaecol 1994; 101: 64–65

78 Brites D, Rodrigues CMP, Oliveira N, Cardoso MD, Graca LM. Correction of maternal serum bile acid profile during ursodeoxycholic acid therapy in cholestasis of pregnancy. J Hepatol 1998; 28: 91–98

79 Palma J, Reyes H, Ribalta J et al. Effects of ursodeoxycholic acid in patients with intrahepatic cholestasis of pregnancy. Hepatology 1992; 15: 1043–1047

80 Davies MH, Dasilva RCMA, Jones SR, Weaver JB, Elias E. Fetal mortality associated with cholestasis of pregnancy and the potential benefit of therapy with ursodeoxycholic acid. Gut 1995; 37: 580–584

81 Giuseppe M, Rizzo N, Azzaroli F et al. Ursodeoxycholic acid administration in patients with cholestasis of pregnancy: effects on primary bile acids in babies and mothers. Hepatology 2001; 33: 504–508

82 Floreani A, Paternoster D, Melis A, Grella PV. S-adenosylmethionine versus ursodeoxycholic acid in the treatment of intrahepatic cholestasis of pregnancy: preliminary results of a controlled trial. Eur J Obstet Gynecol Reprod Biol 1996; 67: 109–113

83 Frezza M, Pozzato G, Chiesa L, Stramentinoli G, Di Padova C. Reversal of interhepatic cholestasis of pregnancy in women after high dose S-adenosyl-L-methionine administration. Hepatology 2001; 4: 274–278

84 Nicastri PL, Diaferia A, Tartagni N, Loizzi P, Fanelli M. A randomised placebo-controlled trial of ursodeoxycholic acid and S-adenosylmethionine in the treatment of intrahepatic cholestasis of pregnancy. Br J Obstet Gynaecol 1998; 105: 1205–1207

85 Frezza M, Centini G, Cammareri G, Le Grazie C, Di Padova C. S-adenosylmethionine for the treatment of intrahepatic cholestasis of pregnancy. Results of a controlled clinical trial. Hepatogastroenterology 1990; 37: 122–125

86 Ribalta J, Reyes H, Gonzalez MC et al. S-adenosyl-l-methionine in the treatment of patients with intrahepatic cholestasis of pregnancy – a randomized, double-blind, placebo-controlled study with negative results. Hepatology 1991; 13: 1084–1089

87 Roncaglia N, Locatelli A, Arreghini A et al. A randomised controlled trial of ursodeoxycholic acid and S-adenosyl-L-methionine in the treatment of gestational cholestasis. Br J Obstet Gynaecol 2004; 111: 17–21

88 Hirvioja M, Tuimala R, Vuori J. The treatment of intrahepatic cholestasis of pregnancy by dexamethasone. Br J Obstet Gynaecol 1992; 99: 109–111

89 Gorelik J, Shevchuk AI, Diakonov I et al. Dexamethasone and ursodeoxycholic acid protect against the arrhythmogenic effect of taurocholate in an *in vitro* study of rat cardiomyocytes. Br J Obstet Gynaecol 2003; 110: 467–474

90 Reyes H, Radrigan ME, Gonzalez MC et al. Steatorrhea in patients with intrahepatic cholestasis of pregnancy. Gastroenterology 1987; 93: 584—590

91 Sadler LC, Lane M, North R. Severe fetal intracranial hemorrhage during treatment with cholestyramine for intrahepatic cholestasis of pregnancy. Br J Obstet Gynaecol 1995; 102: 169–170

92 De Vree JML, Jacquemin E, Sturm E et al. Mutations in the MDR3 gene cause progressive familial intrahepatic cholestasis. Proc Natl Acad Sci USA 1998; 95: 282–287

93 Jacquemin E, Crestell D, Manouvrier S, Boute O, Hadchouel M. Heterozygous non-sense mutation of the MDR3 gene in familial intrahepatic cholestasis of pregnancy. Lancet 1999; 353: 210–211

94 de Pagter AG, van Berge Henegouwen GP, ten Bokkel Huinink JA, Brandt KH. Familial benign recurrent intrahepatic cholestasis. Interrelation with intrahepatic cholestasis of pregnancy and from oral contraceptives. Gastroenterology 1976; 71: 202—207

Judith Hyde Emma Treloar Robert Fox

4

Gestational diabetes mellitus re-appraised

Gestational diabetes mellitus (GDM) is essentially the development of diabetes in pregnancy with a return to normal glucose tolerance after delivery. Virtually all new cases of diabetes in pregnancy are a transient form of type 2 diabetes (T2DM). A small proportion of cases of *de novo* diabetes are found to persist after pregnancy. Most of these are true T2DM; however, rarely, type 1 diabetes (T1DM) will arise during pregnancy simply as a matter of coincidence. In contrast to true GDM, T1DM is a symptomatic condition typified by ketoacidosis.

For many years, there was is no universal consensus on the definition of GDM with confusion over the distinction between impaired glucose tolerance (GIGT) and frank diabetes (GDM). What has been agreed is that more severe forms of gestational glucose intolerance are linked to adverse outcome (Table 1). In a desire to prevent perinatal death and serious morbidity, screening/ intervention programmes became widespread beyond the mid 1970s; by 1999, 89% of UK maternity units were screening for GDM.[1] For many clinicians, the benefit of screening for gestational diabetes was self-evident but, in truth, screening was popularised before considerations of evidence-based practice came onto the health scene. In 1993, Jarrett, a clinical epidemiologist, described GDM as a non-entity which did not achieve the major criteria for a worthwhile screening programme.[2] He pointed out that screening for GDM had failed to gain support from several national organisations including the Cochrane collaboration, the Canadian Task Force on Diabetes, the Center for Disease

Judith Hyde MB MRCOG
Specialist Registrar, Southmead Hospital, Westbury-on-Trym, Bristol, UK

Emma Treloar MB MRCOG
Specialist Registrar, Gloucester Royal Infirmary, Gloucester, UK

Robert Fox MB MRCOG
Consultant Obstetrician, Division of Obstetrics, Gynaecology & Paediatrics, Taunton & Somerset Hospital, Taunton TA1 5DA, UK (for correspondence, E-mail: indigofoxbat@hotmail.com)

Table 1 Adverse outcomes associated with gestational diabetes

Maternal problems
   Pregnancy
      Anxiety
      Abnormal weight gain in pregnancy
      Pre-eclampsia
      Birth trauma (secondary to macrosomia)
      Increased rate of Caesarean section
   Later life
      Increased rate of T2DM in later life
      Increased rate of hypertension and cardiovascular disease

Problems in offspring (fetal/neonatal/adult life)
   Fetal life
      ?Malformation
      Intra-uterine death
      Macrosomia
      Shoulder dystocia/hypoxia-acidosis/Erb's palsy
      Iatrogenic prematurity
   Neonatal life
      Hypoglycaemia
      Polycythaemia
      Hyperbilirubinaemia
      Hypocalcaemia
      Cardiomyopathy
   Adult life
      Obesity
      Increased rate of T2DM in later life
      Increased rate of hypertension and cardiovascular disease
      ?Breast cancer

Control in Atlanta, and the World Health Organization. In a later article, he asserted that screening for gestational glucose intolerance conferred no benefit to the mother or baby but that there were identifiable disadvantages that included the inopportune acquisition of disease status during pregnancy and an increased risk of Caesarean section.[3]

In the 10 years since Jarrett wrote his original treatise, there have been more than 200 research publications posted on the Medline database. In this paper, we have attempted to review these new areas of research and critically re-appraise the role of screening for GDM in maternity care.

ASSOCIATED ADVERSE OUTCOMES

Abnormal fetal growth

The picture of the rotund, plethoric baby of the diabetic mother is surely known to all midwives and obstetricians. The definition of macrosomia is subject to much debate; however, with criteria including birth weight above the 90th centile for gestational age, birth weight exceeding 2 SD of an appropriate normative population (above the 97.75th percentile), birth weight above 4000 g regardless of gestational age or sex, or organ weight disproportionately great in relation to body weight.[4] The recommended

Fetal death and occult GDM

It is generally agreed that there is a higher perinatal mortality rate in pregnancies affected by GDM; 10-fold higher than background rates in some studies.[22] Given that a significant proportion of cases of GDM pass undetected it seems likely that some cases of intra-uterine death occur in women with occult GDM. This will often not be recognised at the time of the fetal death because gestational glucose intolerance quickly reverts to normal and glycated blood components such as HbA_{1c} and fructosamine are usually normal in GDM. In addition, fetal post-mortem evidence of maternal diabetes such as pancreatic cell hypertrophy and beta-cell hyperplasia is often absent because of rapid autolysis within the pancreas.

Some groups have speculated that occult gestational diabetes contributes to a large proportion of unexplained late intrauterine deaths. Robson *et al.*[23] recently undertook a systematic study of glucose tolerance in pregnancies that followed unexplained stillbirth in South Australian women. They found a much higher rate of gestational diabetes in subsequent pregnancies in comparison with well matched controls (OR, 4.29; CI, 2.5–7.1). This finding does not of itself justify screening. Moreover, some have suggested that the link between fetal death and GDM is indirect and simply reflects advanced maternal age.

Long-term health problems for offspring

The immediate effects of intra-uterine death, birth trauma and neonatal hypoglycaemia have been well documented. What is now coming to light is that the offspring of women with GDM are more likely to develop obesity, diabetes, and cardiovascular disease.[24] There are also data which show a link between high birth weight and breast cancer.[25]

Some of this may be the result of a genetic predisposition but it is interesting to note that gestational diabetes is transmitted preferentially (though not exclusively) through the maternal line.[26] There is speculation that the uterine milieu leads to metabolic imprinting which influences the risk of certain diseases in adulthood. This raises the possibility that therapeutic modulation of maternal glycaemic state might prevent the fetus from developing certain diseases in later life. Once more, as yet this is little more than conjecture.

Maternal long-term health problems

It has been shown that women with a history of GDM have about a 30% risk of developing T2DM in later life.[27] This compares with a rate of 8% in the general population. Given the rising incidence of T2DM and earlier age at onset, it seems likely that this risk is set to increase. This constitutes a significant health risk with higher rates of cardiovascular disease and premature death. In 1997, in a debate on the case for screening for gestational diabetes, de Soares and colleagues proposed that screening was justified because of the ability to identify future diabetes.[28] At that stage, however, there was no evidence that medical or life-style intervention in individuals with pre-diabetes resulted in health gain.[3] Two recent intervention trials have challenged that view. Tuomilehto and colleagues[29] in Finland studying subjects with impaired glucose tolerance found a 50% reduction of risk of progression to diabetes (11% versus 23%) after dietary modification. The Diabetes Prevention Research Group[30] in Washington studied life-style modification and metformin therapy in individuals identified as being at high risk of T2DM. Their studies revealed that life-style modification alone reduced the risk of diabetes by 58% and metformin therapy reduced it by 31%.

On the face of it, these data appear to justify screening for gestational diabetes but there are problems with both their interpretation and implementation. First, the average period of follow-up in both studies was relatively short, being 3 years in one and 2.8 years in the other. Second, life-style modification was generally intense particularly with regard to exercise which in the Finnish study consisted of 150 min of activity each week. Finally, the support and supervision offered to the subjects was at a level which is probably not currently available to individuals through most public health services.[31] Evidence from a longer term UK study showed that without support patients returned to their previous life-style and weight was regained.[32]

Clearly, disease prevention is a laudable aim but it remains to be shown that screening for GDM has a positive long-term effect on the lives of those women with abnormal glucose tolerance in pregnancy. Moreover, beyond any arguments about resources and effectiveness, there is a more fundamental issue of whether pregnancy is a good time to be testing women for chronic diseases which might engender unnecessary alarm and so undermine any enjoyment of the newborn child. It should not be forgotten that only one-third of such women go onto develop T2DM. Nor that other equally powerful predictors of T2DM exist outside of pregnancy including central obesity, family history, hypertriglyceridaemia, elevated blood insulin/glucose ratios, and abnormal serum C-peptide concentrations. These tests scan be applied to all (consenting) adults, after careful counselling as to the benefits and disadvantages, and not just to unsuspecting pregnant women.

MANAGEMENT ISSUES

Screening tests

In addition to any controversy over the clinical advantage of detecting GDM, there are arguments as to which is the most effective test for screening, when in pregnancy screening should be undertaken, and to whom it should be applied.

For the most part, GDM is an asymptomatic condition so it can only be detected by screening. Whilst the 75 g oral glucose tolerance test (OGTT) using WHO criteria is now used almost universally throughout the world as the gold standard test for diagnosing GDM, there is no such agreement on the best practice for screening. Numerous tests are available with varying degrees of evidence as to their efficacy as screening tests (Table 3). The confusion which abounds is reflected in the variation in recommendations (Table 4) produced by some national organisations: Diabetes UK,[33] American Diabetic Association[33] the Scottish Intercollegiate Group Network (SIGN),[33] the Society of Obstetricians & Gynaecologists of Canada,[34] and the National Institute for

Table 3 Screening tests used for gestational diabetes

Urine tests	
	Glycosuria
Blood tests	
	Random blood glucose (RBG)
	Fasting blood glucose (FBG)
	1-h 50 g glucose challenge test (GCT)
	2-h 50 g glucose challenge test
	75 g glucose tolerance test (GTT)
	Fructosamine
	Glycated haemoglobin

Clinical Excellence. Interestingly, the Canadian group recommends methods of screening but also states that it is acceptable not to screen because it is of uncertain benefit. It is also worthy of note that a survey of current UK maternity units published in 1999 demonstrated that practice even varies within units by showing that 84% of UK hospitals that screened for GDM used more than one method.[1]

As well as being both sensitive and specific, any test should be simple, cheap and convenient to perform. Most previous work had been done in relation to the glucose challenge test (GCT) and random blood glucose measurement (RBG). Of the two, the GCT had been demonstrated to have the higher sensitivity but it is poorly tolerated as it tends to induce nausea. It is also time consuming and, therefore, expensive. More recently, fasting blood

Table 4 Recommendations of national groups

Diabetes UK[33] – Routine screening
    Urine testing at every ANC visit
    RBG at booking, at 28 weeks and if glycosuria
    A 75 g GTT if RBG > 6.1 mmol/l fasting or > 7.0 mmol/l within 2 h of food

American Diabetic Association (ADA)[33] – Selective screening
    Age > 25 years
    Overweight before pregnancy
    Ethnic group with high prevalence GDM
    Diabetes in first-degree relative
    History of abnormal glucose tolerance
    History of poor obstetric outcome
Screening with 50 g GCT, confirmation with 100 g GTT

Scottish Intercollegiate Guidance Network (SIGN)[33] – Routine screening
    Urine and RBG at every ANC visit

Society of Obstetricians and Gynaecologists of Canada[34]

Each of the following approaches is considered acceptable
    Routine screening at 24–28 weeks with 50 g GCT with cut off 7.8 mmol/l
    No screening as no definitive evidence to support
    High risk diagnostic test as early as possible with repeat at 24–28 weeks

National Institute for Clinical Excellence
    No routine screening

Table 5 Risk factors for selective screening

Maternal age
Family history of type 2 diabetes
Non-white ethnic origin
Obesity
Smoking
Increased weight gain in early childhood
Polycystic ovary syndrome
Previous large infant (> 97th centile)
Previous unexplained still-birth

glucose measurement (FBG) has been shown to have great value as a screening test. Perucchini et al.[35] showed that FBG with a cut off of 4.8 mmol/l yielded a sensitivity of 81% and specificity of 76%. This compared with 69% and 91%, respectively, for the GCT with a cut off of 7.8 mmol/l. With FBG as the primary test, 30% of the population were screened as positive and required a definitive diagnostic test (GTT). As well as having a high sensitivity and relatively good specificity, the FBG test is eminently suitable for screening because it is easier, cheaper and probably more acceptable to the screened population.

For reasons of cost and convenience, many units apply a selective policy by testing only high-risk women (Table 5), but this has the disadvantage of missing up to 50% of cases. For similar reasons, screening is often seen as a one-off test at 28 weeks though, in fact, some of the negative effects on the fetus may have already taken hold. The characteristic of FBG allows it to be applied to all gravid women rather than selectively, and to be applied more than once during pregnancy.

Blood glucose monitoring

Good control of blood glucose with a combination of a careful diet and insulin is seen as the key to effective care before and during pregnancy for pre-existing T1DM. Self-tested blood glucose values using hand-held digital read-out devices and glycated haemoglobin are used to assess the adequacy of care and allow adjustments to be made. For T1DM, blood glucose measurements are undertaken before meals. Fasting and preprandial blood glucose values are often normal in GDM even before treatment, however, and so it is now advised that women with GDM are monitored using 1-h postprandial measurements. de Veciana[36] found that postprandial monitoring resulted in improved glycaemic control compared with conventional assessment, with a concomitant decreased in the risk of macrosomia, Caesarean section, and neonatal hypoglycaemia. Not all have found improved outcomes with postprandial monitoring, however, and further work is justified.[37]

Management of macrosomia

There is much controversy as to how gestational diabetes should be managed to attain optimal birth weight, in particular to prevent fetal macrosomia and its associated risks of fetal and maternal birth trauma, particularly shoulder dystocia and hypoxia.

Screening for macrosomia

Both clinical and conventional ultrasonographic methods of estimating fetal weight are inaccurate with an error of 10–20% even in skilful hands. Reece *et al.*[38] found ultrasonography for the diagnosis of macrosomia to show huge variation in sensitivity 24–88% and specificity 60–98%. The downfall of ultrasound is that fetal body composition and shoulder width cannot be reliably assessed. Serial measurement of abdominal circumference (AC) in the third trimester is currently the best single measurement in detection of macrosomic fetuses. Five novel methods have been proposed to detect excessive fetal growth – cheek-to-cheek diameter, fetal thigh subcutaneous tissue at the level of the femoral diaphysis, thigh soft tissue/femur length (FL) ratio, upper arm soft tissue thickness, and estimated weight derived from a formula incorporating AC, FL and upper arm soft tissue thickness. Unfortunately, when compared to clinical and routine sonographic measurement, they were not found superior.[39]

Prevention of macrosomia

Initial treatment of gestational diabetes is based on dietary manipulation through nutritional education. The American Diabetes Association recommends individualisation of treatment based on maternal height and weight to provide adequate calories and nutrients to meet the needs of the pregnancy and minimise maternal hyperglycaemia.[40] Daily calorific needs in the second half of pregnancy are 30–32 kcal/kg body weight, with a further restriction to 25 kcal/kg in obese women (BMI > 30 kg/m^2) with restriction of carbohydrates to 35–40% of calories. Many regimens also recommend gentle aerobic exercise such as walking for 20–30 min after meals.[41] Although there is no maternal glycaemic threshold for fetal risk, frequent aggressive blood glucose monitoring is also commenced; the aim is to maintain blood glucose concentrations in the range for normal pregnancy. Insulin therapy is commenced in women who fail to maintain sufficient glycaemic control on diet alone.[11–13,15]

The optimal gestational age by which good glycaemic control should be achieved has been questioned. Sameshima *et al.*[42] found that, in a Japanese population, there was a significant reduction in macrosomia in gestational diabetics achieving adequate control before 32 weeks' gestation, but in women achieving control after this time there was no decline in the rate of macrosomia. As in other studies, there was no evidence that good glycaemic control reduced the Caesarean section rate or the risk of shoulder dystocia.[2]

Some groups are using fetal size as an indicator for insulin therapy. In a recent pilot study,[43] Kjos *et al.* questioned the traditional management of gestational diabetes based on maternal glycaemic criteria alone. This group proposed that as only a minority of fetuses (20–30%) are at risk of macrosomia in pregnancies affected by gestational diabetes; normalising glucose levels in all affected pregnancies may result in overuse of insulin therapy and, in some cases, lead to intra-uterine growth restriction. Participants were randomised into two groups either to receive standard insulin therapy, or treatment dependent on fetal abdominal circumference. In the experimental group, women were prescribed insulin if the fetal abdominal circumference was > 70th centile either on initial scan (between 14 and 34 weeks' gestation) or on monthly assessment of fetal growth, whereas in those with normal growth, treatment was by diet alone unless the fasting blood glucose exceeded 120 mg/dl, when insulin was commenced. Out of 48 women in the experimental group, only 30 (62%) required insulin therapy. Both groups were comparable by age, parity, BMI, gestation at which diagnosis made and entered into study, and blood glucose levels. After randomisation, the standard group had lower FBG levels than the experimental group, there was no difference in the rate of macrosomia between groups and all LGA infants measured > 70th centile at entry to the study and there was no significant difference in perinatal morbidity. However, there was a difference in the rate of growth restriction with no affected infants in the experimental group, but three in the group undergoing standard treatment based on blood sugar alone (there were no additional risks for IUGR). If further studies confirm these findings, management of gestational diabetes may take a more fetus-centred approach.

Delivery of the macrosomic fetus

If the fetus is suspected to be large, the timing and mode of delivery must be considered in order to prevent shoulder dystocia. One trial of routine induction of labour at 38 weeks for women with diabetes showed a lower rate of macrosomia (10% versus 23%), a lower Caesarean section rate (25% versus 30%) and no increase in the chance of shoulder dystocia (0% versus 3%).[44] This small study was not simply of women with macrosomic babies, however, and the possibility of uneven segregation on random allocation cannot be excluded. The known association between induction of labour and shoulder dystocia is also cause for concern. Nevertheless, further study is probably justified.

The alternative is to consider elective Caesarean section. Any such decision needs to be taken carefully in a group of women who are not infrequently morbidly obese. Rouse and colleagues[45] calculated that for every three cases of brachial plexus injury prevented by elective section for (non-diabetic) babies greater than 4500 g, 3695 operations would be undertaken and one mother would die. Although the costs are likely to be less for women with diabetes, the number needed to prevent (NNP) is still likely to be very high. It should not be forgotten that Caesarean delivery of the macrosomic fetus is not without risk of birth trauma.

Treatment with oral hypoglycaemic agents

Until recently, the medical management of women with GDM consisted of dietary advice, blood glucose monitoring, and insulin if required. Historically, oral hypoglycaemic agents have been avoided in pregnancy because of evidence that early agents crossed the placenta and stimulated fetal insulin secretion, which was thought to cause fetal macrosomia and severe hyperinsulinaemic hypoglycaemia in neonates. An association with major congenital malformations was also found in animal studies.[46] The use of oral hypoglycaemic agents in pregnancy would potentially have a number of benefits, however, if they could be shown to be effective in terms of glycaemic control and without incurring risks to the fetus. The main obvious advantages to the patient being able to continue their existing treatment, patient compliance with the ease of tablet administration over insulin injection, ease of storage, convenience, and cost. Patient anxiety is also a factor to consider in relation to insulin injections, particularly if in the abdominal wall when pregnant. The issue of safe needle disposal and, therefore, infection risk would also be avoided, particularly for countries with high HIV carrier rates. Oral hypoglycaemic agents are currently not recommended for use in pregnancy. The British National Formulary recommends that women with T2DM who become pregnant are converted to insulin in pregnancy because of theoretical risks to the fetus. Despite this, some research groups are currently re-evaluating the effectiveness and safety of oral hypoglycaemic agents in pregnancy.

Pharmacology

There are a number of different types of oral hypoglycaemic agents that are available for use in the management of type 2 diabetes (T2DM).

Sulfonylureas – This group includes and chlorpropamide, tolbutamide, glyburide (glibenclamide), and glicazide. They act by augmenting insulin secretion by the pancreas and consequently are effective only when some pancreatic β-cell activity is present. With long-term administration they also have an extra pancreatic action. They can cause hypoglycaemia and they encourage weight gain (maternal weight gain in pregnancy has been shown to be a risk factor in macrosomia). Their side-effects otherwise are generally mild and infrequent. They consist mostly of gastrointestinal disturbances such as nausea, vomiting, diarrhoea and constipation.

Biguanides – Metformin is the only available biguanide. It exerts its effect mainly by decreasing gluconeogenesis and by increasing peripheral utilisation of glucose. It acts only in the presence of insulin and so is effective as single agent therapy only if there is still endogenous insulin production but it can be used in conjunction with exogenous insulin as well. At therapeutic doses, hypoglycaemia does not occur when used in isolation but it may exert a hypoglycaemic action when given in overdose. There is a lower incidence of weight gain and weight loss may occur. Gastrointestinal side-effects are common initially but these usually settle within a few days. It can lead to vitamin B_{12} deficiency and it may also provoke lactic acidosis, but the latter is extremely rare and probably only occurs in those with vascular disease and in renal patients.[47] This might be important for women patients with pre-eclampsia.

Acarbose – is an inhibitor of intestinal glucosidases, which delays the digestion and absorption of starch and sucrose. Its use has not been reported for use in pregnancy.

Guar gum – Similarly results in a lowering of postprandial plasma glucose concentrations in diabetes mellitus probably by retarding carbohydrate absorption. Again its use has not been reported for use in pregnancy.

Thiazolidinediones – Pioglitazone and rosiglitazone reduce peripheral insulin resistance, possibly by reducing the production of the hormone resistin from adipose tissue. They are only licensed in combination with metformin or a sulphonylurea. There are no reports of their use in pregnancy.

Treatment of GDM

Sulfonylureas – Early studies investigated the first generation drugs such as chlorpropramide but these drugs crossed the placenta and caused profound sustained neonatal hypoglycaemia.[48] More recently, *in vitro* studies using isolated placental cotyledons have shown minimal maternal–fetal transfer of the second generation drug glyburide.[49] To date, there seems to have been a single clinical study comparing glyburide with insulin in GDM.[50] Langer and colleagues studied 404 women in a random allocation trial. Glyburide was not detected in the cord serum of any infant. Maternal glycaemic control was similar for both treatment groups and they demonstrated no difference in the rate of fetal macrosomia. Neonatal hypoglycaemia, lung complication rates and admissions to neonatal intensive care units were also similar. Patient acceptability was not studied, but one would expect tablets to be preferred to injections.

Biguanides – In contrast to glyburide, metformin does cross the placenta. There have been three studies examining its use in GDM but the accumulated experience with metformin is smaller with less than 200 women treated. And there have already been some disappointing outcome data. The first report from South Africa in 1979 showed a favourable perinatal mortality rate but the comparison was with untreated patients for whom the PNMR was 146/1000.[51] It is difficult to know how these results relate to the UK and similar countries. The authors reported an increase in neonatal jaundice. In the second study, metformin was compared with tolbutamide. Glycaemic control was comparable to insulin-treated patients in both groups but metformin was associated with a 3-fold increase in the incidence of pre-eclampsia and an increased perinatal mortality rate compared with those on tolbutamide and insulin.[52] A third (pilot) study comparing metformin administration with insulin found both similar ability to control hyperglycaemia as insulin but metformin was associated with a higher Caesarean delivery rate and more neonatal hypoglycaemia.[53] These outcomes may well reflect small study sizes but the safety of metformin is not established and it is advocated that it should not be used for this purpose outside of well designed research studies.[54]

Prevention of GDM

It has always been interesting to note that the recurrence risk of GDM in subsequent pregnancies is relatively low. The reason for this is not precisely known. It might relate to variation placental (insulin antagonist) hormone production between pregnancies but one other possibility is that alteration in maternal life-style before conception or early on in any new pregnancy reduces the risk of glucose intolerance. This may have important implications for pre-conceptual counselling in women with a history of GDM who, in contrast to those women with T1DM, receive little care in preparation for pregnancy.

The prospective of care before pregnancy is a potentially important one as theoretically it may help prevent miscarriage, fetal malformation, and the development of diabetes. Some recent research raises possibilities for preventing GDM using pharmacological agents. Studies on the use of metformin therapy before and during pregnancy in women with polycystic ovary syndrome (PCOS), a condition associated with a high rate of GDM, have revealed interesting results. Glueck *et al.*[55] demonstrated a 10-fold reduction in the development of gestational diabetes in PCOS women treated with metformin compared to no treatment. In particular, it was noted that a reduction was seen in those women who had developed gestational diabetes in previous pregnancies. Follow-up studies of these infants to 6 months of life have shown no adverse effects on height, weight and motor and social development. In other studies, the same group have shown a statistically significant reduction in the incidence of first trimester spontaneous miscarriage compared with control groups, and an increased live birth rate with no increase in fetal abnormalities or evidence of teratogenicity.[56–59]

The differences between the results for the prevention and treatment of GDM are of interest. Although the finding may represent nothing more than the size and quality of the studies, it is possible that they reflect different responses because of different pathophysiologies of prediabetes and GDM. It seems that prevention may be better than control.

SUMMARY

GDM appears to be associated with a higher rate of fetal malformation as well as the known risks of macrosomia, birth trauma and neonatal hypoglycaemia. It has also been shown that there is also a high rate of GDM in women with a previously unexplained intra-uterine death. There is no clear evidence that knowledge of gestational glucose intolerance helps in the management of these problems, or any other obstetric problem such as macrosomia, and there is some evidence to suggest screening may be disadvantageous (increased caesarean section rate).

In addition to these immediate risks, it is becoming ever more evident that the diabetic intra-uterine environment predisposes the fetus to a number of diseases later in life, but there have been no intervention studies to show that these can be prevented. Longer term health risks to the mother have been confirmed. Although there are some data from studies of other patient groups with prediabetes which suggest that T2DM can be prevented with life-style modification (with or without metformin), these interventions are not without problems of implementation. Furthermore, even if it were so that change in diet and physical activity reduced morbidity and mortality, one has to question whether pregnancy is the best time to impart the news of long-term health problems.

If screening for GDM were shown to be of certain benefit, then fasting blood glucose measurement is both highly sensitive and simple to implement. Assuming that an immediate benefit of tight control of blood glucose to the mother and baby could be proven, the introduction of oral hypoglycaemic agents presents a potentially valuable advance in care if only for ease of use and cost. Their potential for the prevention of GDM with pre-conceptual therapy is also a particularly exciting prospect. At present, however, the accumulated number of patients studied remains low; before the use of these agents is adopted more widely, much larger trials are needed to examine their safety in this setting.

That gestational diabetes is associated with immediate and long-term adverse events for mother and baby is not doubted. There has been a vast amount of research in the last 40 years but, unfortunately, the scientific literature is bedevilled with underpowered clinical trials (mostly with less than 100 subjects) which rely too heavily on surrogate end points. As a consequence, the case for screening remains unproven but not disproved. Surely the time has come for large multicentre trials of screening and intervention. With the ever rising tide of obesity, the need is both great and urgent.

References

1   Mires GJ, Williams FLR, Harper V. Screening practices for gestational diabetes mellitus in UK obstetric units. Diabetes Med 1999; 16: 138–141
2   Jarrett RJ. Gestational diabetes: a non-entity. BMJ 1993; 306: 37–38
3   Jarrett RJ. Should we screen for gestational diabetes? BMJ 1997; 315: 736–737
4   Potter EL, Craig JM. Pathology of the Fetus and the Infant, 3rd edn. Chicago: Yearbook Medical, 1975; 23–29
5   Schwartz R, Teramo KA. What is the significance of macrosomia? Diabetes Care 1999; 22: 1201–1205
6   Pederson J. The Pregnant Diabetic and her Newborn, 2nd edn. Baltimore: Williams and Wilkins, 1977; 211–220
7   O'Sullivan JB, Gellis SS, Dandrow RV, Tenney BO. The potential diabetic and her treatment during pregnancy. Obstet Gynecol 1966; 27: 683–689
8   Sermer M, Naylor CD, Gare DJ et al. Impact of increasing carbohydrate intolerance on maternal-fetal outcomes in 3637 women without gestational diabetes: the Toronto Tri-Hospital Gestational Diabetes Project. Am J Obstet Gynecol 1995; 173: 146–156
9   Ray JG, Vermeulen MJ, Shapiro JL, Kenshole AB. Maternal and neonatal outcomes in pregestational and gestational diabetes mellitus, and the influence of maternal obesity and weight gain: the DEPOSIT study. Q J Med 2001; 94: 347–356
10 Adams KM, Hongzhe L, Nelson RL, Ogburn Jr PL, Danilenko-Dixon DR. Sequelae of unrecognised gestational diabetes. Am J Obstet Gynecol 1998; 178: 1321–1332
11 Knopp RH, Magee MS, Walden CE, Bonet B, Benedetti TJ. Prediction of infant birth weight by GDM screening tests: importance of plasma triglyceride. Diabetes Care 1992; 15: 1605–1613
12 Nolan CJ, Riley SF, Sheedy MT, Walstab JE, Beischer NA. Maternal serum triglyceride, glucose tolerance and neonatal birth weight ratio in pregnancy. Diabetes Care 1995; 18: 1550–1556
13 Kjos SL, Buchanan TA. Gestational diabetes mellitus. N Engl J Med 1999; 341: 1749–1756
14 Waller DK, Keddie AM, Canfield MA, Scheuerle AE. Do infants with major congenital anomalies have an excess of macrosomia? Teratology 2001; 64: 311–317
15 Schaefer UM, Songster G, Xiang A, Berkowitz K, Buchanan TA, Kjos SL. Congenital malformations in offspring of women with hyperglycaemia first detected during pregnancy. Am J Obstet Gynecol 1997; 177: 1165–1171
16 Aberg A, Westbom L, Kallen J. Congenital malformations among infants whose mothers had gestational diabetes or pre-existing diabetes. Early Hum Dev 2001; 61: 85–95
17 Sheffield JS, Butler-Koster EL, Casey BM, McIntire DD, Leveno KJ. Maternal diabetes mellitus and infant malformations. Obstet Gynecol 2002; 100: 925–930
18 Mironiuk M, Kietlinska Z, Jexierska-Kasprzyk K, Peikosz-Orzechowski B. A class of diabetes in mother, glycemic control in early pregnancy and occurrence of congenital malformations. Clin Exp Obstet Gynecol 1997; 24: 193–197
19 Farrell T, Neale L, Cundy T. Congenital anomalies in the offspring of women with type 1, type 2 and gestational diabetes. Diabetes Med 2002; 19: 322–326
20 Fox R, James M. Diabetic embryopathy in a woman with potential diabetes. J Obstet Gynaecol 1995; 15: 108–109
21 Steel JM, Johnstone FD, Hepburn DA, Smith AF. Can prepregnancy care of diabetic women reduce the risk of abnormal babies? BMJ 1990; 301: 1070–1074
22 Rudge MVC, Calderon IMP, Ramos MD, Abbade JF, Rugolo LMS. Perinatal outcome of pregnancies complicated by diabetes and by maternal daily hyperglycaemia not related to diabetes. Gynecol Obstet Invest 2000; 50: 108–112

23 Robson S, Chan A, Keane RJ, Luke CG. Subsequent birth outcomes after an unexplained stillbirth: preliminary population-based retrospective cohort study. Aust NZ J Obstet Gynaecol 2001; 41: 29–35

24 Sattar N, Greer IA. Pregnancy complications and maternal cardiovascular risk. BMJ 2002; 325: 157–160

25 McCormack VA, dos Santos Silva I, de Stavola BL, Mohsen R, Leon DA, Lithell HO. Fetal growth and subsequent risk of breast cancer. BMJ 2003; 326: 248–251

26 Knowler W, Pettitt DJ, Kunzelman CL, Everhart J. Genetic and environment determinants of NIDDM. Diabetes Res Clin Pract 1985; 1 (Suppl): S309

27 Kaufmann RC, Schleynhahn FT, Huffman DG, Amankwah KS. Gestational diabetes diagnostic criteria: long-term maternal follow-up. Am J Obstet Gynecol 1995; 172: 621–625

28 de Soares J, Dornhorstt A, Beard RW. The case for screening for gestational diabetes. BMJ 1997; 315: 737–739

29 Tuomilehto J, Lindstrom J, Eriksson JG et al. Finnish Diabetes Prevention Study Group. Prevention of type 2 diabetes mellitus by changes in lifestyle among subjects with impaired glucose tolerance. N Engl J Med 2001; 344: 1343–1350

30 Knowler WC, Barrett-Connor E, Fowler SE et al. Diabetes Prevention Program Research Group. Reduction in the incidence of type 2 diabetes with lifestyle intervention or metformin. N Engl J Med 2002: 346: 393–403

31 Swinburn B, Egger G. Prevention of type 2 diabetes. BMJ 2001; 323: 997

32 Swinburn BA, Metcalf PA, Ley KJ. Long term effects of a reduced fat diet intervention in individuals with glucose intolerance. Diabetes Care 2001; 24: 619–624

33 Scott DA, Loveman E, McIntyre L, Waugh N. Screening for gestational diabetes: a systematic review and economic evaluation. Health Technology Assessment 2002; Vol. 6: No. 11

34 Sermer M. Does screening for gestational diabetes mellitus make a difference? CMAJ 2003; 168; 429–431

35 Perucchini D, Fischer U, Spinas GA, Huch R, Huch A, Lehmann R. Using fasting plasma glucose concentrations to screen for gestational diabetes mellitus: prospective population-based study. BMJ 1999; 319: 812–815

36 de Veciana M, Major CA, Morgan MA et al. Postprandial versus preprandial blood glucose monitoring in women with gestational diabetes mellitus requiring insulin therapy. N Engl J Med 1995; 333: 1281–1283

37 Homko CJ, Sivan E, Reece EA. Self-monitoring in the management of gestational diabetes. Diabetes Care 1998; 21 (Suppl 2): B118–B122

38 Reece EA, Friedman AM, Copel J, Kleinman CS. Prenatal diagnosis and management of deviant fetal growth and congenital malformations. In: Reece EA, Coustan DR. (eds) Diabetes Mellitus in Pregnancy, 2nd edn. New York: Churchill Livingstone, 1995; 222–226

39 Chauhan SP, West DJ, Scardo JA, Boyd JM, Joiner J, Hendrix NW. Antepartum detection of macrosomic fetus: clinical versus sonographic, including soft-tissue measurements. Obstet Gynecol 2000; 95: 639–642

40 American Diabetes Association. Gestational Diabetes Mellitus. Diabetes Care 2003; 26 (Suppl 1): S103–S105

41 Homko CJ, Sivan E, Reece EA. Is self-monitoring of blood glucose necessary in the management of gestational diabetes mellitus? Diabetes Care 1998; 21 (Suppl 2): B108–B112

42 Sameshima H, Kamitomo M, Kajiya S, Kai M, Furukawa S, Ikenoue T. Early glycaemic control reduces large-for-gestational-age infants in 250 Japanese gestational diabetes pregnancies. Am J Perinatol 2000; 17: 371–376

43 Kjos SL, Schaeffer-Graf U, Sardesi S et al. A randomised controlled trial using glycaemic plus fetal ultrasound parameters vs. glycaemic parameters to determine insulin therapy in gestational diabetes with fasting hyperglycaemia. Diabetes Care 2001; 24: 1904–1910

44 Kjos SL, Henry OA, Montoro M, Buchanan TA, Mestman JH. Insulin-requiring diabetes in pregnancy. A randomised trial of active induction of labour and expectant management. Am J Obstet Gynecol 1993; 169: 611–615

45 Rouse DJ, Owen J, Goldenburg RL, Cliver SP. The effectiveness and costs of elective

Cesarean section delivery for fetal macrosomia diagnosed by ultrasound. JAMA 1996; 276: 1480–1486

46 Greene MF. Oral hypoglycaemic drugs for gestational diabetes. N Engl J Med 2000; 343: 1178–1179

47 Jones GC, Macklin JP, Alexander WD. Contraindications to the use of metformin. BMJ 2003; 326: 4–5

48 Zucker P, Simon G. Prolonged symptomatic neonatal hypoglycaemia associated with maternal chlorpropramide. Pediatrics 1968; 42: 824–825

49 Garcia-Bournissen F, Feig DS, Koren G. Maternal-fetal transport of hypoglycaemic drugs. Clin Pharmacokinet 2003; 42: 303–313

50 Langer O, Conway DL, Berkus MD, Xenakis EM-J, Gonzales O. A comparison of glyburide and insulin in women with gestational diabetes mellitus. N Engl J Med 2000; 343: 1134–1138

51 Coetzee EJ, Jackson WP. Diabetes newly diagnosed during pregnancy: A 4 year study at Groote Schuur hospital. S Afr Med J 1979; 56: 467–475

52 Hellmuth E, Damm P, Molsted-Pedersen L. Oral hypoglycaemic agents in 118 diabetic pregnancies. Diabetes Med 2001; 18: 604–605

53 Hague WM, Davoren PM, Oliver J, Rowan J. Metformin in pregnancy. BMJ 2003; 326: 762–763

54 Dornan T, Hollis S. Critical appraisal of published research evidence: treatment of gestational diabetes. Diabetes Med 2001; Suppl 3: 1–5

55 Glueck CJ, Wang P, Goldenberg N, Sieve-Smith L. Pregnancy outcomes among women with polycystic ovary syndrome treated with metformin. Hum Reprod 2002; 17: 2858–2864

56 Glueck CJ, Phillips H, Cameron D, Sieve-Smith L, Wang P. Continuing metformin throughout pregnancy in women with polycystic ovary syndrome appears to safely reduce first trimester spontaneous abortion: a pilot study. Fertil Steril 2001; 75: 46—52

57 Jakubowicz DJ, Iuorno MJ, Jakubowicz S, Roberts KA, Nestler JE. Effects of metformin on early pregnancy loss in the polycystic ovary syndrome. J Clin Endocrinol Metab 2002; 87: 524–529

58 Glueck CJ, Wang P, Kobayashi S, Phillips H, Sieve-Smith L. Metformin therapy throughout pregnancy reduces the development of gestational diabetes in women with polycystic ovary syndrome. Fertil Steril 2002; 77: 520–525

59 Coetzee EJ, Jackson WP. Oral hypoglycaemics in the first trimester and fetal outcome. S Afr Med J 1984; 65: 635-637.

Eugene Oteng-Ntim Martin Lupton
Sharon Mensah Elizabeth N. Anionwu Philip Steer

Sickle cell disease and pregnancy

Almost every obstetric department in the UK has patients whose ethnic backgrounds put them at risk of sickle cell disease.[1] In the UK today, this disease affects approximately 1 in 625 African-Caribbeans.[2,3] Most women with sickle cell disease now survive to reproduce. However, the pregnancies of women with severe sickle haemoglobinopathies are associated with a high incidence of maternal and perinatal morbidity and mortality.[4] Table 1 shows maternal death from the disease in the UK since 1964 from the *Confidential Enquires into Maternal Deaths* series.

The clinical syndrome of sickle cell disease was first described in 1910[5] and in 1949 was the first condition to be identified as having a molecular basis by Pauling.[6,11] Sickle cell disorders result from a problem with the quality of the β-globin chains rather than quantity. Homozygous sickle cell anaemia (HbS-S) is the most common of the more than 100 serious haemoglobinopathies described in the literature. This disease, along with its common variants – haemoglobin S-C disease (HbS-C), sickle cell β+-thalassaemia and sickle cell β0-thalassaemia –

Eugene Oteng-Ntim MBBS MRCOG
Consultant Obstetrician, Guy's and St Thomas' Hospital, London, UK

Martin Lupton MA MRCOG
Consultant Obstetrician and Gynaecologist, Chelsea and Westminster Hospital, 369 Fulham Road, London SW10 9NH, UK

Sharon Mensah RGN SCM
Haemoglobinopathy Specialist Nurse Counsellor, Ealing Sickle Cell and Thalassaemia Service, Southall, Windmill Lodge, Uxbridge Road, Southall, London UB1 3EU, UK

Elizabeth N. Anionwu RN NV Tutor PhD CBE
Head, Mary Seacole Centre for Nursing Practice, Faculty of Health and Human Sciences, Thames Valley University, Westel House, 32–38 Uxbridge Road, Ealing, London W5 2BS, UK Honorary Professor, London School of Hygiene and Tropical Medicine, London, UK
(for correspondence, E-mail: elizabeth.anionwu@tvu.ac.uk)

Philip Steer MD FRCOG
Professor of Obstetrics and Gynaecology, Chelsea and Westminster Hospital, 369 Fulham Road, London SW10 9NH, UK

Table 1 Reported maternal deaths from sickle cell disease (Confidential Enquiry into Maternal Death)

CEMD	Number of deaths from SCD	Complication of SCD causing the death
1952–1954	Not reported	Not reported
1955–1957	Not reported	Not reported
1958–1960	Not reported	Not reported
1961–1963	Not reported	Not reported
1964–1966	4	4 SC crises
1967–1969	3	2 SC crises, 1 aplastic anaemia
1970–1972	3	3 SC crises
1973–1975	2	CVA due to SC crisis
1976–1978	4	4 SC crises
1979–1981	1	1 SC crisis
1982–1984	–	–
1985–1987	1	Carrier AS: GA complication (stroke)
1988–1990	–	–
1991–1993	3	2 SC crises and 1 liver sequestration
1994–1996	–	–
1997–1999	1	SC crisis

occurs almost exclusively among those of African, Caribbean, Mediterranean and Middle-Eastern descent and is associated with a shorter life-span, widespread organ damage and numerous medical and perinatal complications. In the heterozygous form of HbS, some protection against *Plasmodium falsiparum* occurs and thus it is found commonly in areas where malaria is endemic consistent with Darwinian theory of natural selection.[7] Table 2 illustrates some carrier frequencies in some ethnic groups.

With improved medical care, the frequency of sickle cell crises has decreased significantly; however, they may still occur at any time in pregnancy and constitute an obstetric emergency. Thus, it is important for every obstetrician to be familiar with the condition.

NORMAL HAEMOGLOBIN

Normal haemoglobin is composed of four subunits, with a single haem group (which binds to and subsequently, releases oxygen) and 4 species-specific

Table 2 Examples of some carrier frequencies of sickle haemoglobinopathies in some ethnic groups

Haemoglobin type	Ethnic group	Estimated carrier frequency
Sickle cell trait	Afro-Caribbeans	1 in 10
	West-Africans	1 in 4
	Cypriots	1 in 100
	Pakistanis, Indians	1 in 100
C Trait	Afro-Caribbeans	1 in 30
	Ghanaians	Up to 1 in 6
D trait	Pakistanis, Indians	1 in 100
	White British	1 in 1000

Source – London: Department of Health, 1993.

globin chains. The haem consists of an iron molecule attached to four pyrrole rings. Two pairs of globin chains (2 α and 2 β) attach to the pyrrole rings and form haemoglobin. The physiological functioning of the haemoglobin molecule depends not only on the integrity of the haem moiety, but also on the amino-acid sequence, which determines the structure of the globin chains, and the interaction between the four subunits of the haemoglobin.[8]

In the normal human, from 6 months of age, 95–97% of the total haemoglobin is haemoglobin A. The two pairs of globin chains in its molecule are called α and β chains. The remaining haemoglobin consists of HbA_2 (which has two α and two δ globin chains) and fetal haemoglobin (with two α and two γ globin chains). The former normally comprises some 2% of the total while the latter constitutes less than 1.5%. The amino-acid sequences of these four different polypeptide chains have been determined, the α chain (identical in each of these three types of haemoglobin molecule) has 141 amino-acid residues and its genetic loci is located on chromosome 16 while the β, δ and γ chains each have 146 residues and their genetic loci reside on chromosome 11.[9]

SICKLE HAEMOGLOBINOPATHY

There are four principal genotypes of sickle cell disease in the population: homozygous sickle cell (SS) disease, sickle cell haemoglobin C (SC) disease, sickle cell $β^+$-thalassaemia and sickle cell $β^0$-thalassaemia. The latter two conditions are relatively uncommon and most experience in pregnancy has been gained caring for mothers with SS disease and SC disease.[2]

Structural changes in the haemoglobin molecule, most commonly a substitution in one or more amino acids in the globin chains, are responsible for the majority of sickle cell haemoglobinopathies. Haemoglobin S, the most common of the structural haemoglobin variants occurs when the negatively charged glutamic acid is replaced by a neutral amino acid, valine, at the sixth position from the N-terminus in the β-chain. Haemoglobin C (HbC) is formed when glutamic acid is replaced by lysine. These structural changes are inherited as an autosomal recessive.

PATHOPHYSIOLOGY

The major complications of sickle cell disease are chronic anaemia and intravascular thrombosis leading to 'crises'.

Chronic anaemia

In the oxygenated state, the solubility of HbS is nearly equal to that of HbA and its oxyhaemoglobin form has the ability to function in a physiological manner. However, in the deoxygenated state, its solubility falls to 1/50th that of HbA[10] resulting in aggregation to form liquid crystals.[11] This causes the erythrocyte to assume the classical 'sickle shape'. Re-oxygenation can restore these erythrocytes to their normal shape. Repetitive cycles of agglutination and polymerisation lead to membrane rigidity and eventually irreversible sickle cells are formed. These permanently damaged erythrocytes are then cleared by the reticulo-endothelial system. Thus, the average life-span of red blood cells of sickle cell patients is 17 days as compared to the 120-day life-span for normal erythrocytes. This results in a chronic compensated anaemia (haemoglobin, 6.5–9.0 g/dl) as the marrow's capacity to generate new red blood cells is limited. As the red blood cells are removed, their concentration falls, reducing the rate of destruction until it just balances the maximal rate of red blood cell production by the marrow. Thus bone marrow aspirate will show erythroid hyperplasia while the blood film will show sickle-shaped red blood cells. Often, there is an associated splenomegaly and gallstone formation, both secondary to excessive red blood cell destruction.

Sickle cell crises

The term sickle cell crisis can be used to describe many of the acute events that occur in individuals with sickle cell disease. While there are two major types of crises – the vaso-occlusive and the haematologic crises – most crises during pregnancy are vaso-occlusive, occurring most often in the latter half of pregnancy or in the peurperium.

Vaso-occlusive crises and end-organ damage

The factors involved in the pathophysiology of the sickle cell vaso-occlusive crises can be explained by the classical Virchow's triad.[12] First, cells with sickle haemoglobin have an altered motion through the microvasculature because of the distorted erythrocyte membranes.[13] This results in vascular stasis and hypoxia which, in turn, creates metabolic acidosis. These adverse events further accelerate deoxygenation resulting in a cycle that continually increases the amount of sickling in the microvascular circulation, further aggravating tissue hypoxia and end-organ damage. Second, because of the interaction of sickled erythrocytes with the capillary endothelial membrane, microvascular injury may occur which creates a pro-thrombotic state resulting in infarction and ischaemic necrosis of various organs. Finally, the stasis of sickled cells in the microcirculation results in aggregation around phagocytic cells which increases the blood viscosity and further aggravates the sickle cell crises cycle. The culmination of these events is a painful, vaso-occlusive sickle cell crisis that often results in end-organ damage.

Acute chest syndrome

This life-threatening complication arises due to sickling in the lungs, possibly combined with infection.[14–16] It is amongst the commonest cause of maternal death (Table 1). The symptoms include fever, coughing, chest pain, shortness of breath and worsening anaemia with audible crackles and/or bronchial breathing on examination with often florid changes on the chest X-ray. The patient may need assisted or mechanical ventilation. While there are thought to be many causes, the underlying features are not totally understood and treatment is often inadequate, although early detection and treatment may reduce the severity and prevent death.[16] Dramatic improvements have been noted following exchange blood transfusions, intravenous heparin and antibiotics.[17]

Haematological crises

Although rare in clinical obstetric practice, an aplastic crisis is the most common haemotologic crisis occurring during pregnancy.[18] It is often associated with infection (in the UK most notably parvovirus) and is characterised by a rapidly falling haematocrit secondary to an aplastic bone marrow. Clinical symptoms include weakness and pallor. Most aplastic crises in pregnancy are mild. However, if left untreated, a severe episode can develop eventually leading to cardiac failure. Another type of haemotologic crisis that can occasionally occur in pregnancy, is a megaloblastic crisis, characterised by increasing mean corpuscular volume and anaemia, precipitated by folate deficiency. Although rare, it can occur with multiple pregnancy (also common in the ethnic groups at risk of sickle cell disease) and malnutrition. This problem can often be avoided by the prophylactic use of folic acid. Splenic sequestration occurs mainly in childhood but can occur in adults if splenic auto-infarction has not taken place.[19]

PROBLEMS IN PREGNANCY

It is only in the last half of the 20th century that women with sickle cell disease have survived to child-bearing age in significant numbers. Early experience with sickle cell disease and pregnancy was a cause for pessimism. The first report of a successful pregnancy in a woman with sickle cell disease was in 1931.[20] The first major review, in 1941, reported a 50% fetal loss.[21] Since that time, there have been a number of observational reports on maternal mortality rates.[22,23] The initiation of early aggressive prenatal care has dramatically improved perinatal outcome and reduced maternal mortality to less than 1%.[23] In general, pregnancy events are determined by the severity of the patient's anaemia.[3] However, sickle cell crises, infection, pre-eclampsia and thrombo-embolic events are also important causes of mortality and morbidity. It is now accepted that, with intensive prenatal care, many women can look forward to a successful pregnancy outcome. However, pregnancies associated with major sickle haemoglobinopathies must be considered high risk and should be managed as such.

Screening

The National Screening Committee defines screening as 'a public health service in which members of a defined population, who do not necessarily perceive they are at risk of, or are already affected by, a disease or its complications, are asked a question or offered a test to identify those individuals who are more likely to be helped than harmed by further tests or treatment to reduce the risk of disease or its complications'.[23]

Use of ethnicity as a screening criterion
Currently, there is low completion and questionable quality of ethnic data collection within the NHS (*i.e.* accuracy of ascertainment is poor),[24,25] and this complicates the situation when screening for haemoglobinopathies.[26] Practitioners, for example, often guess a person's ethnic origin when deciding whom to test.[27,28] A survey of UK antenatal screening practice by Bain and Chapman[28] revealed that, out of 38 localities involved in selective screening, only 23 requested information on ethnic origin. Of these, only four received this information on request forms for more than 20% of patients. Midwives are

the key front-line staff in determining which pregnant woman to screen – their knowledge of haemoglobinopathies has been found to be wanting.[29] Second, 7% of patients with AS and 3% of women with AC will not be from the targeted ethnic group (Africans, African-Caribbeans and Asians).[30]

The alternative is universal screening. However, there is uncertainty about the prevalence level at which universal antenatal and neonatal screening would be cost-effective. More important than this may be how to ensure best coverage, geographical equity and the practicality of screening methods.[28] These factors should inform policy decisions on the approach to be taken to the implementation of screening across the country. The NHS Plan includes a commitment that by 2004 there will be a national linked antenatal and neonatal screening programme for sickle cell disease and thalassaemia.[2]

For women who are tested positive, appropriate counselling should be offered and haemoglobinopathy screening offered to their partners. Prenatal diagnosis can then be offered to those women at risk of having an affected fetus. This can be achieved by chorionic villus sampling, amniocentesis or fetal blood sampling.

Antepartum management

Pregnant women suffering from sickle cell disease must be regarded as high risk. At present, there is no effective long-term method of reducing the chance of sickling. At the first antenatal visit, an extensive medical history should be taken with particular emphasis on previous crises and their pattern. The past obstetric history is relevant. Any medical conditions should be identified and appropriately treated. Dating of the pregnancy is important, as sickle cell women are prone to having intra-uterine growth restricted babies. A baseline full blood count and recticulocyte count, a serum iron, liver and renal function tests should be obtained. Screening for hepatitis and HIV is also essential because they are likely to have had previous blood transfusions.

All women with sickle cell disease should be advised to take a supplement of 1 mg of folic acid per day. The traditional teaching that iron deficiency is uncommon in sickle cell disease is not borne out by some studies looking at iron stores in the bone marrow.[31,32] Routine antenatal administration of iron entails a negligible theoretical risk of iron overload for a substantial benefit.[2] Thus, iron supplements should be given in the same way as to other pregnant women at risk of anaemia. In addition, all patients should be taking penicillin V 250 mg twice daily as asplenism is common in sickle cell patients and hence encapsulated organisms pose a risk of overwhelming sepsis. Patient should be encouraged to remain well hydrated and report any signs of infection.

Women with sickle cell disease are at risk of premature birth, pre-eclampsia and placental abruption; thus, the signs and symptoms of these complications should be reviewed with the patient at each visit to allow early detection and appropriate obstetric management. Prenatal care in the first and second trimester should consist of 2-weekly visits with close liaison with the haematologist and haemaglobinopathy nurse specialist. At each clinic visit, as well as routine assessment of blood pressure and urinalysis, a full blood count and urinary microscopy and culture should also be performed. Gestational age is confirmed by early ultrasound scan and serial growth scans should be performed. If intra-uterine growth restriction is suspected or a co-morbid medical condition is present, then biophysical profile assessment including liquor volume and umbilical artery Doppler velocimetry is recommended.[33] In the absence of an obstetric indication, spontaneous labour at term should be awaited.

Sickling crises

The therapeutic goal for sickle cell patients in crisis is directed toward abating sickle cell pain, treating any infectious process, restoring adequate oxygenation, correcting metabolic acidosis and stabilising the erythrocyte volume.[34] Liberal use of parenteral analgesia, usually an opiate derivative, is indicated during these crises. Pethidine should only be used in exceptional circumstances because of the risk of seizures. The pain may persist until the cycle of vaso-occlusion, tissue infarction and necrosis is reversed. A persistent and vigilant effort to identify any infectious process is important in these patients with the lungs and urinary tract being the most common sites of infection; however, an infection can occur in any organ. Oxygen and hydration continue to be the cornerstone of treatment and are vitally important in the reversal of metabolic acidosis and tissue hypoxia associated with sickle cell crisis. In those situations where the vaso-occlusive crises are unresponsive to conservative management, exchange transfusion may be indicated.[35] Recently, high-dose intravenous methylprednisolone has been tried in children and adolescents and this may serve as an adjunct to supportive therapy at the time of painful crises (although experience of this therapy in pregnancy has not been reported).

Transfusion therapy

Controversially, increasing numbers of obstetric units have adopted prophylactic transfusion regimens even though the benefit of such regimens remains to be established.[36] The basis for exchange transfusion is to decrease the concentration of haemoglobin S, thus increasing the overall oxygen carrying capacity of the blood, thereby reducing the amount of sickling and hence tissue damage. The disadvantages of exchange transfusions are transfusion reaction, allo-immunisation and exposure to infections. The conservative approach uses transfusions only for women with life-threatening illness or when the crises does not respond after 48 h of conservative therapy. The major advantage of conservative therapy is a reduction in the patient's exposure to blood products. Prophylactic transfusion is probably best used on an individualised basis depending on the physician's experience, type of facilities available and the severity of sickle cell disease among women in that region.

Intrapartum

Generalised and supportive measures involving stress reduction during labour appear to have a beneficial effect. It is important to avoid dehydration, hypoxia, sepsis and acidosis. In order to limit the increase in cardiac demand during painful contractions, the liberal use of epidural analgesia is encouraged. However, nitrous oxide (which is a mixture with 50% oxygen) via a face-mask can be used for short-term pain without the risk of precipitating a sickling crisis. Continuous fetal heart rate monitoring is highly recommended to detect fetal hypoxia, which is more common in the fetus of sickle cell patients, particularly those with intra-uterine growth restriction or oligohydramnios.[37] The mode of delivery should be vaginal unless there is an obstetric indication for operative intervention. In the event of Caesarean section, the haematologist should be contacted for advice. Blood should be grouped and saved in case cross-match is needed. Regional block is to be preferred over general anaesthetic because it largely avoids the risk of iatrogenic hypoxia.

Post-partum

The immediate post-partum period is a time of critical importance for patients with sickle cell disease. During this time, there is an increased risk of infections, thrombo-embolism and vaso-occlusive crises. Early ambulation, thrombo-embolic deterrent stockings and appropriate hydration and oxygenation are encouraged. Prophylactic subcutaneous heparin is advisable until the patient is fully ambulant. Adequate analgesia is essential. Breast-feeding is encouraged but adequate hydration and appropriate caloric intake is required. Ensure cord blood has been sent for haemoglobin electrophoresis and, if not, notify the paediatrician so that arrangements are made for sending neonatal samples. In equivocal cases, repeat electrophoresis should be performed at 6 weeks of age. Prophylactic penicillin therapy beginning at the third month is advised for all infants who have sickle cell disease. This is done to decrease the incidence of pneumonia in affected infants.[38]

Contraception

Controversy has affected the recommendations for contraception in sickle cell disease patients. However, family planning is an important issue in these patients as multiple pregnancies in a short time can increase the incidence of haematologic crises. The use of low-dose contraceptive pills is not contra-indicated in these patients and the highly effective protection against unwanted pregnancy conferred by the combined contraceptive pill is a positive advantage.[2] The other option of hormone-based contraception is depot medroxyprogesterone acetate. In addition to being effective contraception, a controlled study of medroxyprogesterone acetate demonstrated beneficial effects on the haematology as well as bone pain.[39] Full counselling and instructions must be provided before the use of these methods. The risk of uterine and tubal infections with the use of the intra-uterine contraceptive device, particularly in nulliparous women, makes their use relatively contra-indicated in sickle cell disease, but may be required in special circumstances for those in whom other methods are considered unsuitable. There is some evidence to suggest that levonorgestrel IUS use is associated with lower rate of pelvic infection than copper IUD use. Barrier methods are widely used, but carry a higher risk of unwanted pregnancies as compared to other methods. Upon completion of child-bearing, sterilisation should be considered taking into account the woman's desired family size, and the risk of genetic transmission.

SUMMARY

Sickle haemoglobinopathies are among the most common genetically transmitted conditions and have a world-wide distribution. During the last three decades, it has been shown that patients with major sickle haemoglobinopathies can have a satisfactory reproductive outcome.[40] This has been achieved through appropriate counselling, intensive prenatal care and effective intervention by providers with a high index of suspicion for predisposing factors to untoward outcomes. Controversy surrounds prophylactic transfusion. Its use needs to be tailored to individual patients depending on the patient's circumstances and provider's experience. The increasing numbers of people with sickle cell disease living in the UK and surviving to reproductive age means that, as healthcare professionals, we will have to become more aware of their problems and familiar with the techniques for their medical care in pregnancy.

References

1   Atkin K, Ahmad WI, Anionwu EN. Screening and counselling for sickle cell disorders and thalassaemia: the experience of parents and health professionals. Soc Sci Med 1998; 47: 1639–1651

2   Streetly A. A national screening policy for sickle cell disease and thalassaemia major for the United Kingdom. Questions are left after two evidence based reports. BMJ 2000; 320: 1353–1354. See also <www.kcl-phs.org.uk/haemscreening/>

3   American College of Obstetricians and Gynecologists. Hemoglobinopathies in Pregnancy. ACOG Technical Bulletin, No. 185, October 1993

4   Dickerhoff R. Sickle cell disease and pregnancy. Geburtshilfe Frauenheilkd 1990; 50: 425–428

5   Herrick JB. Peculiar elongation and sickle shaped red blood corpuscles in a case of severe anaemia. Arch Intern Med 1910; 6: 577–621

6   Pauling L, Itano HA, Singer SJ, Wells IC. Sickle cell anaemia, a molecular disease. Science 1949; 110: 543

7   Schneider RG, Hightower B, Husty TS. Abnormal haemoglobins in a quarter million people. Blood 1976; 48: 629

8   Bunn HF, Forget BG, Ranney HM. Human Haemoglobins. Philadelphia: WB Saunders, 1977

9   Ranney HM, Sharma V. Structure and function of haemoglobin. In: Beutler E, Lichtman MA, Coller BS, Kipps TJ. (eds) Williams' Hematology, 5th edn. New York: McGraw-Hill, 1995; 417

10 Chernoff AI. The amino acid composition of haemoglobin. IV The preparation of pure polypeptide chains of human haemoglobin. J Chromatogr 1965; 17: 140–148

11 Neel JV. The inheritance of sickle cell anaemia. Science 1949; 110: 64–66

12 Jaffe RH. Die Sichelzellenanamie. Virch Arch Pathol Anat 1927; 265: 452–471

13 Ballas SK, Larner J, Smith ED, Surrey S, Schwartz E, Rappaport EF. Rheologic predictors of the severity of the painful sickle cell crises. Blood 1988; 72: 1216

14 Haynes JJ, Manci E, Voelkel N. Microvascular haemodynamics in the sickle red blood cell perfused isolated rat lung. Am J Physiol 1993; 264(2 pt2):H48 4–9

15 Vichinsky EP, Styles LA, Colangelo LH, Wright EC, Castro O, Nickerson B. Acute chest syndrome in sickle cell disease: clinical presentation and course. Cooperative Study of Sickle Cell Disease. Blood 1997; 89: 1787–1792

16 Quinn CT, Buchanan GR. The acute chest syndrome of sickle cell disease. Paediatrics 1999; 135: 416–422

17 Nelson-Piercy C. Handbook of Obstetric Medicine. Second Edition. 2002

18 Martin Jr JN, Files J, Morrison JC. Sickle cell crises. In: Clark SL, Cotton DB, Hankins GDV, Phelan JP. (eds) Critical Care Obstetrics, 2nd edn. Cambridge, MA: Blackwell 1991; 212

19 Beutler E. The sickle cell diseases and related disorders. In: Beutler E, Lichtman MA, Coller BS, Kipps TJ. (eds) Williams' Hematology, 5th edn. New York: McGraw-Hill, 1995; 616

20 Tuck S, White JM. Sickle cell disease. In: JWW Studd (ed) Prog Obstet Gynaecol 1981; 1: 70–79

21 Kobak AJ, Stein Pjand Daro AE. Sickle cell anaemia in pregnancy. A review of the literature and report of six cases. Am J Obstet Gynecol 1941; 41: 811—821

22 Blake PG, Martin Jr JN, Perry Jr KG. Disseminated intravascular coagulation, autoimmune thrombocytopenic purpura and haemoglobinopathies. In: Knuppel RA, Drukker JE. (eds) High-risk Pregnancy. A Team Approach, 2nd edn. Philadelphia: WB Saunders, 1993; 561

23 National Screening Committee. Second Report of the UK National Screening Committee. London: Department of Health, 2002

24 Aspinall PJ. The mandatory collection of data on ethnic group of in-patients' experience of NHS trusts in England in the first reporting years. Public Health 2000; 114: 254–259

25 Aspinall PJ, Anionwu EN. The role of ethnic monitoring in mainstreaming race equality and the modernisation of the NHS: a neglected agenda? Crit Public Health 2002; 12: 1–15

26 Aspinall PJ, Dyson SM, Anionwu EN. The feasibility of using ethnicity as a primary tool for antenatal selective screening for sickle cell disorders: pointers from the research evidence. Soc Sci Med 2003; 56: 285–297

27 Atkin K, Ahmad WIU, Anionwu EN. Screening and counselling for sickle cell disorders and thalassaemia: the experience of parents and health professionals, Soc Sci Med 1998; 47: 1639–1651

28 Bain J, Chapman C. A survey of current United Kingdom practice for antenatal screening for inherited disorders of globin chain synthesis. J Clin Pathol 1998; 51: 382–389

29 Dyson S, Fielder A, Kirkham M. Haemoglobinopathies, antenatal screening and the midwife. Br J Midwif 1996; 4: 319–322

30 Rowley PT, Loader S, Sultera CJ, Walden M, Korzyra A. Prenatal screening for haemoglobinopathies. A prospective regional trial. Am J Hum Genet 1991; 48: 439

31 Anderson MF. The iron status of pregnant women with haemoglobinopathies. Am J Obstet Gynecol 1972; 113: 895–900

32 Oluboyede OA. Iron studies in pregnant and non-pregnant with haemoglobin SS or SC disease. Br J Obstet Gynaecol 1980; 87: 989–996

33 Anyaegbunam A, Langer O, Brustman L, Witty J, Merkatz IR. Third-trimester prediction of small-for-gestational-age infants in pregnant women with sickle disease. N Engl J Med 1994; 330: 733

34 Orion A, Rust MD, Kenneth G, Perry JR. Pregnancy complicated by sickle haemoglobinopathy. Clin Obstet Gynaecol 1995; 18: 472–484

35 James N, Martin Jr JN, Morrison JC. Managing the parturient with sickle cell crises. Clin Obstet Gynaecol 1984; 27: 39–49

36 Mohamed K. Prophylactic versus selective blood transfusion for sickle cell anaemia during pregnancy. Cochrane Review 2000(2): Cd000040

37 National Institute of Clinical Exvellence (NICE) The use of electronic fetal monitoring: The use and interpretation of cardiotocography in intrapartum fetal surveillance. May, 2001.

38 Gaston MH, Verter JI, Woods G. Prophylaxis with oral penicillin in children with sickle cell anaemia: a randomized : a randomized trial. N Engl J Med 1986; 314: 1593

39 Deceulaer K, Gruber C, Hayes RJ, Serjeant GR. Medroxyprogesterone acetate and homozygous sickle-cell disease. Lancet 1982; 2: 229–231

40 Serjeant GR. Historical review. The emerging understanding of sickle cell disease. Br J Haematol 2001; 112: 3–18

Reeba Oliver Ronald F. Lamont

Role of cytokines in spontaneous preterm labour and preterm birth

Spontaneous preterm labour (SPTL) and preterm birth (PTB) are the major causes of perinatal mortality[1] and morbidity[2] in the industrialised world and are a huge burden on the cost of healthcare provision.[3,4] The aetiology of preterm labour is multifactorial but there is overwhelming evidence to implicate infection as a major cause,[5] accounting for about 40% of all cases of SPTL and PTB.[6]

In the amniotic fluid of women in SPTL of infectious aetiology, significantly increased levels of pro-inflammatory proteins (cytokines) can be detected which is in contrast to those women in SPTL of non-infectious aetiology.[7] Babies born preterm in the presence of such cytokines are more likely to suffer lung and white matter tissue damage resulting in bronchopulmonary dysplasia (BPD)[8] and periventricular leukomalacia (PVL).[9] In addition, those babies born in the presence of increased concentrations of white blood cells and cytokines such as interleukin (IL)-6 and IL-8 in amniotic fluid, and in the presence of funisitis (inflammation of the umbilical cord vessels) are significantly more likely to be found to have cerebral palsy at long-term follow-up.[10]

Spontaneous preterm labour and PTB is either a physiological process occurring too early in pregnancy or a pathological process following an abnormal signal. The earlier in pregnancy that labour occurs, the more likely this is to be due to a pathological signal such as infection. While the final end common pathway with respect to the physiology, biochemistry, endocrinology and paracrinology of term and preterm labour may be the same, SPTL and PTB appear to be the result of a heterogeneous group of variables known as the fetal inflammatory syndrome.[7]

Reeba Oliver MBBS MRCOG
Clinical Research Fellow, Department of Obstetrics and Gynaecology, Northwick Park Hospital and St Mark's Hospital, Watford Road, Harrow HA1 3UJ, UK

Ronald F. Lamont BSc MB ChB MD FRCOG
Consultant and Honorary Reader, Department of Obstetrics and Gynaecology, Northwick Park and St Mark's Hospital and Division of Paediatrics, Obstetrics and Gynaecology, Imperial College, London HA1 3UJ, UK (for correspondence, E-mail: Pauline.mills@nwlh.nhs.uk)

It follows that, if we are to understand the link between infection and SPTL and PTB, we must understand the role of cytokines and their interaction between the physiological and pathological processes that take place in feto–maternal tissues as part of the inflammatory process that leads to labour and delivery.

THE INFLAMMATORY PROCESS

Inflammation is defined as the cascade of events in vascularised tissue designed to eliminate a cause of injury as well as the necrotic cells and tissue resulting from the original injury. Any stimuli that damage the tissues lead to an inflammatory reaction and the commonest stimuli are infections. Acute inflammation is characterised by neutrophilic infiltrate, while chronic inflammation is characterised mainly by macrophage infiltration.

Cellular mediators of inflammation

Neutrophils (polymorphonuclear leukocytes) accumulate in areas of acute inflammation, and are the first line of defence against pathogens by the process of phagocytosis. Macrophages also phagocytose organisms and cellular debris. Microbial adherence followed by ingestion occurs through specialised receptors. B and T lymphocytes are involved in cell-mediated as well as humoral (antibody-mediated) immunity. T lymphocytes are classified into T-helper (Th) cells; Th1 cells have a pro-inflammatory effect and Th2 cells have an anti-inflammatory effect. B cells differentiate into plasma cells that secrete antibodies. Mast cells have a similar function to basophils with degranulation of their granules resulting in the release of chemical mediators. Although platelets are mainly involved in blood clotting, following injury, platelets release substances that result in increased capillary permeability and attraction of leukocytes. Natural killer (NK) cells recognise and kill virus infected cells and they play an important part in cell-mediated immunity.

Chemical mediators of inflammation

Vasoactive amines result in increased vascular permeability and dilatation. The major vasoactive amines are histamine released mainly from mast cells and serotonin released by platelets. Plasma proteases mediate many of the effects of inflammation through three plasma derived factors – the kinins, the clotting system and the complement system. The kinin system leads to the formation of bradykinin. Bradykinin causes increased vascular permeability, arteriolar dilatation and bronchial smooth muscle contraction. In the clotting system, factor Xa causes increased vascular permeability and leukocyte migration and thrombin enhances leukocyte adhesion to the endothelium. The complement system consists of a cascade of proteins that mediate vascular permeability, leukocyte adhesion, chemotaxis and phagocytosis. Arachidonic acid metabolites are mainly prostaglandins, leukotrienes and lipoxins. Arachidonic acid metabolism has two major pathways: cyclooxygenase, synthesising prostaglandin and thromboxanes, and lipoxygenase, synthesising leukotrienes and lipoxins. All these metabolites cause vasodilatation or vasoconstriction, increased vascular permeability, chemotaxis and leukocyte adhesion. Cytokines are polypeptide products of many different cell types that modulate the function of other cell types. Interferons (IFNs) are cytokines, which have mainly anti-viral properties, and chemokines are cytokines that have specific chemotactic activity for various leukocytes. Opsonins are molecules such as antibodies that promote phagocytosis of bacteria by the leukocytes, which is the process by which particulate matter is ingested by cells. Opsonins coat the bacterium helping it to attach to the phagocytic leukocyte.

Acute inflammation

Acute inflammation is the immediate and early response to injury. Acute inflammation leads to localised and systemic effects.

Local effects

There are five cardinal signs of inflammation: redness (rubor), swelling (tumor), heat (calor), pain (dolor) and loss of function (functio laesa). Three physiological changes occur with these cardinal signs: hyperaemia, increased vascular permeability and transmigration and recruitment of leukocytes.

Hyperaemia – During inflammation chemical mediators such as histamine and prostaglandin cause smooth muscle relaxation and arteriolar dilatation. This leads to increased blood flow facilitating the recruitment of leukocytes to the site of inflammation.

Increased vascular permeability – Chemical mediators mainly histamine, leukotrienes and prostaglandin act on the endothelial cells causing them to contract and form gaps in the integrity of the endothelial lining of the vessels. This increased permeability leads to oedema (exudate or transudate) and contributes to the swelling seen at inflammatory sites.

Leukocyte transmigration – Initially, leukocytes accumulate at the periphery of vessels (margination). The relatively loose and transient adhesions involved in margination are due to adhesion molecules called selectins, expressed on endothelial cells and leukocytes. Adhesion molecules are molecules on the surface of the cells that assist leukocytes to adhere. Eventually, through the action of endothelial adhesion molecules such as intercellular adhesion molecule (ICAM) neutrophils stick firmly to the endothelial surface (adhesion). Finally, the leukocyte escapes into the extracellular space through the gaps in the vascular endothelium (diapedesis).

Leukocyte recruitment and activation – After extravasation, leukocytes migrate towards sites of injury on a chemical gradient provided by chemokine activity. Chemotactic factors also induce leukocyte activation.

Phagocytosis and degranulation – Phagocytosis consists of three distinct steps: recognition and attachment of the particle causing injury to the leukocyte, engulfment with subsequent formation of a phagocytic vacuole and killing and degradation of the ingested material. Macrophages are recruited to the injured tissue to ingest and clear the cellular debris and facilitate healing.

Systemic effects

Severe inflammation results in systemic changes known as the acute phase response or acute phase reaction. The acute phase response is mediated by cytokines and the symptoms include:

Fever – Pyrogens are substances that cause a rise in temperature (*e.g.* IL-1 and TNF-α). A rise in temperature is the result of the resetting of the hypothalamic thermostat. This is effected by prostaglandin, which is released by the increased concentrations of cytokines. The rise in temperature has been postulated to inhibit the growth of certain bacteria.

Elevated white blood cell (WBC) count – The bone marrow contains reserve stores of neutrophils, which are released into the circulation during inflammation resulting in a raised WBC count. In severe acute phase response, the marrow releases neutrophils before they are fully mature. These band forms of neutrophils signify a severe systemic reaction.

Breakdown of muscle protein – Cytokine-stimulated prostaglandin production acts on myometrial cells, which induces breakdown of myometrial protein.

Production of acute phase proteins by the liver – Cytokines (mainly IL-1) induce liver cells to produce a variety of proteins for wound healing and the inflammatory process. These are classified as group I proteins (*e.g.* fibrinogen and proteins necessary for the complement cascade), and group II proteins (*e.g.* C-reactive protein necessary for opsonisation).

Chronic inflammation

Chronic inflammation occurs if the inflammatory response is not able to eliminate the injury and is of prolonged duration. Macrophages accumulate at the site of infection and may cause further tissue damage. There is proliferation of blood vessels, new vessel formation (angiogenesis) and fibrosis. Macrophages form epithelioid cells, which may fuse to form giant cells. Increased fibrosis is an attempt to wall-off the injury or infection to prevent it from spreading to the surrounding healthy tissue.

Tissue repair

Even as cell injury and death is occurring, the repair mechanisms are set in motion. The repair process begins early in the inflammatory process and involves two major processes: regeneration of injured tissue and replacement by connective tissue (fibrosis). Fibrosis involves angiogenesis, migration and proliferation of fibroblasts, deposition of the extracellular matrix and finally maturation and reorganisation of the fibrous tissue (remodelling).

INTRODUCTION TO CYTOKINES

Cytokines are proteins and peptides, secreted by cells, which act as humoral regulators to modulate the intercellular actions of the cell.[11] They are pleiotropic effectors with diverse actions ranging from growth factors (B-cell growth factors), chemotaxis (chemokines) and angiogenesis factors as well as paracrine and autocrine functions. Specific membrane receptors expressed on the cell surface mediate the biological activity of each cytokine by activating intracellular pathways, which act mainly on the functional activities of the immune cells. These humoral regulators help to establish and maintain pregnancy by co-ordinating the immune response against invading micro-organisms. Since cytokines are the result of enhanced leukocytic activity for immunosurveillance, they play a protective part in shielding the fetus from an adverse environment. Pro-inflammatory cytokines orchestrate the events, which lead to the inflammatory reaction in response to infections, but this can also have detrimental effects on the fetus and the pregnancy. Antigen-specific immunity develops later in life and neonates depend initially upon natural (innate) immunity. Cytokines, especially chemokines, induce cell activation and chemotaxis to sites of acute inflammation both locally and systemically.

STRUCTURE AND FUNCTION OF CYTOKINES

In addition to their well-documented pro-inflammatory functions, some cytokines have an anti-inflammatory function.

Pro-inflammatory cytokines

Interleukin-6 (IL-6)
IL-6 is a glycosylated protein molecule mainly produced by the Th2 lymphocytes but also by monocytes and macrophages. IL-6 is the major physiological mediator of the acute phase reaction.[12] Increased expression correlates with an infectious process and so can be used as a diagnostic indicator of infections and inflammation. IL-6 activates B cells to stimulate antibody secretion by inducing them to differentiate into plasma cells and also induces the differentiation of mature and immature T cells into cytotoxic T cells.

TNF-α
TNF-α is a non-glycosylated protein of 17 kDa and a length of 157 amino acids, which forms dimers and trimers. TNF-α production is stimulated by bacterial lipopolysaccharides (LPSs) and is mainly produced by T-helper cells, monocytes, macrophages and neutrophils.[13] The synthesis of TNF-α is stimulated by interferons, immune complexes and bradykinins. TNF-α is a neutrophilic chemo-attractant and increases the adherence of neutrophils to endothelium. TNF-α also acts as a growth factor for fibroblasts and promotes the synthesis of collagenase and prostaglandin E_2 by the fibroblasts.

Interleukin-1 (IL-1)
IL-1 is a protein of 17 kDa and a length of 159 amino acids, the β-form of which predominates in human tissues. Monocytes are the main source, but IL-1 is also produced by activated macrophages and peripheral neutrophil granulocytes. Originally described as T-cell activation factor, IL-1 is secreted by a number of cells such as macrophages, dendritic cells and mainly monocytes.

The main biological activity is induction of Th1 lymphocytes to produce IL-2.[14] IL-1 plays an important role in inflammation by acting as an endogenous pyrogen and increasing the expression of cell adhesion molecules in the endothelium. An increased level of IL-1 is indicative of an infective process since the major stimulus for IL-1 production by macrophages is the presence of microbial products. As a result, IL-1 is often used as a diagnostic indicator of the presence of an infective process.

Interleukin-2 (IL-2)

IL-2 is a protein of 133 amino acids which is secreted primarily by T-helper cells following activation by antigens, and which acts both on NK and T cells. IL-2 is a growth factor of all subpopulations of T lymphocytes. The autocrine activity of IL-2 results in antigen primed T cell proliferation and by activating B cells results in B cell proliferation.[15]

Interleukin-8 (IL-8)

IL-8 is a non-glycosylated protein of 8 kDa, which is secreted by macrophages, and monocytes, which have been stimulated by IL-1 and TNF-α. The main action of IL-8 is chemotaxis of neutrophils to adhere to endothelium, following which there is diapedesis and recruitment to sites of inflammation. This action of IL-8 is essential in fetal innate immunity as neutrophils are the first immune cells to appear at the site of infection, allowing time for T cells to mount their antigen specific immunity.

Interleukin-12 (IL-12)

IL-12 is a heterodimeric glycoprotein secreted by macrophages and mainly B cells, which activate cytotoxic T cells.[16] IL-12 induces NK and Th1 cell proliferation, and induces the synthesis of IFN-γ, TNF-α and IL-2 by Th1 lymphocytes. This is particularly important with respect to the host immune response against intracellular pathogens.[17]

Other pro-inflammatory cytokines

Recently, previously unrecognised cytokines such as IL-18,[18] IL-16[19] and IL-15[20] have been identified in increased concentrations in the amniotic fluid of women in SPTL in the presence of intra-uterine infections.

Anti-inflammatory cytokines

Interleukin-10 (IL-10)

IL-10 is a homodimeric protein, anti-inflammatory cytokine with subunits, which have a length of 160 amino acids. IL-10 is secreted by T lymphocytes and monocytes following cell activation by bacterial LPS. IL-10 down-regulates Th1 helper T cell function by inhibiting cytokine production by the macrophage.[17] In the choriodecidual unit, IL-10 inhibits the synthesis of IL-1, IL-6, TNF-α and the production of prostaglandin E$_2$.[21]

Interleukin-4 (IL-4)

Originally called B-cell stimulating factor, IL-4 is a protein of 129 amino acids, which is secreted mainly by the Th2 lymphocytes, but also by the non-T/non-B-cells of mast cell lineage. The action of IL-4 on B cells results in B-cell activation and proliferation. IL-4 inhibits decidual prostaglandin production and decreases pro-inflammatory cytokine- induced secretion of prostaglandin in trophoblast cultures.[22]

Site of production

Cytokines are produced in all tissues of the body. The placenta and membranes have been shown to secrete a large number of pro- and anti-inflammatory cytokines and chemokines.[23] In labour, TNF-α is secreted from macrophages in placental tissue, while IL-1β and IL-6 are released from the placental endothelial cells.[24] Stimulation with LPS induces decidual cells to produce IL-1[25] and TNF-α[26] and other *in vitro* studies have established the capacity of decidua and the chorio-amnion to secrete cytokines following stimulation with IL-1, TNF-α or LPS.[23] Decidual cells have been shown to produce significant amounts of chemokines, mainly IL-8, in response to bacterial cell wall components.[27]

MECHANISM OF NORMAL LABOUR AND SPTL OF INFECTIOUS AETIOLOGY

The mechanisms of the onset of labour remain uncertain despite extensive research and involve mainly three physiological processes: (i) remodelling of the connective tissue of the cervix allowing it to soften and dilate; (ii) initiation of uterine myometrial contractions; and (iii) disruption of membrane integrity leading to weakening and rupture.

Molecular mechanism of normal labour

The initiation and control of labour at the molecular level is mainly the interaction between the regulation of prostaglandin production, cytokines and the tissue remodelling by matrix metalloproteinases (MMPs).

Arachidonic acid is the obligate precursor of prostaglandin synthesis and is essential for the initiation and maintenance of labour. Phospholipases are responsible for release of arachidonic acid from glycerophospholipids in the cell membrane following which arachidonic acid is converted to prostaglandin H_2 by prostaglandin H_2 synthase (PGHS). Specific prostaglandin synthases convert prostaglandin H_2 to primary prostaglandin and then to prostaglandin E_2 and prostaglandin $F_{2\alpha}$, which are potent stimulators of myometrial contractility. Prostaglandins are metabolised into inactive metabolites through the action of 15-hydroxyprostaglandin dehydrogenase (PGDH). Progesterone is synthesised from pregnenolone by placental syncytiotrophoblasts and by chorionic trophoblasts. Progesterone has a suppressive action on uterine contractility and also regulates the expression of PGDH in the chorion. During pregnancy, progesterone inhibits the stimulation of prostaglandin by inducing high expression of PGDH. RU486 (a synthetic inhibitor of progesterone) induced blockade of progesterone receptors results in a pro-inflammatory cascade *in utero*, which leads to labour.[28–30]

Cytokines up-regulate PGHS and increase prostaglandin production. IL-1β and TNF-α stimulate arachidonic acid release, which activates the phospholipid metabolic pathway and increases the production of prostaglandin by the myometrium.[31]

Matrix metalloproteinases are zinc-dependent enzymes, which play a central role in the digestion and breakdown of extracellular matrix. The MMP family consist of more than 20 members with action on different substrates. They are mainly collagenases (MMP-1, MMP-8, MMP-13), which cleave collagen, stromelysins (MMP-3, MMP-7, MMP-10), which cleave proteoglycan, and fibronectin, and gelatinases (MMP-2, MMP-9), which act on elastin. Most MMPs have been found to have some action on most of the substrates. Cervical stromal cells and neutrophils produce distinct MMPs, and all leukocytes are major sources of MMPs. The activity of MMPs is inhibited by tissue inhibitors of metalloproteinases (TIMP). The local balance of MMP expression and activation versus the level of TIMP governs the tissue remodelling mediated by the MMP. The MMP function is modulated by cytokines. Cytokine activation of cells lead to increased expression of MMP and cytokines and their receptors can also be substrates for MMP action.

Molecular mechanism of SPTL of infectious aetiology

In vitro studies have demonstrated the capacity of bacteria to invade rapidly the intra-uterine cavity by permeating the chorio-amniotic membranes.[32] Leukocytes recruited to the site of inflammation release cytokines which in turn activates the release of MMP. Cytokine levels in amniotic fluid associated with SPTL and PTB are markedly elevated and increased expression of the chemokine class genes have been shown in fetal membranes in the presence of chorio-amnionitis.

Women with intra-amniotic infection tend to be refractory to the use of tocolytics.[33] In the presence of elevated cytokine levels, this may be predictive of the success of treatment and the continuation of the pregnancy. Inflammatory cells and activated immune cells migrate though the amnion into the amniotic fluid and stimulate the production of cytokines. Incubation of amnion cells with bacterial products has been shown to significantly increase production of prostaglandin E_2,[34,35] IL-6 and IL-8.[36] The amniotic fluid concentrations of cytokines are higher in women with SPTL in the presence of intra-amniotic infection than those without evidence of infection[37,38] and increased levels of IL-6, IL-8 and TNF-α have been detected in the cervicovaginal fluid of women in SPTL associated with intra-uterine infections.[39,40] In the presence of intra-uterine infection, the primary cellular source of cytokines is the leukocyte, especially the neutrophil. The multiple actions of cytokines in inducing preterm labour is summarised in Figure 1.

The anti-inflammatory actions of IL-10 and IL-4 oppose the pro-inflammatory cytokine actions leading to a decreased likelihood of SPTL, PTB and preterm prelabour rupture of membranes (PPROM). IL-10 decreases LPS-stimulated prostaglandin E_2 production by the membranes as well as cytokine and prostaglandin production by the choriodecidual tissues.[41,42] Terrone *et al.*[43] reported the prevention of LPS-induced SPTL and PTB in rats treated with IL-10. IL-10 has also been shown to inhibit gelatinases, which reduce the incidence of PPROM.[44] Lung inflammation in preterm infants increases as they

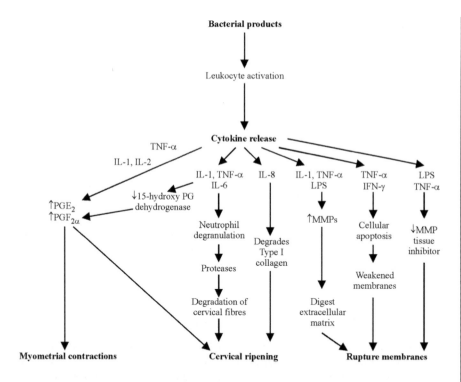

Fig. 1 Mechanism of SPTL of infectious aetiology: multiple mechanisms of cytokine induced preterm labour, triggered by bacterial infections.

become unable to activate IL-10 and lose the inhibitory effect of this cytokine. IL-4 induces increased production of the IL-1 receptor antagonist IL-1RA,[22] which leads to decreased concentration of active IL-1, which in turn leads to decreased prostaglandin production. IL-4 also inhibits PGHS production in the amnion which results in decreased prostaglandin production in SPTL associated with infection.[45] Paradoxically, IL-4 has been shown to increase production of prostaglandin E_2 in the amnion by inducing the enzyme cyclooxygenase-2 (COX-2).[46]

Myometrium

In pregnancy, towards term, there is an up-regulation of factors which increase myometrial contractility. At term, activity of PGHS rises leading to increased production of prostaglandin. Prostaglandin increases myometrial activity and intra-uterine tissues produce increased amounts prior to the onset of labour and PGDH concentrations fall during labour. At term, there is an increased production of IL-6, IL-8, IL-1β and TNF-α.[47] Many of the pro-inflammatory cytokines (mainly IL-1β and TNF-α) have been shown to act on the prostaglandin biosynthetic pathway. IL-1β and TNF-α have been shown to decrease the expression of PGDH[48] leading to increased prostaglandin levels. The increase in COX-2 and prostaglandin E_2 caused by IL-1β, in conjunction with the increased intracellular calcium concentrations of the myometrial cells caused by prostaglandin E_2, stimulate uterine contractions. Cytokines also increase the production of prostaglandin $F_{2\alpha}$, which induces cervical ripening and uterine contractility.[49,50] Cytokines such as IL-2[51] and IL-6[52] act directly on the decidual stromal cells and increase myometrial contractility. The action of IL-6 in stimulating uterine contractions is mainly through its effect on oxytocin secretion and receptor function.[53] IL-6 increases myometrial expression of oxytocin receptors and their responsiveness to oxytocin. IL-6 also increases oxytocin secretion by myometrial cells and at high concentrations stimulates prostaglandin production by amnion and decidua.

The role of prostaglandin in the initiation of SPTL in the presence of intra-uterine infection is well established.[54,55] Bry and Hallman[56] reported a synergistic effect on prostaglandin E_2 production by IL-1, TNF-α and products from activated granulocytes. A role has been postulated for IL-1 in the initiation of SPTL associated with intra-amniotic infection by the positive correlation between IL-1 and prostaglandin concentrations in the amniotic fluid[57] as well as IL-1 induced production of TNF-α, prostaglandin E_2 and prostaglandin $F_{2\alpha}$ resulting in myometrial contractions.[58] Amnion-derived prostaglandin E_2 increases during term and preterm labour[54] and stimulation of prostaglandin production by pro-inflammatory cytokines (mainly IL-6) has been reported.[59,60] TNF-α stimulates uterine activity by increasing the production of prostaglandin by amnion cells[61] in SPTL of infectious aetiology. IL-2 accelerates prostaglandin production, decreases progesterone levels[62] and attenuates the stimulatory actions of IL-1β on prostaglandin E_2 production by amnion cells[63] leading to SPTL. The direct action of cytokines on uterine stromal cells and their indirect actions via modulation of the prostaglandin-synthesis pathway identifies cytokines as central to the initiation of labour in response to an inflammatory stimulus.

Cervix

Towards term, there is an increase in the proteolytic enzyme activity which leads to softening of, and a decrease in, the amount of collagen in the cervix. Cervical ripening is essential for the onset of labour and involves remodelling of the extracellular matrix of the cervix. The main factors involved in cervical ripening are invasion of leukocytes, remodelling of extracellular matrix and proteolytic enzyme activity. At term, there is an influx of leukocytes, mainly neutrophils, into the cervix[64] leading to increased production of IL-6, IL-8, IL-1β and TNF-α.[47] These pro-inflammatory cytokines, through a number of mechanisms result in cervical softening and dilatation.[65] IL-1β increases the production of MMP-1, MMP-3 and MMP-9 and down-regulates TIMP, which leads to increased production of MMP-2. IL-1β also increases PGHS and prostaglandin E_2, which result in cervical dilatation. Prostaglandin E_2, in turn, increases production of proteases and increase vascular permeability leading to increased leukocyte recruitment. Prostaglandin also has a direct action on the cervix by remodelling the cervical connective tissue. IL-6 stimulates macrophages and neutrophils to produce pro-inflammatory cytokines. IL-8 induces neutrophils to release MMP-8 and neutrophil elastase resulting in digestion of the cervical extra cellular matrix. PGDH expression in fetal membranes overlying the internal os is decreased by the action of the pro-inflammatory cytokines during active labour leading to increased prostaglandin concentrations promoting cervical effacement and dilatation.

In SPTL of infectious aetiology, cytokines play a major part in the cervical changes. IL-8 is the main cytokine causing cervical ripening by degradation of type I collagen[66] that predisposes to preterm labour.[67,68] Concomitant with the increase in IL-8 levels during cervical ripening, leukocyte infiltration and increased concentrations of MMP occur.[69] Cytokines synergistically increase the inflammatory response to an infectious agent through IL-1β by activating the lower uterine segment fibroblasts to produce increased amount of IL-8.[70] The neutrophil is the predominant immune active cell found in the placenta and cervix during SPTL of infectious aetiology[71] and neutrophilic chemotactic factors have been implicated in cervical ripening.[72] Increased concentrations of pro-inflammatory cytokines (mainly TNF-α and IL-1β) in the lower uterine segment in response to an infectious stimuli, increase the adhesiveness of capillary endothelium resulting in extravasation of neutrophils. Degranulation of neutrophils causes the release of proteases and further degradation and softening of the cervix. Prostaglandin E_2 induces cervical ripening by stimulating IL-8 production[73] and, synergistically, cytokines increase prostaglandin E_2 production by their action on the prostaglandin-synthesis pathway. Pro-inflammatory cytokines through their action on the extracellular matrix of the cervix via MMP and by inducing neutrophilic degranulation play a significant role in cervical ripening in SPTL of infectious aetiology.

Membranes

Rupture of the membranes is an essential part of normal parturition. Weakening of the membranes over the internal cervical os occurs with thinning and subsequent rupture. MMP degrade the collagen extracellular matrix and lead to rupture of the membranes.[74,75] During labour, the production of IL-6, IL-8, IL-1β and TNF-α by the fetal membranes is increased.[76] IL-1β, IL-8 and TNF-α increase the amniotic production of MMP-9 and also decrease the production of TIMP. The increased activity of these collagenases result in weakening of the membranes and rupture. IL-1β and TNF-α also increase PGHS and prostaglandin E_2 levels which leads to increased concentrations of MMP-9.[77] Both IL-8 production and MMP activity in the fetal membranes are increased by mechanical stretching. Apoptosis of fetal membrane cells contribute to weakening of the membranes and TNF-α and prostaglandin E_2 induce apoptosis and cell necrosis of fetal membrane cells which leads to rupture.

Premature rupture of the membranes accounts for 30% of all SPTL and is associated with increased risk of SPTL and PTB, intra-uterine infection and neonatal mortality and morbidity.[78] MMPs are postulated to digest the fetal membrane extracellular matrix, which leads to PPROM. Intra-uterine infection has been shown to be associated with higher levels of MMP-9 in amniotic fluid[79] and various pro-inflammatory cytokines have been shown to increase the production of MMP in the fetal membranes. IL-1α increases MMP synthesis in the chorion[80] and IL-1β has been shown to induce apoptosis in the amniochorion with infections, which decreases the integrity of the fetal membranes, which makes them prone to rupture.[81]

LPS and TNF-α increase MMP production as well as decreasing the release of TIMP,[82,83] which increases the likelihood of PPROM. TNF-α, in conjunction with IFN-γ, induces apoptosis of trophoblasts, which leads to weakening of the fetal membranes especially the chorion, prior to rupture.[84,85] Due to this disruption of the integrity of the membranes, increased levels of TNF-α in the lower genital tract is predictive of subsequent preterm delivery.[86] Increased cytokine concentration in fetal membranes suggests an inflammatory process[87] and IL-1 and IL-6 secretion is initiated by inflammation in the membranes.[57] Women with intra-amniotic infection are more likely to develop PPROM[88] and the increased levels of these cytokines are predictive of future rupture of the fetal membranes. The actions of MMP and apoptosis are the primary mechanisms by which cytokines predispose to rupture of the fetal membranes in SPTL of infectious aetiology.

LONG-TERM NEONATAL SEQUELAE

Infection affecting an immunocompromised host like the fetus may cause tissue damage and long-term sequelae such as BPD,[8,89] PVL,[9,90] and cerebral palsy.[10,90] Bacterial infections are the major cause of mortality and morbidity in preterm infants. The capacity to synthesise IL-12 in response to LPS is reduced in the neonatal period, which decreases the capacity of the neonate to combat infection.[91] Despite antibiotic therapy, the mortality rate following neonatal sepsis remains at 15–20% and chorio-amnionitis accounts for 50% of the long-term neurological morbidity associated with SPTL and PTB.[92] Preterm and low birth-weight infants exposed to amniotic fluid infections respond by mounting an inflammatory response involving cytokines.[93,94] This inflammatory response may cause tissue damage, which contributes to neonatal mortality and morbidity as much as immaturity *per se*.[95] The fetal inflammatory response has been implicated as a major factor in the morbidity associated with SPTL and PTB such as BPD, PVL, respiratory distress syndrome,[96] intraventricular haemorrhage, cerebral palsy[90] and necrotising enterocolitis and cerebral palsy which are far more common in preterm than in term infants.

Chronic lung disease is the long-term result of the pro-inflammatory cytokine mediated tissue damage and elevated amniotic fluid levels of IL-6, IL-8, IL-1β and TNF-α appear to be predicative of the development of chronic lung disease.[8,89,97] Elevated Levels of IL-1β, IL-6, IL-8 and TNF-α are associated with an increased risk of developing BPD and has been found to be related to antenatal exposure to infection.[98,99] Histological studies have confirmed a severe infiltration of macrophages, neutrophils and lymphocytes in fetal lungs in association with chorio-amnionitis.[100]

Elevated levels of IL-6, IL-8 and MMP-8 have been found in association with an increased risk of developing cerebral palsy[10,101] and 50% of cases of cerebral palsy occur in neonates born before 28 weeks' gestation which is 60 times more common than in term infants.[102] PVL is an important predictor of cerebral palsy and mental retardation.[103] IL-6 levels have been found to be higher in umbilical cord blood of infants born with white matter lesions associated with PVL, indicating an inflammatory aetiology.[9] The highest levels of cytokines were found in infants who subsequently developed hypoxic ischaemic encephalopathy and seizures.[104] High levels of pro-inflammatory cytokines have been shown to be associated with development of intracerebral haemorrhage in preterm infants.[105]

The inflammatory response mounted by the fetal immune system to the pro-inflammatory cytokine activity may adversely affect the fetal organs causing damage and long-term morbidity.

GENETIC PREDISPOSITION TO SPTL OF INFECTIOUS AETIOLOGY

In early pregnancy, nearly 20% of women have abnormal genital tract flora yet only 16% of these will deliver before 34 completed weeks of gestation.[106] Within this 20%, there must be a subgroup that has additional factors present which potentiates their risk of SPTL and PTB. These additional factors may be the presence of a particularly uncommon virulent organism or virulent strains of commonly isolated micro-organisms (increased exposure). Alternatively, the feto–maternal unit may be at increased risk due to a genetic predisposition to initiate a host immune response, which renders the pregnancy at increased risk of SPTL and PTB (increased susceptibility). This balance between susceptibility and exposure has been termed the gene–environment interaction and the genetic control of the inflammatory response in the context of microbiological invasion has recently been elegantly addressed.[107]

Signs of inflammation in vaginal secretions are a risk factor for SPTL and PTB.[108] Women with more than 5 polymorphs per high-power field have an OR of 1.6 (95% CI, 1.1–2.1) for preterm birth before 32 weeks' gestation and this OR reaches 2.9 (95% CI, 2.0–4.3) if there exists evidence of adverse changes in genital tract flora.[109]

Following exposure to antigen, the immune system mounts an inflammatory response (*vide supra*) which should be balanced and appropriate resulting in the recruitment of defensive cells, production of antimicrobial chemical agents, phagocytes, clearance of micro-organisms, cellular debris and followed by the healing process. Unfortunately, some individuals may not provide a balanced and appropriate response, but vary in their genetic predisposition to produce an excessive or inadequate response. Hyper-responders may produce an excessive local and/or systemic inflammatory response leading to tissue damage and potentially more serious conditions such as multi-organ failure and septic shock. In contrast, hyporesponders may, in a similar way to immunosuppressed patients develop overwhelming infection. The optimal host is the mother who is capable of producing a measured and proportionate inflammatory response.

Hyporesponders (women with low levels of IL-1, IL-6 and IL-8) in early pregnancy are much more likely to develop chorio-amnionitis than those with cytokine concentrations above the 25th centile suggesting that these women are at increased risk of invasion of micro-organisms and ascending intra-uterine infection.[110] Equally, hyper-responders (IL-6 concentration > 90th centile in cervicovaginal secretions) are at an increased risk of SPTL and PTB.[111] TNF-α production varies: (i) between individuals; (ii) is under genetic control; (iii) has been impaired in; and (iv) is an excellent example of the role of the cytokines in the mechanism of SPTL and PTB of infectious aetiology. The role of TNF-α in this context is taken from Romero[107] and is shown in tabulated form in Table 1.

Using this information, it might be predicted that those women who have abnormal genital tract flora and who are also genetically predisposed to produce an excess of TNF-α will be at increased risk of SPTL and PTB. In a group of women who suffered SPTL and PTB, environmental exposure was assessed by the detection of bacterial vaginosis using Amsel criteria.[112] Susceptibility was assessed by demonstration of the TNF-α-2 allele. Bacterial vaginosis was associated with an increased risk of SPTL and PTB (OR, 3.3; 95% CI, 1.8–5.9). Those women who carried the TNF-α-2 allele were also at increased risk of SPTL and PTB (OR, 2.7; 95% CI, 1.7–4.5). In women with both bacterial vaginosis and the TNF-α-2 allele, the OR for SPTL and PTB was 6.1 (95% CI, 1.9–2.1), suggesting that a gene–environmental interaction predisposes to SPTL and PTB.[113]

PREDICTION AND PREVENTION OF SPTL AND PTB

By the time a woman is admitted in SPTL, the knowledge that this may be due to infection is largely unhelpful since by this time there may already irreversible changes in the uterine cervix, which renders futile those attempts to reverse the process. The appreciation that infection is a major cause of SPTL and PTB may be of more help in the prediction and the prevention of SPTL and PTB and readers are referred to more detailed reviews of the subject.[114,115]

Abnormal genital tract flora in early pregnancy is predictive of subsequent late miscarriage and SPTL and PTB and this has recently been reviewed.[114,115] In addition, the earlier in pregnancy at which abnormal genital tract flora is detected, the greater is the risk of an adverse outcome. A positive result at 26–32 weeks was associated with a statistically significant 1.4–1.9-fold increased risk of SPTL and PTB. In contrast, a positive result from screening in the second trimester was associated with a 2.0–6.9-fold increased risk of an

---

Table 1 Evidence supporting the role of TNF-α in spontaneous preterm labour and preterm birth of infectious aetiology

TNF-α stimulates prostaglandin production by amnion, decidua and myometrium

Human decidua produces TNF-α in response to bacterial products

Amniotic fluid levels of TNF-α are elevated in women in SPTL with IAI

In women with PPROM and IAI, TNF-α is higher when SPTL commences

In animal studies, TNF-α can induce SPTL and PTB when administered systemically

TNF-α can stimulate the production of MMPs, which are intrinsically involved in PPROM and cervical ripening

TNF-α application to the cervix induces changes that resemble cervical ripening

---

IAI, intra-amniotic infection; MMP, matrix metalloproteinases; PPROM, preterm premature rupture of the membranes; PTB, preterm birth; SPTL, spontaneous preterm labour.
Adapted from Romero.[107]

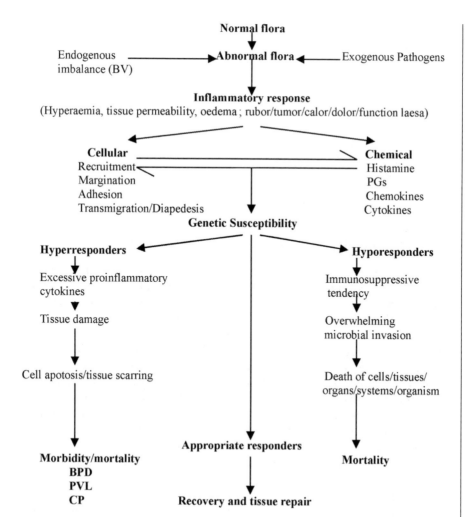

Fig. 2 Schematic view of the progression from normal vaginal flora through abnormal flora, inflammation, infection, tissue damage, host response and outcome of pregnancy. BV, bacterial vaginosis; BPD, bronchopulmonary dysplasia; PVL, periventricular leukomalacia; CP, cerebral palsy.

adverse outcome. It follows that, if interventional antibiotics are to be of help in the prevention of preterm birth, these should be administered early in pregnancy.[116,117] This is re-inforced by the fact that 24% of women with abnormal flora in early pregnancy who subsequently reverted to normal flora experienced an adverse outcome of pregnancy (late miscarriage, PTB, PPROM, *etc.*)[118] which was similar to those with bacterial vaginosis who received placebo as part of a randomised, double-blind placebo controlled trial.[117]

Assuming the process of infection leading to SPTL and PTB involves abnormal genital tract flora progressing to invasive tissue damage and death or handicap, it would seem logical that if antibiotics are to be of help in the prevention of SPTL and PTB and the associated mortality and morbidity, these should be administered as early as possible in the process before inflammatory cytokines cause tissue damage (Fig. 2). Figure 2 might explain why prophylactic antibiotics administered in early pregnancy,[116,117] before tissue damage might occur, were of help, when compared to those studies, criticised for using antibiotics late in pregnancy[119] at which time the inflammatory tissue damage may have already occurred, with the result that no benefit was observed.[120,121]

DIAGNOSTIC POTENTIAL OF CYTOKINES

IL-6 has been the focus of most studies examining and assessing the diagnostic potential of cytokines in SPTL and PTB. Amniotic fluid IL-6 levels positively and consistently correlate with intra-amniotic infection, SPTL[122] and PTB.[123] Elevated amniotic fluid concentration of IL-6 were associated with SPTL and PTB even in the absence of clinical infection and also appeared to predict the failure of tocolysis.[123] A comparative study by Romero et al.[124] found amniotic fluid concentration of IL-6 levels to be the most sensitive test for the detection of microbial invasion of the amniotic cavity and was the only test to predict amniocentesis-to-delivery interval and neonatal complications. Increased amniotic fluid levels of IL-6 indicate microbial invasion of the amniotic cavity in SPTL with intact membranes[125] and indicates the severity of chorio-amnionitis.[126] Low levels of amniotic fluid IL-6 in the third trimester of pregnancy correlates with pre-eclampsia and fetuses which are small for gestational age.[127] IL-6 concentration in umbilical cord blood is higher in infants born in the presence of funisitis[128] and fetal plasma IL-6 concentrations greater than 11 pg/ml are associated with a significantly higher rate of funisitis and vasculitis. Umbilical cord levels of IL-6 have been used to predict infants who develop early sepsis and many studies have shown a positive significant correlation with sepsis[129] as well as the severity of placental inflammation. Umbilical vein IL-6 levels have been shown to increase with increasing gestational age reflecting maturation of the fetal immune response. Significantly elevated levels of IL-6 have been used a diagnostic marker for the fetal inflammatory response syndrome[7] and have been found to be elevated in neonates with white matter lesions in the brain. This might help to identify those neonates who might require early treatment to prevent the sequelae associated with the fetal inflammatory response syndrome. Greci et al.[130] have amended a mathematical model using maternal serum IL-6 levels to quantify the interval to PTB in women in SPTL. The IL-6 concentration in cervicovaginal fluid was a useful marker following PPROM for the likelihood of developing neonatal infection[131] and acted as a prognostic factor for fetal morbidity and the likelihood of subsequent PTB.[111]

Many other pro-inflammatory cytokines have been investigated for their diagnostic potential.

Maternal serum TNF-α levels are increased in SPTL without signs of clinical chorio-amnionitis[132] and the rise in the levels of TNF-α is a sensitive diagnostic marker for an on-going infective process. Elevated amniotic fluid IL-1 levels have been shown to be a significant indicator of subclinical intra-uterine infection.[133] Serum IL-2 levels have been used to diagnose sepsis in neonates with negative blood cultures.[134] IL-12 levels in amniotic fluid are increased in SPTL in the presence of oligohydramnios[135] reflecting immune-cell activation in conditions which are threatening to the fetus. Elevated levels of IL-8 and its gene expression in cord blood are indicative of neonatal infection[136] as well as chorio-amnionitis in association with PTB. Amniotic fluid IL-8 levels are of value in diagnosing intra-amniotic infection[137] and are diagnostic of chorio-amnionitis. Elevated IL-8 levels in cervical secretions predict intra-uterine infection in women in SPTL with intact membranes.[138] Elevated levels of IL-8 are also found in increased concentrations in the amniotic fluid of women whose infants subsequently develop BPD.[139] Discriminatory levels of IL-6 and IL-8 have been shown to predict the success of tocolysis, with elevated levels being most predictive of PTB within 48 h.[140] Amniotic fluid IL-10 concentrations are not increased in SPTL or in association with chorio-amnionitis, reflecting its anti-inflammatory role.[141]

Other, less well-studied cytokines have been examined for their potential role in predicting SPTL and PTB. Granulocyte-colony stimulating factor,[142] RANTES (regulated on activation, normal T cell expressed and secreted),[143] pre-B-cell colony-enhancing factor,[144] macrophage inflammatory protein-1α (MAP-1α),[145] and monocyte chemotactic protein-1 (MCP-1)[146] have all been found to be elevated in association with SPTL of infectious aetiology.

There exists good evidence for the diagnostic effectiveness of umbilical cord blood, amniotic fluid and maternal plasma cytokine levels in predicting intra-uterine infections, SPTL and failure of tocolysis. The potential of other clinical samples such as cytokines in cervicovaginal secretions for the diagnosis of SPTL have been investigated in relatively fewer studies. The sensitivity and specificity of cytokine concentrations is greater than traditional tests such as histology, microbial culture and C-reactive protein levels.

FUTURE TRENDS

Early diagnosis and intervention

Clinical predictors of PTB are accurate only in the later stages of the pathological process when this has gathered momentum such that preventive measures may be ineffective (Fig. 2). By identifying changes using non-invasive tests, which are of no risk to the fetus, prior to the onset of clinical symptoms, it might be possible to introduce effective preventative measures. Maternal plasma and umbilical cord blood cytokine levels provide potential indicators of fetal compromise from samples obtained without any feto–maternal risk. Bedside strip testing for the detection of IL-6 has been developed; in the study by Trebeden et al.,[147] the strip test was twice as sensitive as reverse transcription-polymerase chain reaction (RT-PCR). RT-PCR is a sensitive technique available for detection of RNA, and the measure of RNA is used to detect the cytokine in question. Similar rapid bedside testing would be an important adjunct to the diagnosis of infection and, if available immediately, might permit early intervention.

The therapeutic potential of cytokines

IL-1 receptor antagonist has been shown to reduce IL-1 induced prostaglandin production by the fetal membranes.[148] Similarly, IL-4 has been shown to have an inhibitory effect on prostaglandin production by decreasing PGHS production in the amnion.[149] The use of anti-inflammatory cytokines to manipulate the physiologically protective mechanisms or defences may turn out to be the most effective method of preventing the onset of SPTL.

CONCLUSIONS

Cytokines through their interactions with MMP and prostaglandin play an essential role in the mechanisms of normal labour. As part of their role in the normal immune response to infection, it is possible that infection triggers release of cytokines, which leads to the cascade of myometrial contractions, substantive cervical changes and rupture of the fetal membranes which are an essential part of normal labour. To understand the relationship between abnormal genital tract flora, SPTL, PTB and neonatal tissue damage with long-term morbidity and mortality, it is essential to appreciate the role that cytokines play in the induction and modulation of immune responses and cellular changes, which result in these adverse outcomes.

ACKNOWLEDGEMENTS

We are grateful to Dr Andy Stagg of the Antigen Presentation Research Group at the Northwick Park Hospital for his help in the preparation of the manuscript. We are also grateful to the Clementine Churchill BMI Hospital which provides the salary for Dr Oliver.

References

1   Magowan BA, Bain M, Juszczak E *et al*. Neonatal mortality amongst Scottish preterm singleton births. Br J Obstet Gynaecol 1998; 105: 1005–1010
2   Woods NS, Marlow N, Costeloe K *et al*. Neurologic and developmental disability after extremely preterm birth. EPICURE Study Group. N Engl J Med 2000; 343: 378–384
3   Kierse M. New perspectives for the effective treatment of preterm labor. Am J Obstet Gynecol 1995; 173: 618–628
4   Petrou S. Economic consequences of preterm birth and low birthweight. Br J Obstet Gynaecol 2003; 110 (Suppl 20): 17–23
5   Lamont RF, Fisk NM. The role of infection in the pathogenesis of preterm labour. Prog Obstet Gynaecol 1993; 10: 135–158
6   Lettieri L, Vintzileos AM, Rodis JF *et al*. Does 'idiopathic' preterm labor resulting in preterm birth exist? Am J Obstet Gynecol 1993; 168: 1480–1485
7   Romero R, Gomez R, Mazor M *et al*. The preterm labor syndrome. In: Elder MG, Lamont RF, Romero R. (eds) Preterm Labor. New York: Churchill Livingstone, 1997; 29–49
8   Yoon BH, Romero R, Jun JK *et al*. Amniotic fluid cytokines (interleukin-6, tumor necrosis factor alpha, interleukin-1 beta and interleukin-8) and the risk for the development of bronchopulmonary dysplasia. Am J Obstet Gynecol 1997; 177: 825–830
9   Yoon BH, Romero R, Yang SH *et al*. Interleukin-6 concentrations in umbilical cord plasma are elevated in neonates with white matter lesions associated with periventricular leukomalacia. Am J Obstet Gynecol 1996; 174: 1433–1440
10 Yoon BH, Romero R, Park J *et al*. Fetal exposure to an intraamniotic inflammation and the development of cerebral palsy at the age of three years. Am J Obstet Gynecol 2000; 182: 675–681
11 Baggiolini M, Dewald B, Moser B. Human chemokines: an update. Annu Rev Immunol 1997; 15: 675–705

12 Le JM, Vilcek J. Interleukin 6: a multifunctional cytokine regulating immune reactions and the acute phase protein response. Lab Invest 1989; 61: 588–602

13 Tracey KJ, Ceremi A. Tumor necrosis factor: an updated review of its biology. Crit Care Med 1993; 21: S415–S422

14 Dinarello CA. Biological basis for interleukin-1 in disease. Blood 1996; 87: 2095–2147

15 Williams TM, Fox KR, Kant JA. Interleukin 2: basic biology and therapeutic use. Hematol Pathol 1991; 5: 45–55

16 Anderson R, MacDonald I, Corbett T et al. Construction and biological characterization of an interleukin 12 fusion protein (flexi 12): delivery to acute myeloid leukemic blasts using adeno associated virus. Hum Gene Ther 1997; 8: 1125–1135

17 Quesniaux VF. Interleukins 9, 10, 11 and 12 and kit ligand: a brief overview. Res Immunol 1992; 143: 385–400

18 Pacora P, Romero R, Maymon E et al. Participation of the novel cytokine interleukin-18 in the host response to intra-amniotic infection. Am J Obstet Gynecol 2000; 183: 1138–1123

19 Athayde N, Romero R, Maymon E et al. Interleukin-16 in pregnancy, parturition, rupture of fetal membranes, and microbial invasion of the amniotic cavity. Am J Obstet Gynecol 2000; 182: 135–141

20 Fortunato SJ, Menon R, Lombardi SJ. IL-15, a novel cytokine produced by human fetal membranes is elevated in preterm labour. Am J Reprod Immunol 1998; 39: 16–23

21 Sato TA, Keelan JA, Mitchell MD. Critical paracrine interactions between TNF-alpha and IL-10 regulate lipopolysaccharide-stimulated human choriodecidual cytokine and prostaglandin E$_2$ production. J Immunol 2003; 170: 158–166

22 Bry K, Hallman M. Transforming growth factor-beta opposes the stimulatory effect of interleukin-1 and tumor necrosis factor on amnion cell prostaglandin E2 production: implication for preterm labour. Am J Obstet Gynecol 1992; 167: 222–226

23 Bowen JM, Chamley L, Mitchell MD et al. Cytokines of the placenta and extra-placental membranes: Biosynthesis secretion and roles in establishment of pregnancy in women. Placenta 2002; 23: 239–256

24 Steinborn A, Von Gall C, Hildenbrand R et al. Identification of placental cytokine-producing cells in term and preterm labour. Am J Obstet Gynecol 1998; 91: 329–335

25 Romero R, Wu YK, Mazor M et al. Human deciduas: a source of interleukin-1. Obstet Gynecol 1989; 73: 31–34

26 Casey ML, Cox SM, Beutler B et al. Cachectin/tumor necrosis factor-± formation in human deciduas. Potential role of cytokines in infection-induced preterm labour. J Clin Invest 1989; 83: 430–436

27 Dudley DJ, Edwin SS, Van Wagoner J et al. Regulation of decidual cell chemokine production by group B streptococci and purified bacterial cell wall components. Am J Obstet Gynecol 1997; 177: 666–672

28 Padayachi T, Norman RJ, Moodley J et al. Mifepristone and induction of labour in second half of pregnancy. Lancet 1988; 1: 647

29 Wolf JP, Sinosich M, Anderson TL et al. Progesterone antagonist (RU 486) for cervical dilatation, labor induction, and delivery in monkeys: effectiveness in combination with oxytocin. Am J Obstet Gynecol 1989; 160: 45–47

30 Cabrol D, Bouvier D'Yvoire M, Mermet E et al. Induction of labour with mifepristone after intrauterine fetal death. Lancet 1985; 2: 1019

31 Molnar M, Romero R, Hertelendy F. Interleukin-1 and tumor necrosis factor stimulate arachidonic acid release and phospholipid metabolism in human myometrial cells. Am J Obstet Gynecol 1993; 169: 825–829

32 Gyr TN, Malek A, Mathez LF et al. Permeation of human chorioamniotic membranes by *Escherichia coli in vitro*. Am J Obstet Gynecol 1994; 170: 223–237

33 Duff P, Kopelman JN. Subclinical intra-amniotic infection in asymptomatic patients with refractory preterm labour. Obstet Gynecol 1987; 69: 756–759

34 Lamont RF, Rose M, Elder MG. Effect of bacterial products on prostaglandin E production by amnion cells. Lancet 1985; 2: 1331–1333

35 Lamont RF, Anthony F, Myatt L et al. Production of prostaglandin E$_2$ by human amnion *in vitro* in response to addition of media conditioned by microorganisms associated with chorioamnionitis and preterm labor. Am J Obstet Gynaecol 1990; 162: 819–825

36 Reisenberger K, Egarter C, Schiebel I et al. *In vitro* cytokine and prostaglandin production by amnion cells in the presence of bacteria. Am J Obstet Gynecol 1997; 176: 981–984

37 Gomez R, Ghezzi F, Romero R et al. Preterm labour and intra-amniotic infection. Clinical aspects and role of the cytokines in diagnosis and pathophysiology. Clin Preg 1995; 22: 281–342

38 Romero R, Salafia CM, Athanassiadis AP et al. The relationship between acute inflammatory lesions of the placenta and amniotic fluid microbiology. Am J Obstet Gynecol 1992; 166: 1382–1388

39 Rizzo G, Capponi A, Rinaldo D et al. Interleukin-6 concentrations in cervical secretions identify microbial invasion of the amniotic cavity in patients with preterm labour and intact membranes. Am J Obstet Gynecol 1996; 175: 812–817

40 Inglis SR, Jeremias J, Kuno K et al. Detection of tumor necrosis factor-alpha, interleukin-6 and fetal fibronectin in the lower genital tract during pregnancy: Relation to outcome. Am J Obstet Gynecol 1994; 171: 5–10

41 Wang P, Wu P, Siegel M et al. Interleukin (IL)-10 inhibits nuclear factor kappa-B (NF-kappa-B) activation in human monocytes: IL-10 and IL-4 suppress cytokine synthesis by different mechanisms. J Biol Chem 1995; 270: 9558–9563

42 Spencer S, Edwin SS, Mitchell MD et al. Interleukin-10 (IL-10) inhibits prostaglandin E_2 (PGE_2) and interleukin-6 production in human decidual cells: a potential role in preterm labour. J Invest Med 1995; 43: 186–191

43 Terrone DA, Rinehart BK, Granger JP et al. Interleukin-10 administration and bacterial endotoxin-induced preterm birth in a rat model. Obstet Gynecol 2001; 98: 476–480

44 Fortunato SJ, Menon R, Lombardi SJ et al. Interleukin-10 inhibition of gelatinases in fetal membranes: therapeutic implications in preterm premature rupture of membranes. Obstet Gynecol 2001; 98: 284–288

45 Keelan JA, Sato TA, Hansen WR et al. Interleukin-4 differentially regulates prostaglandin production in amnion-derived WISH cells stimulated with pro-inflammatory cytokines and epidermal growth factor. Prostaglandins Leukot Essent Fatty Acids 1999; 60: 255–262

46 Spanziani EP, Lantz ME, Benoit RR et al. The induction of cyclooxygenase-2 (COX-2) in intact human amnion tissue by interleukin-4. Prostaglandins 1996; 51: 215–223

47 Steinborn A, Kuhnert M, Halberstadt E. Immunmodulating cytokines induce term and preterm parturition. J Perinat Med 1996; 24: 381–390

48 Mitchell MD, Goodwin V, Mesnage S et al. Cytokine-induced coordinate expression of enzymes of prostaglandin biosynthesis and metabolism: 15-hydroxyprostaglandin dehydrogenase. Prostaglandins Leukot Essent Fatty Acids 2000; 62: 1–5

49 Mitchell MD, Dudley DJ, Edwin SS et al. Interleukin-6 stimulates prostaglandin production by human amnion and decidual cells. Eur J Pharmacol 1991; 192: 189–191

50 Witkin S, McGregor JA. Infection-induced activation of cell-mediated immunity: possible mechanism for preterm birth. Clin Obstet Gynecol 1991; 34: 112–121

51 Kimatrai M, Oliver C, Abadia-Molina AC et al. Contractile activity of human decidual stromal cells. J Clin Endocrin Metab 2003; 88: 844–849

52 Lechner W, Bergant A, Marth C et al. Effect of interleukin-6 on uterine contractility in the human *in vivo*. Z Geburtshilfe Neonatol 1998; 202: 10–13

53 Rauk PN, Friebe-Hoffman U, Winebrenner LD et al. Interleukin-6 up-regulates the oxytocin receptor in cultured uterine smooth muscle cells. Am J Reprod Immunol 2001; 45: 148–153

54 Gibb W. The role of prostaglandins in human parturition. Ann Med 1998; 30: 235–241

55 Kniss DA. Cyclooxygenases in reproductive medicine and biology. J Soc Gynecol Invest 1999; 6: 285–292

56 Bry K, Hallman M. Synergistic stimulation of amnion cell prostaglandin E_2 synthesis by interleukin-1, tumor necrosis factor and products from activated human granulocytes. Prostaglandins Leukot Essent Fatty Acids 1991; 44: 241–245

57 Romero R, Brody DT, Oyarzun E et al. Infection and labour, III: interleukin-1: a signal for the onset of parturition. Am J Obstet Gynecol 1989; 160: 1117–1123

58 Baggia S, Gravett MG, Witkin SS et al. Interleukin-1 beta intra-amniotic infusion induces tumor necrosis factor-alpha, prostaglandin production, and preterm contractions in pregnant rhesus monkeys. J Soc Gynecol Invest 1996; 3: 121–126

59 Ishihara O, Khan H, Sullivan MHF et al. Interleukin-1α stimulates decidual stromal cell

cyclo-oxygenase enzyme and prostaglandin production. Prostaglandin 1992; 44: 43–52

60 Bry K, Hallman M, Lappalainen U. Cytokines released by granulocytes and mononuclear cells stimulate amnion cell prostaglandin E_2 production. Prostaglandin 1994; 48: 389–399

61 Hansen WR, Sato T, Mitchell MD. Tumour necrosis factor-alpha stimulates increased expression of prostaglandin endoperoxide H synthase Type 2 mRNA in amnion-derived WISH cells. J Mol Endocrinol 1998; 20: 221–231

62 Ohno Y, Kasugai M, Kurauchi O et al. Effect of interleukin-2 on the production of progesterone and prostaglandin E_2 in human fetal membranes and its consequences for preterm uterine contractions. Eur J Endocrinol 1994; 130: 478–484

63 Coulam CH, Edwin SS, LaMarche S et al. Actions of interleukin-2 on amnion prostaglandin biosynthesis. Prostaglandins Leukot Essent Fatty Acids 1993; 49: 959–961

64 Osmann I, Young A, Ledingham MA et al. Leukocyte density and pro-inflammatory cytokine expression in human fetal membranes, deciduas, cervix, and myometrium before and during labor at term. Mol Hum Reprod 2003; 9: 41–45

65 Peltier MR. Immunobiology of term and preterm labor. Reprod Biol Endocrinol 2003; 1: 122

66 Lopez BA, Hansell DJ, Khong TY et al. Prostaglandin E production by the fetal membranes in unexplained preterm labour and preterm labour associated with chorioamnionitis. Br J Obstet Gynaecol 1989; 96: 1133–1139

67 Sennstrom MK, Brauner A, Lu Y et al. Interleukin-8 is a mediator of the final cervical ripening in humans. Eur J Obstet Gynecol Reprod Biol 1997; 74: 89–92

68 Chwalisz K, Benson M, Scholz P et al. Cervical ripening with the cytokines interleukin 8, interleukin 1 beta and tumor necrosis factor alpha in guinea-pigs. Hum Reprod 1994; 9: 2173–2181

69 Osmers RGW, Adelmann-Grill BC, Rath W et al. Biochemical events in cervical ripening dilatation during pregnancy and parturition. J Obstet Gynaecol 1995; 21: 185–194

70 Winkler M, Rath W, Fischer DC et al. Regulation of interleukin-8 synthesis in human lower uterine segment fibroblasts by cytokines and growth factors. Obstet Gynaecol 2000; 95: 584–588

71 Cherouny P, Pankuch G, Romero R et al. Neutrophil attractant/activating peptide-1/interleukin-8: association with histological chorioamnionitis, preterm delivery, and bioactive amniotic fluid leukoattractants. Am J Obstet Gynecol 1993; 169: 1299–1303

72 Maradny EE, Kanayama N, Halim A et al. Effects of neutrophil chemotactic factors on cervical ripening. Clin Exp Obstet Gynecol 1995; 22: 76–85

73 Ekman G, Granstrom L, Malmstrom A et al. Cervical fetal fibronectin correlates to cervical ripening. Acta Obstet Gynaecol Scand 1995; 74: 698–701

74 Mitchell MD, Branch DW, Lundin-Schiller S et al. Immunological aspects of preterm labour. Semin Perinatol 1991; 15: 210–224

75 Winkler M, Rath W. The role of cytokines in the induction of labour, cervical ripening and rupture of the fetal membranes. Z Geburtshilfe Perinatol 1996; 200: 1–12

76 Young A, Thomson AJ, Ledingham MA et al. Immunolocalization of proinflammatory cytokines in myometrium, cervix, and fetal membranes during human parturition at term. Biol Reprod 2002; 66: 445–449

77 McLaren J, Taylor DJ, Bell SC. Prostaglandin E_2-dependent production of latent matrix metalloproteinase-9 in cultures of human fetal membranes. Mol Hum Reprod 2000; 6: 1033–1040

78 Bryant-Greenwood GD, Millar LK. Human fetal membranes: their preterm premature rupture. Biol Reprod 2000; 63: 1575–1579

79 Draper D, McGregor J, Hall J et al. Elevated protease activities in human amnion and chorion correlate with preterm premature rupture of membranes. Am J Obstet Gynecol 1995; 173: 1506–1512

80 Katsura M, Ito A, Hirakawa S et al. Human recombinant interleukin-1 alpha increases biosynthesis of collagenase and hyaluronic acid in cultured human chorionic cells. FEBS Lett 1989; 244: 315–318

81 Fortunato SJ, Menon R. IL-1β is a better inducer of apoptosis in human fetal membranes than IL-6. Placenta 2003; 24: 922–928

82 Fortunato SJ, Menon R, Lombardi SJ. Amniochorion gelatinase-gelatinase inhibitor imbalance in vitro: a possible infectious pathway to rupture. Obstet Gynecol 2000; 95: 240–244

83 So T. The role of matrix metalloproteinases for premature rupture of the membranes. Acta Obstet Gynaecol Jpn 1993; 45: 227–233

84 Garcia-Lloret MI, Yui J, Winkler-Lowen B *et al*. Epidermal growth factor inhibits cytokine-induced apoptosis of primary human trophoblasts. J Cell Physiol 1996; 167: 324–332

85 Runic R, Lockwood CJ, LaChapelle L *et al*. Apoptosis and Fas expression in human fetal membranes. J Clin Endocrinol Metab 1998; 83: 660–666

86 Inglis SR, Jeremias J, Kuno K *et al*. Detection of tumor necrosis factor-alpha, interleukin-6 and fetal fibronectin in the lower genital tract during pregnancy: relationship to outcome. Am J Obstet Gynecol 1994; 171: 5–10

87 Keelan JA, Marvin KW, Sato TA *et al*. Cytokine abundance in placental tissues: evidence of inflammatory activation in gestational membranes with term and preterm parturition. Am J Obstet Gynaecol 1999; 181: 1530–1536

88 Wahbeh CJ, Hill GB, Eden RD *et al*. Intra-amniotic bacterial colonization in premature labour. Am J Obstet Gynecol 1984; 148: 739–743

89 Yoon BH, Romero R, Kim KS *et al*. A systemic fetal inflammatory response and the development of bronchopulmonary dysplasia. Am J Obstet Gynecol 1999; 181: 773–779

90 Yoon BH, Jun JK, Romero R *et al*. Amniotic fluid inflammatory cytokines (interleukin-6, interleukin-1beta, and tumor necrosis factor-alpha), neonatal brain white matter lesions, and cerebral palsy. Am J Obstet Gynecol 1997; 177: 19–26

91 Upham JW, Lee PT, Holt BJ *et al*. Development of interleukin-12 producing capacity throughout childhood. Infect Immun 2002; 70: 6583–6588

92 Goldenberg RL, Hauth JC, Andrews WW. Intrauterine infection and preterm delivery. N Engl J Med 2000; 342: 1500–1507

93 Eschenbach DA. Amniotic fluid infection and cerebral palsy. Focus on the fetus. JAMA 1997; 278: 247–248

94 Romero R, Gomez R, Ghezzi F *et al*. A fetal systemic inflammatory response is followed by the spontaneous onset of preterm parturition. Am J Obstet Gynecol 1998; 179: 186–193

95 Hitti J, Tarczy-Hornoch P, Murphy J *et al*. Amniotic fluid infection, cytokines, and adverse outcomes among infants at 34 weeks' gestation or less. Am J Obstet Gynecol 2001; 98: 1080–1088

96 Hitti J, Krohn MA, Patton DL *et al*. Amniotic fluid tumor necrosis factor-alpha and risk of respiratory distress syndrome among preterm infants. Am J Obstet Gynecol 1997; 177: 50–56

97 Lyon A. Chronic lung disease of prematurity. The role of intra-uterine infection. Eur J Pediatr 2000; 159: 798–802

98 Watterberg KL, Demers LM, Scott SM *et al*. Chorioamnionitis and early lung inflammation in infants in whom bronchopulmonary dysplasia develops. Pediatrics 1996; 97: 210–215

99 Ozdemir A, Brown MA, Morgan WJ. Markers and mediators of inflammation in neonatal lung disease. Pediatr Pulmonol 1997; 23: 292–306

100 Schmidt B, Cao L, Mackensen-Haen S *et al*. Chorioamnionitis and inflammation of the fetal lung. Am J Obstet Gynecol 2001; 185: 173–177

101 Moon JB, Kim JC, Yoon BH *et al*. Amniotic fluid matrix metalloproteinase-8 and the development of cerebral palsy. J Perinat Med 2002; 30: 301–306

102 Hagberg H, Wennerholm UB, Savman K. Sequelae of chorioamnionitis. Curr Opin Infect Dis 2002; 15: 301–306

103 Krageloh-Mann I, Petersen D, Hagberg G *et al*. Bilateral spastic cerebral palsy: MRI pathology and origin. Analysis from a representative series of 56 cases. Dev Med Child Neurol 1995; 37: 379–397

104 Shalak LF, Laptook AR, Jafri HS *et al*. Clinical chorioamnionitis, elevated cytokines, and brain injury in term infants. Pediatrics 2002; 110: 673–680

105 Tauscher MK, Berg D, Brockmann M *et al*. Association of histologic chorioamnionitis, increased levels of cord blood cytokines, and intracerebral hemorrhage in preterm neonates. Biol Neonate 2003; 83: 166–170

106 Hay PE, Lamont RF, Taylor-Robinson D *et al*. Abnormal bacterial colonisation of the genital tract as a marker for subsequent preterm delivery and late miscarriage. BMJ 1994; 308: 295–298

107 Romero R, Chaiworapongsa T, Kuivaviemi H *et al*. Bacterial vaginosis, the inflammatory response and the risk of preterm birth: a role for genetic epidemiology in the prevention of preterm birth. Am J Obstet Gynecol 2004; 190: 1509–1519

108 Donders GG, Odds A, Vereecken A, Van Bulck B *et al.* Abnormal vaginal flora in the first trimester, but not full-blown bacterial vaginosis, is associated with preterm birth. Prenat Neonat Med 1998; 3: 588–593

109 Simhan HN, Caritis SN, Krohn MA *et al.* Elevated vaginal pH and neutrophils are associated strongly with early spontaneous preterm birth. Am J Obstet Gynecol 2003; 189: 1150–1154

110 Simhan HN, Caritis SN, Krohn MA *et al.* Decreased cervical pro-inflammatory cytokines permit subsequent upper genital tract infection during pregnancy. Am J Obstet Gynecol 2003; 189: 560–567

111 Goepfert AR, Goldenberg RL, Andrews WW *et al.* The preterm prediction study: association between cervical interleukin-6 concentration and spontaneous preterm birth. National Institute of Child Health and Human Development Maternal-Fetal Medicine Units Network. Am J Obstet Gynecol 2001; 184: 483–488

112 Amsel R, Totten P, Speigel CA *et al.* Non-specific vaginitis: diagnostic criteria and microbial and epidemiological associations. Am J Med 1983; 74: 14–22

113 Macones G, Parry S, Elkousy M *et al.* A polymorphism in the promoter region of TNF and bacterial vaginosis: preliminary evidence of gene-environmental interaction in the etiology of spontaneous preterm birth. Am J Obstet Gynecol 2004; 190: 1504–1508

114 Lamont RF. Infection in preterm labour. In: MacLean A, Regan L, Carrington D. (eds) Infection and Pregnancy. Proceedings of the 40th Study Group of the Royal College of Obstetricians and Gynaecologists. London: RCOG Press, 2001; 305–317

115 Lamont RF. Bacterial vaginosis. In: Critchley H, Thornton S, Bennett P. (eds) Preterm Birth. Proceedings of the 46th Study Group of the Royal College of Obstetricians and Gynaecologists. London: RCOG Press, 2004; 163–180

116 Ugwumadu A, Manyonda I, Reid F *et al.* Effect of early oral clindamycin on late miscarriage and preterm delivery in asymptomatic women with abnormal vaginal flora and bacterial vaginosis: a randomised controlled trial. Lancet 2003; 361: 983–988

117 Lamont RF, Duncan SLB, Mandal D *et al.* Intravaginal clindamycin cream to reduce preterm birth in women with abnormal genital tract flora. Obstet Gynecol 2003; 101: 516–522

118 Rosenstein IJ, Morgan DJ, Lamont RF *et al.* Effect of intravaginal clindamycin cream on pregnancy outcome and abnormal vaginal microbial flora of pregnant women. Infect Dis Obstet Gynecol 2000; 8: 158–165

119 Lamont RF. Antibiotics for the prevention of preterm birth. N Engl J Med 2000; 342: 581–583

120 Carey JC, Klebanoff MA, Hauth JC *et al.* Metronidazole to prevent preterm delivery in pregnant women with asymptomatic bacterial vaginosis. National Institute of Child Health and Human Development Maternal-Fetal Medicine Units Network. N Engl J Med 2000; 342: 534–540

121 Kenyon SL, Taylor DJ, Tarnow-Mordi W. Broad-spectrum antibiotics for spontaneous preterm labour: the oracle II randomised trial. ORACLE Collaboration Group. Lancet 2001; 357: 989–994

122 Bielecki M, Zdrodowska J, Bielecki DA *et al.* Maternal plasma and amniotic fluid interleukin-6 levels in imminent preterm labour. Ginekol Pol 2000; 71: 719–723

123 El-Bastawissi AY, William M, Riley DE *et al.* Amniotic fluid interleukin-6 and preterm delivery: a review. Am J Obstet Gynecol 2000; 95: 1056–1064

124 Romero R, Yoon BH, Mazor M *et al.* A comparative study of the diagnostic performance of amniotic fluid glucose, white blood cell count, interleukin-6, and gram stain in the detection of microbial invasion in patients with preterm premature rupture of membranes. Am J Obstet Gynecol 1993; 169: 839–851

125 Coultrip LL, Lien JM, Gomez R *et al.* The value of amniotic fluid interleukin-6 determination in patients with preterm labour and intact membranes in the detection of microbial invasion of the amniotic cavity. Am J Obstet Gynecol 1994; 171: 901–911

126 Tsuda A, Ikegami T, Hirano H *et al.* The relationship between amniotic fluid interleukin-6 concentration and histological evidence of chorioamnionitis. Acta Obstet Gynecol Scand 1998; 77: 515–520

127 Silver RM, Schwinzer B, McGregor JA. Interleukin-6 levels in amniotic fluid in normal and abnormal pregnancies: preeclampsia, small-for-gestational age fetus, and premature labour. Am J Obstet Gynecol 1993; 169: 1101–1105

128 Yoon BH, Romero R. The relationship among inflammatory lesions of the umbilical cord

(funisitis), umbilical cord plasma IL-6 concentration, Amniotic fluid infection and neonatal sepsis. Am J Obstet Gynecol 2000; 183: 1124–1129

129 Smulian JC, Vintzileos AM, Lai YL *et al.* Maternal chorioamnionitis and umbilical vein interleukin-6 levels for identifying early neonatal sepsis. J Matern Fetal Med 1999; 8: 88–94

130 Greci LS, Gilson GJ, Nevils B *et al.* Is amniotic fluid analysis the key to preterm labour? A model using interleukin-6 for predicting rapid delivery. Am J Obstet Gynecol 1998; 179: 172–178

131 Matsuda Y, Kouno S, Nakano H. The significance of interleukin-6 concentrations in cervicovaginal fluid: its relation to umbilical cord plasma and the influence of antibiotic treatment. J Perinatol Med 2000; 28: 129–132

132 Gucer F, Balkanli-Kaplan P, Yuksel M *et al.* Maternal serum tumor necrosis factor-alpha in patients with preterm labour. J Reprod Med 2001; 46: 232–236

133 Putz I, Lohbreyer M, Winkler M *et al.* Appearance of inflammatory cytokines interleukin-1 beta and interleukin-6 in amniotic fluid during labour and in intrauterine pathogen colonization. Z Geburtshilfe Neonatol 1998; 202: 14–18

134 Spear ML, Stefano JL, Fawcett P *et al.* Soluble interleukin-2 receptor as a predictor of neonatal sepsis. J Pediatr 1996; 128: 445–446

135 Lemancewicz A, Urban R, Urban J *et al.* Evaluation of interleukin concentrations in amniotic fluid in preterm and term parturition and in oligohydramnios. Med Sci Monit 2001; 7: 924–927

136 Dembinski J, Behrendt D, Heep A *et al.* Cell associated IL-8 in cord blood of term and preterm infants. Clin Diag Lab Immunol 2002; 9: 320–323

137 Puchner T, Egarter C, Wimmer C *et al.* Amniotic fluid interleukin-8 as a marker for intraamniotic infection. Arch Gynecol Obstet 1993; 253: 9–14

138 Rizzo G, Capponi A, Vlachopoulou A *et al.* Ultrasonographic assessment of the uterine cervix and interleukin-8 concentrations in cervical secretions predict intrauterine infection in patients with preterm labour and intact membranes. Ultrasound Obstet Gynecol 1998; 12: 86–92

139 Ghezzi F, Gomez R, Romero R *et al.* Elevated interleukin-8 concentrations in amniotic fluid of mothers whose neonates subsequently develop bronchopulmonary dysplasia. Eur J Obstet Gynecol Reprod Biol 1998; 78: 5–10

140 Albert JR, Naef 3rd RW, Perry Jr KG *et al.* Amniotic fluid interleukin-6 and interleukin-8 levels predict the success of tocolysis in patients with preterm labour. J Soc Gynecol Invest 1994; 1: 264–268

141 Dudley DJ, Hunter C, Mitchell MD *et al.* Amniotic fluid interleukin-10 (IL-10) concentrations during pregnancy and with labour. J Reprod Immunol 1997; 33: 147–156

142 Boggess KA, Greig PC, Murtha AP *et al.* Maternal serum granulocyte-colony stimulating factor in preterm birth with subclinical chorioamnionitis. J Reprod Immunol 1997; 33: 45–52

143 Athayde N, Romero R, Maymon E *et al.* A role for the novel cytokine RANTES in pregnancy and parturition. Am J Obstet Gynecol 1999; 181: 989–994

144 Ognjanovic S, Bryant-Greenwood GD. Pre-B-cell colony-enhancing factor, a novel cytokine of human fetal membranes. Am J Obstet Gynecol 2002; 187: 1051–1058

145 Dudley DJ, Hunter C, Mitchell MD *et al.* Elevations of amniotic fluid macrophage inflammatory protein-1α concentrations in women during term and preterm labour. Obstet Gynecol 1996; 87: 94–98

146 Jacobsson B, Holst RM, Wennerholm UB *et al.* Monocyte chemotactic protein-1 in cervical and amniotic fluid: relationship to microbial invasion of the amniotic cavity, intra-amniotic inflammation, and preterm delivery. Am J Obstet Gynecol 2003; 189: 1161–1167

147 Trebeden H, Goffinet F, Kayem G *et al.* Strip test for bedside detection of interleukin-6 in cervical secretions is predictive for impending preterm delivery. Eur Cytokine Netw 2001; 12: 359–360

148 Romero R, Sepulveda W, Mazor M *et al.* The natural interleukin-1 receptor antagonist in term and preterm parturition. Am J Obstet Gynecol 1992; 167: 863–872

149 Keelan JA, Sato TA, Hansen WR *et al.* Interleukin-4 differentially regulates prostaglandin production in amnion-derived WISH cells stimulated with pro-inflammatory cytokines and epidermal growth factor. Prostaglandins Leukot Essent Fatty Acids 1999; 60: 255–262

Diaa M. El-Mowafi

Management of breast cancer during pregnancy

Pregnancy and cancer result in two diametrically opposing emotional reactions in young women. The first leads usually to a joyous elation, whilst the other to dismay and horror. When the two occur together, the patient is inevitably distraught and terrified, whilst her obstetrician and medical advisers are faced with a therapeutic dilemma involving surgical, perinatal, obstetric, psychological and moral issues.

Breast cancer occurring during pregnancy or within the first year after delivery is considered to be pregnancy-associated breast cancer (PABC).[1] Some researchers have distinguished between malignancy occurring during pregnancy and during lactation. Because of the variability in the length of lactation, cancer occurring up to 1 year after delivery has been accepted as standard definition in most articles.[2,3]

Breast cancer is the most common cancer encountered in pregnant women occurring in about 1 in 3000 pregnancies. This incidence is expected to increase as more women choose child-bearing at a later age. It is estimated that the obstetrician attending 250 deliveries per year would need to accumulate 40 years of clinical experience to encounter 2–3 cases of PABC.[4] This may lead to erroneous perception that PABC is rare. If the probable latent or preclinical time period of breast cancer is considered, it becomes likely that larger numbers of women with breast cancer have been pregnant at sometime during the course of the disease, despite the fact that they do not meet the criteria for PABC. When women delay their first pregnancy until the age of 35 years or more, the risk of breast cancer increases 3-fold compared to those women who initially conceive prior to the age of 20 years.[5] Diagnosis and treatment of breast cancer during pregnancy encompasses many diagnostic and therapeutic dilemmas. The engorgement of the breasts in this period may hinder detection

Diaa M. El-Mowafi MD
Professor, Obstetrics and Gynecology Department, Benha Faculty of Medicine, Egypt; Educator and Researcher, Wayne State University, Detroit, Michigan USA; and Fellow of Geneva University, Switzerland; Consultant and Head of Obstetrics & Gynaecology Department, King Khalid General Hospital, Hafr El-Batin 31991, Saudi Arabia.(E-mail: dmowafi@yahoo.com)

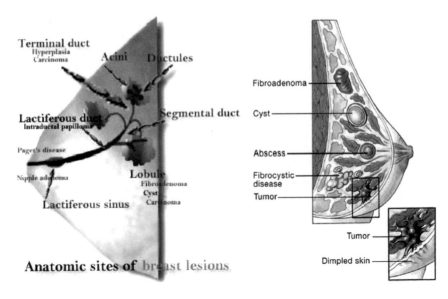

Fig. 1 Anatomical sites of breast lesions.

of masses and delays in diagnosis are common. This delay in addition to the young age can explain that overall survival of pregnant women generally worse than in non-pregnant women.[6] Mammography has a limited value in diagnosis due to increased breast density during pregnancy. Chemotherapy and radiotherapy are contra-indicated. Still, two questions have to be answered: (i) should pregnancy terminated when breast cancer is diagnosed? and (ii) if and when this lady can get pregnant again?

ANATOMY

The paired hemispheres of breast tissue are attached on their planoconcave surface against the fascia of the ventral chest wall from the parasternal to the anterior axillary line covering the second through the seventh ribs. The adult female breast has two components. These are the epithelial elements responsible for milk formation and transport, namely the acini and ducts, and the supporting tissues, muscle, fascia and fat. The epithelial elements consist of twenty or more lobes. Each lobe drains into a mammary duct, each of which ends separately at the nipple. The lobe consists of lobules, the number of which is very variable. Each lobule is a collection of between ten and hundred acini grouped around, and converging on a collecting duct (Fig. 1).

The breast is contained in a fascia envelope, its superficial layer being subcutaneous and its deep layer adjacent to the fascia of the chest wall muscles. Fascial septa separate each lactiferous lobe into a separate entity. These fascial partitions extend from the deep to the superficial fascial envelope. In the superior aspect of the breast, these fascial supports are thickest, presumably because of gravity traction, and are called Cooper's ligament.

The fat of the breast composes a significant proportion of the breast volume. It occurs as a 1–3 cm layer between the skin and the superficial fascia. The fatty tissue in the most dependent portion of the breast often becomes oedematous and indurated as a function of gravity and dependency. This indurated area is known as the inframammary ridge. Vascular supply is from the axillary vessels through the upper outer quadrants and through perforating internal mammary vessels via the parasternal and intercostal spaces.

The lymphatics of the breast drain mostly to the axilla and then medially along the axillary vein. Most of these lymphatics drain around and under the pectoral muscles, although some pathways do exist through and between the musculature (Rotter's nodes). The medial and centromedial areas of the breast contain lymphatics that course toward the sternum, perforate the intercostal spaces, and drain into the internal mammary chain inside the thorax. Lesser pathways of drainage include epigastric, supraclavicular, and anterior cervical lymphatics.

PHYSIOLOGICAL CHANGES IN THE BREAST DURING PREGNANCY

Pregnancy induces both proliferation and differentiation of the mammary epithelium. Both lobular and alveolar growth occur. Differentiation of the alveoli into mature milk-producing cells requires the stimulus of cortisol, insulin, and prolactin.[7] Prolactin is the major stimulus for galactopoiesis, and prolactin levels are markedly elevated during the later trimesters of pregnancy and lactation. The weight of the breasts approximately doubles with a 180% increase in blood flow. The increase in size, weight, vascularity, and density makes detection of mass lesions difficult both clinically and mammographically.

GENETIC FACTORS IN BREAST CANCER

The occurrence of breast cancer early in life, bilaterally or with tumours of other organs (particularly the ovary) suggests an underlying genetic susceptibility. In women with hereditary breast cancer, both mutated P53 and the BRCA1 gene have been identified. The BRCA1 gene, located on chromosomal region 17q12-q23, has previously been associated with early-onset breast cancer. This gene is estimated to account for about 45% of families with several cases of breast cancer and up to 67% of such families where the age at onset of the cancers is less than 45 years.[8] Almost all families with epithelial ovarian cancer in addition to several cases of breast cancer carry the BRCA1 gene.[9] However, it has to be said that only a small proportion of breast cancers (5%) are caused by dominant genes.[8]

DIFFERENTIAL DIAGNOSIS OF BREAST CARCINOMA

Benign lesions unique to pregnancy and lactation

Conditions that present as a dominant lump in the breast include carcinoma, fibrocystic disease, fibro-adenomas, sarcomas, fat necrosis, and other uncommon breast lesions. These include galactoceles, sebaceous cysts, histiocytomas, leiomyomas, lipomas, adenolipomas, granular cell tumours, neurofibromas, sarcoidosis, and tuberculosis (Fig. 1).

Although most of the benign lesions seen in pregnancy are the same as those seen in the non-gravid state (*e.g.* fibro-adenomas, lipomas, papillomas), they may be altered in size or consistency as well as histological appearance by the hormonal stimulation of pregnancy and lactation. About 30% of breast masses are lesions unique to pregnancy, such as lactating adenomas, galactoceles, mastitis, and infarcts.[10]

The lactating adenoma (nodular lactational hyperplasia or lactating nodule) is a benign breast lesion unique to pregnancy and lactation. Histologically, it is characterised by florid lactational changes with a tubulo-alveolar appearance to the glands. There is considerable variability in size.[11]

Infarction of a fibro-adenoma, lactating adenoma, or hypertrophied breast tissue can occur during pregnancy. The typical lesion presents with increase in size and tenderness of a pre-existing mass or as a new tender mass. Histological examination may reveal extensive necrosis with few or no residual glandular elements.[15]

Galactoceles are single or multiple nodules that contain retained milk. Anything that obstructs the ductal system during lactation may cause a galactocele. Most commonly, these lesions occur with the cessation of lactation when milk is allowed to stagnate in the ducts. The presentation may be delayed for months after the cessation of nursing. These palpable lesions are usually located peripherally in the breast. Sometimes, fluctuance is elicited upon palpation, and firm pressure on the mass may express milk. Aspiration can be both diagnostic and curative if the lesion does not recur. The findings on mammography are highly suggestive of this lesion owing to the mixed water and fat densities. Mammography is usually not necessary, as the clinical presentation is usually characteristic. Occasionally, a benign or malignant tumour is the cause of obstruction. Excision is advised if the lesion recurs after aspiration or if a mass persists.

Lactational mastitis may rarely progress to breast abscess. Although inflammatory carcinoma of the breast is no more common in PABC than in the non-gravid state, its incidence is high enough to recommend biopsy of the abscess wall when a breast abscess is drained.[12]

Bloody nipple discharge during pregnancy and lactation

Bloody nipple discharge is a relatively common occurrence during pregnancy and lactation. This finding *per se* does not necessarily portend serious consequences. Although bloody nipple discharge may occur with malignancy, it is usually associated with a palpable mass. Cytologically, bloody nipple secretions commonly demonstrate desquamated epithelial cells similar to those seen in intraductal papillomas. Pregnancy induces changes in the ducts, which lead to the formation of delicate intraductal epithelial spurs that are easily traumatised and shed, thus resulting in a bloody discharge.[12] Although cytological study of the bloody discharge is indicated, it may be difficult to interpret because the proliferative changes associated with pregnancy may confound the diagnosis of a malignant process.[14]

If a bloody discharge is not accompanied by a palpable mass and if the cytology is not suggestive of malignancy, it is appropriate to observe the patient clinically for several months postpartum. If the bloody discharge persists for more than 2 months after delivery, is localised to one duct, or is associated with a palpable mass, mammography and biopsy may be indicated. The presence of blood is not a contra-indication to breast-feeding. Bloody discharges may commonly be associated with the initiation of breast-feeding and usually cease after breast-feeding.[15]

CLINICAL PRESENTATION OF BREAST CANCER IN PREGNANCY

Carcinoma usually presents as a painless, firm, deep-seated mass. Of these masses, 90% are detected by self-breast examination.[15] Any breast mass warrants prompt attention, and every effort must be made to reduce the delay between signs, symptoms, and diagnosis in PABC. Local infiltration may cause fixation of the tumour to the chest wall. This is elicited by adduction of the arm to set the pectoralis muscle and fascia. Fixation or oedema of the skin are other signs of advancing malignancy, altered vascularity and increased metabolism of the tumour produce increased heat as measured by thermography or skin erythema after alcohol application. Although a thorough breast examination must be an integral part of the initial prenatal examination, this examination ideally should be performed prior to the development of physiological breast changes (Fig. 2). An enlarging mass that persists without regression and other primary or secondary signs malignancy such as nipple retraction, fixation of a mass to skin, skin thickening, dimpling, or development of axillary adenopathy should be considered indications of possible malignancy, and a diagnostic work-up should be initiated.

DELAY IN DIAGNOSIS OF BREAST CANCER IN PREGNANCY

Diagnosis of breast cancer in pregnancy is usually delayed 5–7 months due to physiological changes that take place with pregnancy.[17] This will lead to discovery of the breast cancer in a relatively advanced stage. The increased vascularity and lymphatic drainage from the gravid or lactating breast is

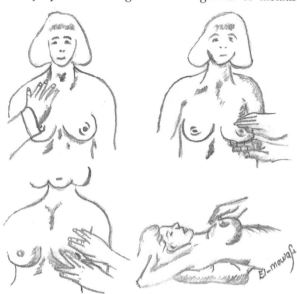

Fig. 2 Initial prenatal examination.

another factor that aids metastatic spread. Difficulty in evaluating the mass lesions in the pregnant and lactating breast, a reluctance to perform biopsy, false diagnosis as an inflammatory mass that fails to respond to treatment can be established, and inadequate flow up by patient and physician have all been reported. Physical examination may be difficult because the breasts are hypervascular, engorged, and nodular. A discreet mass is often difficult to palpate during lactation and malignancy may be mistaken with mastitis.

Over 75% of pregnant women diagnosed with breast cancer have nodal metastases, far more than the general population. Nettleton and colleagues[18] created a mathematical model to infer the risk of nodal metastases with PABC. If the tumour doubling time is assumed to be 65 days, a delay of 6 months in diagnosis raises the probability of nodal metastases by more than 10%.

TECHNIQUES OF EVALUATING BREAST LUMPS

Friction-free examination

The breast skin can be rendered friction free by the use of powder, thin lubricating jelly, or warm soap and water, thus improving an appreciation of breast structures by palpation. Subareolar prominences can be distinguished as a circular ring of uniform structures. The hot rinse after the soap and water examination serves two purposes. The soap is removed to avoid an itchy aftermath, and the hot compress effect tends to promote nipple discharge and will improve the yield of nipple discharge samples that can be tested for occult blood. Bloody or sticky yellow nipple secretions should be further evaluated.[19]

Mammography

The increase in size, vascularity and glandular density of the breasts during pregnancy is characterised by an increase in radiographic density, thus limiting the sensitivity of mammography. Mammography, therefore, should be used as a screening test during pregnancy or lactation. However, mammography should not be avoided, if indicated, because with abdominal shielding the radiation exposure to the fetus is negligible.[20] There are no reports of untoward effects of mammography on the mother and fetus.

Ultrasound may be a useful diagnostic modality, and several series have shown increased accuracy in confirming the presence of palpable masses in PABC.[3]

Ultrasonography accurately depicts the difference between solid and cystic masses and is being subjected to extensive trials of its accuracy in diagnosing early malignant disease in the breast. It is used as an adjunct to mammography since combinations of the two modalities have been shown in some reports to be better than either alone.[21] Calcification, asymmetric density, axillary lymphadenopathy, skin and trabecular thickening are helpful for diagnosis of PABC. Sonographic findings of a solid mass with posterior acoustic enhancement and a marked cystic component are somewhat different from the appearance of breast cancer in non-pregnant women, possibly because of the physiological changes of pregnancy and lactation.

Magnetic resonance imaging (MRI) is of great help to delineate the soft tissue lesions in the breast.

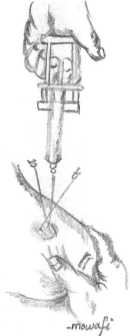

Fig. 3 Needle aspiration of the breast.

Aspiration cytology

Needle aspiration of the breast is a simple procedure. The mass or area of suspicion is held between two fingers of the left hand. Cutaneous spray with ethyl chloride until the skin is blanched provides adequate anaesthesia for this puncture. A 20-gauge needle attached to a 10-ml syringe is quickly thrust into the centre of the area. This syringe and needle are previously prepared by aspirating a small amount of Ringer's lactate into the dead space of the syringe and needle lumen. After insertion of the needle, vigorous suction is applied to the syringe while multiple small tracts are made in the breast tissue (Fig. 3).

Aspirated cyst fluid is spread thinly on an albumin-coated or a totally frosted slide, sprayed with cytological fixative and submitted as a Papanicolaou smear.

Thermography

Many thermographers have resorted to an innovation known as liquid crystal thermography, a type of brachthermometry, in the course of which the breasts are pressed directly against a thermosensitive plate lined with cholesteric crystals. The resulting thermographic film depicts the skin of the breast and contrasting colours that represent the underlining thermal pattern. The equipment with which this is accomplished is relatively less expensive and has been widely advertised for use in free-standing breast clinics and private offices. Although some authors recommended thermography as a helpful tool in diagnosis of breast cancer,[22] others have stated that it is seldom employed for that purpose.[23]

Breast biopsy

Complete evaluation of any lump in the breast requires an excisional biopsy and histological examination of the tissue. In women over the age of 50 years, any dominant breast lump is an indication for immediate excision. In younger patients, especially if menstruation is still occurring, re-examination should be scheduled after the next menstrual period and excision performed if the mass remains or becomes larger. Abnormal biopsy material should be submitted in ice for determination of oestrogen and progesterone-binding protein of the tumour.

DIAGNOSTIC WORK-UP IN WOMEN WITH A PALPABLE MASS

Masses discovered during routine examination or detected by the patient require evaluation. Significant physician delay has been noted in virtually all series of PABC. Mammography is of limited value. Ultrasound may be of help in differentiating cystic versus solid masses and may confirm the presence of a mass when physical examination is equivocal and the woman complains of pain or tenderness. The decision to observe the mass in the pregnant woman is fraught with danger as physical examination becomes progressively more difficult with increasing breast enlargement and vascularity as pregnancy progresses. A mass may seem to disappear when, in fact, it is enlarging and simply has become buried in the surrounding breast tissues. Since at least 25% of mammograms in pregnancy may be negative in the presence of cancer, a biopsy is essential for the diagnosis of any palpable mass. Diagnosis may be safely accomplished with a fine-needle aspiration or excisional biopsy under local anaesthesia. Fine-needle aspiration cytology is the initial procedure of choice for evaluating breast masses detected during pregnancy and lactation. The cytopathologist must be informed that the patient is pregnant or lactating because the physiological changes of pregnancy and lactation induce proliferation in the normal breast that can be confused with malignant change. Fine-needle aspiration cytology is useful in distinguishing benign breast masses of pregnancy from those with marked cytological atypia requiring surgical biopsy and minimise the delay in diagnosis of carcinoma associated with pregnancy.[24]

Although breast biopsy is one of the most common surgical procedures performed during pregnancy, it is reserved for masses in which fine-needle aspiration cytology is non-diagnostic. Because most breast masses associated with pregnancy and lactation are benign and with the more extensive use of fine-needle aspiration cytology, the number of open breast biopsies performed during pregnancy will be small. Breast biopsy may be performed under local or general anaesthesia. Procedures using local anaesthesia are usually without risk to the fetus.

The nursing mother should be advised to stop breast-feeding and to allow milk production to cease prior to biopsy. The cessation of lactation will decrease the risk of milk fistula and vascularity of the breast. Milk fistulas are more likely to occur when central lesions are excised. If milk fistula occurs, meticulous attention to local cleanliness and dressing changes is important to decrease the incidence of secondary infection and possible abscess formation. The fistula will generally close spontaneously when breast-feeding is stopped. The development of breast infection with or without an abscess following biopsy is more common in lactating women because of the nutrient value of the milk.

Although inflammatory breast carcinoma is not more common in PABC than in the general population with breast cancer, an incidence of 1.4%–4% has been reported.[12] For this reason, all abscesses that are surgically drained should have a biopsy of the wall and any suspicious area.

If the patient insists on continuing breast-feeding, she must be informed of the risks of milk fistula and the increased incidence of postoperative infection and abscess. The breast-feeding woman should express as much milk as possible prior to surgery.

PATHOLOGY OF BREAST CANCER

Carcinoma of the breast is either spheroidal cell or adenocarcinoma.[25]

Spheroidal cell carcinoma

Spheroidal cell carcinoma (90% of cases) consists of groups of spheroidal cells embedded in a fibrous stroma.

Atrophic scirrhous carcinoma

The amount of fibrous tissue exceeds much the number of cells. It grows slowly, affecting postmenopausal women with atrophic breasts. The tumour is small and very hard.

Scirrhous carcinoma

This is the commonest variety (65%), affecting middle-aged females. The tumour is small, hard, and fixed. When cut with a knife, a gritty sensation is felt, it retracts when cut and the cut surface becomes concave. The tumour is greyish in colour with areas of degeneration, necrosis and haemorrhage. It has no capsule and infiltrates surrounding structures.

Encephaloid carcinoma

This occurs in well-developed breasts in young females. It may reach a large size, grows rapidly and disseminates early. The cut section is brain-like with areas of haemorrhage and necrosis. Histologically, it appears as masses of highly malignant cells with minimal delicate vascular stroma.

Mastitis carcinomatosa

This occurs during pregnancy and lactation. The breast becomes swollen and painful with dilated veins, with red hot oedematous skin; the picture is similar to acute mastitis. Differentiation can be by clinical test using antibiotics. Histologically, it is a rapidly proliferating anaplastic cell with very little fibrous tissue stroma.

Adenocarcinoma

Duct carcinoma

Duct carcinoma arises in the larger milk ducts either on top of duct papilloma or *de novo*. It occurs in elderly females and spreads less rapidly than spheroidal cell carcinoma.

Intracystic papilliferous carcinoma
Intracystic papilliferous carcinoma is rare.

Paget's disease of the nipple

This is rare, affecting middle-aged and elderly females. It is a malignant eczema eroding the nipple and spreading peripherally. It is usually followed after 2 years by the appearance of scirrhous carcinoma within the breast. Histologically, there is hyperplasia of all layers of epidermis with the appearance of vacuolated Paget cells among the basal cells.

STAGING SYSTEM FOR BREAST CANCER

The staging system for breast cancer is summarised in Table 1.

TERMINATION OF PREGNANCY AND BREAST CANCER

Hormonal factors appear to play an important role early in the development of breast cancer; however, pregnancy itself does not appear to influence the outcome of an established breast cancer.[17]

Through the 1950s and 1960s, concerns regarding hormonal stimulation of tumour growth, poor survival, and the lack of effective systemic therapy for breast cancer led many clinicians to advocate therapeutic abortions when breast cancer was diagnosed during pregnancy. Subsequent series demonstrated that therapeutic abortion not only failed to improve survival but might be detrimental.[16,26] The finding of a high percentage of oestrogen receptor (ER)- and progesterone receptor (PR)-negative tumours in most series of PABC give little theoretical grounds for pregnancy termination. Most series of PABC reporting on receptor status indicate that as many as 80% of lesions are ER- and PR-negative.[3] Studying histopathological parameters and immunoreactivity of the oestrogen and progesterone receptors, c-erbB-2 and c-erbB-4 showed low frequency of hormone receptors, BRCA1, p27, cyclin E, D1 and high expression of c-erbB-2.[25,26] These findings gave the impression that PABC is an aggressive tumour.

The sole advantage of pregnancy termination is that full and complete treatment of aggressive or advanced disease with chemotherapy, radiotherapy, and surgery may be instituted without consideration of the effects on the fetus.

It is difficult to interpret some of the data indicating a worse prognosis associated with pregnancy termination because there may be considerable selection bias (abortions were performed only in women with more advanced or more aggressive tumours).[29]

The medical recommendation to terminate a pregnancy should be based on whether pregnancy will present a significant obstacle to effective therapy and whether the fetus will sustain harm as a result of therapy. Because pregnancy has no effect upon the course of disease, the termination of pregnancy does not ameliorate disease. Spontaneous abortions and prematurity are not increased in pregnant women with malignancy. As chemotherapy can not be given before 14–15 weeks of pregnancy, therapeutic abortions may be considered in

Table 1 The staging system for breast cancer

T		Primary tumour measurement
T0		No tumour
TIS		Pre-invasive carcinoma (CIS), non-infiltrating intraductal carcinoma or Paget's disease of nipple and no demonstrable tumour
T1		Tumour size 2 cm
	T1a	No fixation to pectoral fascia and/or muscle
	T1b	Fixation to pectoralis fascia and/or muscle
T2		Tumour size 2–5 cm
	T2a	No fixation to pectoralis fascia and/or muscle
	T2b	Fixation to pectoralis fascia and/or muscle
T3		Tumour size more than 5 cm
	T3a	No fixation to pectoralis fascia and/or muscle
	T3b	Fixation to pectoralis fascia and/or muscle
T4		Tumour of any size with direct extension to chest wall or skin (not including skin dimpling or nipple retraction)
	T4a	Fixation to chest wall
	T4b	Oedema, infiltration or ulceration of the skin (including peau d'orange), or satellite nodules confined to the same breast
	T4c	Both (T4a and T4b)
N		Regional lymph nodes
N0		No palpable homolateral axillary nodes
N1		Movable homolateral axillary nodes
	N1a	Metastasis not suspected
	N1b	Metastasis suspected
N2		Fixed homolateral axillary nodes
N3		Homolateral supraclavicular or infraclavicular nodes or oedema of the arm
M		Distant metastases
M0		No evidence of distant metastasis
M1		Distant metastases present, including skin involvement beyond the breast area

Stage-grouping

TIS Carcinoma *in situ*

Invasive carcinoma

Stage I	T1a, N0	or N1a	M0
	T1b, N0	or N1a	M0
Stage II	T0, N1b		
	T1a, N1b		
	T1b, N1b		
	T2a, N0	or N1a	M0
	T2b, N0	or N1a	
	T2a, N1b		
	T2b, N1b		
Stage III	Any T3	with any N	
	Any T4	with any N	M0
	Any T	with N2	
	Any T	with N3	
Stage IV	Any T,	any N	with M1

the first or second trimester so that metastatic disease can be treated promptly, particularly if the patient is ER-positive.[30]

TREATMENT OF PREGNANCY-ASSOCIATED BREAST CANCER

Perhaps no aspect of breast cancer care is more challenging than the treatment of the pregnant patient. In addition to the usual complexities of treatment decisions, one must add the incalculable factors related to the importance of child-bearing, and the potential for side effects upon the fetus or child through exposure to chemotherapy or radiotherapy. It is very difficult to make general comments about treating such patients. Each individual will weigh the potential risks and benefits differently, and may reach different decisions. Patients are invariably best served by multimodality team approaches, with co-ordinated efforts of surgeons, medical oncologists, and obstetricians trained in high-risk maternal–fetal medicine.

Breast conservation requires radiation therapy. Generally, this is not administered during pregnancy because of the potential for radiation exposure to the fetus. Surgery can usually be performed safely during pregnancy with minimal risk to the fetus and mother, particularly in the second and third trimesters. When compared with radiation therapy and chemotherapy, surgery is least likely to affect the pregnancy. Thus the usual treatment for technically operable breast cancer is modified radical mastectomy. This operation entails the preservation of the pectoralis major and minor muscles, providing better arm motion and thoracic outline and reducing the incidence of postoperative lymphoedema of the arm. It is probably the procedure most frequently used today for breast cancer.[20] Following modified radical mastectomy, radiotherapy to the chest wall, internal mammary lymph nodes, and the dissected axilla was customary for patients whose final pathological report indicated the presence of lymph node metastases. This approach has been superseded because radiotherapy has not been effective in controlling lymph node metastases or hematogeneous spread. Staging studies are performed selectively, and an individualised decision regarding subsequent chemotherapy is made. Women with advanced or technically inoperable disease may require palliative chemotherapy or radiotherapy.

In general, the metastatic work-up should be limited to those patients in whom there is a high clinical suspicion of metastatic disease and in whom documentation of disease would alter management. The fetal radiation exposure from a chest radiograph obtaining with abdominal shielding is minimal. The alkaline phosphatase level is normally elevated during pregnancy and is, therefore, an unreliable indicator of metastatic disease. Ultrasound of the lever is preferable to CT scanning. MRI may be indicated if ultrasound is non-diagnostic. Radiography of the long bones and skull can be performed in a symptomatic woman, but a complete skeletal survey exposes the fetus to an unnecessary large dose of radiation. A general bone scan is avoided because of low yield. However, if bony metastases are strongly suspected, a bone scan with [99m]technetium is preferable to a skeletal survey. Because this agent was used for placental scanning before the availability of ultrasound, there is a sufficient experience with its use in the second and third trimesters. Adequate hydration prior to and during the scan facilitates rapid washout of the isotope from the blood. Draining the bladder with a Foley catheter during the procedure and for 8–12 h after the scan avoids an accumulation of the isotope within the pelvis.[31]

RADIOTHERAPY OF BREAST CANCER

In general, radiation therapy is contra-indicated during pregnancy. An external irradiation dose of 5000 cGy to the breast exposes the fetus to at least 10–15 cGy. The part of the fetus located immediately below the diaphragm late in pregnancy is exposed to several hundred centigrays.[32] Because much of this dose comes from internal scatter of radiation within the body of the mother, abdominal shielding is only partially effective. The fetal dose depends on the total dose administered, the distance from the fetus to the field source, the field size, and the energy source. The fetal dose varies and must be calculated for each case. A general guideline is to limit the total fetal dose to 5 cGy.[33] Radiation therapy is rarely used if other alternatives exist.

BREAST-CONSERVING SURGERY DURING PREGNANCY

Because breast-conserving surgery (lumpectomy or quadrantectomy) generally employs postoperative radiotherapy, this modality is discouraged. Although this surgery can be performed during pregnancy, the radiation therapy required to complete local therapy for the breast must be delayed until after delivery. This is most suitable when PABC is diagnosed during the late third trimester.[34]

It has been suggested that delays of as much as 8 weeks from diagnosis to definitive therapy may allow safe delivery of the infant.[35] However, delaying radiation therapy may result in an increased incidence of local failure. Evidence suggests that selected patients who undergo breast-conservation therapy may benefit from chemotherapy prior to radiation therapy.[36] Based on that, it is prudent to limit breast-conserving therapy to those women who desire breast preservation, are otherwise suitable candidates, and are diagnosed late in pregnancy.

Mitchell[22] described the operation to be done by placing self-retaining retractor in the wound and grasping the tissue immediately overlying the lesion with an Allis clamp or tooth forceps. Minor bleeding, which can obscure the field, must be controlled at each step by cautery. Although it is possible to perform the operation alone, an assistant is very helpful in keeping the field clear and providing countertraction. Maintaining traction on the tissue to be resected, the surgeon enucleates it with small, curved scissors.

Blunt dissection is of little help, since there are no well-defined tissue planes. Frequent pauses are necessary to evaluate the scope of the dissection and to avoid cutting into the lesion or removing too much normal lobular tissue. The instrument elevating the lesion is shifted around its periphery as the dissection progresses to provide better exposure of the underside.

After removal of the tumour, the defect is closed with fine absorbable suture material, taking care that these sutures do not cause retraction or dimpling of the overlying skin. Some surgeons prefer to drain the area. All bleeding must be controlled before closure. When there is a large residual defect, as after segmental resection, a plastic type of closure for a satisfactory cosmetic result, and suction drainage may be used to avoid the postoperative accumulation of fluid. The skin is closed with either subcuticular stitch of fine absorbable suture material or interrupted 5/0 nylon. A pressure dressing for the first 24 h is desirable but may not be necessary in relatively minor cases. The sutures should be removed in not more than 6 days to prevent scarring, and steristrips are applied as necessary.

When a bloody nipple discharge suggests the likelihood of an intraductal papilloma, sharp dissection is carried medially from a circumareolar incision placed in the breast quadrant that pressure tests have indicated in most likely to be the source of bleeding. Directly beneath the nipple, the main ducts are encountered and placed on traction with a small hook. The ducts are followed downward until the lesion is found, usually not more than 3–4 cm from the surface.

Papillomas are dark red and soft and may be multiple. Generous portion of the duct system around the diseased area is resected and the severed ends are ligated. Usually there is a relatively small defect that need not be closed, and care must be taken not to cause retraction of the nipple by suturing. Inverting the nipple and scraping all ductal tissue from the under surface has been advocated but seems unnecessary in most cases.

CHEMOTHERAPY

Generally speaking, all chemotherapeutic agents are theoretically teratogenic and mutagenic. Their use may result in fetal growth restriction, fetal malformation, spontaneous abortion, or fetal death. It is important to differentiate teratogenic and mutagenic effects from those related to a suboptimal uterine environment or to maternal toxicity, such as neutropaenia, infection, thrombocytopaenia, or myocardial toxicity. Chemotherapy should be given only after 14–15 weeks' gestational age. The first trimester is the most critical time period with respect to exposure to chemotherapy. The blastocyst is resistant to teratogens in the first 2 weeks of life. If it is not destroyed, a surviving blastocyst exposed during the first 2 weeks will not manifest any abnormalities from a chemotherapeutic agent. The third to the eighth week of development, 5–10 weeks' gestational age, is the period of maximal susceptibility to teratogenic agents. With the exception of brain and gonadal tissue, organogenesis is complete by 13 weeks' gestation.

If chemotherapy induces severe damage early in gestation, spontaneous abortion results. If, however, sublethal damage occur between the second and the tenth week of gestation, teratogenesis may occur. After organogenesis is complete, the risk for birth defects induced by chemotherapy is decreased, and intra-uterine growth restriction becomes the dominant effect. About 10–20% of infants exposed to cytotoxic agents during the first trimester have major malformations as compared with a rate of 3% in the general population. The underlying rates of spontaneous abortion and birth defects in the general population are large enough to confound the data from small series. In general, chemotherapy should be delayed whenever possible until after the first trimester.

Most series of PABC that report the ER and PR status indicate that as many as 80% of patients are ER- and PR-negative.[3] During the first trimester, the combination of cyclophosphamide, methotrexate and 5-fluorouracil (CMF) should not be used owing to the toxicity of folate antagonists. If chemotherapy must be administered during the first trimester, the combination of cyclophosphamide, doxorubicin (Adriamycin), and 5-fluorouracil (CAF) should be considered. CMF can be used safely during the second and third trimesters.[34]

Chemotherapy is contra-indicated in lactating women as many chemo-therapeutic agents including cyclophosphamide, doxorubicin, methotrexate, hydroxyurea, and cisplatin are secreted in breast milk. Otherwise, breast-feeding should be stopped before initiating the chemotherapy. All other modalities of treatment are available during lactation. If surgery is planned, breast-feeding should be stopped to reduce size and vascularity.

ANTI-OESTROGEN AND OOPHORECTOMY

Tamoxifen has been considered inappropriate due to concerns over possible teratogenesis and lack of efficacy. In a case report, Isaacs et al.[37] reported that the use of tamoxifen in pregnancy is complex, but is not necessarily associated with fetal harm and may be considered a therapeutic option in selected cases. Theoretically, advanced disease may be helped by oophorectomy; however, as this is not proven and if the patient is still in the child-bearing period, hormonal manipulation by anti-oestrogens is more practical depending on receptor status of the tumour.

GENERAL TREATMENT PLAN

Generally speaking, the treatment is individualised according to the circumstances of each case including: (i) the gestational age at which the cancer was discovered; (ii) surgical staging; (iii) the pathology of the tumour; (iv) hormonal receptor status; (v) involvement of lymph nodes; and (vi) the number of children the lady has. Stages I and II are operable and are treated by modified radical mastectomy with or without postoperative irradiation, hormone therapy or chemotherapy. Stages III and IV are inoperable and are treated by simple mastectomy as palliative measure for pain and fungation followed by palliative chemotherapy, hormone therapy or irradiation.

First and second trimester

Termination of pregnancy could be the choice to allow a free hand in dealing with the cancer, especially in late stages and positive lymph nodes sampling. Those cases will need postoperative radiation and/or chemotherapy. Both are contra-indicated in that period of pregnancy.

Third trimester

Surgical treatment should be applied without delay; pregnancy should be terminated once the fetal maturity allows. Postpartum radiotherapy and chemotherapy can be given with prevention of lactation in case of chemotherapy.

METASTASIS OF BREAST CANCER TO CONCEPTION

Metastatic spread to the placenta has been reported but is extremely rare.[38] Placental metastasis has generally been reported in association with wide-spread metastatic disease. Spread to the fetus has never been reported, although such spread has been reported for melanoma, haematopoietic malignancies, hepatoma, and choriocarcinoma. Careful histological examination of the placenta is required even if the placenta is grossly normal. The fear that breast cancer may spread to the fetus is a major concern of patients.

PROGNOSIS

Breast cancer is generally believed to carry a worse prognosis during pregnancy because of the potential adverse effects of anticancer treatment on the fetus and of pregnancy-related hormonal and immunological modifications on the disease.[38] Also, most studies indicate that PABC tends to be more advanced at initial presentation because pregnancy-related changes in the breasts obscure clinical and radiological manifestations. Actually, breast cancer has equivalent prognosis in pregnant and non-pregnant women when matched by age and stage at diagnosis at the same institution during the same time period.[3,4,35,39]

DOES PREGNANCY PROTECT FROM BREAST CANCER?

Interruption of the first pregnancy will remove the protective effect of that first full-term pregnancy and subject the woman to a small, but real, increased risk of developing breast cancer in the future compared to the risk she would have if she carried the pregnancy. According to the US National Cancer Institute, there is an overall 50% increase in the subsequent risk of breast cancer following an induced abortion. If a woman has a mother, sister, aunt or grandmother with breast cancer, she will increase her chance of getting breast cancer by 80%, if she is under 18 years, she will double her chance of getting breast cancer, and if both conditions pertain, her risk is much higher.[40]

PREGNANCY AFTER TREATMENT

Chemotherapeutic agents significantly affect subsequent fertility. The risk of premature ovarian failure induced by chemotherapy can be estimated from the women's age, the agent used, and the total dose.[41] Alkylating agents such as cyclophosphamide cause amenorrhoea through direct ovarian depression. The severity of the depression seems to be a function of the number and activity of the follicles present at the initiation of the chemotherapy. Prepubertal ovaries, not yet under cyclic hormonal control, seem protected against destruction from chemotherapy. The younger the patient, the larger the reserve of oocytes that can be recruited after chemotherapy. Although cyclophosphamide is a major cause of ovarian failure, methotrexate and 5-fluorouracil are not. About 50% of women less than 35 years of age resume menses after a full course of adjuvant chemotherapy.

As a general rule, cancer identified prior to conception should be adequately treated with appropriate follow-up before pregnancy is attempted. Once successfully treated, few malignant diseases absolutely preclude future pregnancy. There are no prospective studies evaluating the effects of subsequent pregnancy on breast cancer. Although most recurrences are seen within 2 years, many women have later recurrences. No studies have shown an adverse effect of subsequent pregnancy even in patients with positive axillary nodes and in those in whom the pregnancy occurs earlier than 2 years after treatment.[37] Several studies have suggested that women who become pregnant after treatment for breast cancer demonstrate a trend toward improved prognosis when compared with women not subsequently pregnant.[42,43] Abortion does not improve survival, and termination of pregnancy is considered only in women with recurrent disease. It is recommended that patients wait two or three years after diagnosis before attempting to conceive.

SUMMARY

Breast cancer is the most common cancer in pregnant and postpartum women, occurring in about 1 in 3000 pregnancies. The average patient is between 32–38 years of age and, with many women choosing to delay child-bearing, it is likely that the incidence of breast cancer during pregnancy will increase. There is no evidence to implicate pregnancy or lactation in either the aetiology or the progression of breast cancer. The increase in size, weight, vascularity, and density of the breasts in pregnancy hinder the early detection of the breast masses either clinically or by mammography. Most of the benign lesions seen in pregnancy are the same ones in the non-gravid state. Most of pregnancy associated breast cancer (PABC) present as painless masses, and as many as 90% of these masses are detected by breast self-examination. Women with PABC generally have more advanced disease with larger tumours, a higher percentage of inoperable lesions, and a higher percentage of nodal involvement. As most PABC presents with a palpable mass, the role of imaging modalities in the evaluation of these patients remains limited. Fine-needle aspiration cytology is the initial procedure of choice for evaluating breast masses during pregnancy and lactation. Induction of abortion does not improve survival. Operable disease in the first 6–7 months of pregnancy should be treated by modified radical mastectomy, as irradiation is contra-indicated. Late in pregnancy, a lumpectomy and axillary dissection can be done, with irradiation being delayed until after delivery. General anaesthesia is safe if the usual precautions are taken to compensate for the physiological changes induced by pregnancy. Adjuvant chemotherapy can be considered in the second and third trimesters but is better delayed until after delivery. In patients with locally advanced or metastatic cancer diagnosed early in pregnancy, for whom both chemotherapy and radiation therapy would be indicated, consideration must be given to termination of pregnancy. Unfortunately, delay in diagnosis is common and 70–89% of patients with operable primary lesions have positive axillary lymph nodes. Late stage appears to be the only reason for the generally worse prognosis in these patients as, stage for stage, they have a course similar to that of non-pregnant patients. No studies have shown an adverse effect of a subsequent pregnancy even in patients with positive axillary nodes and patients get pregnant earlier than 2 years after treatment. In spite of that, it is advised to postpone pregnancy for 2 years to allow proper diagnosis and management of recurrences. In addition, recurrences may influence the decision to be a mother.

References

1 Rugo H. Management of breast cancer diagnosed during pregnancy. Curr Treat Options Oncol 2003; 4: 165–173

2 Hoover H. Breast cancer during pregnancy and lactation. Surg Clin North Am 1990; 70: 1151–1163

3 Petrek J. Pregnancy-associated breast cancer. Semin Surg Oncol 1991; 7: 306–310

4 Marchant D. Breast cancer in pregnancy. Clin Obstet Gynecol 1994; 37: 993–997

5 Shepherd J. Cancer in pregnancy. Prog Obstet Gynaecol 1996; 12: 219–234

6 Mignot L. Cancer of the breast and pregnancy: the point of view of the breast cancer specialist. Bull Cancer 2002; 89: 772–778

7 Danforth Jr DN. How subsequent pregnancy affects outcome in women with a prior breast cancer. Oncology 1991; 5: 23–30

8 Evans D, Fentiman I, McPherson K, Asbury D, Ponder B, Howell A. Familial breast cancer. BMJ 1994; 308: 183–187

9 Narod S, Feunteum J, Lynch H. Familial breast-ovarian cancer locus on chromosome 17q12-q23. Lancet 1991; 338: 82–83

10 Sorosky J, Scott-Conner C. Breast disease complicating pregnancy. Obstet Gynecol Clin North Am 1998; 25: 353–363

11 Slavin J, Billson V, Oster A. Nodular breast lesions during pregnancy and lactation. Histopathology 1993; 22: 481–485

12 Olsen C, Gordon Jr R. Breast disorders in nursing mothers. Am Fam Physician 1990; 41: 1509–1516

13 Kline T, Lash S. The bleeding nipple of pregnancy and postpartum. Acta Cytol (Phila) 1984; 8: 336–340

14 Healy C, Dijkstra B, Kelly L, McDermott E, Hill A, O'Higgins N. Pregnancy-associated breast cancer. Ir Med J 2002; 95: 51–54

15 Dequanter D, Hertens D, Veys I, Nogaret J. Breast cancer and pregnancy. Review of the literature. Gynecol Obstet Fertil 2001; 29: 9–14

16 Keleher A, Theriault R, Gwyn K et al. Multidisciplinary management of breast cancer concurrent with pregnancy. J Am Coll Surg 2002; 194: 54–64

17 Moore H, Foster Jr R. Breast cancer and pregnancy. Semin Oncol 2000; 27: 646–653

18 Nettleton J, Long J, Kuban D. Breast cancer during pregnancy: quantifying the risk of treatment delay. Obstet Gynecol 1996; 87: 414–418

19 Chaudary M. Nipple discharge: the diagnostic value of testing for occult blood. Ann Surg 1982; 196: 651–658

20 Gwyn K, Theriault R. Breast cancer with pregnancy. Oncology 2001; 15: 39–46

21 Ahn B, Kim HH, Moon W et al. Pregnancy- and lactation-associated breast cancer: mammographic and sonographic findings. J Ultrasound Med 2003; 22: 491–497

22 Mitchell G. Benign and malignant diseases of the breast. In: Thompson J, Rock J. (eds) Te Linde's Operative Gynecology. J.B. Lippincott, 1993; 979–999

23 Shirley R. The breast. In: Ryan K, Berkowitz R, Barbieri R. (eds) Kistner's Gynecology, Principles and Practice. Year Book Medical Publisher, 1999; 305–319

24 Novotony D, Maygardin S, Shermer R. Fine-needle aspiration of benign and malignant breast masses associated with pregnancy. Acta Cytol 1991; 35: 676–686

25 Preece P. The breast. In: Cuschieri et al. (eds) Essential Surgical Practice. London: Wright, 1982; 811

26 Espie M, Cuvier C. Treating breast cancer during pregnancy. What can be taken safely? Drug Safety 1998; 18: 135–142

27 Reed W, Hannisdal E, Skovlund E, Thoresen S, Lilleng P, Nesland J. Pregnancy and breast cancer: a population-based study. Virchows Arch 2003; 20: 234–244

28 Reed W, Sandatad B, Holm R, Nesland J. The prognostic impact of hormone receptors and c-erbB-2 in pregnancy-associated breast cancer and their correlation with BRCA1 and cell cycle modulators. Int J Surg Pathol 2003; 11: 65–74

29 Clark R, Chua T. Breast cancer and pregnancy: the ultimate challenge. Clin Oncol 1989; 1: 11–18

30 Newcomb P, Storer B, Longnecker MP. Pregnancy termination in relation to risk of breast cancer. JAMA 1996; 275: 282–288

31 International Commission on Radiological Protection. Summary of the Current ICRP

Principles for Protection of the patient in Diagnostic Radiology. Oxford: Pergamon, 1993; ix–x

32 Liberman L, Giess C, Dershaw D. Imaging of pregnancy associated breast cancer. Radiology 1994; 191: 245–248

33 Miller R. Intrauterine radiation exposure and mental retardation. Health Phys 1988; 55: 295–298

34 Gwyn K, Theriault R. Breast cancer during pregnancy. Curr Treat Options Oncol 2000; 1: 239–243

35 Barnavon Y, Wallack M. Management of the pregnant patient with carcinoma of the breast. Surg Gynecol Obstet 1990; 171: 347–352

36 Rect A, Come S, Henderson I. The sequencing of chemotherapy and radiation therapy after conservative surgery for early stage breast cancer. N Engl J Med 1996; 334: 1356–1361

37 Isaacs R, Hunter W, Clark K. Tamoxifen as systemic treatment of advanced breast cancer during pregnancy: case report and literature review. Gynecol Oncol 2001; 80: 405–408

38 Eltorky M, Khare V, Osborne P. Placental metastasis from maternal carcinoma: a report of three cases. J Reprod Med 1995; 40: 339–403

39 Barrat J, Marqpeau L, Demuynck B. Breast cancer and pregnancy. Rev Fr Gynecol Obstet 1993; 88: 544–549

40 Moore H, Foster R. Breast cancer and pregnancy. Semin Oncol 2000; 27: 646–653

41 Reichman B, Green K. Breast cancer in young women: effect of chemotherapy on ovarian function, fertility, and birth defects. Monogr Natl Cancer Inst 1994; 16: 125–129

42 Von Schoultz E, Johanwson H, Wilking N. Influence of prior and subsequent pregnancy on breast cancer prognosis. J Clin Oncol 1995; 12: 430–434

43 Upponi S, Ahmed F, Whitaker I, Purushotham A. Pregnancy after breast cancer. Eur J Cancer 2003; 39: 736–741

Asma Khalil Pat O'Brien

Operative vaginal delivery

Obstetric history is littered with accounts of instruments designed to deliver women in obstructed labour. The Chamberlen family invented the modern obstetric forceps 400 years ago, and for the first time there was a reasonable expectation of delivering the baby alive in this situation. Their attempts to keep their invention hidden ultimately failed, and forceps have been in common use ever since.[1] James Simpson, Professor of Midwifery in Edinburgh, is widely credited with inventing the first vacuum extractor in the 1840s, but the most widely used cup over the last 30 years is the Bird-modification type.[2] Over the years, there have been many modifications of both instruments, but the basic principles remain the same. It is only in the past 20 years that scientific evaluation of their risks and benefits has taken place. This chapter summarises the current evidence used to guide best practice.

PATTERNS OF USE

Overall, instrumental delivery rates world-wide are around 10%, but vary widely from 1.5% of deliveries in the Czech Republic to 15% in Canada.[3] Even within a single country, the range is wide (*e.g.* in Scotland, from 4% to 26% in primiparous women).[4] In most countries, the overall rate is reasonably constant, but there is a gradual move away from forceps towards ventouse. This trend is largely due to a perception that the ventouse is easier and safer to use. It is conceivable that instrumental delivery rates may fall over the next decade because of several factors. There is a general tendency to less intervention because of the realisation that the length of the second stage is not

Asma Khalil MB BCh
Senior Resident in Obstetrics and Gynaecology, Ain Shams University Hospital, Cairo, Egypt

Pat O'Brien MB BCh MRCOG MFFP
Consultant in Obstetrics and Gynaecology, Obstetric Hospital, University College London Hospitals, Huntley Street, London WC1E 6AU, UK (for correspondence, E-mail: patrick.obrien@uclh.org)

as critical as previously thought; studies of almost 36,000 women found no relationship with infant mortality or morbidity.[5-7] In addition, the increasing use of the 'mobile' epidural mix is likely to be associated with less intervention for 'failure to progress'.

INDICATIONS AND CONTRA-INDICATIONS

Either instrument may be used when the second stage is prolonged, or where there is a need to shorten the second stage, for example when there is presumed fetal compromise (abnormal CTG or scalp pH), antepartum haemorrhage, or maternal exhaustion or cardiac disease.

The woman should have adequate analgesia, and the membranes ruptured. Full dilatation is a prerequisite for attempting forceps; but, in experienced hands, ventouse delivery is possible from 7 cm dilation. The fetal position should be identified; the vertex should be at least at the level of the ischial spines, and none of the head palpable abdominally. Signs of cephalo-pelvic disproportion should be sought and instrumental delivery attempted only if there is a good chance of success. Adequate contractions are needed when attempting ventouse delivery, but are less critical for forceps.

Morales et al.[8] found no increased neonatal morbidity in preterm babies weighing 1500–2499g delivered by ventouse. In spite of this, there remains a reluctance to use this instrument to deliver before 36 weeks' gestation; the argument is that the forceps may better protect the soft fetal skull and delicate brain at this stage.

There have been some case reports of haemorrhage in babies delivered by ventouse following fetal scalp blood sampling (FBS).[9] However, larger series[10,11] have not borne this out, and FBS does not appear to be a contra-indication.

FORCEPS DELIVERY VERSUS VACUUM EXTRACTION

Failure is more likely with ventouse than with forceps (RR, 1.69; 95% CI, 1.31–2.19).[12] This is presumably because it is not possible to pull with as much force as when using forceps. Because the ventouse cup is less invasive and takes up less room than forceps, it is associated with less pain for the mother; meta-analysis has found less requirement for regional or general anaesthesia, and less pain at delivery and 24 h later.[12]

Maternal injury

Serious maternal perineal trauma is less common with ventouse (OR, 0.4; 95% CI, 0.3–0.5). Anal sphincter damage seems more likely after forceps delivery;[13] Sultan[14] reported an incidence of 81% compared with 36% after ventouse.

However, the situation with regard to persistent urinary stress and anal incontinence is not as clear-cut. A link has been suspected for many years because of the recognition that forceps delivery can damage the anal sphincter and pelvic floor, either directly or by compromising the nerve supply. However, more recent studies[15-17] show no difference between forceps and ventouse delivery in terms of long-term incidence of urinary or anal incontinence (follow-up ranged from 9 months to 5 years). Interestingly,

Mason *et al.*[17] found a high incidence of urinary stress incontinence at 34 weeks' gestation, but 8 weeks after delivery there was no difference in urinary incontinence rates between those women who had spontaneous vaginal or instrumental delivery.

It seems clear that the greater the perineal damage, the greater the risk of long-term incontinence, both urinary and faecal. But there are no good quality studies with long-term follow-up, which control for factors such as size of the baby, malposition, length of labour, type of analgesia, pre-existing incontinence, *etc.* Until such studies are carried out, this issue will remain unresolved.

Neonatal injury

The ventouse is associated with an increased incidence of cephalhaematoma, caused by shear stress to the fetal scalp. Although these collections are often impressive, they are rarely of serious consequence to the baby. Serious injuries can occur after either forceps or ventouse delivery, but thankfully they are rare. Towner *et al.*[18] reported the outcome of over half a million vaginal deliveries. They showed a higher rate of intracranial haemorrhage (ICH) after ventouse compared with spontaneous vaginal delivery (RR, 2.22). Interestingly though, they found no significant difference between the rates of ICH in those delivered by ventouse (0.15 per 1000), forceps (0.26 per 1000), or Caesarean section in labour (0.25 per 1000), suggesting that the bleed may be due to the events of labour rather than the delivery itself.

Sub-galeal haemorrhage is a serious complication, which is fatal in up to 20% of cases. It has been reported after both ventouse and forceps delivery, but is rare; its true incidence is uncertain. It has not been reported in a recent meta-analysis,[12] suggesting that with modern silastic cups, and heroic instrumental deliveries becoming increasingly uncommon, its occurrence is rare.

Scalp lacerations are more common during forceps delivery, as is facial nerve palsy (4.5 per 1000 compared with 0.46 per 1000 after ventouse).[18] Jaundice requiring phototherapy is equally common (4%). The incidence of retinal haemorrhage is greater after ventouse (50% compared with 30%) but this does not seem to be of any clinical significance.

There are few long-term neurodevelopmental studies of children born by instrumental delivery.[15,34,35] Re-assuringly, these studies found no difference in school achievement, speech skills, neurological status or cognitive development between those delivered by ventouse or forceps and those who had spontaneous vaginal delivery.

TECHNIQUE

A detailed description of the technique of instrumental delivery is beyond the scope of this chapter, but some topical issues are worthy of discussion. There has been some debate about the relative merits of silicone and metal vacuum cups. Johanson summarised the evidence in a Cochrane Review which included 9 trials.[21] He found that there is an increased chance of failure with the soft cup (OR, 1.65; 95% CI, 1.2–2.3); this is likely to be due to the poor suction achieved with this cup when there is significant caput. Consistent with this finding, fetal trauma is less common in association with the soft cup (OR,

0.45; 95% CI 0.15–0.6). However, serious neonatal trauma is re-assuringly rare (though case reports are common, more often reporting on trauma caused by the metal cup). There is no difference in the incidence of **maternal** trauma with either type of vacuum cup. Overall, the consensus is that in cases of mal-position (occipito-posterior or -transverse), potentially difficult occipito-anterior deliveries, or when there is significant caput, the metal cup is preferable. In all other cases, the silastic cup should be the first choice. A recent addition to the armamentarium is a hand-held disposable vacuum cup, which has the advantage of convenience and speed, and is perhaps less intimidating for the woman; initial assessments suggest it is as effective as more traditional cups.

With regard to the technique of ventouse application, there have been several interesting studies recently. Lim *et al.*[22] compared rapid (negative pressure increased to a maximum of 0.8 kg/cm^2 without interruption) versus step-wise application of the vacuum. He found no difference in the rate of cup detachment or fetal scalp trauma. In the 'rapid application' group, total ventouse time was 8 min compared with 14 min in the 'step-wise' group. Bofill and colleagues[23] compared continuous with intermittent vacuum, but found no differences in outcome. Vacca[24] has shown the importance of correct cup application over the 'flexion point'.

There are no randomised controlled trials addressing the safety of prolonged ventouse cup application. Consequently, recommendations come from a consensus of experts,[25] based on observational studies which report low rates of fetal injury.[12,15,21,24,26–33] The cup should be attached for no more than 4 contractions, over a maximum of 20 min. There should be no more than 2 cup detachments, and there should be progressive descent with each contraction.

Recent reports have suggested a possible increased incidence of intracranial haemorrhage (RR, 3.4; 95% CI 1.7–6.6) associated with the sequential use of different instruments (*i.e.* ventouse followed by forceps or vice versa).[18] If one instrument fails, careful assessment for possible unrecognised cephalo-pelvic disproportion is essential. Any attempt at delivery with a second instrument must be made only by an experienced operator. Similarly, any trial of instrumental delivery should be attempted only by an experienced obstetrician who feels there is a good chance of success. The trial should be in theatre, with preparations already in place for emergency Caesarean section, should the trial fail.

TRAINING

Until recent years, training of junior doctors in the use of forceps and ventouse was inadequate – very much of the 'see one, do one, teach one' school. Thankfully, the situation has now changed. It is important that obstetricians learn these skills, not on patients, but in a skills laboratory, using models tailor-made for this purpose. A programme of structured training and supervision should be in place on the delivery suite to ensure that they achieve the appropriate level of competence.

CONCLUSIONS

Despite the body of evidence referred to above, many questions and uncertainties remain around the use of ventouse and forceps. Further large good-quality randomised trials are needed to address some of the issues raised above, and long-term follow-up of mothers and babies is essential. These instruments are for the most part safe for both mother and baby, but the obstetrician needs to remain constantly mindful of the potential harm they may cause if used without appropriate care and attention.

References

1 Hibbard BM. Forceps delivery. In: Turnbull A, Chamberlain G. (eds) Obstetrics. London: Churchill Livingstone, 1989; 833–834

2 Bird GC. Modification of Malmstrom's vacuum extractor. BMJ 1969; 3: 526

3 Stephenson PA. International differences in the use of obstetrical interventions, WHO.EUR/ICP/MCH 112. Copenhagen: World Health Organization, 1992

4 Middle C, Macfarlane A. Labour and delivery of 'normal' primiparous women: analysis of routinely collected data. Br J Obstet Gynaecol 1996; 102: 970–977

5 Cohen WR. Influence of the duration of second stage labor on perinatal outcome and puerperal morbidity. Obset Gynecol 1977; 49: 266–269

6 Albers LL, Schiff M, Gorwoda JG. The length of active labor in normal pregnancies. Obstet Gynecol 1996; 87: 355–359

7 Menticoglou SM, Manning F, Harman C, Morrison I. Perinatal outcome in relation to second-stage duration. Am J Obstet Gynecol 1995; 173: 906–912

8 Morales R, Adair CD, Sanchez-Ramos L, Gaudier FL. Vacuum extraction of preterm infants with birth weights of 1500–2499 grams. J Reprod Med 1995; 40: 127–130

9 Roberts IF, Stone M. Fetal hemorrhage, complication of vacuum extractor after fetal blood sampling. Am J Obstet Gynecol 1978; 132: 109

10 Lee KH. Vacuum extraction after fetal blood sampling. Aust NZ J Obstet Gynecol 1970; 10: 205

11 Johanson RB, Rice C, Doyle M, et al. A randomised prospective study comparing the new vacuum extractor policy with forceps delivery. Br J Obstet Gynaecol 1993; 100: 524–530

12 Johanson RB. Vacuum extraction versus forceps delivery for assisted vaginal delivery. The Cochrane Database of Systematic Reviews 1999; 2: 1–12

13 Groutz A, Fait G, Lessing JB et al. Incidence and obstetric risk factors of postpartum anal incontinence. Scand J Gastroenterol 1999; 34: 315–318

14 Sultan AH, Kamm MA, Bartram CI, Hudson CN. Anal sphincter trauma during instrumental delivery. Int J Obstet Gynecol 1993; 43: 263–270

15 Johanson RB, Heycock E, Carter J et al. Maternal and child health after assisted vaginal delivery: five-year follow up of a randomised controlled study comparing forceps and ventouse. Br J Obstet Gynaecol 1999; 106: 544–549

16 Zetterstrom JP, Lopez A, Anzen B et al. Anal incontinence after vaginal delivery: a prospective study in primiparous women. Br J Obstet Gynaecol 1999; 106: 324–330

17 Mason L, Glenn S, Walton I, Appleton C. The prevalence of stress incontinence during pregnancy and following delivery. Midwifery 1999; 15: 120–128

18 Towner D, Castro MA, Eby-Wilkens E, Gilbert WM. Effect of mode of delivery in nulliparous women on neonatal intracranial injury. N Engl J Med 1999; 341: 1709–1714

19 Ngan H, Miu P, Ko L, Ma H. Long-term neurological sequelae following vacuum extractor delivery. Aust NZ J Obset Gynecol 1990; 30: 111–114

20 Carmody F, Grant A, Mutch L et al. Follow up of babies delivered in a randomized controlled comparison of vacuum extraction and forceps delivery. Acta Obstet Gynecol Scand 1986; 65: 763–766

21 Johanson R, Merton V. Soft versus rigid vacuum extractor cups for vaginal assisted delivery. The Cochrane Database of Systematic Reviews 1999; 1–4

22 Lim FTH, Holm JP, Schuitemaker NWE, Jansen FHM, Hermans J. Stepwise compared with rapid application of vacuum in ventouse extraction procedures. Br J Obstet Gynaecol 1997; 104: 33–36

23 Bofill JA, Rust OA, Sehorr SJ et al. A randomized prospective trial of vacuum extraction technique [abstract]. Am J Obstet Gynecol 1996; 174: 353

24 Vacca A. Handbook of vacuum extraction in obstetrical practice. London: Edward Arnold, 1992

25 O'Grady JP, Pope CS, Patel SS. Vacuum extraction in modern obstetric practice: a review and critique. Curr Opin Obstet Gynecol 2000; 12: 475–480

26 Bofill JA, Rust OA, Sehorr SJ et al. A randomized prospective trial of the obstetric forceps versus the M-cup vacuum extractor. Am J Obstet Gynecol 1996; 175: 1325–1330

27 Bofill JA. Rust OA, Schorr SJ et al. A randomized trial of two vacuum extraction techniques. Obstet Gynecol 1997; 89: 758–762

28 Vacca A, Grant A, Wyatt G, Chalmers I. Portsmouth operative delivery trial: a comparison of vacuum extraction and forceps delivery. Br J Obstet Gynaecol 1983; 90: 1107–1112

29 Sjostedt JE. The vacuum extractor and forceps in obstetrics. A clinical study. Acta Obstet Gynecol Scand 1967; 46 (Suppl 10): 1–208

30 O'Grady JP. Instrumental delivery: a critique of current practice. In: Nichols D, Clarke-Pearson D. (eds) Gynecologic, obstetric and related surgery. St Louis: Mosby 2000; 1081–1105

31 Berkus MD, Ramamurthy RS, O'Connor PS et al. Cohort study of silastic obstetric vacuum cup deliveries: I Safety of the instrument. Obstet Gynecol 1985; 66: 503–509

32 Berkus MD, Ramamurthy RS, O'Connor PS et al. Cohort study of silastic obstetric vacuum cup deliveries: II Unsuccessful vacuum extraction. Obstet Gynecol 1986; 68: 662–666

33 Johanson R, Pusey J, Livera N, Jones P. North Staffordshire/Wigan assisted delivery trial. Br J Obstet Gynaecol 1989; 96: 537–544

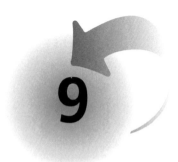

Andrew D. Weeks

The retained placenta

Post-partum haemorrhage is a significant cause of maternal mortality in the non-industrialised world. Many cases of post-partum haemorrhage are associated with retained placenta, a condition that affects 0.6–3.3% of normal deliveries.[1-3] Where there is easy access to hospital care and transfusion, mortality from this condition is very low. In the UK, the death rate from retained placenta has shown impressive falls since the triennial reviews started in 1952. Indeed, between 1969 and 1996 there were no deaths from haemorrhage related to simple retained placenta in the UK – all deaths occurred as a result of placental inversion, placenta accreta or complications of treatment. The most recent triennial report describes a death from post-partum haemorrhage secondary to retained placenta for the first time in 30 years.[4] From these data, the estimated death rate from retained placenta in the UK is 1 in every 1.5 million deliveries, or an estimated 1 death for every 30,000 retained placentae.

In many parts of the non-industrialised world, however, the case fatality rate is high. In an observational study from rural India in which traditional birth attendants delivered the majority of women at home, there were 2 deaths (9%) from the 22 women who had placental retention of over 60 min.[2] In a large northern Nigerian hospital, the mortality was 3% amongst 894 women treated for retained placenta over a 3.5-year period.[5] The cause of death is usually haemorrhage. This is more frequent when facilities for manual removal of placenta (MROP) is not immediately available or when travelling times to hospital are long. Clearly, an effective medical treatment could have major implications for the reduction of maternal mortality.[6]

Andrew D. Weeks MD MRCOG
Clinical Lecturer in Obstetrics and Gynaecology, Department of Obstetrics and Gynaecology,
Liverpool Women's Hospital, Crown Street, Liverpool L8 7SS, UK (E-mail: aweeks@liverpool.ac.uk)

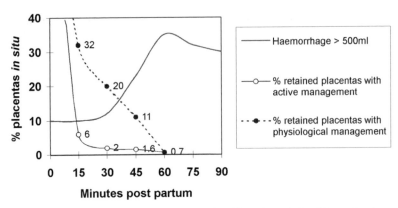

Fig. 1 Natural history of retained placentae. Blood loss data derived from Combs and Laros.[1] The natural history of the third stage is derived from the length of third stage from the active versus control arms of the trials of active management of labour for 20 and 40 min, and the expectant management arms from the trials the umbilical oxytocin as a treatment for retained placenta.[9,11]

CURRENT EPIDEMIOLOGY

There is no consensus as to the length of the third stage after which a placenta should be called 'retained'. Various authorities have suggested anything between 20 min and 2 h.[7] In the US, the average time after which manual removal is conducted is often very short; in one study, it averaged only 20 min.[8] This probably occurs as a result of the impatience of the private attendants rather than anything else. Indeed, there is no increase in the haemorrhage rate until 30 min have elapsed (Fig. 1),[1] whilst large numbers of placentae will deliver spontaneously during this time. In the control arms of trials of umbilical oxytocin for the treatment of retained placenta, 42% of placentae delivered spontaneously without any intervention in the 30 min following recruitment (which was mainly 15–30 min after delivery[9]). In contrast, in the only randomised trial to recruit ar 60 min post partum, the spontaneous delivery rate in the control group (in this case saline injection) was 0% over the subsequent 30 min.[10]

The use of prophylactic oxytocics has marked effects on the length of the third stage. In the Cochrane Review, the mean length of the third stage in those who had physiological management was 15.5 min compared with 8.8 min in those who had active management.[11] This also translates into a reduction in the number of placentae still *in situ* at 20 and 40 min. When the numbers who actually need manual removal is compared, however, there is no difference between the two groups.

These overall results disguise major differences between the individual trials within the meta-analysis. It is debatable as to whether all the trials should be analysed together as there is considerable variation between the oxytocic used for the third stage. The Dublin trial[12] is the only trial that compares intravenous ergometrine to expectant management, and the results are markedly different to those of the other trials. It is the only trial that shows an increase in the need for MROP with the oxytocic (relative risk, 19.5; 95% CI, 2.6–145.4). In addition (and in contrast to the other trials) the mean length of

Table 1 Factors associated with prolonged third stage;[1] note that 'Asian origin' is a negative association

Factor	Adjusted odds ratio (95% CI)
Gestational age < 36 weeks (versus > 36 weeks)	3.81 (2.89–5.02)
Delivery in a labour bed (versus delivery room)	2.17 (1.71–2.76)
Pre-eclampsia	1.76 (1.17–2.67)
Augmented labour	1.47 (1.17–1.85)
Nulliparity (versus parous)	1.45 (1.16–1.81)
Midwife delivery (versus physician)	1.36 (1.02–1.80)
Maternal age > 30 years (versus < 30 years)	1.36 (1.09–1.70)
Previous abortion	1.35 (1.09–1.67)
Asian origin (versus non-Asian)	0.60 (0.43–0.84)

the third stage is no different to that of those managed expectantly. The range of values, however, are wide suggesting that although many placentae were retained, a large number were also delivered more quickly than with placebo. Ergometrine, in contrast to oxytocin, causes a powerful tonic uterine contraction. When given intramuscularly, the onset is only after 10 min. With intravenous administration, however, the onset is immediate and this tends to close the cervix at the same time as the placental detachment occurs, thus trapping the placenta behind a closed cervix. The association of retained placenta with the use of ergometrine was supported by data from a population study in Sweden.[13] The retained placenta rate in 10 centres which routinely used methylergometrine 0.2 mg was 2.7% compared to 1.8% in those that used oxytocin 5 or 10 units alone ($P < 0.001$).

The aetiological factors for a prolonged third stage were studied in a series of 13,000 deliveries by Combs and Laros.[1] Logistic regression identified 9 factors that were independently associated with a third stage of over 30 min (Table 1). The strongest association was with gestational age. Dombrowski *et al.*[8] studied this in more detail and produced gestation specific rates for

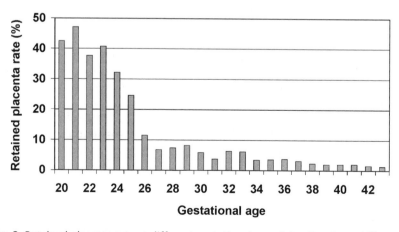

Fig. 2 Retained placenta rate at different gestational ages (after Dombrowski[8]).

retained placenta (Fig. 2). The high rate of retained placenta in premature deliveries may relate to the continued production of myometrial inhibitors by the immature placenta (see later). In a case-control study from Saudi Arabia, 114 women with retained placenta were compared to 116 with normal third stages.[14] Logistic regression analysis showed significant associations of retained placenta with multiparity, induced labour, small placenta, high blood loss, high pregnancy number, previous uterine injury and pre-term labour.

It has also been suggested that uterine abnormalities may be an aetiological factor for retained placenta. Indeed, in a series of 63 pregnancies in women with Mullerian duct fusion abnormalities, 11 (17%) had retained placentae.[15] However, given the rarity of these abnormalities in the general population (0.2%), it would not seem necessary to investigate every woman with a retained placenta for uterine abnormalities. Indeed in the Green and Harris series,[15] the chance of any one woman with a retained placenta having a Mullarian duct abnormality would only have been 1.5%, assuming a retained placenta rate of 2%. Subtle abnormalities may, however, be more common. Golan et al.[16] conducted routine hysteroscopy 6 weeks after MROP in 48 women; they found an incomplete uterine septum in 15%.

Following a retained placenta in one pregnancy there is a recurrence rate of 6.25%.[17]

PATHOPHYSIOLOGY

It has long been recognised that the term 'retained placenta' covers a number of pathologies. Some placentae are simply trapped behind a closed cervix (the 'trapped' or 'incarcerated' placenta), some are adherent to the uterine wall but easily separated manually ('placenta adherens'), whilst others are pathologically invading the myometrium (placenta accreta). Attempts to separate out the different causes suggest that around 53% of retained placentae are, in fact, separated but trapped behind the cervix (Fig. 3).[18] Placenta accreta is thought to have an incidence of 1: 2510,[19] although this does not include the many placentae in which a clear plane of separation cannot be identified at MROP and in whom the placenta is removed piecemeal. It is likely that in most of these there is a small area of accreta. The close association of placenta accreta with both previous Caesarean section and placenta praevia means that it rarely

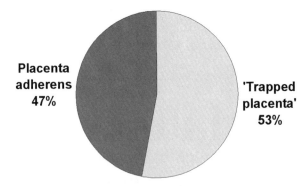

Fig. 3 Retained placenta divided by pathophysiology (after Rogers et al.[18]). Placenta accreta makes up less than 0.25% of cases.

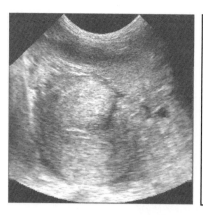
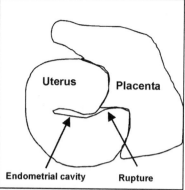

Fig. 4 An unusual case of retained placenta. A low transverse abdominal ultrasound view of a Ugandan woman with retained placenta showing the placenta extruded through the uterine rupture. At presentation, she was in great pain with shock and vaginal bleeding and the cord was hanging from the vagina. She recovered well following a subtotal hysterectomy.

presents as a retained placenta after vaginal delivery. In the series of 62 cases by Millar,[19] all but 7 were associated with placenta praevia and they were all delivered by Caesarean section. In the absence of placenta praevia, therefore, the placenta accreta rate was 1 in 22,000. Assuming a retained placenta rate of 2%, this suggests that less than 1 in 400 women with a retained placenta following vaginal delivery will have placenta accreta.

A very rare cause of retained placenta is a ruptured uterus with the placenta expelled into the peritoneal cavity (Fig. 4).

The importance of the retro-placental myometrium

Ultrasound studies

As long ago as 1933, Brandt[20] described the necessity of a uterine contraction to cause detachment of the placenta from the decidual bed. This has recently been confirmed using ultrasound where examination of the immediate post-partum uterus has clarified the process of both the normal and abnormal third stage of labour. Herman *et al.*[21] first demonstrated ultrasonographically that a retro-placental myometrial contraction is mandatory in order to produce shearing forces upon the interface between the placenta and myometrium and lead to its detachment. He divided the third stage into 4 phases according to the ultrasound appearances. In the **latent** phase, which immediately follows delivery of the fetus, all the myometrium contracts except for that behind the placenta which remains relaxed (see Fig. 5). In the **contraction** phase, the retro-placental myometrium contracts leading to the **detachment** phase where the placenta is sheared away from the decidua. In the **expulsion** phase, the placenta is expelled from the uterus by uterine contraction. Contractions occurring prior to delivery are insufficient to cause placental detachment as in the presence of the fetus, the myometrium is unable to achieve the necessary strain for detachment.[22]

These ultrasound studies also shed light on the aetiology of the retained placenta. They demonstrate that the duration of the third stage of labour is

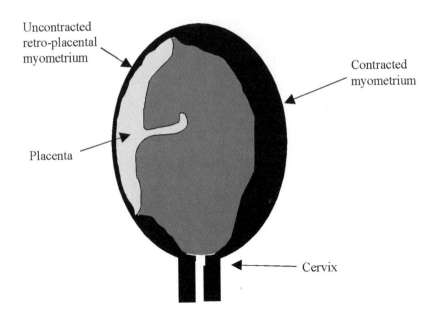

Fig. 5 Diagram of uterus and placenta in the latent phase of the third stage of labour. Although the majority of the myometrium has contracted, the retro-placental myometrium remains relaxed. When it contracts, it will shut off the spiral arteries and shear off the placenta leading to detachment.

dependent on the length of the latent phase and a prolonged third stage is due to contractile failure in the retro-placental area.[21] In the 5 cases of retained placenta in which they conducted serial ultrasonographic myometrial thickness measurements, these authors found a universal failure of retro-placental contraction. Doppler studies confirm that, in these women, blood flow continues through the myometrium to the placenta irrespective of whether the cause is placenta accreta or prolongation of the latent phase.[23] This provides a scientific explanation for the increased rates of haemorrhage during MROP when compared with spontaneous delivery.[24] It also explains why partial or forced detachment of the placenta prior to onset of the contraction phase is associated with high rates of haemorrhage.

Association with dysfunctional labour
The finding that the basic abnormality in women with non-accreta retained placenta (or placenta adherens) is a failure of the contraction phase raises a number of issues. It is unlikely that this retro-placental contractile failure is limited to the post-partum period. It is likely to have occurred throughout labour. This may explain the fact that retained placenta and dysfunctional labour have been shown to be closely associated,[1] even though all women with severe dysfunctional labour are delivered by Caesarean section. Indeed, in a small case control study from the UK, the need for MROP at the time of Caesarean section was found to be higher in women having Caesarean section for 'failure to progress' than for other reasons (Weeks, unpublished observations). In 10 cases having emergency Caesarean sections for failed

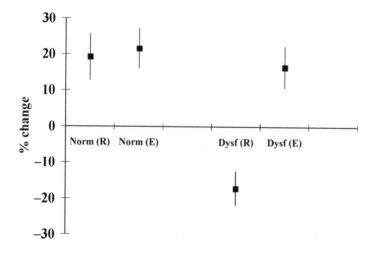

Fig. 6 The changes in myometrial thickness that occurs during a contraction (% of original thickness ± SEM). On the left, the changes that occur in normally progressing labours in the retro-placental (R) and the extra-placental (E) myometrium. On the right, the changes in the dysfunctional labours. Note the thinning of the retro-placental myometrium during contractions in the dysfunctional labours (data from Weeks[25]).

induction or 'failure to progress', 3 required MROP whilst none of the 10 having Caesareans for other indications needed MROP.

An attempt has also been made to compare the 'retro-placental' and 'extra-placental' myometrial contractility during labour using the increase in myometrial thickness during contractions (measured using ultrasound) as a measure of the strength of local myometrial contractility. In 10 women in whom labour was progressing normally, there was no difference in contractility between the two sites. In the 10 women with dysfunctional labour, however, whilst the extra-placental myometrium showed normal thickening, the retro-placental myometrium thinned during contractions (Fig. 6).[25] This suggests a localised failure of contractility. The thinning is thought to occur as a result of stretching of the relaxed myometrium by the raised intra-uterine pressure.

The relative lack of contractile strength in the retro-placental myometrium may make evolutionary sense for both the mother and fetus. During strong contractions, it not only prevents inadvertent placental detachment, but also allows good blood flow to the placenta to be maintained.

Pathophysiological mechanisms for retained placenta
The second issue raised is the nature of the biochemical abnormality that produces the failure of retro-placental contractility. The localised nature of the contractile failure suggests that it is the placenta that is responsible, rather than the underlying myometrium. It has been known for many years that the placenta is important in determining the onset of labour and it is likely that this occurs as a result of the loss of an inhibitory factor of placental origin. The association of retained placenta with both preterm delivery and the need for

induction[1,8] suggests that it may be the same placental factor that is responsible for both. The role of the feto–placental unit in the regulation of uterine contractility is complex with a finely controlled balance between stimulatory and inhibitory factors.[26] This balance can be likened to a set of scales with inhibitory and stimulatory factors on either side. Loss of inhibition may result in the onset of labour (as with the administration of anti-progesterones) as may an increase in the stimulatory factors (as with the administration of exogenous oxytocin or prostaglandins). It could be hypothesised that if the pro-contractile stimuli were strong enough, then successful labour could occur even in the presence of persisting, localised placental inhibition. In this situation, there would be a high risk of retained placenta due to the persistent inhibition of retro-placental myometrial contractility by the placenta.

There are a number of candidates for the identity of this localised inhibitor. The placenta has a role in inhibiting myometrial contractions through the production of progesterone and possibly nitric oxide (NO). Progesterone is an important inhibitor of myometrial contractility in many animals, but the situation in humans is yet to be fully clarified. The anti-progesterone mifepristone is a powerful sensitiser of the myometrium to exogenous prostaglandins, and it is effective for induction of human labour in all trimesters of pregnancy.[27–29] Attempts to identify the mechanism for this, however, have so far been unsuccessful as, unlike in animal models, a reduction in serum progesterone is not seen prior to labour.[30] Recent evidence, however, suggests that its effect may occur through a reduction in progesterone metabolites.[31] If persistent progesterone inhibition is the cause of the failure of retroplacental contractility, then we would expect those treated with mifepristone at term to have low rates of retained placenta (and possibly dysfunctional labour).

Nitric oxide is also a powerful smooth muscle relaxant that is produced in large quantities by nitric oxide synthase (NOS) in the placenta[32] and, to a lesser extent, in the myometrium.[33] As it is rapidly oxidised following its production, its effect is very localised. Ramsay et al.[34] showed decreases in villous trophoblast NOS activity through pregnancy, but Thompson et al.[35] showed no change in placental NOS activity before and after labour. However, all the placentae studied came from women who had Caesarean sections. The indication for most of these operations in the labouring group was 'failure to progress' (Thompson, personal communication) and this is the very group who may have excessive NOS activity. This study, therefore, does not disprove the hypothesis that a reduction in placental NO is necessary for the onset of normal labour. Indeed, a change in the production of placental NO could explain the fact that exogenous NO appears to relax myometrium, but that infusion of NOS inhibitors (which may not reach the placenta) have no effect of myometrial quiescence in animal models.[36]

The detail of how these various factors combine to initiate and sustain labour, as well as the pathological mechanisms that cause dysfunctional contractions and post-partum myometrial contractile dysfunction, are clearly complex. The study of women with retained placenta in which there is a clear inhibitory effect of the placenta on myometrium may allow some of the mechanisms underlying dysfunctional labour as well as retained placenta to be elucidated.

Implications for directed treatment

From the ultrasound studies above, it is clear that contractile failure of the retroplacental myometrium is a major cause of retained placenta. That being

Placenta adherens

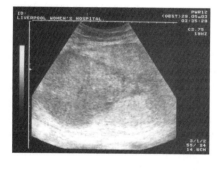
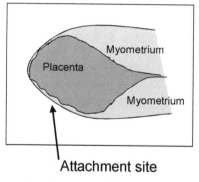

Attachment site

Trapped placenta

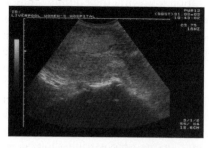
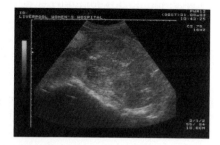

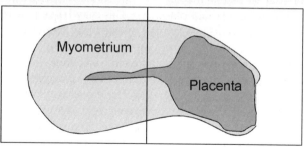

Fig. 7 Ultrasound pictures (saggital midline view) of placenta adherens and a trapped placenta.

so, the problem of retained placenta (and possibly dysfunctional labour) could be solved by stimulating contractions in this area. This could either be achieved through removing the inhibitor (*e.g.* by treatment with an anti-progesterone) or by stimulation with oxytocics. Delivery of the oxytocin through the placenta via the umbilical vein has been suggested as a way of delivering a localised stimulus to the retro-placental myometrium and will be discussed further below.

MANAGEMENT

Diagnosis

The differentiation between a placenta that is 'trapped', or adherent (placenta adherens) or accreta is not easy unless ultrasound is used. Placenta accreta is very rare in women having a vaginal delivery, and an attempt at manual removal should always be made unless a definitive diagnosis has been made prior to delivery. Clues to a trapped placenta will be if the fundus feels small and contracted, or if the edge of the placenta is palpable through a tight cervical os. Alternatively, Herman et al.[21] suggest that ultrasound should be used to differentiate between a trapped and adherent placenta. With a trapped placenta, the myometrium is seen to be thickened all around the uterus and a clear demarcation is often seen between the placenta and the myometrium. In contrast, with an adherent placenta, the myometrium will be thickened in all areas except where the placenta is attached where it will be very thin or even invisible (Fig. 7).

If the placenta is 'trapped' then the use of tocolytics (such as glyceryl trinitrate [GTN]) may be attempted to release the placenta (see below). The woman should be kept under close observation following their administration as haemorrhage may follow uterine relaxation.

Systemic oxytocics

The role of systemic oxytocics in the management of retained placentae is controversial. Oxytocics given prophylactically at the time of delivery increase the number of placental deliveries at 20 and 40 min, but have no effect on the number of placentae that eventually need manual removal.[11] The only randomised trial to assess the use of intravenous ergometrine showed an increase in the rate of retained placenta.[12] This may have occurred as a result of myometrial spasm distal to a fundally-placed placenta leading to its forced retention (see above).

The finding that prophylactic oxytocin injections (which last in the circulation for only 10 min) increase the number of placentae delivered in the first 30 min following delivery, provides the theoretical basis for the use of oxytocics to try and deliver the remainder. Midwives have recommended nipple stimulation for many years to stimulate the production of endogenous oxytocin to deliver the placenta, but this has never been formally evaluated for this indication. Bullough et al.[37] conducted a randomised trial to assess the benefits of nipple stimulation in a rural African setting to prevent post-partum haemorrhage. With only 4227 women in the trial, it was insufficiently powered to detect any changes in the retained placenta rate, but it is interesting to note that there were only 2 retained placentae in each of the study and control groups (the retained placenta rate in this trial was only 1 per 1000, but with a case fatality rate of 25%).

The use of an intravenous infusion of oxytocin has never been subjected to a randomised trial, but it has been suggested that it (or intramuscular ergometrine) may prevent haemorrhage during transfer or preparation for theatre.[38,39] Its use is wide-spread throughout the world in this situation. Oxytocin is given in the form of a continuous infusion of 5–10 IU/h as this increases the overall tone of the myometrium as well as stimulating strong phasic contractions. Ergometrine, which produces a long continuous contraction for up to 90 min, is less frequently used. However, because it is widely available and does not require an intravenous infusion, it is often used in rural areas whilst transfer is arranged. Misoprostol, an orally active prostaglandin E$_1$ analogue, has an effect similar to that of an oxytocin infusion, producing increases in both background tone and contraction strength for around 90 min.[40] Its cost, tolerance to heat and oral availability make it an excellent drug for rural African use where electricity and trained health workers may be scarce. However, results of trials in which it was being tested as a prophylactic agent to prevent post-partum haemorrhage found that there was no difference in retained placenta rate after its use compared to when oxytocin 10 IU had been given.[41] As it lasts in the circulation for 90 min (compared to the 10 min of oxytocin), it is unlikely that it would have any beneficial effect if given to a woman with retained placenta. This question has, however, not been specifically addressed by research trials and, in the absence of an alternative, it would be wise to give 1000 µg of misoprostol rectally to prevent haemorrhage during transfer.

Umbilical vein injection

Oxytocin

The notion that oxytocin may be delivered directly to the retro-placental myometrium by injecting it into the placental bed via the umbilical vein has stimulated a lot of interest. This technique allows the treatment to be directed specifically at the area with the contractile failure, whilst sparing the remainder. Results from trials of this treatment have been mixed. A recent Cochrane Review[9] concluded that the use of umbilical oxytocin is effective in the management of retained placenta, despite the fact that the meta-analysis showed the reduction in retained placenta rates not to be significantly different to that obtained with expectant management (RR, 0.86; 95% CI, 0.72–1.01). The

Table 2 Success rates of placental filling using different techniques. Radio-opaque dye was injected into the umbilical vein or artery of a delivered placenta using a variety of techniques. The placenta was the X-rayed and the filling of the cotyledons and capillaries assessed visually. The most successful techniques were when 30 ml of the dye was either injected down a catheter, or when it was injected into the vein and then milked down the cord towards the placenta (from Pipingas et al.[42]).

			Umbilical vein						Umbilical artery	
	Catheter		Short cannula							
			Cord bled		Cord not bled		Cord 'milked'			
	20 ml (n = 5)	30 ml (n = 5)	20 ml (n = 5)	30 ml (n = 5)	20 ml (n = 5)	30 ml (n = 5)	20 ml (n = 5)	30 ml (n = 5)	20 ml (n = 5)	30 ml (n = 5)
No. of capillaries demonstrated	4	5	4	5	1	3	2	5	3	5
No. of cotyledons demonstrated	5	5	0	1	0	3	1	5	0	1

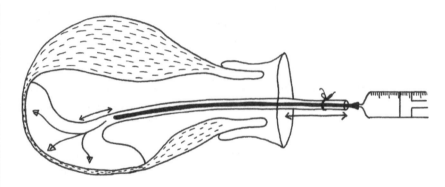

Fig. 8 The Pipingas technique. A nasogastric tube is threaded down the umbilical vein to the placental bed, and then withdrawn by 5 cm and tied; 30 ml of solution is then injected down the catheter. This technique achieved optimal filling of the placental bed capillaries in the trial by Pipingas et al.[42]

basis for this conclusion was data from trials in which umbilical oxytocin was compared to placebo which showed a significant reduction in need for MROP with umbilical oxytocin injection (RR, 0.79; 95% CI, 0.69–0.91).

The inconclusive results from randomised trials may be due to inadequate delivery of the oxytocin to the retro-placental myometrium. Pipingas et al.[42] compared various methods of intra-umbilical injection, using injections of radio-opaque dye into the delivered placenta to enable radiological comparisons. They found that the method of injection used in most trials (injection of oxytocin diluted in 20–30 ml saline and injected directly into the umbilical vein) only resulted in capillary filling in 20–60% of cases (Table 2). As a result of their studies, they proposed that the oxytocin should be diluted in 30 ml of saline and injected down an infant nasogastric feeding tube which has been passed along the umbilical vein (Fig. 8). They suggested that, after re-cutting the cord (in order to achieve a clean end for insertion of the tube), a size 10 nasogastric tube be passed along the vein until resistance is felt. The tube is then withdrawn by 5 cm to allow for any divisions of the vein prior to its insertion into the placenta. This method resulted in complete filling of the placental bed capillaries in all patients studied. An alternative (and equally successful) method *in vitro* is to inject 30 ml directly into the cord, but then 'milk the cord' so as to flush the solution up into the placenta. In clinical settlings, however, when the placenta is still intra-uterine, the majority of the cord is intravaginal making access to it for 'milking' difficult or impossible. The milking technique may, therefore, not produce the same success in practice as was achieved in the experiments.

A further problem with the previous trials has been an inconsistency regarding the dose of oxytocin. There are no comparative studies that assess different doses of oxytocin and the choice of dosage has, therefore, largely been empirical. Trials to date have mainly used a dose of 10–20 IU oxytocin, although doses of up to 100 IU have been reported.[43] The published trials that have used higher dosages of oxytocin have, on the whole, found higher success rates (Fig. 9).

Clinicians are wary of using high doses as an intravenous injection of as little as 5 IU of oxytocin can produce significant changes in maternal blood pressure.[44] Although oxytocin can clearly pass through the placenta, the data are unclear as to how quickly this occurs or whether it is complete.[45] In a recent pilot study in Uganda, 10 women with retained placentae for a mean of 3 h (range, 1.5–12 h) were given intra-umbilical injections of 50 IU oxytocin by the Pipingas technique. There was no significant effect on maternal blood pressure or pulse (Weeks, unpublished observations; Fig. 10). Of the 4 cases in which the injection was unsuccessful, in only 1 could the placenta be easily removed at MROP. The remainder required piecemeal removal suggesting some placenta accreta.

Further evidence for the efficacy of higher doses comes from a recent observational study of 30 women with retained placenta for over 1 h who were injected with 100 IU oxytocin diluted in 30 ml of saline via an infant feeding tube as suggested by Pipingas.[42] In this group, a 93% delivery rate of retained placentae was achieved within 5 min of injection.[46] Clearly, there is a need for a randomised

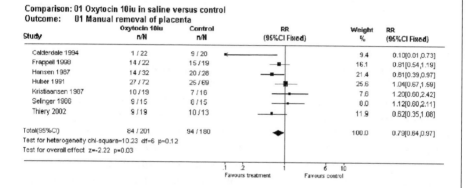

Fig. 9 Success rates of umbilical vein injection when injected with various doses of oxytocin compared with control. From top to bottom, graphs show results with 10 IU oxytocin, 20 IU oxytocin and > 20 IU oxytocin. In all trials, the control group was saline injection except for the Thiery trial where it was expectant management.[10,43,47,62–69]

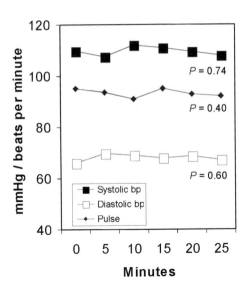

Fig. 10 Changes in mean blood pressure and pulse following an injection of 50 IU oxytocin into the placenta by the Pipingas method. *P* values obtained using ANOVA test.

trial in which high dose intra-umbilical injection by the Pipingas technique is compared to placebo.

Prostaglandins

There is only one trial to assess the benefit of an intra-umbilical injection of prostaglandins. Bider et al.[10] randomised 17 women with retained placenta after 60 min to receive either 20 mg of prostaglandin $F_2\alpha$ in 20 ml saline or saline alone (there was also an oxytocin group). The technique was successful in all 10 who received prostaglandin, whilst all those injected with saline alone required manual removal. This would appear a very promising technique, but more trials are needed. Misoprostol, as well as being soluble in saline, is much cheaper and easier to use than the other prostaglandins, and would appear to be an excellent candidate for study.

MANUAL REMOVAL OF PLACENTA (MROP)

Timing of removal

The most common treatment for a retained placenta is its manual removal under anaesthetic. During this procedure, the woman is exposed to anaesthetic risks as well as the infective risk that comes from inserting a hand into the uterus. Both risks are higher in non-industrialised countries where the prevalence of infections is high and personnel skilled in obstetrics and anaesthesia are in short supply. The time that is allowed to lapse before manual removal varies, but many authorities suggest a delay of 30–60 min in the absence of haemorrhage. This is because there is no increase in haemorrhage until at least 30 min post-partum (see Fig. 1[1]), and because of the finding that between 30 and 60 minutes a further 40% of placentae will spontaneously deliver with the loss of an average of only 300 ml of blood.[47]

Technique of manual removal

Adequate analgesia is vital for effective MROP. This can be achieved through regional or general anaesthetic. Although general anaesthetic helps to relax the uterus, it is associated with higher complication rates than regional anaesthesia (from failed intubation and inhalation of vomit). Regional anaesthesia, if available, is therefore the ideal technique. If the uterus is very contracted, nitrates can be used for relaxation (see below). Irrespective of the type of analgesia used, MROP is best conducted in theatre where aseptic technique is more easily achieved and where any complications (haemorrhage, placenta accreta or perforation) may be rapidly dealt with in association with the anaesthetist. Because of the risk of haemorrhage, at least 2 units of blood should be available before the procedure is commenced.

After obtaining informed consent, the woman should be placed in lithotomy position with her legs in stirrups. Ideally, the surgeon should use long sterile gloves (gauntlets). After cleaning, draping and catheterising the woman, the surgeon should identify the interface between the uterus and maternal surface of the placenta. This is best done by following the umbilical cord through the vagina up to its insertion into the placenta. This will give a basic idea of the position of the placenta within the uterus and allow an exploration of the cavity. The other hand is used to steady the fundus of the uterus through the woman's abdomen. Once the rough, velvety interface between the uterus and placenta is identified, the plane is gently dissected using a side-to-side motion of the fingers. This process should be continued, seeking out the areas where dissection is simple, and using the other hand on the abdomen to feel the position of the dissecting hand. If removal proves difficult, it may be necessary to remove the placenta in pieces ('piecemeal removal'). Beware of haemorrhage in this situation – have strong oxytocics ready. For placentae implanted on the right side of the uterus, the manual removal may be difficult for the right-handed surgeon (and *visa versa*). In this situation, the surgeon may find it easier to swap hands and conduct the removal with his/her left hand.

At the end of the process, it is not unusual to find a small area where the placenta is very adherent to the uterus. This can usually be dealt with by patient, persistent working at the interface with the fingers, slowly identifying a plane of separation and easing the placenta away. The plane of dissection is often partially through the placenta at this stage, leaving some placenta adherent to the decidua and myometrium. This is not a problem so long as the uterus can obtain sufficient contraction afterwards to obstruct the blood flow through the radial arteries to the placental fragments. Strong oxytocics (*e.g.* ergometrine 0.5 mg) should be used to obtain this contraction, and the woman closely observed for 2 days afterwards for further haemorrhage. Sharp curettage should be avoided as the myometrium may be very thin at the point of adherence and there is high risk of perforation. If further haemorrhage occurs, then further gentle attempts at uterine evacuation may be necessary, or even hysterectomy.

Placenta accreta

If wide-spread placental adherence is found when manual removal is attempted (this occurs in less than 1 in 400 cases), then there are a number of management options. Often a partial removal is achieved manually and curettage is used to remove as much as possible of the remaining tissue. So long as haemorrhage is controlled with this method and the uterus remains well contracted, then this is usually adequate to prevent continued haemorrhage. The remaining trophoblast is usually re-absorbed spontaneously, although levels of β-HCG take longer to return to normal.[48] Further curettage may be needed if haemorrhage continues. In the case of placenta percreta, blood will continue to flow through the area of invasion when the bulk of the placenta is removed due to the absence of the myometrial physiological ligature which would normally stem the flow.[23] If discovered at Caesarean section, then haemostasis may be achieved through the use of sutures placed deep into the myometrial bed, resection of the affected area (if small), or through ligation of the uterine or internal iliac arteries.[49,50] Uterine packing or balloon tamponade may also be useful in this situation. A hysterectomy is, however, usually required. If the diagnosis of placenta percreta can be made before any of the placental tissue is removed (as may be achieved antenatally using ultrasound) then the patient could be treated conservatively, so long as she accepts the attendant risks of haemorrhage. This involves delivering the baby as normal but leaving the placenta *in situ*. The levels of β-HCG are followed and manual removal and curettage performed when they become undetectable.[51] Methotrexate may be beneficial in this situation at a dose of 50 mg slow intravenous on alternate days.[52,53]

Preventing infection

MROP carries with it an increased risk of endometritis. In a retrospective study of 1052 women whose placentae were removed manually, 6.7% developed clinical endometritis compared with only 1.8% in those who delivered their placenta spontaneously.[54] None of the women received prophylactic antibiotics. This is similar to data from studies comparing infection rates in women who had their placentae delivered manually or spontaneously during Caesarean section.[55]

Because of the increased rate of post-partum endometritis following manual removal, it is important to take measures to prevent infection. Full aseptic procedures should, therefore, be followed and a prophylactic broad-spectrum antibiotic used.

Facilitating manual removal with tocolytics

The frequent use of ergometrine or oxytocin infusions to try and deliver a retained placenta may lead to a difficult manual removal due to closure of the cervix. Opening of the cervix is usually conducted manually, forming the fingers into a cone shape to forcibly dilate the cervix. The other hand is placed on the maternal abdomen to steady the uterus and provide counter-pressure. This can be a difficult and tiring procedure, and is made easier by the use of uterine relaxants. If a general anaesthetic is used, then relaxation will be provided for by any of the commonly used inhalation agents such as isofluorane or halothane.

If a spinal or epidural anaesthetic has been used, then nitrates may be used to relax the uterus. The commonest is nitroglycerin (also known as glyceryl trinitrate, GTN or glyceryl nitrate) given intravenously in a dose of 50–500 µg.[56–58] The initial report by Peng *et al.*[56] was of 15 women needing MROP who were treated with a 500 µg intravenous bolus of nitroglycerin. They reported that this treatment made the manual removal easier and that in 'several cases' the placenta was expelled spontaneously after the cervix opened. These were presumably the 'trapped placentae' (see above). They also reported that the mean systolic blood pressure was decreased by 8% and the mean diastolic blood pressure was decreased by 5%, although there were no adverse clinical effects of this. DeSimone *et al.*[57] reported the use of a dose of only 50 µg injected intravenously in 22 women. They found no changes in blood pressure, but marked uterine relaxation after 30–40 s in all but one (who required a second dose). The uterus recovered its tone after 1 min. Although these studies both used intravenous nitroglycerin, glyeryl trinitrate (GTN) sublingual spray (two 400 µg puffs) or GTN tablets (two 300 µg tablets) may also be effective.[59]

It is important to remember that following the use of tocolytics for MROP, the uterus may contract poorly leading to further haemorrhage. Oxytocics should, therefore, be given immediately after removal of the placenta and a careful check made to ensure that haemostasis has been achieved before finishing the procedure.

Complications of MROP

Haemorrhage is clearly a risk at the time of MROP and either oxytocin or ergometrine should be routinely used following manual removal to ensure a good uterine contraction. In the event of failure, this could be augmented with

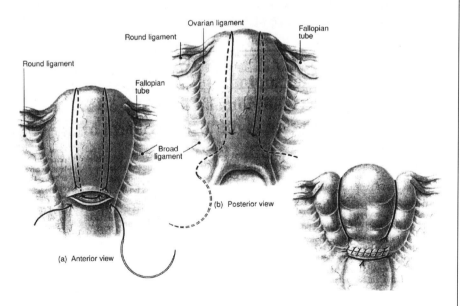

Fig. 11 The B-Lynch suture. An absorbable suture is passed through both sides of a low transverse uterine incision and then looped over the fundus whilst an assistant compresses the uterus manually. It is fixed posteriorly opposite the uterine incision before being passed back over the uterus again. The suture is finally tied anteriorly. (Diagrams from B-Lynch[60] with permission.)

carboprost 250 μg (Haemobate®) or misoprostol 1000 μg per rectum. At times, uterine packing, balloon tamponade or surgery may also be required. The B-Lynch suture (Fig. 11) has proved very useful in clinical practice for the atonic uterus.[60]

Infection in the form of endometritis is also a risk as discussed above. There are anecdotal reports of trauma or perforation of the uterine wall caused by the hand during manual removal. This may occur with the fingers through the fundus, but is more likely to occur through an old uterine scar. Setubal et al.[61] reported a case in which a woman developed a vesico-uterine fistula following an uncomplicated labour and apparently uneventful MROP. The authors warn that a thin lower segment in women with previous Caesarean sections may be susceptible to perforation.

SUMMARY

For industrialised countries

The retained placenta is a very rare cause of maternal mortality and morbidity throughout the industrialised world. Although it complicates 2% of all deliveries, the estimated case fatality rate for it in the UK is only 1 per 30 million deliveries.

Ultrasound studies have provided fresh insights into the mechanism of the third stage of labour and the aetiology of the retained placenta. Following delivery of the baby, the retro-placental myometrium is initially relaxed. It is only when it contracts that the placenta shears away from the placental bed and is detached. This leads to its spontaneous expulsion. Retained placenta occurs when the retro-placental myometrium fails to contract. There is evidence that this may also occur during labour leading to dysfunctional labour. It is likely that this is caused by the persistence of one of the placental inhibitory factors that are normally reduced prior to the onset of labour, possibly progesterone or nitric oxide.

After a placenta is retained, it is worth initially waiting for 1 h as 40% will be delivered spontaneously during this time without increases in haemorrhage. An ultrasound examination will reveal whether the placenta is detached or not. If detached, then sublingual GTN (two 400 μg puffs sublingually) may be used to relax the uterus allowing the placenta to be delivered by controlled cord traction. If, however, the placenta is seen to be attached, then an injection of 50 IU in 30 ml saline through a nasogastric tube inserted into the umbilical vein should be attempted. If this is unsuccessful, then MROP should be carried out under anaesthetic. GTN can be used to facilitate the process if the cervix is tightly constricted. A strong oxytocic should be used following manual removal to ensure effective myometrial contraction, and prophylactic antibiotics should be used to prevent infection. The recurrence rate in subsequent pregnancies is 6%.

For non-industrialised countries

The retained placenta is a significant cause of maternal mortality and morbidity throughout the non-industrialised world. It complicates 0.5% of all deliveries and has a case mortality rate of around 10% in rural areas.

Retained placenta is associated with the use of intravenous ergometrine as prophylaxis against post-partum haemorrhage, as well as with premature, induced or augmented labour. Other prophylactic oxytocics are not associated with retained placenta.

If adequate monitoring facilities are available, then it is worth initially waiting for 1 h after delivery as 40% of retained placentae will be delivered spontaneously during this time without increases in haemorrhage. Following this, an injection of 50 IU in 30 ml saline through a nasogastric tube inserted into the umbilical vein should be attempted. Alternatively, if no nasogastric tube is available, then the injection may be given directly into the cord and the cord massaged to encourage the drug up the cord into the placental bed. If this is unsuccessful after 30 min, then a MROP should be carried out under anaesthetic. A strong oxytocic should be used following manual removal to ensure effective myometrial contraction, and prophylactic antibiotics should be used to prevent infection. If MROP is difficult due to a closed cervix, then halothane may be helpful to relax the uterus. The technique of umbilical vein oxytocin injection should be taught to all midwifery and medical staff so that it can be used in rural areas, especially where theatre facilities are unavailable.

The recurrence rate in subsequent pregnancies is 6% and women should, therefore, be encouraged to attend hospital for future deliveries.

KEY POINTS FOR CLINICAL PRACTICE

- Retained placenta affects 1–2% of all deliveries

- The mortality rate of this condition is up to 10% if left untreated

- The usual reason for retained placenta is failure of the retro-placental myometrium to contract, thus preventing detachment

- The risk of major haemorrhage rises after 30 min of placental retention

- Ultrasound can distinguish between a 'trapped' placenta and an 'adherent' placenta, allowing the former to be treated with glyceryl trinitrate (two 400 mg puffs sublingually) and controlled cord traction

- For 'adherent' placentae injection of 50 IU oxytocin (in 30 ml saline) down the umbilical cord by the Papingas method is a worthwhile first-line option

- If this is unsuccessful after 30 min, then manual removal should be carried out under antibiotic cover

ACKNOWLEDGEMENT

Thanks to Dr Christian Fiala for permission to use the ultrasound image of the ruptured uterus (Fig. 4).

References

1 Combs CA, Laros RK. Prolonged third stage of labour: morbidity and risk factors. Obstet Gynecol 1991; 77: 863–867
2 Gordon JE, Gideon H, Wyon JB. Midwifery practices in rural Punjab, India. Am J Obstet Gynecol 1965; 93: 734–742

3 Tandberg A, Albrechtsen S, Iverson OE. Manual removal of placenta. Acta Obstet Gynecol Scand 1999; 78: 33–36

4 Confidential Enquiries into Maternal Deaths (CEMD). Why Mothers Die. 1997–1999. London: RCOG Press, 2001

5 Harrison KA. Childbearing, health and social priorities: survey of 22,774 consecutive hospital births in Zaria, Northern Nigeria. Br J Obstet Gynaecol 1985; 92 (Suppl 5): 100–115

6 Weeks AD, Mirembe FM. The retained placenta – new insights into an old problem (editorial). Eur J Obstet Gynecol Reprod Biol 2002; 102: 109–110

7 Enkin MW, Keirse MJNC, Renfrew MJ, Neilson JP. A Guide to Effective Care in Pregnancy and Childbirth, 2nd edn. Oxford: Oxford University Press, 1995

8 Dombrowski MP, Bottoms SF, Saleh AA, Hurd WW, Romero R. Third stage of labor: analysis of duration and clinical practice. Am J Obstet Gynecol 1995; 172 : 1279–1284

9 Carroli G, Bergel E. Umbilical vein injection for management of retained placenta (Cochrane Review). In: The Cochrane Library, Issue 1, 2003. Oxford: Update Software

10 Bider D, Dulitzky M, Goldenberg M, Lipitz S, Mashiach S. Intraumbilical vein injection of prostaglandin F_2alpha in retained placenta. Eur J Obstet Gynecol Reprod Biol 1996; 64: 59–61

11 Prendiville WJ, Elbourne D, McDonald S. Active versus expectant management of the third stage of labour (Cochrane Review). In :The Cochrane Library, Issue 1, 2003. Oxford: Update Software

12 Begley CM. A comparison of 'active' and 'physiological' management of the third stage of labour. Midwifery 1990; 6: 3–17

13 Hammar M, Boström K, Borgvall B. Comparison between the influence of methylergometrine and oxytocin on the incidence of retained placenta in the third stage of labour. Gynecol Obstet Invest 1990; 30: 91–93

14 Adelusi B, Soltan MH, Chowdhury N, Kangave D. Risk of retained placenta: multivariate approach. Acta Obstet Gynecol Scand 1997; 76: 414–418

15 Green LK, Harris RE. Uterine abnormalities. Frequency of diagnosis and associated obstetric complications. Obstet Gynecol 1976; 47: 427–429

16 Golan A, Raziel A, Pansky M, Bukovsky I. Manual removal of the placenta – its role in intrauterine adhesion formation. Int J Fertil Menop Stud 1996; 41: 450–451

17 Hall MH. Halliwell R. Carr-Hill R. Concomitant and repeated happenings of complications of the third stage of labour. Br J Obstet Gynaecol 1985; 92: 732–738

18 Rogers J, Wood J, McCandlish R, Ayers S, Truesdale A, Elbourne D. Active versus expectant management of third stage of labour: the Hinchingbrooke randomised controlled trial. Lancet 1998; 351: 693–699

19 Miller DA, Chollet JA, Goodwin TM. Clinical risk factors for placenta previa-placenta accreta. Am J Obstet Gynecol 1997; 177: 210–214

20 Brandt ML. The mechanism and management of the third stage of labour. Am J Obstet Gynecol 1933; 25: 662–667

21 Herman A, Weinraub Z, Bukovsky I et al. Dynamic ultrasonographic imaging of the third stage of labor: new perspectives into third stage mechanism. Am J Obstet Gynecol 1993; 168: 1496–1499

22 Deyer TW, Ashton-Miller JA, Van Baren PM, Pearlman MD. Myometrial contractile strain at uteroplacental separation during parturition. Am J Obstet Gynecol 2000; 183: 156–159

23 Krapp M, Baschat AA, Hankeln M, Gembruch U. Gray scale and color Doppler sonography in the third stage of labor for early detection of failed placental separation. Ultrasound Obstet Gynecol 2000; 15: 138–142

24 Wilkinson C, Enkin MW. Manual removal of placenta at caesarean section (Cochrane Review). In: The Cochrane Library, Issue 1, 2003. Oxford: Update Software

25 Weeks AD. Placental influences on the rate of labour progression: a pilot study. Eur J Obstet Gynecol Reprod Biol 2003; 106: 158–159

26 Lye SJ, Ou C-W, Teoh T-G et al. The molecular basis of labour and tocolysis. Fetal Mat Med Rev 1998; 10: 121–136

27 Weeks AD, Stewart P. The use of low dose mifepristone and vaginal misoprostol for first trimester termination of pregnancy. Br J Fam Plan 1995; 21: 85–86

28 Weeks AD, Stewart P. The use of mifepristone in combination with misoprostol for second trimester termination of pregnancy. Br J Fam Plan 1995; 21: 43–44

29 Neilson JP. Mifepristone for induction of labour (Cochrane Review). In: The Cochrane Library, Issue 1, 2003. Oxford: Update Software

30 Schellenberg JC, Liggins GC. Initiation of labour: uterine and cervical changes, endocrine changes. In: Chard T, Grudzinskas JG. (eds) The Uterus. Cambridge: Cambridge University Press, 1994

31 Thornton S, Terzidou V, Clark A, Blanks A. Progesterone metabolite and spontaneous myometrial contractions in vitro. Lancet 1999; 353: 1327–1329

32 Ledingham M-A, Thompson AJ, Greer IA, Norman JE. Nitric oxide in parturition. Br J Obstet Gynaecol 2000; 107: 581–593

33 Weeks AD, Massmann AG, Monaghan JM et al. Decreasing estrogen in nonpregnant women lowers uterine myometrial type I nitric oxide synthase protein expression. Am J Obstet Gynecol 1999; 181: 25–30

34 Ramsay B, Sooranna SR, Johnson MR. Nitric oxide synthase activities in human myometrium and villous trophoblast throughout pregnancy. Obstet Gynecol 1996; 87: 249–253

35 Thompson A, Telfer JF, Kohnen G et al. Nitric oxide synthase activity and localisation do not change in uterus and placenta during human parturition. Hum Reprod 1997; 12: 2546–2552

36 Sladek SM, Magness RR, Conrad KP. Nitric oxide and pregnancy. Am J Physiol 1997; 272: R441–R463

37 Bullough CH, Msuku RS, Karonde L. Early suckling and postpartum haemorrhage: controlled trial in deliveries by traditional birth attendants. Lancet 1989; 8662: 522–525

38 Donald I. Postpartum haemorrhage. In: Practical Obstetric Problems by Donald I. London: Lloyd-Luke Ltd, 1976

39 McDonald S. Physiology and management of the third stage of labour. In: Bennett VR, Brown LK. (eds) Myles Textbook for Midwives, 13th edn. Edinburgh: Churchill Livingstone, 1999

40 Danielsson KG, Marions L, Rodriguez A, Spur BW, Wong PYK, Bygdeman M. Comparison between oral and vaginal administration of misoprostol on uterine contractility. Obstet Gynecol 1999; 93: 275–280

41 Gulmezoglu AM, Villar J, Ngoc NT et al. WHO multicentre randomised trial of misoprostol in the management of the third stage of labour. Lancet 2001; 358: 689–695

42 Pipingas A, Hofmeyr GJ, Sesel KR. Umbilical vessel oxytocin administration for retained placenta: in-vitro study of various infusion techniques. Am J Obstet Gynecol 1993; 168: 793–795

43 Wilken-Jensen C, Strom V, Nielsen MD, Rosenkilde-Gram B. Removing placenta by oxytocin – a controlled study. Am J Obstet Gynecol 1989; 161: 155–156

44 Hendricks CH, Brenner WE. Cardiovascular effects of oxytocic drugs used post partum Am J Obstet Gynecol 1970; 108: 751

45 Patient C, Davison JM, Charlton L, Baylis PH, Thornton S. The effect of labour and maternal oxytocin infusion on fetal plasma oxytocin concentration. Br J Obstet Gynaecol 1999; 106: 1311–1313

46 Chauhan P. Volume and site of injection of oxytocin solution is important in the medical treatment of retained placenta. Int J Obstet Gynecol 2000; 70(Suppl 1): A83

47 Carroli G, Belizan JM, Grant A, Gonzalez L, Campodonico L, Bergel E for the Grupo Argentino de Estudio de Placenta Retenida. Intra-umbilical vein injection and retained placenta: evidence from a collaborative large randomised controlled trial. Br J Obstet Gynaecol 1998; 105: 179–185

48 Reyes FI, Winter JSD, Faiman C. Postpartum disappearance of chorionic gonadotrophin from the maternal and neonatal circulations. Am J Obstet Gynecol 1985; 153: 486–489

49 Morken NH, Henriksen H. Placenta percreta – two cases and review of the literature. Eur J Obstet Gynecol Reprod Biol. 2001; 100: 112–115

50 Johanson RB. Mechanism and management of placental non-separation. In: Kingdom J, Jauniaux E, O'Brien S. (eds) The Placenta: Basic Science and Clinical Practice. London: RCOG Press, 2000

51 Dunstone SJ, Leibowitz CB. Conservative management of placenta praevia with a high risk

of placenta accreta. Aust NZ J Obstet Gynaecol 1998; 38: 429–433

52 Arulkumaran S, Ng CSA, Ingemarsson I, Ratnam SS. Medical treatment of placenta accreta with methotrexate. Acta Obstet Gynecol Scand 1986; 65: 285–286

53 Gupta D, Sinha R. Management of placenta accreta with oral methotrexate. Int J Gynecol Obstet 1998; 60: 171–173

54 Ely JW, Rijhsinghani A, Bowdler NC, Dawson J. The association between manual removal of the placenta and postpartum endometritis following vaginal delivery. Obstet Gynecol 1995; 86: 1002–1006

55 Atkinson MW, Owen J, Wren A, Hauth JC. The effect of manual removal of the placenta on post-Cesarean endometritis. Obstet Gynecol 1996; 87: 99–102

56 Peng AT, Gorman RS, Shulman SM, DeMarchis E, Nyunt K, Blancato LS. Intravenous nitroglycerin for uterine relaxation in the postpartum patient with retained placenta. Anesthesiology 1989; 71: 172–173

57 DeSimone CA, Norris MC, Leighton BL. Intravenous nitroglycerin aids manual extraction of a retained placenta. Anesthesiology. 1990; 73: 787

58 Axemo P, Fu X, Lindberg B, Ulmsten U, Wessen A. Intravenous nitroglycerin for rapid uterine relaxation. Acta Obstet Gynecol Scand 1998; 77: 50–53

59 Greenspoon JS, Kovacic A. Breech extraction facilitated by glyceryl trinitrate sublingual spray. Lancet 1991; 338: 124–125

60 B-Lynch C, Coker A, Lawal AH, Abu J, Cowen MJ. The B-Lynch surgical technique for the control of massive postpartum haemorrhage: an alternative to hysterectomy? Five cases reported. Br J Obstet Gynaecol 1997; 104: 372–375

61 Setubal A, Clode N, Bruno-Paiva JL, Roncon I, Graça LM. Vesicouterine fistula after manual removal of placenta in a woman with previous Cesarean section. Eur J Obstet Gynecol Reprod Biol 1999; 84: 75–76

62 Calderale L, Dalle NF, Franzoi R, Vitalini R. Éutile la somministrazione di ossitocina nella vena ombilicale per il trttamento della placenta ritenuta? G Ital Ostet Ginecol 1994; 16(5): 283-286. Quoted in: Carroli G, Bergel E. Umbilical vein injection for management of retained placenta (Cochrane Review). In: *The Cochrane Library*, Issue 1, 2003. Oxford: Update Software

63 Frappell JM, Pearce JM, McParland P. Intra-umbilical vein oxytocin in the management of retained placenta: a random, prospective, double blind, placebo controlled study. J Obstet Gynaecol 1988; 8: 322–324

64 Gazvani MR, Luckas MJM, Drakeley AJ, Emery SJ, Alfirevic Z, Walkinshaw SA. Intraumbilical oxytocin for the management of retained placenta: a randomized controlled trial. Obstet Gynecol 1998; 91: 203–207

65 Hansen P, Jorgensen L, Dueholm M, Hansen S. Intraumbilical oxytocin in the treatment of retained placenta. Ugeskr Laeger 1987; 149: 3318-3319. Quoted in: Carroli G & Bergel E. Umbilical vein injection for management of retained placenta (Cochrane Review). In: *The Cochrane Library*, Issue 1, 2003. Oxford: Update Software

66 Huber MGP, Wildschut HIJ, Boer K, Kleiverda G, Hoek FJ. Umbilical vein administration of oxytocin for the management of retained placenta: It is effective? Am J Obstet Gynecol 1991; 164: 1216–1219

67 Kristiansen FV, Frost L, Kaspersen P, Moller BR. The effect of oxytocin injection into the umbilical vein for the management of retained placenta. Am J Obstet Gynecol 1987; 156: 979–980

68 Selinger M, Mackenzie IZ, Dunlop P, James D. Intra-umbilical vein oxytocin in the management of retained placenta. A double blind placebo controlled study. J Obstet Gynaecol 1986; 7: 115–117

69 Thiery M. Management of retained placenta with oxytocin injection into the umbilical vein. Personal communication quoted in: Carroli G, Bergel E. Umbilical vein injection for management of retained placenta (Cochrane Review). In: *The Cochrane Library*, Issue 1, 2003. Oxford: Update Software

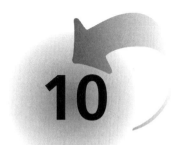

Keerthy R. Sunder Debra L. Bogen
Katherine L. Wisner

Contemporary issues in peripartum depression

Maternal morbidity due to psychiatric disorders is common. Suicide is the leading cause of maternal death in the UK.[1] World-wide, depression during pregnancy and the postpartum period remains the least recognised complication of childbearing, with tragic outcomes for the family and society.

EPIDEMIOLOGY

The *Diagnostic and Statistical Manual of Mental Disorders* (4th edn; DSM-IV) defines postpartum depression as a major depressive episode that occurs within 4 weeks of delivery,[2] although epidemiological studies suggest 3 months after delivery as the period of elevated risk for new onset depressive episodes.[3] Postpartum emotional disturbances that last beyond 2-weeks post-birth suggest depression rather than 'baby blues'. The term 'baby blues' refers to a mild, self-limiting condition characterised by tearfulness and lability of mood in the first 2-weeks post-birth.

Affective disorders are twice as common in women as in men and the prevalence of depression is less than 20% in women in the general population.[4] Large cross-sectional studies that use screening tools consistently find high rates of pregnancy and postpartum depressive symptoms. Marcus *et al.*[5] found that 20% of pregnant women scored above the threshold of 16 on the Center for

Keerthy R. Sunder MD MS DRCOG
Senior Resident Physician in Psychiatry, Magee Women's Hospital and Western Psychiatric Institute and Clinic/University of Pittsburgh Medical Center, 3811 O'Hara Street, Pittsburgh, PA 15213, USA (for correspondence, E-mail: sunderkr@upmc.edu)

Debra L. Bogen MD FAAP
Assistant Professor of Pediatrics, Children's Hospital of Pittsburgh, University of Pittsburgh Medical Center, Pittsburgh, PA 15213, USA

Katherine L. Wisner MD MS
Professor of Psychiatry, Obstetrics and Gynecology and Reproductive Sciences, and Epidemiology, Director, Women's Behavioral HealthCARE, Western Psychiatric Institute and Clinic/University of Pittsburgh Medical Center, Pittsburgh, PA 15213, USA

Epidemiological Studies-Depression scale (CES-D). In a British study that involved 14,000 pregnant women, Evans et al.[6] found that 13.5% and 9.1% of women scored above the threshold for depression at 32 weeks of pregnancy and at 8 weeks postpartum, respectively. A score of $\geq$ 13 on the Edinburgh Postnatal Depression Scale (EPDS) was used in this study.

AETIOLOGY

At least three possible aetiologies have been suggested to explain depression and depressive symptoms among pregnant and postpartum women, including reproductive hormones, thyroid hormones and social stress.

Reproductive hormones

Reproductive hormonal fluctuations modulate central affective function. Oestrogen-modulated N-methyl-D-aspartate receptors induce the formation of new synapses. This observation suggests a pivotal role for oestrogen in the plasticity of the nervous system.[7]

Exposure to and withdrawal from the neurosteroidal metabolite of progesterone, allopregnanolone,[8] influence a principal regulator of cognitive function and affect, the GABA-A receptor. Selective serotonin re-uptake inhibitors (SSRIs), such as fluoxetine and paroxetine, increased brain concentrations of allopregnanolone in rats, which may explain their antidepressant efficacy in depressed patients mediated via GABAergic receptor activity.[9] Additionally, the SSRI sertraline prevents postpartum depression while the tricyclic antidepressant nortriptyline does not. This phenomenon may be explained by the fact that SSRIs increase brain levels of neuroactive steroids, which may decrease the risk for depression in the postpartum milieu.[10]

The long-standing assumption that gonadal steroid hormone withdrawal plays a role in the pathophysiology of puerperal affective disorders was supported by data from Bloch and colleagues.[11] These investigators induced hypogonadism in 16 women with a gonadotropin-releasing hormone agonist and then administered oestrogen and progesterone to mimic a pregnancy state. An analogue of the puerperium was attained by an abrupt replacement of hormones with placebo. Of eight women with a prior history of postpartum depression, four developed depression which provides direct evidence that a subpopulation of women with a history of postpartum depression is differentially sensitive to the mood-destabilising effects of sex steroid fluctuations.[11]

Thyroid hormones

Postpartum thyroid dysfunction occurs in 5–10% of women within 1 year following delivery and may predispose a woman to affective dysregulation.[12] Simultaneous treatment of both the thyroid dysfunction and the affective disorder is usually essential for optimum treatment results.[13]

Social stress

Prior depressive episodes are strong predictors of postpartum depression. Antepartum depression, marital discord, and stressful life events are added risk factors for postpartum depression. Breast-feeding, parity and advanced maternal age are not associated with increased risk for peripartum depression.[14–16]

MATERNAL DEPRESSION AND REPRODUCTIVE TOXICITY

Behavioural perinatology investigators have examined the maternal, fetal and infant effects of peripartum mood disorders along the following domains.

Fetal growth

Prenatal stress has been implicated as a developmental teratogen in animal studies with effects on maternal–fetal physiology (placental CRH activity), gestational age (preterm labour) and fetal growth (growth retardation and low birth weight).[17] A significant association between increased uterine artery resistance and maternal anxiety in the third trimester has been demonstrated that suggests its role in fetal growth restriction and pre-eclampsia.[18,19]

Preterm labour

In neuroendocrine studies of major depressive disorder (MDD), HPA axis dysfunction remains one of the most reproducible findings.[20] Elevated placental corticotropin-releasing hormone (CRH) levels derived from an activated HPA axis are associated with spontaneous preterm labour.[21] Several studies confirm significantly elevated levels of CRH in cases of preterm labour compared to gestational age-matched controls.[18,22]

Pre-eclampsia

A population-based study that involved 623 nulliparous women with singleton pregnancies demonstrated that depression, anxiety, or both were associated with increased risk for pre-eclampsia.[23] Altered excretion of vasoactive hormones or neuroendocrine transmitters during stress and depression may be responsible for the increased risk for hypertension.[24,25]

Paediatric effects

Maternal depression is associated with excessive crying in newborns,[26] and depressed mothers discontinue breast-feeding earlier than non-depressed controls.[27] A life-time history of depression is twice as common in children of depressed mothers relative to children of never-depressed mothers. This increased risk occurs after brief (1–2 months) exposure to maternal major depression.[28] Suboptimal cognitive and emotional development of the child has been related to difficulties in the early mother–infant relationship.[29] The children from families with mothers who suffered depressive symptoms at 2 months postpartum showed less persistence in play, and less joy in re-union after separation from their mothers compared with children of non-depressed mothers at 15–18 months.[30]

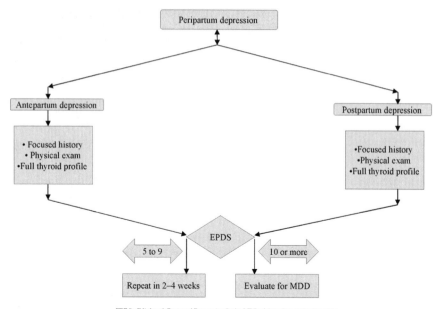

EPDS= Edinburgh Postnatal Depression Scale; MDD= Major Depressive Disorder

Fig. 1 Peripartum depression screening algorithm.

DETECTION OF PERIPARTUM DEPRESSION

An algorithm for screening peripartum depression is given in Figure 1.

Obstetric settings

Contrary to popular belief, pregnancy does not confer protection against depressive illness nor enhance the rate of its detection by professionals. Given the routine investment in time and resources for peripartum care, the role of sensitive history taking and screening for depression by obstetric staff cannot be overestimated.[31] In a depression screening survey by non-clinical staff on 3472 pregnant women across 10 obstetric clinics, Marcus et al.[5] obtained significant (90%) response rates from women in completing the survey.

Paediatric settings

Paediatric well-baby visits, which usually occur 6 times during the first year of life, provide another opportunity to screen mothers. Of 338 eligible mothers who participated in a screening survey for postpartum depression, 77% of the surveys were completed by the child's designated paediatric provider.[32] However, the reluctance among health-care professionals and mothers alike about screening for depression in traditional peripartum settings remains a continuing challenge.

The Edinburgh Postnatal Depression Scale (EPDS)

The EPDS is a user-friendly, 10-item self-report measure validated for antepartum and postpartum use.[33,34] An EPDS score of >10 identified 100% of

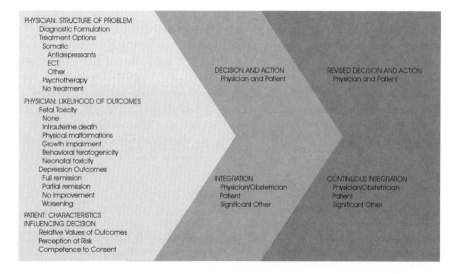

Fig. 2 Model for decisions regarding treatment of depression during pregnancy.[37] Copyright (2000), The American Psychiatric Association <http://psychiatryonline.org>; reprinted with permission.

women who became depressed in a British community sample comprising 86 recently delivered mothers.[35] Cox *et al.*[36] have suggested a cut-off of >12 to provide the best compromise between false-positives and false-negatives. A score between 5 and 9 on the EPDS should be followed by a re-evaluation in 2–4 weeks to determine whether depression has evolved following birth.[3] A diagnostic interview should follow a positive screen. Any positive score on the self-harm item 10 of EPDS is serious and a systematic inquiry for suicidal thoughts and infanticidal thoughts is warranted.[36] Urgent psychiatric consultation is recommended in these cases. The EPDS is presented in Appendix 1.

REPRODUCTIVE PHYSIOLOGY, PHARMACOLOGY AND TOXICITY

Established treatments for depression include antidepressant medication, psychotherapy and electro-convulsive therapy (ECT). However, physicians need to take into account multiple factors before recommending treatment strategies. Wisner *et al.*[37] described a model that used case vignettes to frame the approach to risk–benefit decision-making (Fig. 2).

Peripartum pharmacokinetics

Reproductive physiology
Increased activity of the cytoplasmic P4502D6 isoenzyme during pregnancy[38] and proliferation of the hepatic endoplasmic reticulum during the last 3 months of pregnancy have been demonstrated.[39] Also, enhanced hepatic metabolism, increased distribution volume, decreased protein-binding capacity, progesterone-induced decrease in gastrointestinal motility and increased glomerular filtration changes all contribute to progressive increases in antidepressant dose requirements during pregnancy.[40]

Reproductive pharmacology

The dosage of SSRIs needs to be increased to maintain antidepressant efficacy during pregnancy.[41] Suboptimal treatment may occur due to the tendency to keep doses low during pregnancy coupled with an increased clearance rate, especially during the latter half of pregnancy.[42] Heikkinen et al.[43] showed a 2.4-fold mean increase in the metabolic ratio of norfluoxetine/fluoxetine in late pregnancy with proportionately low serum concentrations of fluoxetine. Pharmacotherapy in the postpartum period requires a judicious approach. Diminished metabolism of tricyclic antidepressants during the early postpartum period[44] would require cautious follow-up and dose adjustments during the first 8 weeks after delivery. Comparable postpartum data for SSRIs are not available.

Reproductive toxicity

The categorical format (A, B, C, D, X) of teratogenic risk as classified by the Food and Drug Administration is under revision.[45] The sophistication of risk–benefit decision analysis has improved with the incorporation of multiple domains of reproductive toxicity.[46] Intra-uterine fetal death, morphological teratogenicity, growth impairment, neonatal toxicity and neurobehavioural teratogenicity represent these five domains.[46]

Intra-uterine death

Intra-uterine death is not associated with exposure to fluoxetine,[47–50] sertraline, paroxetine, citalopram and fluvoxamine,[48,50,51] venlafaxine,[52] or tricyclic antidepressants.[47–49]

Morphological teratogenicity

Minor malformations (which by definition have no functional or cosmetic significance) have been reported after first trimester fluoxetine exposure.[50] Major malformations have not been reported with tricyclics, the SSRIs, venlafaxine or the phenylpiperazine antidepressants, trazadone and nefazadone.[47–53]

Growth impairment (low birth-weight, small for gestational age infants and preterm labour)

In small cohort studies, comparable antenatal growth and birth weights occurred in infants exposed to tricyclics, newer SSRIs, venlafaxine, trazadone and nefazadone relative to non-depressed controls.[47,48,51–53] In a study that involved 969 pregnant women, the mean birth weight in a specific pregnancy week was greater in infants of mothers who were on antidepressants compared with non-depressed controls.[49] Chambers et al.[50] reported significantly lower birth weights related to lower maternal weight gain after fluoxetine exposure in the third trimester.

Simon et al.[48] reported a 2-fold increase in preterm labour after SSRI exposure that was not limited to infants exposed late in pregnancy. However, they did not report the specific dosing or timing of treatment during pregnancy to justify the negative attributions to the SSRI exposure. Obstetrical factors were not excluded and depressive symptoms were not assessed directly. The active (state) effects of depression and the residual (trait) effects (changes in maternal physiology which remain even when the mother is asymptomatic) could affect pregnancy outcome negatively. Thus, the negative outcomes attributed to the SSRI may well have been related to either unremitting depression or the interaction of depression with SSRI exposure.[51]

Chambers et al.[50] also reported an increased risk for preterm birth (14.3%) in infants whose mothers took fluoxetine in the third trimester compared to infants whose mothers discontinued fluoxetine before the third trimester (4.1%) as well as controls (5.6%). Compared to a combined group of infants whose mothers took paroxetine during the first and second trimesters as well as controls, increased preterm birth in infants whose mothers took paroxetine in the third trimester has been reported.[54]. Firm conclusions based on these early observations await further robust studies.

Neonatal toxicity

Both withdrawal symptoms and direct pharmacological toxic effects can occur after prenatal exposure to any antidepressant. Simon et al.[48] recently reported lower APGAR scores after third trimester SSRI exposure. Anticholinergic stimulation causing bladder distension and gastrointestinal stasis in newborns has been described.[55] Serotonin overstimulation (myoclonus, restlessness, tremor, shivering, hyper-reflexia, incoordination, rigidity) with fluoxetine,[56,57] paroxetine,[58–60] and sertraline has also been reported.[61]

The risk of withdrawal reactions may be greater with short half-life drugs such as paroxetine and venlafaxine when compared with fluoxetine.[62] The half-lives of paroxetine and sertraline are similar at 24 h but the largely inactive metabolite of sertraline, desmethylsertraline, is eliminated slowly,[66] which prevents occurrence of frequent withdrawal reactions.[62] It has been suggested that a dose taper before delivery will minimise the fetal drug load at birth.[63] However, predicting labour is rarely accurate; therefore, this decision requires clinical judgement based on a risk–benefit analysis.

Behavioural teratogenicity

Antepartum exposure to agents that affect the central nervous system can impact the neurology and behaviour of the infant in the postpartum period.[64] Oberlander et al.[65] examined pain sensitivity in SSRI-exposed neonates relative to controls and found attenuated acute pain response in the SSRI-exposed group that persisted at 2 months of age. Increased tremulousness, increased sleep times and REM sleep in newborns exposed to SSRIs relative to unexposed newborns has been recently reported.[66] The long-term significance of these findings remains to be established. In a 7-year follow-up study, Nulman et al.[67,68] reported that global IQ, verbal comprehension, expressive language development, temperament and general behaviour were similar in children exposed at any time in pregnancy to tricyclics or fluoxetine compared with controls. Similar studies on newer drugs are not available.

TREATMENTS AND PROPHYLAXIS

Clinical trials in postpartum depression

In the only published randomised controlled trial of pharmacotherapy in postpartum depression, significant antidepressant effects measured as mean scores on the EPDS were seen with both fluoxetine and six sessions of cognitive behavioural counselling with no additive effect of the two treatments.[69] Postpartum depression may be more responsive to SSRIs (79%) than to tricyclics (67%) as demonstrated in an open trial.[70]

Lactation

Based on multiple case series evaluating its safety profile, sertraline is recommended as the SSRI of choice in lactating mothers.[71] Weismann *et al.*[72] conducted a meta-analysis of data from 1966 to August 2001 and examined antidepressant levels in lactating mothers, breast-milk and nursing infants. Fluoxetine (29.4%) produced the highest proportion of infant levels elevated above 10% of the average maternal level, followed by citalopram (16.7%) and sertraline (7.6%). Infant levels of nortryptiline and paroxetine were undetectable. Levels of venlafaxine and its active metabolite were low or unquantifiable in three nursing mother/infant pairs.[73]

The long-term effects of breast feeding on the physical and cognitive development of infants of depressed mothers who take antidepressants remain unknown. Infant levels are highly correlated with maternal dose and breast milk level for citalopram and fluoxetine, but current data do not support measuring breast milk levels or serum levels except in premature or sick infants as a measure of exposure.[72,73]

Alternative treatments

Interpersonal therapy (IPT)
Women with postpartum depression were 2–3 times more likely to recover when randomly assigned to 12 sessions of interpersonal therapy (IPT) compared to the wait list control.[74] In a group intervention study based on IPT during pregnancy, Zlotnick *et al.*[75] successfully prevented postpartum depression in at-risk women while 33% of the treatment as usual control group developed major depressive disorder.

Electro-convulsive therapy (ECT)
Electro-convulsive therapy (ECT) administration is recommended as first-line treatment if psychotic symptoms are present[76] and as an effective alternative to untreated depression in the peripartum period. However, uterine tocodynamometry and fetal cardiotocography monitoring to detect premature uterine activity and fetal arrhythmias are recommended precautions during ECT administration.

Oestrogen therapy
Endogenous oestrogenic steroids exert both genomic and non-genomic activational effects on brain function.[77] Gregoire *et al.*[78] studied the antidepressive properties of transdermal oestrogen (17β-oestradiol) in 61 women with chronic treatment-resistant postpartum depression. The mean EPDS scores improved rapidly during the first month of treatment when compared with controls with an overall treatment effect of 4.38 points on the EPDS (95% CI, 1.89–6.87). Although sustained over 5 months, the oestradiol

antidepressant effect was confounded by the co-administration of antidepressants in half the population.

Bright light therapy

The effectiveness of bright light therapy for antepartum depression was provided in a small controlled trial. Ten pregnant women were randomised to 5 weeks of 7000-lux box (active) or a 500-lux (placebo) box. At 10 weeks, there was a significant treatment effect; phase advancement of melatonin circadian rhythm on measured salivary melatonin levels was correlated with the treatment effect.[79]

Essential fatty acids

Hibbeln[80] and Otto et al.[81] demonstrated a significant association between low docasahexaenoic acid (DHA) levels, an ω-3 essential fatty acid, and the occurrence of postpartum depression. In an open-label trial of ω-3 essential fatty acids, 7 depressed women at least 16 weeks pregnant were prescribed between 0.93 and 2.8 g/day of eicosapentaenoic and docosahexaenoic acid (EPA/DHA).[82] Five of the seven patients experienced a decrease of > 40% on the EPDS scores which were > 12 at the beginning of the study. This approach merits further studies because of its safety and tolerability.

Acupuncture

Manber et al.[83] randomised 61 women to active acupuncture, valid control acupuncture that did not address depression symptoms and massage for 8 weeks. Responders were provided treatment until 10 weeks postpartum. The active acupuncture group achieved a 43.8% remission in symptoms compared with 21.1% in the control group and 31.6% in the massage group.[83] This novel study provides preliminary efficacy data for acupuncture treatment in antepartum depression and warrants further trials.

Prevention trials in postpartum depression

Women who have experienced postpartum depression have a 25% risk of recurrence with a subsequent pregnancy.[84] Thus, women with a history of postpartum depression should be at a minimum closely monitored with established screening tools. Preventive pharmacotherapy should also be considered after delivery. Effective prophylaxis may require treatment for 6 months using the drug that previously provided a good response or from an SSRI.[84,85] Following the treatment phase, a gradual taper of the antidepressant dose at a rate of 33% per week is recommended to prevent the onset of a discontinuation syndrome.[86]

THE FUTURE

The US Surgeon General's report[87] proclaims that 'mental health is fundamental to health'. Cross-specialty collaboration in real-world peripartum settings has already begun. Translational research holds promise in helping mothers access effective evidence-based treatments. It is imperative that physicians take the lead in destigmatising this burdensome but easily recognised and treated complication of childbearing. Web-based public educational tools such as Postpartum Support

International (<www.postpartum.net>), Depression after Delivery (<http://www.depressionafterdelivery.com/>) and WomensbehavioralhealthCARE (<www.womensbehavioralhealth.org>) should be popularised in diverse health settings to heighten our efforts to recognise and address this treatable condition.

ACKNOWLEDGEMENT

The authors wish to thank Dr Eydie Moses-Kolko MD for her constructive suggestions in the preparation of this manuscript.

References

1   National Institute for Clinical Excellence (NICE). Why Mothers Die 1997–1999: The Confidential Enquiries into Maternal Deaths in the United Kingdom. London: Royal College of Obstetricians and Gynecologists, 2001
2   American Psychiatric Association. Diagnostic and Statistical Manual of Mental Disorders, 4th edn. Washington, DC: American Psychiatric Association, 1994
3   Kendell RE, Chalmers JC, Platz C. Epidemiology of puerperal psychoses. Br J Psychiatry 1987; 151: 135
4   Weissman MM, Klerman GL. Sex differences and the epidemiology of depression. Arch Gen Psychiatry 1977; 34: 98–111
5   Marcus SM, Flynn HA, Blow FC, Barry KL. Depressive symptoms among pregnant women screened in obstetric settings. J Womens Health 2003; 12: 373–380
6   Evans J, Heron J, Francomb H, Oke S, Golding J. Cohort study of depressed mood during pregnancy and after childbirth. BMJ 2001; 323: 257–260
7   Wooley C, McEwen BS. Estradiol regulates hippocampal dendritic spine density via an N-methyl-D-aspartate receptor-dependent mechanism. J Neurosci 1994; 14: 7680–7687
8   Sundstrom PI, Smith S, Gulinello M. GABA receptors, progesterone and premenstrual dysphoric disorder. Arch Womens Mental Health 2003; 6: 23–41
9   Uzunov DP, Cooper TB, Costa E, Guidotti A. Fluoxetine-elicited changes in brain neurosteroid content measured by negative ion mass fragmentography. Proc Natl Acad Sci USA 1996; 93: 599–604
10 Griffin LS, Mellon SH. Selective serotonin reuptake inhibitors directly alter activity of neurosteroidogenic enzymes. Proc Natl Acad Sci USA 1999; 96: 13512–13517
11 Bloch M, Schmidt PJ, Rubinow DR *et al*. Effects of gonadal steroids in women with a history of postpartum depression. Am J Psychiatry 2000; 157: 56–62
12 Mestman JH. Evaluating and managing postpartum thyroid dysfunction. Medscape Womens Health 1997; 2: 3
13 Wisner KL, Stowe ZN. Psychobiology of postpartum mood disorders. Semin Reprod Endocrinol 1997; 15: 77–89
14 O'Hara MW, Swain AM. Rates and risk of postpartum depression: a meta-analysis. Int Rev Psychiatry 1996; 8: 37–54
15 Swendsen JD, Mazure CM. Life stress as a risk factor for postpartum depression: current research and methodological issues. Clin Psychol Sci Pract 2000; 7: 17–31
16 O'Hara MW. Postpartum mental disorders. In: Sciarra JJ. (ed) Gynecology and Obstetrics, vol. 6. Philadelphia: Harper & Row, 1991; 1–17
17 Wadhwa PD. Prenatal stress and life span development. In: Friedman HS. (ed) Encyclopedia of Mental Health, vol. 3. San Diego: Academic Press, 1998; 265–280
18 McLean M, Bisits A, Davies J *et al*. A placental clock controlling the length of human pregnancy. Nat Med 1995; 1: 460–463
19 Teixeira JMA, Fisk MN, Glover V. Association between maternal anxiety in pregnancy and increased uterine artery resistance index: cohort based study. BMJ 1999; 318: 153–157
20 Wisner KL, Stowe ZN. Psychobiology of postpartum mood disorders. Semin Reprod Endocrinol 1997; 15: 77–89
21 Wadhwa PD, Sandman CA, Garite TJ *et al*. The association between prenatal stress and infant birth weight and gestational age at birth: a prospective investigation. Am J Obstet

Gynecol 1993; 169: 858–865

22 Holzman C, Jetton J, Siler-Khodr et al. Second trimester corticotropin-releasing hormone levels in relation to preterm delivery and ethnicity. Obstet Gynecol 2001; 97: 657–663

23 Kurki T, Hiilesmaa V, Ylikorkala O et al. Depression and anxiety in early pregnancy and risk of preeclampsia. Obstet Gynecol 2000; 95: 487–490

24 Sandman C, Wadhwa P, Chicz-DeMet A, Dunkel-Schetter C, Porto M. Maternal stress, HPA activity, and fetal/infant outcome. Ann NY Acad Sci 1997; 814: 266–275

25 Potter W, Manji H. Catecholamines in depression: an update. Clin Chem 1994; 40: 279–287

26 Zuckerman B, Bauchner H, Parker S, Cabral H. Maternal depressive symptoms during pregnancy and newborn irritability. J Dev Behav Pediatr 1990; 11: 190–194

27 Cooper PJ, Murray L, Stein A. Psychosocial factors associated with the early termination of breastfeeding. J Psychosom Res 1993; 37: 171–176

28 Hammen C, Brennan PA. Severity, chronicity, and timing of maternal depression and risk for adolescent offspring diagnoses in a community sample. Arch Gen Psychiatry 2003; 60: 253–258

29 Sinclair D, Murray L. Effects of postnatal depression on children's adjustment to school. Br J Psychiatry 1998; 172: 58–63

30 Edhborg M, Lundh W, Seimyr L, Widstrom AM. The parent-child relationship in the context of maternal depressive mood. Arch Womens Mental Health 2003: 6: 211–216

31 Fergerson SS, Jamieson DJ, Lindsay M. Diagnosing postpartum depression: Can we do better? Am J Obstet Gynecol 2002; 186: 899–902

32 Heneghan AM, Silver EJ, Bauman LJ, Stein REK. Do pediatricians recognize mothers with depressive symptoms? Pediatrics 2000; 106: 1367–1373

33 Murray D, Cox JL. Screening for depression during pregnancy with the Edinburgh depression scale (EPDS). J Reprod Infant Psychol 1990; 8: 99–107

34 Thorpe K. A study of the Edinburgh postnatal depression scale for use with parent groups outside the postpartum period. J Reprod Infant Psychol 1993; 11: 119–125

35 Cox JL, Holden JM, Sagovsky R. Detection of postnatal depression: Development of the 10-item Edinburgh Postnatal Depression Scale. Br J Psychiatry 1987; 150: 782–786

36 Holden JM, Sagovsky R, Cox JL. Counseling in a general practice setting: a controlled study of health visitor intervention in the treatment of postnatal depression. BMJ 1989; 298: 223–226

37 Wisner KL, Zarin DA, Frank E et al. Risk–benefit decision making for treatment of depression during pregnancy. Am J Psychiatry 2000; 157: 1933–1940

38 Wadelius M, Darj E, Frenne G, Rane A. Induction of CYP2D6 in pregnancy. Clin Pharmacol Ther 1997; 62: 400–407

39 Perez V, Gorodisch S, Casavilla F, Maruffo C. Ultrastructure of human liver at the end of normal pregnancy. Isr J Obstet Gynecol 1971; 110: 428–431

40 Cupit GC, Rotmensch HH. Principles of drug therapy in pregnancy. In: Gleicher N. (ed) Principles of Medical Therapy in Pregnancy. New York: Plenum, 1985; 77–90

41 Hostetter A, Stowe ZN, Strader JR, McLaughlin E, Llewellyn A. Dose of selective serotonin uptake inhibitors across pregnancy: clinical implications. Depression Anxiety 2000; 11: 51–57

42 Nulman I, Gargaun S, Koren G. Suboptimal pharmacotherapy for depression in pregnancy. Clin Pharmacol Ther 2003; 73: 28

43 Heikkinen T, Ekblad U, Palo P et al. Pharmacokinetics of fluoxetine and norfluoxetine in pregnancy and lactation. Clin Pharmacol Ther 2003; 73: 330–337

44 Wisner KL, Perel JM, Hanusa BH et al. Effects of the postpartum period on nortriptyline pharmacokinetics. Psychopharmacol Bull 1997; 33: 243–248

45 Center for Drug Evaluation and Research notice of part 15 hearings. Prescription drugs and biological products labeling. 97 Federal Register 20247, 1997

46 Wisner KL, Gelenberg AJ, Leonard H, Appelbaum P, Zarin D, Frank E. Pharmacologic treatment of depression during pregnancy. JAMA 1999; 282: 1264–1269

47 Pastuszak A, Schick-Boschetto B, Zuber C et al. Pregnancy outcome following first-trimester exposure to fluoxetine (Prozac). JAMA 1993; 269: 2247–2248

48 Simon GE, Cunningham ML, Davis RL. Outcomes of prenatal antidepressant exposure. Am J Psychiatry 2002; 159: 2055–2061

49 Ericson A, Kallen B, Wiholm BE. Delivery outcome after the use of antidepressants in early pregnancy. Eur J Clin Pharmacol 1999; 55: 503–508

50 Chambers CD, Johnson KA, Dick LN, Felix RJ, Jones KL. Birth outcomes in pregnant women taking fluoxetine. N Engl J Med 1996; 335: 1010–1015

51 Kulin NA, Pastuszak A, Sage SR. Pregnancy outcome following maternal use of the new selective serotonin reuptake inhibitors. JAMA 1998; 279: 609–610

52 Einarson A, Fatoye B, Koren G et al. Pregnancy outcome following gestational exposure to venlafaxine: a multicenter prospective controlled study. Am J Psychol 2001; 158: 1728–1730

53 Einarson A, Bonari L, Voyer-Lavigne S et al. A multicenter prospective controlled study to determine the safety of trazadone and nefazadone use during pregnancy. Can J Psychol 2003; 48: 106–110

54 Costei MA, Kozer E, Ho T, Ito S, Koren G. Perinatal outcome following third trimester exposure to paroxetine. Arch Pediatr Adolesc Med 2002; 156: 1129–1132

55 Wisner KL, Perel JM. Psychopharmacologic agents and electro convulsive therapy during pregnancy and the puerperium. In: Cohen RL. (ed) Psychiatric Consultation in Childbirth Settings. New York, NY: Plenum, 1998; 165–206

56 Spencer MJ. Fluoxetine hydrochloride (Prozac) toxicity in a neonate. Pediatrics 1993; 92: 721–722

57 Mhanna MJ, Bennet JB, Izatt SD. Potential fluoxetine chloride (Prozac) toxicity in a newborn. Pediatrics 1997; 100: 158–159

58 Dahl ML, Olhager E, Ahlner J. Paroxetine withdrawal syndrome in a neonate. Br J Psychiatry 1997; 171: 391–392

59 Gerola O, Fiocchi S, Rondini G. Antidepressant therapy in pregnancy: a review from the literature and report of a suspected paroxetine withdrawal syndrome in a newborn. Riv Ital Pediatr 1999; 25: 216–218

60 Stiskal JA, Kulin N, Koren G et al. Neonatal paroxetine withdrawal syndrome. Arch Dis Child Fetal Neonatal Ed 2001; 84: F134–F135

61 Kent LS, Laidlaw JD. Suspected congenital sertraline dependence. Br J Psychiatry 1995; 167: 412–413

62 Trenque T, Piednoir D, Germain ML et al. Reports of withdrawal syndrome with the use of SSRIs: a case/non-case study in the French Pharmacovigilance database. Pharmacoepidemiol Drug Safety 2002; 11: 281–283.

63 Lane K, Heikkinen T, Ekblad U, Kero P. Effects of exposure to SSRIs during pregnancy on serotonergic symptoms in newborns and cord blood monoamine and prolactin concentrations. Arch Gen Psychiatry 2003; 60: 720–726

64 Wisner KL. Antidepressant therapy during pregnancy. Primary Psychiatry 1996; 3: 40–42

65 Oberlander TF, Grunau RE, Fitzgerald C et al. Prolonged prenatal psychotropic medication exposure alters neonatal acute pain response. Pediatr Res 2002; 51: 443–453

66 Zeskind PE, Stephens LE. Maternal selective serotonin reuptake inhibitor use during pregnancy and newborn neurobehavior. Pediatrics 2004; 2: 368–375

67 Nulman I, Rovet J, Koren G et al. Neurodevelopment of children exposed in utero to antidepressant drugs. N Engl J Med 1997; 336: 258–262

68 Nulman I, Rovet J, Koren G et al. Child development following exposure to tricyclic antidepressants or fluoxetine throughout fetal life: a prospective controlled study. Am J Psychiatry 2002; 159: 1889–1895

69 Appleby L, Warner R, Whitton A, Faragher B. A controlled study of fluoxetine and cognitive-behavioural counselling in the treatment of postnatal depression. BMJ 1997; 314: 932–936

70 Wisner KL, Peindl KS, Gigliotti TV. Tricyclics vs SSRIs for postpartum depression. Arch Womens Mental Health. 1999; 1: 189–191

71 Altshuler LL, Cohen LS, Docherty JP et al. The expert consensus guideline series. Postgraduate Medicine. March 2001, McGraw Hill

72 Weismann AM, Hartz AJ, Wisner KL et al. Pooled analysis of antidepressant levels in lactating mothers, breast-milk and nursing infants. Am J Psych 2004; 166(6): 1066–1078

73 Weissman AM, Wisner KL, Bentler MS. Venlafaxine levels in lactating mothers, breast milk, and nursing infants. Arch Womens Mental Health. 2003; 6 (Suppl 1): 1–28

74 O'Hara MW, Stuart S, Gorman LL, Wenzel A. Efficacy of interpersonal psychotherapy for postpartum depression. Arch Gen Psychiatry 2000; 57: 1039–1045

75 Zlotnick C, Johnson SL, Miller IW, Pearlstein T, Howard M. Postpartum depression in women receiving public assistance: pilot study of an interpersonal-therapy- oriented group intervention. Am J Psychiatry 2001; 158: 638–640

76 Miller LJ. Use of electro convulsive therapy during pregnancy. Hosp Comm Psychiatry 1994; 45: 444–450

77 Panay N, Studd JWW. The psychotherapeutic effect of estrogens. Gynecol Endocrinol 1998; 12: 353–365

78 Gregoire AJP, Henderson AF, Kumar R, Everitt B, Studd JWW. Transdermal estrogen for treatment of severe postnatal depression. Lancet 1996; 347: 930–933

79 Epperson NC, Terman M, Wisner et al. Randomized clinical trial of bright light therapy for antepartum depression: preliminary findings. J Clin Psychiatry 2004; 65: 421–425

80 Hibbeln JR. Seafood consumption, the DHA content of mother's milk and prevalence rates of postpartum depression: a cross-national ecological analysis. J Affective Disord 2002; 69: 15–29

81 Otto SJ, Groot de RHM, Hornstra G. Increased risk of postpartum depressive symptoms is associated with slower normalization after pregnancy of the functional docasahexaenoic acid status. Prostaglandins Leukot Essent Fatty Acids 2003; 69: 237–243

82 Freeman MP, Wisner KL, Gelenberg AJ, Hibbeln J. Omega-3 fatty acids for depression in pregnancy: an open label trial. Poster presentation. Biological Psychiatry meeting; May 2003

83 Manber R, Schnyer RN, Aller JJB. Does acupuncture hold promise as a treatment for depression during pregnancy? Society of Biological Psychiatry's Annual Convention, San Francisco, CA. May 15, 2003

84 Wisner KL, Perel JM, Rapport D et al. Prevention of recurrent postpartum depression: a randomized clinical trial. J Clin Psychiatry 2001; 62: 82–86

85 Wisner KL, Perel JM, Peindl KS, Hanusa BH, Piontek CM, Findling RL. Prevention of postpartum depression: a pilot randomized clinical trial. Am J Psychiatry 2004; In press

86 Sunder KR, Wisner KL, Hanusa BH, Perel JM. Postpartum depression recurrence versus discontinuation syndrome: observations from a randomized controlled trial. J Clin Psychiatry 2004; In press

87 US Department of Health and Human Services. Mental Health: A report of the Surgeon General-Executive Summary. Rockville, MD: Department of Health and Human Services, National Institute Health, 1999

APPENDIX 1 (see next page)

APPENDIX 1

Edinburgh Postnatal Depression Scale

Please circle the answer that best describes how you have felt over the past 7 days.

1.   I have been able to laugh and see the funny side of things

   0 = as much as I could
   1 = not quite so much now
   2 = definitely not so much now
   3 = not at all

2.   I have looked forward with enjoyment to things

   0 = as much as I ever did
   1 = rather less than I used to
   2 = definitely less that I used to do
   3 = hardly at all

3.   I have blamed myself unnecessarily when things went wrong

   3 = yes, most of the time
   2 = yes, sometimes
   1 = hardly ever
   0 = no, not at all

4.   I have been anxious or worried for no good reason

   3 = yes, very often
   2 = yes, sometimes
   1 = hardly ever
   0 = no, not at all

5.   I have felt scared or panicky for no very good reason

   3 = yes, quite a lot
   2 = yes, sometimes
   1 = no, not much
   0 = no, not at all

6.   Things have been getting on top of me

   3 = yes, most of the time I haven't been able to cope at all
   2 = yes, sometimes I haven't been coping as well as usual
   1 = no, most of the time I have coped quite well
   0 = no, I have been coping as well as ever

7.   I have been so unhappy that I have had difficulty sleeping

   3 = yes, most of the time
   2 = yes, sometimes
   1 = not very often
   0 = no, not at all

8.   I have felt sad or miserable

   3 = yes, most of the time
   2 = yes, quite often
   1 = not very often
   0 = no, not at all

9.   I have been so unhappy that I have been crying

   3 = yes, most of the time
   2 = yes, quite often
   1 = only occasionally
   0 = no, never

10.   The thought of harming myself has occurred to me

   3 = yes, quite often
   2 = sometimes
   1 = hardly ever
   0 = never

Kamal I. Shehata Tahir A. Mahmood

Clinical management of first trimester spontaneous miscarriage

Spontaneous miscarriage is the most common complication of pregnancy, and its incidence varies between 10% and 20% in clinically recognised pregnancies.[1-3] It is estimated that around 80,000 uterine curettage procedures are carried out every year for women with spontaneous miscarriage in the UK.[4] It is also recognised as an adverse life event with negative impact on women's psychological welfare.[5] Therefore, the management of spontaneous miscarriage represent a substantial part of the emergency gynaecological workload for the NHS.

DEFINITIONS AND TERMINOLOGY

Various authors have used different terminologies to describe early pregnancy problems. This needs to be standardised to allow clinicians to compare the outcomes following the use of different management options. The terminology used should provide a clear description of the actual clinical condition to guide further management and should also give a sensitive description of this clinical event experienced by many women in their reproductive years.

Before the introduction of ultrasound imaging, the term 'threatened abortion' was used to describe the clinical findings of any vaginal bleeding during the first half of the pregnancy in the presence of a closed uterine cervix.[6] With the increasing use of ultrasound imaging, it was realised that similar clinical findings can be associated with any of the following conditions: on-

Kamal I. Shehata MRCOG
Senior Specialist Registrar, Department of Obstetrics and Gynaecology, University Hospital of Wales, Heath Park, Heath, Cardiff CF14 4XW, Wales, UK
(for correspondence, E-mail: KamalIbrahim.Shehata@CardiffandVale.wales.nhs.uk)

Tahir A. Mahmood MD FRCOG FRCPI MBA
Consultant Obstetrician and Gynaecologist/Clinical Director, Department of Obstetrics and Gynaecology, Forth Park Hospital, 30 Bennochy Road, Kirkcaldy, Fife KY2 5RA, UK

going pregnancy, non-viable pregnancy (missed abortion), incomplete miscarriage, complete miscarriage and ectopic pregnancy. At present, 'threatened miscarriage' is used to describe an on-going pregnancy with bleeding per-vaginum.[7] However, it is debatable whether an on-going pregnancy can be labelled as 'threatened miscarriage' while the cause of bleeding is usually unknown and in the majority of these cases, the pregnancy would continue to the age of viability.[8]

The term 'missed abortion' was first described by Matthew Duncan in 1874 as a clinical entity in which *the fetus died before viability with no effort at its expulsion by the uterus*.[9] This definition did not stipulate the duration of retention of the dead fetus *in utero*. It inevitably became a point of dispute among different investigators. In order to differentiate between missed abortion, threatened and/or incomplete abortion, various arbitrary limits were set; varying from periods of retention of non-viable products of conception of 4 weeks,[10,11] 8 weeks,[12,13] and up to 2 months.[9] On the other hand, some researchers have designated 'missed abortion' as fetal death *in utero* before the age of viability, regardless of the duration of the retention of the fetus, provided that there was no evidence of spontaneous abortion at the time of the diagnosis.[14]

A non-viable pregnancy diagnosed in the first trimester is also often referred to as a missed abortion.[15] It is, however, very difficult during the first 12 weeks of the pregnancy to justify the classical definition of retention of non-viable products of conception for 8 weeks or more.[16] Therefore, alternative terms have been adopted to describe non-viability at different duration within the first trimester such as chemical pregnancy,[17] blighted ovum,[18] anembryonic gestation,[15] impending abortion,[19] and first trimester intra-uterine fetal demise.[15]

With the availability of higher resolution ultrasound scanning, distinction between blighted ovum and missed abortion has also been disputed. Goldstein[20] suggested that most of these anembryonic pregnancies are not truly without embryos. They simply lose viability before our ability to image them. He also suggested that, in many cases, there is initially early embryonic development with subsequent loss of viability and then embryonic resorption. This then ultimately results in sonographic appearance of empty sac.[20]

The use of the term 'spontaneous abortion' rather than 'miscarriage' has been considered to be inappropriate,[21] because it may lead to negative self-perception in a group of women who already have a sense of guilt and inadequacy because of their unfortunate miscarriage. Other inadequate terminologies (*e.g.* pregnancy failure, abnormal pregnancy, silent miscarriage and delayed miscarriage) need to be replaced by appropriate terminology which describes the exact diagnosis of the clinical condition. We suggest the use of the term 'retained non-viable pregnancy'" as an alternative to the term 'missed abortion'.

DIAGNOSTIC DILEMMAS

One of the difficult areas in the management of women with spontaneous miscarriage is the establishment of the correct diagnosis. Clinical history alone is not always a useful guide to the diagnosis and clinical management of incomplete miscarriage. Therefore, clinicians have been increasingly relying on

Table 1 Ultrasound criteria for incomplete and non-viable pregnancy in the first trimester of pregnancy

Ultrasound criteria described for the diagnosis of incomplete miscarriage

Central cavity echo(s)[108]

Thick irregular echoes in the uterine cavity[118]

Echoes consistent with intrauterine tissues or clots[120]

Endometrial line not present or partly present and the cavity is filled with echogenic products of conception and/or echolucent areas representing blood clots[119]

Endometrial thickness > 5 mm[22,35]

Endometrial thickness > 10 mm[33,120,123]

Endometrial thickness > 15 mm[32]

Recommendations of ultrasound criteria for establishing the death of an embryo[23]

The presence of either an empty gestational sac of > 20 mm in the mean sac diameter is to be considered highly suggestive of the presence of non-viable pregnancy

The presence of an embryo of crown rump length > 6 mm with no evidence of fetal heart beats are to be considered highly suggestive of missed miscarriage

When the gestational sac is < 20 mm or the crown rump length is < 6 mm, then a repeat examination should be performed at least 1 week later to assess the growth of gestational sac and embryo and to establish whether heart activity exists

If the gestational sac is smaller than expected for gestational age, the possibility of incorrect dates should always be considered, especially in the absence of clinical features suggestive of a threatened miscarriage. A repeat scan should be arranged after a period of at least 7 days to be performed by experienced personnel

ultrasound examination to select women suitable for surgical evacuation of retained products of conception.[22]

Various ultrasound features described by different workers for the diagnosis of incomplete and complete miscarriage are summarised in Table 1. These criteria, however, show inconsistencies between the ultrasound findings suggestive of the presence or absence of retained products of conception. For that reason, these diagnostic parameters have not been adopted universally in clinical practice. The clinicians usually use both clinical and ultrasound findings for further management of these cases.

The recognition of cases of non-viable pregnancy is not always a straightforward diagnosis. Misdiagnosis of a normal pregnancy believed to be miscarrying may occur.[23] In 1993, a number of cases were reported in Wales where fetal death was erroneously diagnosed by ultrasound examination. As a consequence, an independent inquiry was set up to investigate the circumstances of these cases and to make recommendations for sound clinical practice. The agreed guidelines of this enquiry are also summarised in Table 1.[23]

Hurd et al.[19] reported their guidelines for the diagnosis of a non-viable pregnancy by the use of ultrasound features alone or in combination with biochemical assays. According to their experience, a non-viable pregnancy was diagnosed without the aid of ultrasound in women of less than 6 weeks' gestation when β-hCG levels were found to be decreasing before reaching 1000 mIU/ml. Over 6 weeks of gestation, the diagnosis of non-viable pregnancy was made if there was no growth in visible gestational sac over a 1-week period and the β-hCG level failed to increase normally (approximately doubling every 48–72 h). In the presence of an increasing β-hCG level, non-viability was also diagnosed when fetal cardiac activity could not be detected with either a gestational sac of > 17 mm in diameter or with a β-hCG level of > 30,000 mIU/ml.[19]

MANAGEMENT

There are different methods of dealing with retained products of conception. Following the publication of several case series during the 1930–1950s,[24-27] which reported a high incidence of maternal morbidity and mortality due to pelvic sepsis in women with retained products of conception, surgical uterine evacuation became the 'gold standard' management of women with spontaneous miscarriage. Although it is invariably accepted as a safe procedure, serious sequelae have also been reported[28,29] which encouraged clinicians to investigate the use of non-surgical options.

In the 1980s and 1990s, preliminary work on the use of medical agents (e.g. RU486 and prostaglandin analogues) for the management of women with spontaneous miscarriage demonstrated efficacy.[30,31] A few years later, reports on expectant management[32,33] of women with spontaneous miscarriage also demonstrated the efficacy and safety of an expectant approach for selected cases of spontaneous miscarriage in the first trimester when compared to surgical uterine evacuation. These reports have generated new interest in exploring these alternative management options in terms of women's acceptability, safety in the short- and long-term, and the health-economic implications.

Surgical management

Surgical uterine evacuation

There are two established surgical methods to evacuate intra-uterine retained products of conception: (i) sharp curettage; and (ii) suction evacuation. Up until the late 1960s and early 1970s, sharp curettage using the curette and the ovum forceps were the only instruments employed for the evacuation of the gravid uterus.[34] It has been suggested that by using sharp curettage, it is not possible to differentiate precisely between the basal and functional layers of the endometrium. Therefore, there is always a possibility of causing damage to the deeper basal layer of the endometrium and the myometrium which could lead to complications such as intra-uterine adhesions, oligomenorrhoea, amenorrhoea, infection and subfertility. This clinical practice has now largely been replaced by suction evacuation of the uterus.

Peretz et al.[27] commented that at suction evacuation, smaller, delicate and blunt instruments were routinely used, and operations could be completed in shorter times as compared to sharp curettage. They reported a reduced blood loss and a reduction in the risk of infection. The other advantages of using suction evacuation were a reduction in the occurrence of uterine perforation, lower risk of haemorrhage, sepsis, or unexpected bleeding.[34] This group also pointed out the limitations of suction evacuation: (i) that the suction tube may not be delicate enough to differentiate fine anatomical changes in the uterine cavity; (ii) the tube can be blocked by the dense placental tissues when pregnancy was > 10 weeks; (iii) the retrieved tissue could lose its anatomical shape; and (iv) that incomplete evacuation of the retained products of conception requires a repeat uterine curettage.

Success rate following surgical management

There is a general agreement about the efficacy of the surgical management of spontaneous miscarriage especially in the first trimester. Several small studies reported a success rate of 89–100% for surgical uterine evacuation of retained products of conception.[29,32,35–40] These studies have been mainly comparisons between sharp curettage and suction evacuation of retained products of conception or between surgical management and other alternative management options. There were no agreed criteria used in these studies to describe, 'failed surgical management' (Table 6). The criteria used for 'failed surgical management' were either the re-evacuation rate of the uterus following surgical management or the incidence of pelvic infection or other complications.

Complications of surgical management

The recognised complications of surgical management can be broadly classified into either anaesthetic complications or traumatic injuries related to the surgical technique. The complications encountered due to the surgical technique are described as follows. The re-evacuation rate of the uterus following surgical management of incomplete miscarriage varied between 1.1% and 2.1%[37–39,41,42] and there was no mention in these reports of the factors responsible for the failed surgical evacuation. Kaunitz et al.,[43] in a large study for elective abortion, reported that the risk of failed surgical abortion was found to be higher among women with one or more previous pregnancies (relative risk [RR] = 2.2), women having an abortion at less than 6 weeks' gestation (RR = 2.9), particularly when: (i) small suction cannulae were used (RR = 11.1); (ii) the procedure was performed by inexperienced medical staff (RR = 2.2); and (iii) the procedure was performed on women with uterine anomalies (RR = 90.6).

The reported postoperative sepsis rate following surgical suction evacuation ranged between 1% and 2.3%,[38,44] compared to higher rates of 4% for conventional sharp curettage.[38,42] Data from studies of termination of pregnancies, however, suggest that infective complications in these cases can be up to 10%. The presence of Chlamydia trachomatis, Neisseria gonorrhea,[48–51] or bacterial vaginosis[48,49] in the lower genital tract at the time of abortion is associated with an increased risk.[50] A randomised trial of prophylactic single intravenous dose of doxycycline (100 mg) administered at curettage for incomplete miscarriage showed no obvious benefits of routine chemoprophylaxis; however, this study was of insufficient power to detect a clinically meaningful change in infectious morbidity following the use of chemoprophylaxis.[51]

Risk of surgical uterine perforation among women undergoing first trimester elective abortion was reported by Hodgson[52] to be less than 1%. But risk of uterine perforation reported in another two studies of pregnancy termination[53,54] ranged from 0.09–19.8/1000 and was much higher (up to 2%) when direct visualisation using laparoscopy was carried out.

The prevalence of intra-uterine adhesions following surgical uterine evacuation has been evaluated in a number of studies,[55-60] by performing either hysterosalpingography,[58] or hysteroscopic examination.[59,61] The investigators reported an incidence of intra-uterine adhesions varying between 16-19% following hysterosalpingography[59,61] and between 15%[58] and 22.7%[55] following hysteroscopic examination. There was no difference in the occurrence of adhesions among women managed by surgical evacuation for missed miscarriage[60,61] when compared to women with incomplete miscarriage, which was opposite to what was previously believed.[62-64] It is also obvious from the reported data that with an increasing number of curettage following miscarriage (> 2), the incidence of intra-uterine adhesions also increased,[57] which can vary between 32% and 47%.[59,60]

Medical management

Various therapeutic agents have been used for medical management of women with spontaneous miscarriage, including: (i) hypertonic fluids;[65-68] rivanol;[69] and (iii) mifepristone, prostaglandins (natural and synthetic) and other oxytocins.[30,70-89] Some of these agents have now been abandoned because of their health hazards,[90] particularly hypertonic solutions[91] and sulprostone.[92]

Medical agents used for first trimester spontaneous miscarriage

Hypertonic fluids: Reports about the use of intra-amniotic injection of hypertonic fluids such as 50% glucose solution and 20% and 10% sodium chloride, were characterised by a high incidence of failures among women with less than 15 weeks of gestation, who eventually required surgical uterine evacuation. Furthermore, warnings were issued when maternal deaths were reported following instillation of hypertonic solution in the amniotic sac for termination of the pregnancy.[91]

Prostaglandins: Karim et al.[83] were the first to report on the successful use of prostaglandins in the management of cases of intra-uterine fetal death. Following this, the use of prostaglandins for the management of missed miscarriage and intra-uterine fetal death has been extensively researched in many trials, where different types of prostaglandin, both natural and synthetic had been used. Natural prostaglandins ($PGF_2\alpha$ or PGE_2) stimulate the pregnant and non-pregnant uterus and have proved to be effective in inducing labour in cases of intra-uterine fetal death and missed miscarriage.[78] The prostaglandin analogues (gemeprost and misoprostol) are more potent,[78] and can be used at a lower dose and by different routes with fewer side effects compared to the natural prototypes. The prostaglandin analogue (PGE_1) gemeprost is relatively expensive and requires refrigeration, while misoprostol (PGE_1) is relatively stable at room temperature and also cheaper than gemeprost. Following the successful use of mifepristone prior to prostaglandin administration for the management of women requesting therapeutic abortion,[93-95] investigators have used similar regimens for the management of women with retained products of conception following spontaneous miscarriage as well.[30,86,99] It should, however, be recognised that misoprostol remains unlicensed to procure medical abortion or to be used in cases of early pregnancy failure.

In the 1970s and early 1980s, investigators administered prostaglandins intra-amniotically,[100,101] extra-amniotically[102] or systemically, either intravenously or intramuscularly, which had been accompanied by higher incidence of side effects when compared with locally administered prostaglandins.

Gasterointestinal symptoms and painful uterine contractions are the most frequent side effects encountered with the use of different prostaglandins. Serious complications following the use of different prostaglandins were also reported (*i.e.* uterine rupture,[103,104] chorioamniontitis,[95] and excessive blood loss[105,106]). A case of maternal death was reported following the use of PGE_2 and sulprostone, which led the manufacturer to withdraw sulprostone from the market.[92,107] Cardiogenic shock was the cause of death in this report, which quoted an incidence related mortality rate of 1.3 (CI 0.025–5.8) per 100,000 abortions.

Medical management of women with incomplete miscarriage

Studies of medical management of cases with retained products of conception following spontaneous miscarriage in the first trimester of pregnancy, showed a wide range of success rates, as summarised in Table 2.

Henshaw *et al.*[31] reported a 95.3% success rate using a single 0.5 mg dose of intramuscular sulprostone or a 400 µg dose of oral misoprostol. Conversely, de Jonge *et al.*,[108] in a randomised trial, reported a success rate of 13% after a single dose of oral misoprostol (400 µg). All other published studies failed to replicate the excellent results reported by Henshaw *et al.*[31] The largest series ($n = 635$) for medical management of women with incomplete miscarriage was reported by Chung *et al.*,[109] where women were randomised to either surgical uterine evacuation ($n = 314$) or to medical treatment to receive misoprostol 400 µg orally every 4 h, to a maximum dosage of 1.2 mg. Although women managed medically in this study had a fewer side effects compared to surgical management, the success rate of the medical management was only 50%.

It has not been possible to compare different studies of the medical management of women with incomplete miscarriage because of the diversity of the data with regard to the population studied, methodology used and outcome measures reported. The mean gestational age of the women recruited into the different studies varied between 9 and 12 weeks of gestation. Oral misoprostol has been the most commonly investigated prostaglandin. Different regimens of misoprostol have been used in different studies,[31,108-112] ranging from a single oral dose of 400 µg to a 4-hourly dose of 400 µg with a maximum of 1.2 mg per day for one or two successive days. Gemeprost was given vaginally up to a maximum of 5 mg and sulprostone was administered

Table 2 Medical treatment of spontaneous miscarriage complicated by incomplete miscarriage

Author(s)	Number of women	Gestational age	Intervention	Success rate	Intervention and medical regimen	Complications and side effects of medical treatment
Pandian et al. (2001)[131]	112	6–13 weeks of gestation	Retrospective analysis	85%	Misoprostol 600 µg x 3 followed by 400 µg/hourly x 2	3 with suspected PID. One woman had a blood loss > 500 ml. 85% received analgesia; 2% received parental opiates
Pang et al. (2001)[113]	103	10.22 (2.0)	Randomised controlled trial	61.1%	Misoprostol 800 µg orally	65.3% diarrhoea
	95	10.6 (2.3)		64.4%	Misoprostol 800 µg vaginally	13.6% diarrhoea
Chung et al. (1999)[109]	321	10.7 (SD 2.5)	Randomised controlled trial	50.3%	Misoprostol 400 µg/4 h given orally (a total of 1.2 mg)	28% had pain, 6% had parenteral analgesia and surgical management had higher rate of complications as compared to medical management
	314	10.8 (SD 2.6)		69%	Surgical evacuation	
Chung et al. (1997)[110]	214		Prospective study	69%	Misoprostol given orally 400 µg up to a total dose of 1.2 mg/ day for two days	27.1% required analgesia compared to only 0.7% from surgical group; 0.8% PID compared to 3.6% from the surgical group
	137			93%	Surgical evacuation	
De Jonge et al. (1995)[108]	23	80 days	Randomised study	13.0%	Misoprostol (400 µg)	26% from misoprostol group and 23% from surgical group required > 1 unit of blood transfusion
	27	80 days		96%	Surgical evacuation	
Chung et al. (1995)[111]	141	9 (6–18) weeks	A prospective observational study	62%	Misoprostol 400 µg orally every 4 h for a total of 1.2 mg	Two (1%) women complained of nausea and vomiting, 5 (4%) of diarrhoea, 3 (2%) of headaches, one felt dizzy and 13 (9%) women developed transient pyrexia (> 37.5°C and one developed hypotension
Chung et al. (1994)[112]	132	9.4 (6–18) weeks	A prospective trial	44%	Gemeprost vaginal pessaries (up to 5 mg total)	Nausea (17.4%), diarrhoea (11.5%) abdominal pain (24.2%) drowsiness (0.7%) and postural hypotension (1.4%)
Henshaw et al. (1993)[31]	43	66 (40–91) days	Prospective study	95.3%	Single dose of 0.5 mg sulprostone intramuscularly or misoprostol 400 µg orally	29.5% required analgesia

TVS, transvaginal scan; PID, pelvic inflammatory disease.

intramuscularly in two different studies. Recently, a study by Pang et al.[113] demonstrated that vaginal misoprostol has a similar efficacy to oral misoprostol with a reduction in the incidence of diarrhoea from 61% with the latter to 13% with the former route of administration.

Medical management of women with non-viable pregnancy

Earlier reports of medical management of cases, where the pregnancy was considered to be non-viable in the first 12 weeks of gestation, have been incorporated with data for the second trimester missed miscarriage and third trimester intra-uterine fetal death.[72,76,78,84,106] Recently, several studies have concentrated on medical management of non-viable pregnancies in the first trimester (Table 3).[30,85,86,89,114,115]

The success rate of medical management in various randomised trials where medical treatment has been compared with either placebo[89] or surgical evacuation[85,115] or conservative management,[99] varied between 76.6–82.5%. A higher success rate was reported with medical management in non-randomised observational studies varying between 83.4–93%. The total number of women involved in randomised reports varied between 46-122, with a variable gestational age between 9-11 weeks of gestation. The number of women included in the non-randomised reports varied between 31-220. The duration following medical management till offering surgical evacuation for 'failed' cases also varied in these reports between a few hours and up to 5 days.

Medical agents used in these reports included mifepristone alone (600 mg orally) with a success rate of 82%,[89] misoprostol (vaginally 800 μg) with a success rate of 82.5%,[105] gemeprost (vaginally 1 mg/3 h) with a maximum dose of 3 mg/day with a success rate of 76.7%,[85] and a combination of mifepristone (400 mg) with misoprostol (400 μg orally) had a success rate of 82%.[99] The medical regimen used in the non-randomised reports were usually a combination of mifepristone (200–600 mg) and misoprostol. However, the route and frequency of administration of misoprostol tablets varied in these reports. Misoprostol was administered sublingually by Wagaarachchi et al.,[116] who reported an overall success rate of 83.4% and this was accompanied by a high incidence of side effects. The same group of investigators reported a similar 84.1% success rate, but a lower incidence of side effects, when the first dose of misoprostol was given vaginally and followed by subsequent doses given either vaginally or orally. Nielsen et al.[86] administered a single dose of vaginal misoprostol, with low incidence of side effects but with a high failure rate of 48%. Similarly, El-Raefy et al.[30] used repeated doses of oral misoprostol for 2 days to achieve a 93% success rate but again reported a high incidence of side effects.

The incidence of side effects for women managed medically in randomised studies was comparable to the incidence of complications in the control groups. The incidence of different complications and side effects with medical management as given in randomised and non-randomised reports were as follows: the need for re-admission (3.6–6%), pelvic infection (0.8–4%), heavy bleeding > 500 ml or requiring blood transfusion (1–26%), the need for analgesia (24.2–85%), the need for parenteral analgesia (2–32.1%), diarrhoea (4–65.3%), nausea and vomiting (1.4–30%), pyrexia (9%) and postural hypotension (1.4%). The variations in the incidence of these side effects were

Table 3 Medical management of women with non-viable pregnancy in the first trimester

Author(s)	Number of women	Gestational age (weeks)	Intervention	Regimen and intervention	Success rate	Complications and side effects of medical management
Wagaarachchi et al. (2002)[116]	56	9.6 (1.84)	Prospective observational study	Mifepristone 200 mg + misoprostol 400 µg sublingually x 3	83.9%	32.1% required parental analgesia and 50% only oral analgesia. 50% had diarrhoea (mild in 2/3). 3.6% required admission, one for prolonged bleeding and one for PID
Demetoulis et al. (2001)[115]	40	10.4 (8–13)	Prospective randomised trial with 85% power	Misoprostol 800 µg vaginally	82.5%	Abdominal pain (53%), 17% received analgesia and duration of pain was longer in women receiving medical management 4.7 (2.4) days. The drop in Hb was comparable between the two groups
	40	9.5 (6–13)		Surgical evacuation	100%	
Wagaarachchi et al. (2001)[114]	220	10.1 (6–13)	Prospective observational study	Mifepristone 200 mg + misoprostol 800 µg + misoprostol 40 µg x 2 vaginally or orally	84.1%	63.5% had pain with 17.4% requiring parental analgesia. Re-admission rate was 6.3%, 1.8% with presumed pelvic infection, 2.2% required surgical evacuation
Nielsen et al. (1999)[99]	60	67 (SD 11)	Randomised controlled study	Mifepristone 400 mg + misoprostol 400 µg orally	82%	66% had pain with medical management as compared to 62% in women managed conservatively
	62	68 (SD 11)		Conservative	76%	
Creinin et al. (1997)[87]	12	≥ 8	Randomised study	Misoprostol 400 µg orally/day for 2 days	25%	30% vomiting, 50% diarrhoea
	8			Misoprostol 800 µg vaginally/day for 2 days	88%	13% vomiting, 38% diarrhoea
Nielsen et al. (1997)[86]	31	77 (12)	Prospective study	400 mg mifepristone orally misoprostol 400 µg vaginally	52%	Two (6%) women had severe pain, 2 (6%) women had severe bleeding and one (3%) woman developed pelvic infection
Egarter et al. (1995)[85]	43	10.1 (8–12)	Randomised controlled study	Gemeprost 1 mg vaginally/3 h up to 3 mg/day for 2 days	76.7%	60% required analgesia
	44			Surgical evacuation	100%	
Lelaider et al. (1993)[89]	23	11 (6.6–14)	Randomised double-blind study	Mefipristone 600 mg orally	82%	4% endometritis, 2 (9%) haemorrhagic expulsion managed by surgical uterine evacuation
	23			Placebo	8%	
El-Refaey et al. (1992)[30]	59	71 (42–110)	Prospective descriptive study	Mifepristone 600 mg (400 + 200) orally + misoprostol. 600 µg x 2	93%	5 given anti-emetic, 7 had diarrhoea, 13 (22%) received oral analgesia and 7 (12%) had parental analgesia. Duration of bleeding varied between 2–22 days

related to the route of administration of prostaglandins and the dose given to induce expulsion of the retained products.

Direct comparisons between the different medical agents are not available. Only one study[87] with small numbers ($n = 20$), compared misoprostol given orally (400 µg daily for 2 days) or vaginally (800 µg daily for 2 days) for the management of early pregnancy failure where the gestational age was 8 weeks or less confirmed by ultrasound and pelvic examination. The success rate in the former group (oral route) was 25% compared to 88% in the latter group (vaginal route). There was also a higher incidence of gastrointestinal side effects when misoprostol was given orally.

Following reviewing the evidence reported in all these studies, it is obvious that the ideal medical regimen for the management of women with non-viable pregnancy is still to be determined. A medical regimen which used combinations of mifepristone with multiple doses of prostaglandins demonstrated higher success rates (82–93%) compared to the use of either of these agents alone (76.5–82%). Furthermore, higher success rate(s) required repeated administration of misoprostol, which was also accompanied by higher incidence of side effects. In general, there is a lack of randomised trials of optimal power and appropriate design to assess the effectiveness of medical treatment against the surgical management. This partially explains the reluctance on the part of medical fraternity of introducing medical management as an option for women with early pregnancy failure.

Conservative management

Investigators have either used the terminology of 'expectant' or 'conservative' management to describe 'the watchful waiting of the occurrence of spontaneous miscarriage' instead of surgical intervention. Tassig[117] was the first to use the term 'expectant' to describe an observational period of care, which was usually followed by surgical evacuation of products of conception and he also used the term 'conservative' to describe any form of care provided to the woman, but surgical management. Another researcher[109] even used the term 'conservative' to describe a non-surgical approach of treating women with a prostaglandin E_1 analogue (misoprostol).

Conservative management of women with complete miscarriage

In the 1980s and the early 1990s, investigators used transabdominal scanning to screen for retained products of conception. They reported their results using descriptive criteria rather than ultrasonically measured diameters to indicate the presence or absence of retained products of conception. The descriptive criteria used[36,108,118,119] were not suitable for routine practice and this may explain the hesitancy of adopting them for the management of women with complete miscarriage.

However, since the introduction of transvaginal scanning into routine clinical practice in the 1990s, investigators have started to measure the endometrial thickness in different planes. Rulin et al.[120] used a single endometrial thickness of < 10 mm to chose women suitable for conservative management. Haines et al.[121] considered a measurement of the endometrial lining < 6 cm² in the saggital plane and of < 5 cm² in the transverse plane to

Table 4 Immediate and short-term outcomes with expectant management of retained products of conception following spontaneous miscarriage

Author(s)	Participants	Intervention	Success rate (conservative group)	Complications (conservative)	Emergency curettage	Infectious morbidity	Other outcome measures
CSO-study (Shehata et al.)*	161 Expectant 122 Surgical	Randomised controlled study	93.2%	6% versus 9.8% for surgical evacuation	1.8% versus 1.6% for surgical evacuation	0% versus 2.4% for surgical evacuation	81.6% had a successful outcome after 2 weeks. Women managed conservatively who had incomplete miscarriage achieved 100% and those with nonviable pregnancy achieved 91.5%
Luise et al. (2002)[124]	451 Expectant	Prospective study	96.7% 70% within 14 days and 81% after 4 weeks 99%	1% versus 2% for surgical group	0.2%		70% chose to have conservative management After 4 weeks 91% for incomplete miscarriage and 76% for missed miscarriage
Sairam et al. (2001)[22]	305 Expectant 235 Surgical	Prospective study	86% after 2 weeks of expectancy	3%	3%	1%	96% for women with incomplete miscarriage and 62% for women with missed miscarriage
Schwarzler et al. (1999)[33]	84 Expectant 240 Surgical	Prospective study	84% after 4 weeks	8% versus 13%	5.8% versus 0% (surgical evacuation)	1% versus 4% (surgical evacuation)	Colour Doppler can be used to select women suitable for conservative management
Jurkovic et al. (1998)[123]	85 Expectant 23 Surgical	Prospective study	87% 25% versus 99% (197/199) for surgical group.	16.5% versus 2% for surgical evacuation	16.5%	0% in both groups	16.5% with complete miscarriage and 58.8% preferred surgical evacuation once experienced the symptoms of miscarriage or because of prolonged follow-up
Hurd et al. (1997)[9]	105 Expectant 136 Surgical	Retrospective cohort study.	91% versus 98% in the surgical group.	9% versus 3% for surgical evacuation	6%	1%	Complications following expectant management occurred only in women with gestational sac > 10 mm. One woman had a uterine perforation in surgical group
Chipchase & James (1997)118	19 Expectant 47 Surgical	Randomised controlled study	95% versus 94% of women managed surgically	5% versus 6% for surgical evacuation	0%	5% versus 6% for surgical evacuation	Pain, duration of bleeding, sick leave, return of menses, satisfaction with management and future reproductive performance were similar for both groups
Nielsen et al. (1995)[32]	103 Expectant 52 Surgical	Randomised controlled trial	79% versus 89% for surgical group	3% versus 11% for surgical evacuation	2%	3% versus 10% for surgical evacuation	The outcome measures were needed for surgical uterine evacuation, risk of genital tract infection, duration of bleeding and pain, sick leave and change in PCV

*CSO-study (Chief Scientist Office) in preparation.; TVS, transvaginal scanning; PCV, packed cell volume.

represent an empty uterine cavity which, therefore, does not require surgical evacuation. These measurements were less than the calculated value of the mean plus 2 SD of the endometrial thickness, which was previously recorded as being representative of an empty uterine cavity following surgical evacuation of the uterus.[121] The reported negative predictive value of transvaginal scanning for detection of the absence of chorionic villi varied between 98% and 100% and a positive predictive value of their presence was 69%.[120] However, these studies did not describe an upper limit of ultrasound measurements where conservative management may not be appropriate.

Conservative management of women with retained products of conception

Nielsen et al.[32] reported the first randomised study describing the conservative management of women with retained products of conception. This study included women with residual intra-uterine tissues representing an endometrial thickness between 15–50 mm in the anteroposterior diameter. Women in this study were managed expectantly for 3 days. Although this study had several methodological problems,[122] the study findings created a lot of interest among clinicians to explore the role of conservative management further.

Of all the studies of conservative management of women with retained products of conception reported so far (Table 4), only 2 were randomised[32,35] and the rest were either observational[22,33,123,124] or were case-control reports.[19] The number of women managed conservatively in these two randomised trials were 19 in Chipchase et al.[35] and 103 in Neilsen et al.;[32] in the non-randomised trials the total numbers varied between 84–478. The number of women with non-viable pregnancies included in the non-randomised reports varied between 85–230. The length of the expectancy period, ranged from 3 days[32] to 49 days.[123]

The success rate reported in the two randomised trials[32,35] for women with incomplete and inevitable miscarriage who were managed conservatively varied between 79% and 100%. The success rate reported in the non-randomised reports varied between 91% and 100%. The success rate for women with incomplete miscarriage varied between 79% and 100% and for women with non-viable pregnancy ranged between 25% and 84%. Recently, the Chief Scientist Office (CSO) at the Scottish Health Department funded a large randomised study ($n = 283$) to compare surgical uterine evacuation against conservative management of women with retained products of conception in the first trimester (unpublished work). The overall success rate for women managed conservatively was 93.5% versus 96.7% for surgical evacuation. The success rate for women with incomplete miscarriage who were randomised to conservative management ($n = 36$) was 100% and for women with non-viable pregnancy ($n = 125$) in the same group was 77% at 2 weeks, which rose to 93% after 7 weeks of conservative management.

A similar incidence of complications was reported in the individual studies following randomisation to either conservative management or surgical evacuation of women with residual intra-uterine tissues. The incidence of different complications for women managed conservatively varied between 1–8% compared to 2–13% reported for women managed by surgical uterine evacuation. The overall incidence of emergency curettage for haemostatic uterine evacuation, suspected genital tract infection or any other complications for women managed conservatively varied between 0.2–5.8%. The reported incidence of pelvic infection was higher among women managed surgically (0–10%) than women managed conservatively (0–3%).

Meta-analysis comparing conservative management and surgical uterine evacuation

A meta-analysis (Fig. 1) of all the studies comparing conservative management with surgical uterine evacuation for different complications did not show any difference between both management strategies (P = 0.72, OR 1.09 [CI 0.68–1.7]). However, a meta-analysis comparing the two management options showed the incidence of pelvic infection to be lower in women managed conservatively as compared to women managed by surgical evacuation (P = 0.03, OR 0.32 [CI 0.11–0.89]).

We have reviewed all published studies describing success rates with three management options in Table 6. The cumulative success rate for women managed expectantly was 87.6%, 68% for those managed medically and 90.4% for those who underwent uterine evacuation.

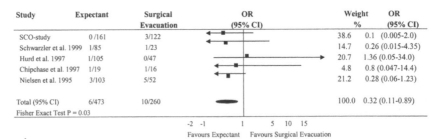

Comparison: Expectant vs Surgical Evacuation

Outcome: Total incidence of different complications

Study	Expectant	Surgical Evacuation	OR (95% CI)	Weight %	OR (95% CI)
SCO-study	10/161	12/122		16.7	0.6 (0.25-1.45)
Luise et al 2002	6/451	5/235		40.2	0.6 (0.18-2.05)
Schwarzler et al. 1999	6/85	3/23		6.3	0.5 (0.11-2.2)
Jurkovic et al. 1998	14/85	3/199		16.7	12.8 (3.59-46.1)
Hurd et al. 1997	9/105	1/47		9.0	4.3 (0.53-35.0)
Chipchase et al. 1997	1/19	1/16		2.0	0.8 (0.047-14.4)
Nielsen et al. 1995	3/103	6/52		9.1	0.23 (0.055-0.96)
Total (95% CI)	49/1009	31/694		100.0	1.09 (0.68-1.7)
Fisher's Exact Test P = 0.72					

-2 -1   1   5   10   15
Favours Expectant   Favours Surgical Evacuation

a

Comparison: Expectant vs Surgical Evacuation

Outcome: Incidence of pelvic infection

Study	Expectant	Surgical Evacuation	OR (95% CI)	Weight %	OR (95% CI)
SCO-study	0 /161	3/122		38.6	0.1 (0.005-2.0)
Schwarzler et al. 1999	1/85	1/23		14.7	0.26 (0.015-4.35)
Hurd et al. 1997	1/105	0/47		20.7	1.36 (0.05-34.0)
Chipchase et al. 1997	1/19	1/16		4.8	0.8 (0.047-14.4)
Nielsen et al. 1995	3/103	5/52		21.2	0.28 (0.06-1.23)
Total (95% CI)	6/473	10/260		100.0	0.32 (0.11-0.89)
Fisher Exact Test P = 0.03					

-2 -1   1   5   10   15
Favours Expectant   Favours Surgical Evacuation

b

Fig. 1 The analysis of the overall incidence of complications showed similar incidence for women managed conservatively and those managed by surgical uterine evacuation (a). Women managed conservatively had a significantly lower incidence of pelvic infection when compared with women with surgical evacuation (b).

Table 5 Studies concerned with reproductive performance following expectant management of spontaneous miscarriages

Author(s)	No. of women	Intervention	Pregnancy rate	Miscarriage rate	Ectopic pregnancy	Other outcome measures
Blohm et al. (1997)[127]	76 Expectant	Randomised study and information collected retrospectively	92%			93% for women managed expect- antly and 91% for those managed expectantly and then required surgical evacuation
	37 Surgical		88%			
Chipchase & James (1997)[118]	19 Expectant 16 surgical	Randomised study	75% vs 67% in the surgical group			The incidence of pelvic sepsis was similar in both groups 5% for con- servative manage- ment versus 6% for surgical evacuation
Kaplan et al. (1996)[126]	161	Prospective descriptive study	73/161	29.7%	1.7%	97% of all women studied did not require surgical intervention. 67.8% within 6 months
Ben-Baruch et al. (1991)[36]	35 Expectant, 52 surgical	Randomised study	74% vs 75% for surgical group	22.9% vs 25%	3% vs 0% for surgical group	100% no immediate complications in both groups

TVS = transvaginal scanning.

The use of colour Doppler imaging of the intervillous space and the uterine artery blood flow has been used to predict the occurrence of successful outcome following conservative management of women with non-viable pregnancy. The blood flow in the former was found to be more useful than the latter in this respect.[33] It was also suggested that the use of serum β-hCG and serum progesterone levels might help in selecting women with retained products of conception who will benefit from surgical evacuation.[125]

Future fertility following expectant management
The possible impairment of future fertility following conservative management of women with spontaneous miscarriage has been one of the main reasons responsible for clinicians' reluctance to encourage women to select expectant management.

Preliminary reports[36,126] on future fertility following conservative management of complete miscarriage were re-assuring in relation to subsequent pregnancy rate, miscarriage rate and the incidence of ectopic pregnancy (Table 5). However, the Ben-Baruch et al.[36] report was of small numbers and the report of Kaplan et al.[126] was not a randomised study either.

Blohm et al.[127] compared future fertility rates among women with incomplete miscarriage managed conservatively in comparison to surgical uterine evacuation. They collected their data retrospectively 2 years later following the publication of the study by Neilsen et al.[32] The cumulative conception rates in women managed expectantly but who later required surgical evacuation were 93%, those managed expectantly 91%, and those managed with primary evacuation 88%.

In summary, the success rate reported for women managed conservatively with incomplete miscarriage was always higher than the success rate reported for women with non-viable pregnancy following similar periods of expectancy. Women with retained products of conception who were managed conservatively had similar incidence of complications and even lower incidence of pelvic sepsis when compared with surgical uterine evacuation under general anaesthesia. Despite these re-assuring reports on future reproductive performance following conservative management, further evidence from prospective randomised studies would be welcomed by women and clinicians.

Table 6 Cumulative success rates reported in all published papers on expectant, medical, and surgical treatment of spontaneous miscarriage

	Expectant		Medical		Surgical	
	Patients (n)	Success (%)	Patients (n)	Success (%)	Patients (n)	Success (%)
CSO study (Shehata et al)[a]	161	93.2	–	–	122	96.7
Luise et al. (2002)	451	81	–	–	208	99
Wagaarachchi et al. (2002)	–	–	56	83.9	–	–
Sairam et al. (2001)	305	86	–	–	–	–
Demetoulis et al. (2001)[a]	–	–	40	82.5	40	100
Wagaarachchi et al. (2001)	–	–	220	84.1	–	–
Pandian et al. (2001)	–	–	118	85.0	–	–
Pang et al. (2001)[a]	–	–	103	61.1	95	64.4
Nielsen et al. (1999)[a]	62	76	60	82	–	–
Chung et al. (1999)[a]	–	–	321	50.3	314	69
Schwarzler et al. (1999)	84	84	–	–	23	87
Jurkovic et al. (1998)	85	99.0	–	–	136	99.0
Chipchase & James (1997)[a]	19	95	–	–	16	94.0
Chung et al. (1997)	–	–	214	69.0	137	93.4
Creinin et al. (1997)[c]	–	–	20	50.0	–	–
Kaplan et al. (1996)	172	96.5	–	–	–	–
Chung et al. (1995)	–	–	141	62.0	–	–
Nielsen et al. (1995)[a]	103	76.7	–	–	52	89.0
Egarter et al. (1995)[a]	–	–	43	76.7	44	100
de Jonge et al. (1995)[a]	–	–	23	13	27	96
Chung et al. (1994)	60	88.3	132	44	–	–
Haines et al. (1994)	32	100	–	–	–	–
Rulin et al. (1993)	49	98.0	–	–	–	–
Henshaw et al. (1993)	–	–	43	95.3	–	–
Leliader et al. (1993)	–	–	82	82.0	–	–
Verkuyl & Crowther (1993)[b]	–	–	–	–	270	95
Mansur (1992)	43	97.7	–	–	–	–
El-Refaey et al. (1992)	–	–	59	93.0	–	–
Ben-Baruch et al. (1991)[a]	46	100	–	–	68	100
Leterie et al. (1991)	21	95.2	–	–	–	–
Kizza & Rogo (1990)	–	–	–	–	585	92
Farrell et al. (1982)	–	–	–	–	111	94
Marshall (1971)	–	–	–	–	86	88
Suter et al. (1970)	–	–	–	–	104	94.2
Tan et al. (1969)	–	–	–	–	89	98.9
Cumulative success rate	1693	87.6%	1675	68%	2527	90.4%

[a]Randomised controlled trials across treatment categories.
[b]Randomised controlled trials comparing types of surgical treatment only.
[c]Randomised controlled trials comparing between medical regimens.

Women's acceptability and satisfaction following management of early pregnancy loss

The psychological impact of management of early pregnancy losses has in the past been ignored or underestimated in clinical trials.[112] Medical termination of pregnancy with misoprostol and mifepristone is generally well tolerated,[93] but this treatment may not be so well tolerated by women with miscarriage. The pain and bleeding of a miscarriage can be severe and some women might prefer an operative treatment. Women's acceptability and quality of life as a reflection of their acceptance to their management should be considered in future trials investigating alternative forms of management of spontaneous miscarriages in comparison to the standard surgical management.

Health economic aspects of the management of early pregnancy loss

Assessment of effectiveness alone is unlikely to determine whether a new treatment makes the best use of available resources. Economic evaluation as part of randomised clinical trials on alternative clinical management is still a rarity, accounting for less than 1% of studies published between 1966 and 1988.[128] Reports on the health–economic implications of medical management of induced abortion suggest that no extra resources are required to provide medical abortion service.[129] It was also reported that it might be possible to generate savings by introducing medical methods in the management of spontaneous early miscarriages, provided that the costs associated with theatre use can be correctly estimated.[130] In case of conservative management, there are potential cost savings with reduction in in-patient care episodes and consequently reductions in acute bed occupancy, as well as potential benefits to the women with natural method of management and more research is required in this area.

CONCLUSIONS

The routine use of ultrasound examination, especially transvaginal ultrasound with high resolution, has become an essential exercise for the management of women with spontaneous miscarriage. This has made the use of routine surgical evacuation of the uterus in women with complete miscarriage unjustifiable and a conservative approach is rather more appropriate.

Among the three options available for the management of women with retained products of conception, surgical uterine evacuation of the uterine cavity is currently accepted as the 'gold standard' management, particularly in the presence of the intact gestational sac. Between the two established methods of surgical evacuation, suction evacuation under general anaesthesia seems to be the preferred method. It is accompanied by lower incidence of complications and requires less operative time compared to sharp curettage. Generally, surgical suction evacuation has a low incidence of immediate complications, such as the need for re-evacuation (1.1–2.1%), infectious morbidity (1–2.3%) and uterine perforation (< 1%). However, the incidence of pelvic infection among women with spontaneous miscarriage following instrumentation of the uterine cavity for surgical evacuation can be up to 10%.

This should alert clinicians to the importance of obtaining routine high vaginal and *Chlamydia* swabs during the course of management of women with retained products of conception. Whether routine antibiotic prophylaxis could be adopted as an alternative to bacteriological screening, remains to be investigated.

As regards medical management of women with spontaneous miscarriage, prostaglandin analogues gemeprost and misoprostol are currently used in the medical management of spontaneous miscarriages. They have a low incidence of side effects compared to their prototypes. The use of mifepristone prior to prostaglandins' administration seems to offer higher success rate compared to the use of either of these drugs alone. However, a wide range of success rates with different medical regimen (25–86%) have been reported; therefore, the optimal regimen for the management of women with incomplete and non-viable pregnancy needs to be determined.

The available evidence confirms the safety and efficacy of a conservative approach in comparison to surgical uterine evacuation for the management of women with spontaneous miscarriage whether incomplete or non-viable pregnancy. Women with retained products of conception had similar incidence of complications and a lower incidence of pelvic infection than women managed by surgical evacuation. The success rate following conservative management for women with incomplete miscarriage was higher when compared with the success rate for women with non-viable pregnancy. Conservative management may represent a sympathetic option for women when the diagnosis of spontaneous miscarriage is made. This approach allows for the results of the bacteriological swabs to become available and also allow women to decide on their preferred method of management. By following this strategy, women can avoid the stress of having to come to the hospital immediately following the diagnosis and also allows them to accept the diagnosis without any regrets or doubts of the possibility that clinicians and sonographers could have made a wrong diagnosis.

Women who are motivated to choose conservative management or those who are not convinced with the diagnosis of spontaneous miscarriage should be provided with telephone contact numbers and followed up regularly until their management is completed. They need to be informed of the symptoms that they might experience during the passage of the products of conception and an ultrasound examination be arranged later on to confirm a complete miscarriage. There are two possible disadvantages of conservative management: first, the length of expectancy period may sometimes be longer than expected; and second, a lack of availability of products of conception for histopathological evaluation. Therefore, future research should aim towards identifying predictors of success of expectant management and to select women suitable for surgical evacuation from the outset. The rare possibility of missing cases of vesicular mole among women managed conservatively be kept in mind, if these women present with recurrent uterine bleeding.

ACKNOWLEDGEMENT

We gratefully acknowledge the secretarial support provided by Mrs Morag Telfer.

References

1 Heritage AT, Rock J, Adams E, Menkin C. Thirty-four fertilized human ova, good, bad and indifferent, recovered from 210 of known fertility. A study of biological wastage in early human pregnancy. Paediatrics 1959; 23: 202–211

2 Jorgenson C, Skjaerris J, Sunden B, Aberg A. Diagnostic ultrasound in threatened abortion and suspected ectopic pregnancy. Acta Obstet Gynecol Scand 1980; 59: 233–235

3 Pandya PP, Snijders RJ, Psara N, Hilbert L, Nicolaides KH. The prevalence of non-viable pregnancy at 10–13 weeks of gestation. Ultrasound Obstet Gynecol 1996; 7: 170–173.

4 Jurkovic D. Modern management of miscarriage: is there a place for non-surgical treatment? Ultrasound Obstet Gynecol 1998; 11: 161–163.

5. Neugebauer R, Kline J, O'Connor P et al. Depressive symptoms in women in the six months after miscarriage. Am J Obstet Gynecol 1992; 106: 104–109.

6 Donald I. Symptoms and Signs of Abortion, 4th edn. Lioyed Link, 1969; 32–35

7 Williams. Williams' Obstetrics, 19th edn. Appleton & Lange, 1993, 675–676

8 Frates MC, Benson CB, Doubilet PM. Pregnancy outcome after a first trimester sonogram demonstrating fetal cardiac activity. J Ultrasound Med 1993; 12: 383–386.

9 Litzenberg JC. Missed abortion. Am J Obstet Gynecol 1921; 1475.

10 Greenhill JP. Obstetrics, 13th edn. Philadelphia: WB Saunders, 1960; 580

11 Dodson MG. Bleeding in pregnancy. In: Aladjems S. (ed) Obstetrical Practice. St Louis: Mosby, 1980; 458

12 Brewer JI, DeCosta GJ. Text of Gynecology, 4th edn). Baltimore: Williams & Wilkins, 1974; 308

13 Lees DH, Singer A. (1982) Missed abortion. In: A Color Atlas of Gynaecological Surgery, vol. 6. Chicago: Year Book Medical, 1982; 45

14 Goldstein, SR. Early pregnancy failure – appropriate terminology. Am J Obstet Gynecol 1990; 163: 1093

15 Pridjian G, Moawad AH. Missed abortion: still appropriate terminology? Am J Obstet Gynecol 1989; 161: 261–262

16 Grimes, DA. Surgical management of abortion. In: Thompson JD, Rock JA. (eds) TeLinde's Operative Gynecology, 7th edn. Philadelphia: JB Lippincott, 1985: 317–342

17 Glastein IZ, Hornstein MD, Kahana MJ, Jackson KV, Friedman AJ. The predictive value of discriminatory human chorionic gonadotrophin levels in the diagnosis of implantation outcome in *in vitro* fertilization cycles. Fertil Steril 1995; 63: 350–356

18 Donald I, Morley P, Barnett E. The diagnosis of blighted ovum by sonar. J Obstet Gynecol Br Cwlth 1972; 79: 304–310

19 Hurd WW, Whitfield RR, Randolph JF, Kercher ML. Expectant management versus elective curettage for the treatment of spontaneous abortion. Fertil Steril 1997; 68: 601–606

20 Goldstein SR. Embryonic death in early pregnancy: a new look at the first trimester. Obstet Gynecol 1994; 84: 294–297

21 Beard RW, Mowbray JR, Pinker GD. Miscarriage or abortion. Lancet 1985; 2: 1122–1123

22 Sairam S, Khare M, Michailidis G, Thilaganathan B. The role of ultrasound in the expectant management of early pregnancy loss. Ultrasound Obstet Gynecol 2001; 17:506–509

23 Hately W, Case J, Campbell B. Establishing the death of an embryo by ultrasound: report of a public inquiry with recommendations. Ultrasound Obstet Gynecol 1995; 5: 353–357.

24 Dunn RD. A five-year study of incomplete abortions at the San Francisco Hospital. Am J Obstet Gynecol 1937; 33: 149–153

25 Hertig AT, Livingstone RG. Spontaneous, threatened and habitual abortion: their pathogenesis and treatment. N Engl J Med 1944; 230: 797–806

26 Russell Jr PB. Abortions treated conservatively: a twelve-year study covering 3,739 cases. S Med J 1947; 40: 314–324.

27 Hartman JW. A comparative study of incomplete abortion at San Francisco Hospital. Stanford Med Bull 1953; 11: 69–70

28 Heisterberg L, Hebjorn S, Anderson LF, Petersen H. Sequelae of induced first trimester abortion. A prospective study assessing postabortal pelvic inflammatory disease and

prophylactic antibiotics. Am J Obstet Gynecol 1986; 155: 76–80

29 Farrell RG, Stonington DT, Ridgeway RA. Incomplete and inevitable abortion: treatment by suction curettage in the emergency department. Ann Emerg Med 1982; 11: 652–658

30 El-Refaey H, Hinshaw K, Henshaw R, Smith N, Templeton AA. Medical management of missed abortion and anembryonic pregnancy. BMJ 1992; 305: 1399

31 Henshaw RC, Cooper K, el-Refaey H, Smith NC, Tempelton AA. Medical management of miscarriage: non-surgical uterine evacuation of incomplete and inevitable spontaneous abortion. BMJ 1993; 306: 894–895

32 Nielsen S, Hahlin M. Expectant management of first trimester abortion. Lancet 1995; 345: 84–86

33 Schwarzler P, Holden D, Nielsen S, Hahlin M, Sladkevicius P, Bourne TH. The conservative management of first trimester miscarriage and the use of colour Doppler sonography for patient selection. Hum Reprod 1999; 14: 1341–1345

34 Peretz A, Grunstein S, Brandes JM, Paldi E. (1969) Evacuation of the gravid uterus by negative pressure (suction evacuation). Am J Obstet Gynecol 1969; 98: 18–22

35 Chipchase J, James D. Randomised trial of expectant versus surgical management of spontaneous miscarriage. Br J Obstet Gynaecol 1997; 104: 840–841

36 Ben-Baruch G, Schiff E, Moran O, Menaohe Y, Mashiach S, Mencger J. Curettage vs. nonsurgical management in women with early spontaneous abortion. The effect on fertility. J Reprod Med 1991; 36: 644–646

37 Tan PM, Ratnam SS, Quek SP. Vacuum aspiration in the treatment of incomplete abortion. J Obstet Gynaecol Br Cwlth 1969; 76: 835–836

38 Verkuyl DA, Crowther CA. Suction versus conventional curettage in incomplete abortion. A randomised controlled trial. S Afr Med J 1993; 83: 13–15

39 Suter PE, Chatfield WR, Kotonya AO. The use of suction curettage in incomplete abortion. J Obstet Gynaecol Br Cwlth 1970; 77: 464–466

40 Kizza AP, Pogo KO. Assessment of manual vacuum aspiration (MVA) equipment in the management of incomplete abortion. E Afr Med J 1990; 67: 812–822

41 Rashid S, Smith P. Suction evacuation of the uterus for incomplete abortion. J Obstet Gynaecol Br Cwlth 1970; 77: 1047–1048

42 Beric BM, Kupresanian M. Vacuum aspiration, using pericervical block, for legal abortion as an outpatient procedure up to the 12th week of pregnancy. Lancet 1971; 2: 619–621

43 Kaunitz AM, Rovira EZ, Grimes DA, Schulz KF. Abortions that fail. Obstet Gynecol 1985; 66: 533–537

44 Filshie GM, Ahluwalia J, Beard RW. Portable Karman curette equipment in management of incomplete abortion. Lancet 1973; 2: 1114–1116

45 Westergaard L, Philipsen T, Scheibel J. Significance of cervical *Chlamydia trachomatis* infection in postabortal pelvic inflammatory diseases. Obstet Gynecol 1982; 60: 322–325

46 Qvigstad E, Skaug K, Jerve F, Fylling P, Ulstrop JC. Pelvic inflammatory diseases associated with *Chlamydia trachomatis* infection after therapeutic abortion. Br J Ven Dis 1983; 59: 189–192

47 Morton K, Regan L, Spring J, Houang E. A further look at infection at the time of therapeutic abortion. Eur J Obstet Gynaecol Reprod Biol 1990; 37: 231–236

48 Hamark B, Forssman L. Postabortal endometritis in *Chlamydia*-negative women – association with preoperative clinical signs of infection. Gynaecol Obstet Invest 1991; 31: 102–105

49 Larsson PG, Platz-Christensen JJ, Thejls H, Forsum U, Pahlson C. Incidence of pelvic inflammatory disease after first trimester legal abortion in women with bacterial vaginosis after treatment with metronidazole: a double-blind, randomised study. Am J Obstet Gynecol 1992; 166): 100–103

50 Penney GC, Thomson M, Norman J et al. A randomised comparison of strategies for reducing infective complications of induced abortion. Br J Obstet Gynaecol 1998; 105: 559–604

51 Prieto JA, Erikson NL, Blanco JD. A randomised trial of prophylactic doxycycline for curettage in incomplete abortion. Obstet Gynecol 1995; 85: 692–696

52 Hodgson JE. Major complications of 20,248 consecutive first trimester abortions: problems of fragmented care. Adv Plann Panat 1975; 9: 52–59

53 Lindell G, Flam F. Management of uterine perforations in connection with legal abortions. Acta Obstet Gynaecol Scand 1995; 74: 373–375

54 Kaali SG, Szigetvari IA, Barttfai GS. The frequency and management of uterine perforation during first trimester abortions. Am J Obstet Gynecol 1989; 161: 406–408

55 Martius G. Prophylaxes und Therapie des Asherman syndroms. In: Martius G. (ed) Gynakologische Operationin: EinLehrbuch fur die facharztiche Aus-und weiterbildung, 2. Stuttgart: Thieme, 1989; 30–31

56. Lancet M, Kessler B. A review of Asherman's syndrome, and results of modern treatment. Int J Fertil 1988; 33: 14–24

57 Schenker JG, Margalioth EJ. Intrauterine adhesions: an updated appraisal. Fertil Steril 1982; 37: 593–610

58 Adoni A, Plati Z, Mildwidsky A. The incidence of intrauterine adhesions following spontaneous abortion. Int J Fertil Steril 1992; 58: 505–510

59 Friedler S, Margalioth EJ, Kafka I, Yaffe H. Incidence of post-abortion intrauterine adhesions evaluated by hysteroscopy – a prospective study. Hum Reprod 1993; 34: 442–424

60 Romer TH. Post-abortion hysteroscopy – a method for early diagnosis of congenital and acquired intrauterine causes of abortions. Eur J Obstet Gynaecol Reprod Biol 1994; 57: 171–173

61 Golan A, Raziel A, Schnieder D, Bukovsky I, Aurech O, Gaspi E. Hysteroscopic findings after missed abortion. Fertil Steril 1992; 58: 508–510

62 Valle RF, Sciarra JJ. Hysteroscopic treatment of intrauterine adhesions. In: Siegler AM, Lindemann HJ. (eds) Hysteroscopy, Principles and Practice. Philadelphia: JB Lippincott, 1984; 193–197

63 Valle RF, Sciarra JJ. Intrauterine adhesions: hysteroscopic diagnosis, classification, treatment and reproductive outcome. Am J Obstet Gynecol 1987; 158: 1459–1470

64 Sugimoto O. Diagnostic and therapeutic hysteroscopy for traumatic intrauterine adhesions. Am J Obstet Gynecol 1978; 131: 539–547

65 Boreo EA. Gynaecol Obstet 1935; 32: 502

66 Brosset A. The induction of therapeutic abortion by means of a hypertonic glucose solution injected into amniotic sac. Acta Obstet Gynaecol Scand 1958; 37: 519–525

67 Wagner G, Kanker H, Fuchs F, Bengtsson LP. Induction of abortion by intra-ovular instillation of hypertonic saline. Dan Med Bull 1962; 9: 137

68 Sciarra JJ, King TM, Steev CM. Induction of labor by the intra-amniotic instillation of hypertonic solutions. Bull Sloane Hosp Women 1964; 10: 48

69 Olund A. Extra-amniotic instillation of rivanol in the management of patients with missed abortion and fetal death. Acta Obstet Gynaecol Scand 1981; 60: 313–315

70 Jaschevatzky OE, Rosenberg RP, Noy Y, Dascclu S, Anderman S, Ballas S. Comparative study of extra-amniotic prostaglandin F_2 alpha infusion and increasing intravenous oxytocin for termination of second trimester missed abortion. J Am Coll Surg 1994; 178: 435–438

71 Fruzzetti F, Melis GB, De Cecco L, Genazzani AR, Fioretti P. The use of 16,16-dimethyl-trans-delta 2-prostaglandin E_1 methyl ester vaginal suppositories for management of missed abortion and fetal death. Int J Obstet Gynecol 1991; 36: 115–119

72 Garcea N, Dargenio R, Panetta V, Moneta E, Tancredi G, Giannitelli A. A prostaglandin analogue (ONO-802) in treatment missed abortion, intrauterine fetal death and hydatiform mole: a dose-finding trial. Eur J Obstet Gynecol Reprod Biol 1987; 25: 15–22

73 Gulisano AS, Pepe F, Panella M, Privetera CD, Pepe G, Piccione G. Intravenous 16-phenoxy PGE_2 methylsulfonylamide for induction of labor in cases of fetal death. Clin Exp Obstet Gynecol 1987; 14: 103–105

74 Thavarasah AS, Almohdzar SA. Prostaglandin (F_2 alpha) in missed abortion. Intravenous, extra-amniotic and intramuscular administration – a randomised study. Biol Res Preg Perinatol 1986; 7: 106–110

75 Christensen NJ, Bygdeman M. The use of prostaglandins for termination of abnormal pregnancy. Acta Obstet Gynaecol Scand Suppl 1983; 113: 153–157

76 Ekman G, Forman A, Ulmsten U, Wingerup L. Termination of pregnancy in patients with missed abortion and intrauterine dead fetuses by a single intracervical application of prostaglandin E_2 in viscous gel. Zentralbl Gynakol 1980; 102: 219–222

77 Ekman G, Uldbjerg N, Wingerup L, Ulmsten U. Intracervical instillation of PGE_2-gel in

patients with missed abortion of intrauterine fetal death. Arch Gynecol 1983; 233: 241–245

78 Mapa MK, Singh PM, Misra I. Management of missed abortion by intramuscular administration of 15(S)15 methyl prostaglandin F$_2$ alpha. Asia J Obstet Gynaecol 1982; 8: 369–372

79 Karim SM, Ratnam SS, Hutabarat H et al. Termination of pregnancy in cases of intrauterine fetal death, missed abortion, molar and anencephalic multicentre study. Ann Acad Med Singa 1982; 11: 508–512

80 Satho K, Kinshita K, Sakamoto S. Clinical trial of Cervagm (ONO-802) for applications in first and second trimester abortions in Japan. In: Karim S. (ed) Cervagem. A new prostaglandin in obstetrics and gynaecology. Lancaster: MTP, 1982; 77–103

81 Naithmith WC, Barr W. Simultaneous intravenous infusion of prostaglandin E$_2$ (PGE$_2$) and oxytocin in the management of intrauterine death of the fetus, missed abortion and hydatidiform mole. J Obstet Gynaecol Br Cwlth 1974; 81: 146–149

82 Filshie GM. The use of prostaglandin E$_2$ in the management of intrauterine death, missed abortion and hydatidiform mole. J Obstet Gynaecol Br Cwlth 1971; 78: 87–90

83 Karim SM. Use of prostaglandin E$_2$ in the management of missed abortion, missed labour and hydatidiform mole. BMJ 1970: 3: 196–197

84 Herabutya Y, O-Pasertsawat. Misoprostol in the management of missed abortion. Int J Gynaecol Obstet 1997; 56: 263–266

85 Egarter C, Lederhilger J, Kurz C, Karas H, Reisenberger K. Gemeprost for the first trimester missed abortion. Arch Obstet 1995; 256: 29–32

86 Nielsen S, Hahlin M, Platz-Christensen JJ. Unsuccessful treatment of missed abortion with a combination of an antiprogesterone and a prostaglandin E$_1$ analogue. Br J Obstet Gynaecol 1997; 104: 1094–1096

87 Creinin MD, Moyer R, Guido R. Misoprostol for medical evacuation of early pregnancy failure. Obstet Gynecol 1997; 89: 768–772

88 Ragusa A, Vignali Jr M, Zanetta G, Norchi S, Zanini A. Pre-operative cervical preparation before first trimester missed abortion a randomised controlled comparison between single and double intracervical administration of PGE$_2$ gel. Prostaglandins Leukot Essen Fatty Acids 1994; 50: 267–269

89 Lelaider C, Baton-Saint-Mleux C, Fernandez H, Bourget P, Frydman R. Mifepristone (RU 486) induces embryo expulsion in first trimester non-developing pregnancies: a prospective randomised trial. Hum Reprod 1993; 8: 492–495

90 Liggins Jr GC. Obstet Gynaecol Br Cwlth 1962; 69: 277

91 Wagatsuma T. Intra-amniotic injection of saline for therapeutic abortion. Am J Obstet Gynecol 1965; 93: 743–745

92 Anonymous. A death associated with mifepristone/sulprostone. Lancet 1991; 337: 969–970

93 UK Multicentre Trial. The efficacy and tolerance of mifepristone and prostaglandin in first trimester termination of pregnancy. Br J Obstet Gynaecol 1990; 97: 481–486

94 World Health Organization Task Force on Postovulatory Methods for Fertility Regulation. Termination of early human pregnancy with RU486 (mifepristone) and prostaglandin analogue sulprostone: a multicentre randomised comparison between two treatment regimens. Hum Reprod 1989; 4: 718

95 World Health Organization. Pregnancy termination with mifepristone and gemeprost: a multicentre comparison between repeated doses and a single dose of mifepristone. Fertil Steril 1990; 56: 132–140

96 Norman JE, Thong KJ, Baired DT. Uterine contractility and induction of abortion in early pregnancy by misoprostol and mifepristone. Lancet 1991; 338: 1233–1236

97 Thong KJ, Lynch P, Baird V. A randomised study of two doses of gemeprost in combination with mifepristone for induction of abortion in the second trimester of pregnancy. Contraception 1996; 54: 97–100

98 Urquhart R, Templeton AA. The efficacy and tolerance of mifepristone and prostaglandin in first trimester termination of pregnancy. Br J Obstet Gynaecol 1996; 97: 480–486

99 Nielsen S, Hahlin M, Platz-Christensen J. Randomised trial comparing expectant with medical management for first trimester miscarriages. Br J Obstet Gynaecol 1999; 106: 804–807

100 Frumar AM, Smith ID, Korba AR. Prostaglandin $F_2\alpha$ for the induction of labour in the pregnancies complicated by intrauterine death anencephaly, chromosomal anomaly. Prostaglandins 1974; 6: 125–135

101 Toppozada MD, Bydgeman M, Wiqvist N. Induction of abortion by intrauterine administration of prostaglandin $F_2\alpha$. Contraception 1971; 4: 293

102 Embrey MP, Calder AA, Hillier K. Extra-amniotic prostaglandins in the management of intrauterine fetal death, anencephaly and hydatiform mole. J Obstet Gynaecol Br Cwlth 1974; 81: 47–51

103 Sandler RZ, Knutzen VK, Milano CM, Geicher N. Uterine rupture with the use of vaginal prostaglandin E_2 suppositories. Am J Obstet Gynecol 1979; 134: 348

104 Schulman H, Salanda L, Lin CC, Randolph G. Mechanism of failed labor after fetal death and its treatment with prostaglandin E_2. Am J Obstet Gynecol 1979; 33: 742–752

105 Baily CDH, Newman C, Ellinas SP, Anderson GG. Use of prostaglandin E_2 vaginal suppositories in intrauterine fetal death and missed abortion. Obstet Gynecol 1975; 45: 110–113

106 Rutland A, Ballard C. Vaginal prostaglandin E_2 for missed abortion and intrauterine fetal death. Am J Obstet Gynecol 1977; 128: 503–506

107 Patterson SP, White JH, Reaves EM. A maternal death associated with the prostaglandin E_2. Obstet Gynecol 1979; 54: 123–124

108 de Jonge ET, Makin JD, Manefeldt E, De Wet GH, Pattinson RC. Randomised clinical trial of medical evacuation and surgical curettage for incomplete miscarriage. BMJ 1995; 311: 662

109 Chung TK, Lee DT, Cheung LP, Haines CJ, Chang AM. Spontaneous abortion: a randomised, controlled trial comparing surgical evacuation with conservative management using misoprostol. Fertil Steril 1999; 71: 1054–1059

110 Chung T, Leung P, Cheung LP, Haines CJ, Chang AM. A medical approach to management of spontaneous abortion using misoprostol. Extending misoprostol treatment to a maximum of 48 hours can further improve evacuation of retained products of conception in spontaneous abortion. Acta Obstet Gynaecol Scand 1997; 76: 248–251

111 Chung TK, Cheung LP, Leung TY, Haines CJ, Chang AMZ. Misoprostol in the management of spontaneous abortion. Br J Obstet Gynaecol 1995; 102: 832–835

112 Chung TK, Cheung LP, Lau WC, Haines CJ, Chang AM. Spontaneous abortion: a medical approach to management. Aust NZ J Obstet Gynaecol 1994; 34: 432–436

113 Pang MW, Lee TS, Chung TKH. Incomplete miscarriage: a randomised controlled trial comparing oral with vaginal misoprostol for medical evacuation. Hum Reprod 2001; 16: 2283–2287

114 Wagaarachchi PT, Ashok PW, Narvekar N, Smith NC, Templeton A. Medical management of early fetal demise using a combination of mifepristone and misoprostol. Hum Reprod 2001; 16: 1849–1853

115 Demetroulis C, Saridogan E, Kunde D, Naftalin A. A prospective randomised trial comparing medical and surgical treatment for early pregnancy failure. Hum Reprod 2001; 16: 365–369

116 Wagaarachchi PT, Ashok PW, Smith NC, Templeton A. Medical management of early fetal demise using sublingual misorprostol. Br J Obstet Gynaecol 2002; 109: 462–465

117 Tassig FJ. Abortion Spontaneous and Induced Medical and Social Aspects, St Louis: Mosby, 1936; 156–184

118 Chipchase I, Campbell S, Grudzinskas JG. Ultrasonic assessment of complications during first trimester of pregnancy. Lancet 1987; 2: 1237–1240

119 Mansur MM. Ultrasound diagnosis of complete abortion can reduce the need for curettage. Eur J Obstet Gynaecol Reprod Biol 1992; 65–69.

120 Rulin MC, Bornstein SG, Campbell JD. The reliability of ultrasonography in the management of spontaneous abortion, clinically thought to be complete: a prospective study. Am J Obstet Gynecol 1992; 168): 12–15

121 Haines CH, Chung T, Leung DYL. Transvaginal sonography and conservative management of spontaneous abortion. Gynecol Obstet Invest 1994; 37: 14–17

122 Ankum WM, Van der Veen H. Management of first-trimester spontaneous abortion. Lancet 1995; 345: 1179–1183

123 Jurkovic D, Ross JA, Nicolaides A. Expectant management of missed miscarriage. Br J Obstet Gynaecol 1998; 105: 670–671

124 Luise C, Karen J, May C, Costello G, Collins WP, Bourne TH. Outcome of expectant management of spontaneous first trimester miscarriage: observational study. BMJ 2002; 324; 873–875

125 Nielsen S, Hahlin M, Oden A. Using logistic model to identify women with first-trimester spontaneous abortion suitable for expectant management. Br J Obstet Gynaecol 1996; 103: 1230–1235

126 Kaplan B, Pardo J, Rabinerson D, Fisch B, Neri A. Future fertility following conservative management of complete miscarriages. Hum Reprod 1996; 11: 92–94

127 Blohm F, Hahlin M, Nielsen S, Milsom L. Fertility after randomisation trial of spontaneous abortion managed by surgical evacuation or surgical management. Lancet 1997; 349: 995

128 Adams ME, McCall NT, Gray DT, Orza MJ, Chalmers TC. Economic analysis in randomised controlled trials. Med Care 1992; 30: 231–243

129 Henshaw RC, Naji SA, Russell IT, Templeton AA. A prospective economic evaluation comparing medical abortion (using mifepristone and gemeprost) and surgical vacuum aspiration. Br J Fam Plan 1994; 20: 64–68

130 Hughes J, Scholar N, Ryan M et al. The costs of treating miscarriage: a comparison of medical management and surgical management. Br J Obstet Gynaecol 1996; 103: 1217–1221

131 Pandian Z, Ashok P, Templeton A. The treatment of incomplete miscarriage with oral misoprostol. Br J Obstet Gynaecol 2001; 108: 213–214

Sharif I. M. F. Ismail

Saline sonohysterography

Saline sonohysterography entails the distension of the endometrial cavity with saline during standard transvaginal ultrasound, delineating focal endometrial lesions and visualising abnormalities of the uterine cavity. This chapter provides a background to the clinical situations in which this investigation can be used and describes how the investigation is performed. Its value in clinical practice is discussed, highlighting the advantages it affords in reducing cost and streamlining patient care.

CLINICAL BACKGROUND

The technique can be used to investigate the endometrium and the endometrial cavity, which is valuable when investigating abnormal uterine bleeding, recurrent miscarriage and preterm labour, amenorrhea as well as prior to assisted conception.

Abnormal uterine bleeding

Abnormal uterine bleeding includes heavy and/or prolonged periods (menorrhagia) as well as those with bleeding in between periods (irregular uterine bleeding).[1] Whilst menorrhagia before the age of 40 years is unlikely to be due to endometrial carcinoma,[2] making its exclusion unnecessary in these patients,[3,4] assessing the endometrium is important in those who do not respond to medical treatment, as they might have polyps[5] as well as those patients above that age. Likewise, ovulation and breakthrough bleeding are considered normal,[1] yet other forms of irregular uterine bleeding necessitate excluding local causes, especially in perimenopausal and postmenopausal patients.[6]

Sharif I. M. F. Ismail MSc MBA MA MMedSci(Ed) LLM MRCOG
Specialist Registrar in Obstetrics and Gynaecology, Singleton Hospital, Sketty, Swansea SA2 8QA, UK
(E-mail: sharif212121@hotmail.com)

The choice often lies between taking an out-patient endometrial pathology and arranging for an ultrasound scan, to measure the endometrial thickness, performing an in-patient hysteroscopy,[7] or arranging for an out-patient hysteroscopy.[8] As will become clear below, saline sonohysterography enhances the value of ultrasound and guides the use of hysteroscopy.

Recurrent pregnancy loss

Recurrent pregnancy loss (miscarriage and preterm labour) can be due to congenital anomalies of the uterine cavity, polycystic ovaries and antiphospholipid syndrome. Hysteroscopy and/or hysterosalpingography has often been used in these cases to establish whether there is uterine septum or not, with hysteroscopic resection preferred to laparotomy.[9,10] As outlined later, saline sonohysterography represents a reliable alternative that can avoid hysteroscopy in those patients without a septum and guides the resection in those with septate uterus.

Amenorrhea

Amenorrhea can result from obliteration of the uterine cavity by adhesions, commonly known as Asherman's syndrome,[11] as well as polycystic ovaries and ovarian failure.[1] The adhesions commonly result from strenuous curretage, usually after miscarriage or delivery and hysteroscopic division of such adhesions is preferred to blind attempts to divide them at dilatation and curettage.[10] Again, saline sonohysterography can avoid the use of hysteroscopy in those without such adhesions and guide resection in those with adhesions.

Assisted conception

Patients undergoing assisted conception (*e.g. in vitro* fertilisation) are often investigated for abnormalities of the uterine cavity, such as fibroid polyps and uterine septae, which need resection to avoid failure of implantation.[12] These patients undergo ultrasound examination for various reasons – detection of fibroids as well as measurement of endometrial thickness and monitoring of ovulation induction. Saline sonohysterography can identify those with abnormalities and guide their resection, with little addition to the scans they usually have to measure the endometrial thickness and monitor ovulation induction.

THEORY

The introduction of saline into the uterine cavity provides a contrast[5] that helps localisation of abnormalities as intracavitary, endometrial or submucosal.[13] Fluid represents an excellent medium for transmission of sound waves and provides a good contrast to examine the endometrial cavity, just as it is better to look at the fetus in cases of polyhydramnios.[14] The saline also distends the endometrial cavity, separating endometrial walls so as to visualise polyps that could be seen as part of the overall endometrial thickness, when both walls are measured together in the standard scan.

NOMENCLATURE

Various names have been used to describe the technique, including saline instillation sonography, transvaginal saline hysterosonography,[15] saline infusion sonography,[5] saline infusion sonohysterosalpingography,[16] saline infusion sonohysterography,[14] saline contrast hysterosonography,[17] and hydrosonography.[18] Hysterography was chosen here because it describes the actual value of the technique in visualising the uterine cavity; 'sono' differentiates it from standard hystero-salpingography and saline distinguishes it from the use of other distension media.[19,20]

TECHNIQUE

Timing

For patients with bleeding, this is best in the proliferative phase when the endometrium is thin to facilitate the detection of polyps.[21] Patients suspected of having fibroids are better examined in the secretary phase, when the thickened endometrium provides a contrast to the hypo-echoic liomyomata, though this could lead to more artefacts from shedding of the thick endometrium as the test catheter is inserted, appearing as polyps. This can be difficult with irregular bleeding. In all cases, pregnancy should be excluded as with hysterosalpingography.[13]

Preparation

As with all forms of uterine instrumentation, the test should only be performed after pelvic infection has been excluded. Patients with history of chronic pelvic infection are given a course of doxycycline.[21] Although some prescribe antibiotics to all patients,[19,22] there is little point in taking swabs or administering antibiotics in asymptomatic patients with no history of previous infection.[14] There was once a case of pelvic inflammatory disease in a patient suspected of having prior infection despite using prophylactic antibiotics.[23] Those with cardiac disease are given prophylactic antibiotics as done with other genito-urinary procedures.[13]

The investigation can cause some pain as a result of introducing catheters, inflating balloons and/or distension of the uterine cavity with saline. This is often similar to period pain and of short duration.[19] It could be reduced by non-steroidal anti-inflammatory drugs[5,13] although some[24] used rectal antispasmodics 1 h prior to the investigation and others[16] needed Entonox (50% nitrous oxide/50% oxygen) for pain experienced upon inflating the balloons of Foley's catheters, bearing in mind that vasovagal response could occur.[14,24,25]

A standard transvaginal scan is carried out initially with an empty bladder. This shows fibroids and adnexal masses[17] and the endometrial thickness is measured. Occasionally, spontaneous fluid is noted within the endometrial cavity which, if of adequate amount, might allow examination of the endometrium without the need for saline instillation.[25] Such collections are likely to be associated with pathology if the surrounding endometrium is thick and/or echogenic,[26] the fluid itself is echogenic (denoting pus or blood), the uterus is enlarged or there are symptoms like pain, bleeding or discharge.[27]

In the absence of such fluid, catheterisation of the cervix will be necessary for the introduction of saline. The transvaginal ultrasound transducer is removed and a speculum is inserted to visualise the cervix. In the absence of infection, the cervix is cleaned with an antiseptic solution and a small catheter is then introduced into the endometrial cavity using forceps. Such catheters should be 25 cm long to enable the injection of saline after the transvaginal probe is re-introduced.[5] Such catheters could be without or with balloons. Catheters without a balloon tend to be cheaper and are readily available as they are used for other purposes (*e.g.* the size 5 F paediatric feeding catheter[13] or the size 5 F insemination catheter[14,22]). These catheters do not occlude a patulous cervix, leading to saline leakage, and thus poor distension of the uterine cavity. Catheters with balloons, such as the 5 Fr hysterosalpingography catheter[21] and the CH 10 Foley's catheter[16] occlude the cervix with their balloons,[15,16,23] thereby avoiding saline leakage. However, these catheters can alter the view of the lower part of the uterus, which will have to be examined as the balloon is deflated to withdraw the catheter[21] and are more expensive.

It is advisable to use non-balloon catheters, as they cause less discomfort,[28] leaving balloon catheters for those with patulous cervix.[29,30] Difficult catheterisation is dealt with by dilating the cervix, using local anaesthesia if necessary, as with out-patient hysteroscopy.[13] Catheters, and balloons should be flushed and connected to saline syringes before they are introduced into the cervix to avoid introducing air bubbles, which could produce artefacts.

The size of syringes used ranged from 1–2 ml[22] and 10 ml[14,23] to 20 ml[25,16] and 60 ml.[5] Ideally, the syringe should allow completion of the examination without the need for refilling with saline to avoid time wastage and loss of the distension pressure. Although some have found small volumes such as 3–30 ml[19,20,25,21,31] of saline sufficient to distend the uterine cavity, others needed larger volumes such as 10–60 ml.[5,15] It might, therefore, be better to use a 20 ml syringe to start with and re-adjust the size in the light of experience.

The sonohysterogram

The transvaginal transducer is re-introduced and saline is injected to reach and maintain uterine distension. The uterus is scanned in the longitudinal axis, from one cornu to the other, then in transverse sections, from the top of the uterus to the cervix.[16] Normal endometrium appears uniform and symmetric all around with no protrusions or filling defects. Although detecting saline in the pouch of Douglas indicates patent tubes,[15] the investigation is not reliable in checking tubal patency for which there is a specialised technique – hysterosalpingo contrast sonography (HyCoSy),[32,33] which deserves separate consideration but is not addressed here. Abnormalities include:

Polyps
Polyps appear as protrusions into the cavity, when examined at their stalks, otherwise they appear as balls of endometrial tissue surrounded by saline (Fig. 2b). Movement upon injecting saline differentiates them from blood clots, which can be displaced anywhere in the uterine cavity.[16] It is important to note the number of polyps, their size, site, margin, areas of increased echogenicity

and whether they have cystic (anechoic) areas or not.[15,25] Colour Doppler shows the vascularity of pedicles and demonstrates atypical blood flow pattern, which might suggest malignancy,[16] though this evaluation is neither specific nor sensitive enough to rely on in diagnosing malignancy.[34]

It is valuable also to examine the stalk of polyps as this will guide their resection.[13] A single polyp with a thin pedicle is easily removed at out-patient operative hysteroscopy whereas multiple polyps and those with a thick pedicle, especially if near the cornu, would require resection under general anaesthesia. Verifying the attachment of polyps enables the localisation of endocervical polyps,[14] bearing in mind that a large endocervical polyp could make it difficult to secure tight seal of catheters to avoid leakage of saline.

The precision of saline hysterosonography in establishing the presence of polyps is of special help in patients on tamoxifen, usually for breast cancer. This treatment can stimulate endometrial hyperplasia and even carcinoma[35,36] and increasingly patients are monitored by regular ultrasound measurement of endometrial thickness.[37] Saline sonohysterography helps the identification of not only polyps in these patients[35] but also detection of sub-endometrial thickening, thought to be due to activation of myometrial adenomyoseal foci that do not need excision. These foci can cause an apparent thickening of the endometrium with cystic changes on a standard scan, only to be rebuked by a hysteroscopy revealing thin inactive endometrium.[14]

Fibroids

Fibroids appear as filling defects with mixed echogenicity[30] that is different to the endometrium with which they are usually covered.[29] They sometimes distort[23] or even fill the uterine cavity such that it can not be distended adequately, especially if they are large and/or multiple.[13] They can be differentiated from polyps[21] and intramural extensions are detected; these can make resection difficult requiring more skill, equipment and time[14] and even multiple-stage resection.[38]

It is especially important to note if fibroids actually extend to the serosal surface of the uterus,[39] as resection should not be attempted in these cases.[14] Such fibroids might appear no different to other polyps at hysteroscopy; even with polyp forceps, they could be difficult to remove or get avulsed with peritoneum, denoting perforation. Incomplete excision and/or perforation of the uterus, with possible thermal damage to abdominal viscera, are obvious risks. Gonadotrophin releasing hormone analogues could shrink these fibroids enough to enable their resection.[38] Alternatively, laparotomy (for hysterectomy or myomectomy) might be a safer option, depending on the patient features.

Focal endometrial thickening

The endometrial thickness of each wall is measured separately,[17] identifying focal thickening[15] which could be specifically biopsied at hysteroscopy (Fig 2a).[13] The surface of the endometrium should be examined for irregularities.[17] Heterogenicity of the endometrium, irregularity of the junction between the endometrium and myometrium,[25] poor distension of the uterine cavity on injecting saline and uniform increased echogenicity of the endometrium[15] should raise the suspicion of malignancy, whilst bearing in mind that these features are not specific nor sensitive enough.[25]

Table 1 Saline sonohysterography

Indications
    Abnormal uterine bleeding
        Endometrial thickness > 5 mm in patients with postmenopausal bleeding
        Endometrial thickness > 8 mm in premenopausal patients with:
            Irregular uterine bleeding
            Heavy and/or prolonged periods aged 40 years or more
            Heavy and/or prolonged periods below the age of 40 years who do not respond to medical treatment
        Cystic, echogenic or heterogeneous endometrium on ultrasonography
        Hyperechoic line around the endometrium
        Failure to visualise the endometrium on ultrasound
    Recurrent pregnancy loss (miscarriage/preterm labour)
    Amenorrhea/oligomenorrhea
    Prior to assisted conception

Advantages
    Reliable in detecting polyps, fibroids, focal endometrial thickening as well as septae and adhesions
    Patient friendly, out-patient and does not cause much pain
    Relies on readily available material
    Cost effective, avoids unnecessary repetition of hysteroscopy
    Guides and informs the use of hysteroscopy
    Delineates subendometrial thickening in patients on tamoxifen
    Supports one-stop out-patient approach to bleeding, infertility and recurrent pregnancy loss

Limitations
    Can not diagnose malignancy
    Risk of infection and pain
    Separate procedures for the checking the uterus and checking the tubes

Abnormalities of the uterine cavity

Intra-uterine adhesions and malformations of the uterine cavity appear as immobile connections between the uterine walls.[30] If there are thick and/or wide-spread adhesions, as in Asherman's syndrome, they might preclude distension of the cavity.[13] Incomplete separation of the anterior and posterior uterine walls, in longitudinal sections of the uterus (sagital), denotes intra-uterine synechiae and can give the uterus a 'bow tie' appearance on transverse (coronal) sections.[13] Malformations of the uterine cavity would cause much thicker connections between the anterior and posterior walls. For example, a V-shaped echogenic midline extension into the endometrial cavity in transverse (coronal) sections of the uterus suggests a septum and the presence of two endometrial cavities, separated by echogenic appearance of myometrium, indicates a bicornuate uterus (see Table 1).[23]

Conclusion of the examination

The transvaginal ultrasound probe is removed at the end of the examination and the patient is allowed to dress before discussing her subsequent management plan. Patients are advised that they can expect spotting after such an investigation and any mild colicky lower abdominal pain is treated with non-steroidal anti-inflammatory drugs. They should contact their general practitioner or the hospital if they notice any continuous or heavy bleeding, unusual or smelling discharge, increasing abdominal pain or fever.[13]

Subsequent management

In one-stop bleeding clinics,[40] patients would be seen by a gynaecologist immediately after the scan. An endometrial biopsy could be obtained at this time, if appropriate, for example in a patient presenting with abnormal uterine bleeding without a focal lesion.[22] Those who try and obtain an endometrial biopsy at the end of out-patient hysteroscopy, when fluid distension media have been used, know well that they may need repeat aspiration to clear most of the fluid used before they can obtain a decent biopsy. Alternatively, an out-patient hysteroscopy could be carried out, when small polyps could be removed.[41]

If saline sonohysterography shows a pathology, such as a polyp or a septum, then operative hysteroscopy is likely to be required, taking note of the information provided, for example by pre-treatment with gonadotrophin releasing hormone analogues. The presence of spontaneous fluid requires examining the cervix digitally and taking a biopsy from it in addition to an endometrial biopsy if the endometrium is thin. Otherwise, an examination under anaesthesia, hysteroscopy and biopsy to rule out cervical as well as endometrial carcinoma if the patient is symptomatic, the fluid is echogenic, the endometrium is thickened and/or echogenic or the uterus itself is enlarged. If no abnormality is detected, then the patient could be re-assured and in cases of bleeding or recurrent miscarriage for example, proceed with subsequent care, like assisted conception, or have further investigations for her condition, as with amenorrhea. If saline sonohysterography fails, then it is better to proceed with operative hysteroscopy, taking note of the tendency of malignancy to be more advanced in these patients,[25] though one might carry out an out-patient hysteroscopy in patients with medical problems rendering them at anaesthetic risk (Fig. 1).

VALUE IN CLINICAL PRACTICE

Accuracy

The accuracy of saline hysterosonography in detecting polyps, fibroids and focal thickening was found to be comparable with that of office hysteroscopy in a large comparison that included 113 patients with abnormal bleeding, with both the hysteroscopist and ultrasonographer blinded to the findings of each other. The technique had sensitivity of 97%, specificity of 93%, positive predictive value of 94% and negative predictive value of 97%. There was no statistically significant difference between the two techniques.[5]

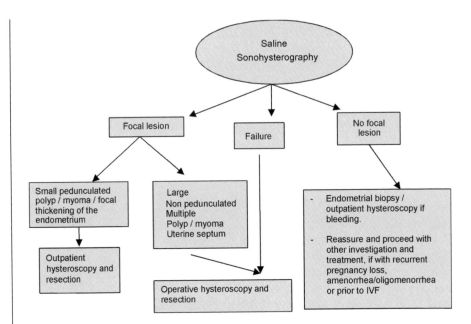

Fig. 1 Algorithm for the care of patients after saline sonohysterography.

Saline sonohysterography is much better than hysterosalpingography and transvaginal sonography in detecting abnormalities of the uterine cavity. When compared to hysterosalpingography in 18 patients with recurrent pregnancy loss,[23] it had a sensitivity and a specificity of 100% in detecting pathology in the uterine cavity, including synechiae, submucosal fibroids, bicornuate uterus and uterine septum, whereas hysterosalingography had a sensitivity of 90% and a specificity of 80%. When compared to hysteroscopy in 38 patients awaiting *in vitro* fertilisation for infertility,[12] it had a sensitivity of 87.5%, 100% specificity, 100% positive predictive value and 91% negative predictive value, whereas the comparable figures for transvaginal sonography were 81%, 95%, 93% and 86%.

Ease of use

Most authors encountered no failures,[13,17,21,23] though some did. Failure rates ranged from 3–8%,[5,12,16,20] though one study reported failure rate of 21%, dropping to 10% in the latter part, suggesting a learning curve,[25] with most cases due to cervical stenosis. These could be managed with cervical dilatation under local anaesthesia, as with out-patient hysteroscopy, bearing in mind that saline sonohysterography causes less pain than hysteroscopy,[5] and is more acceptable to patients.[37] It is to be noted, however, that failed cases tend to have severe degrees of stenosis,[5,12,16,20] or significant intra-uterine adhesions,[5] which might indicate that failure should be followed by operative hysteroscopy.

Cost effectiveness

Apart from the catheters, syringes and saline, the technique does not have any additional requirements other than those needed for a standard transvaginal sonography, which should be available in most hospitals world-wide nowadays. Moreover, it does not require much additional training, above the usual training in gynaecological ultrasound, as well as inserting catheters into the uterus, for radiologists[15] and ultrasonographers.[25] It does not add much time to a standard ultrasound scan, reported figures include 3.5 min[5] to 5–10 min,[17] < 5 min[21] to 15 min.[12]

The technique has the potential of saving cost in the way in which it helps the use of hysteroscopy. It distinguishes those who need an operative hysteroscopy, those who do not need further investigation as well as those in whom an endometrial sample or an out-patient hysteroscopy would be sufficient. It guides the process of resection by giving an idea about adhesions and septa as well as the number, location and size of any polyp, and identifies those who would benefit from gonadotrophin releasing hormone analogues and/or multiple resection.

The technique helped proceeding with operative in-patient hysteroscopy in 66 patients with abnormal bleeding, out of 129 in whom the investigation was carried out (51%),[17] bearing in mind that the investigation could not be carried out in another 10, bringing the percentage of those avoiding repeat hysteroscopy to 47%, which is almost half the work load. Savings become more obvious if one considers hysteroscopy equipment, set-up, theatre time, staff, sterilisation and resterilisation, anaesthesia as well as inpatient admission.

Application

As the technique is best in detecting focal endometrial lesions, describing fibroid polyps as well as identifying abnormalities of the uterine cavity, it should be used in patients with abnormal uterine bleeding that is likely to be due to focal endometrial lesions and/or fibroid polyps, patients receiving assisted conception, in whom polyps need to be excluded, patients suspected of having intra-uterine synechiae or Asherman's syndrome with amenorrhea/oligomenorrhea as well as those with recurrent miscarriage and early preterm labour, that could be attributed to anomalies in the uterine cavity. The technique can also be used for a postoperative check, assessing the success in resecting polyps and fibroids as well as division of adhesions or septa.[13]

The likelihood of focal lesions in patients with abnormal uterine bleeding relates to a number of features that can be detected on the conventional ultrasound scan carried out at the start of the investigation

Endometrial thickness

Whilst the normal limits are 14 mm for premenopausal patients, 8 mm for postmenopausal patients on hormone replacement therapy and 5 mm for postmenopausal patients not on hormone replacement therapy,[15] a cut off level of > 8 mm in premenopausal patients and > 5 mm in postmenopausal ones provides a good sensitivity for detecting benign and malignant pathology.[17] The 5 mm cut level for postmenopausal bleeding, irrespective of the use of hormone replacement therapy, was recommended by a recent meta-analysis[42] and several other studies.[25,43–45]

Appearance of the endometrium

The presence of cystic areas within the endometrium as well as a hyperechoic line around it are characteristic of focal lesions.[29] Increased or mixed echogenicity of the endometrium should raise suspicion of a pathological lesion, even if the total endometrial thickness falls within normal limits.[15,46] There were 3 cases of benign endometrial polyps with an overall endometrial thickness < 5 mm in one study[47] and < 6 mm in another,[48] all having irregular endometrial surface. Likewise, failure to visualise the endometrium, for example due to adhesions, should be considered as a reason for suspicion, as there could be areas of abnormal endometrium in isolated pockets of endometrium.[15]

THE FUTURE

It might be possible one day to increase the value of this investigation in detecting malignancy, through better understanding of Doppler parameters or possibly by changing the distension medium. Concomitant assessment of the uterine cavity and tubal patency might be possible as well, through developing new distension media. Likewise, a single device could be used to inject the distension medium and sample the endometrium at the end, avoiding the need to re-insert a speculum and re-negotiate the cervix.

Saline sonohysterography can reshape one-stop bleeding clinics[40] as a first step in the investigation of bleeding[49] to guide the referral for in-patient hysteroscopy and biopsy, with those not requiring such procedure having an endometrial biopsy at the end of the investigation.

There has been one report comparing the use of intra-uterine sonography as an alternative to saline sonohysterography.[22] Although this technique has been used in examining embryos and detecting anomalies,[50–52] its use in gynaecology remains very limited and future research may lead to a bigger role for this technique.

CONCLUSIONS

Saline hysterosonography entails the use of saline to distend the endometrial cavity during transvaginal ultrasound examination, delineating intra- and peri-endometrial pathology. It can accurately identify polyps, fibroids and focal lesions; short of detecting malignancy; as well as intra-uterine adhesions and malformations of the uterine cavity, avoiding unnecessary hysteroscopies. It provides valuable information about polyps and fibroids, indicating those likely to require special skill and preparation. It is, therefore, helpful in cases of abnormal uterine bleeding likely to be due to an endometrial cause, recurrent pregnancy loss and preterm labour, amenorrhea as well as prior to assisted conception. It can also be used to check completion after resection of polyps, fibroids and septae as well as division of adhesions.

The investigation follows a standard transvaginal scan, checking the uterus, the endometrium and the adnexae. It requires catheterisation of the cervix, using a balloon catheter to occlude patulous cervices. Cervical stenosis is managed by dilating the cervix under local anaesthesia, as with out-patient hysteroscopy. It should not be performed in the presence of local infection;

those with previous infection as well as those with cardiac disease will need prophylactic antibiotics. Fluid collection in the endometrial cavity obviates the need for catheterisation, but necessitates ruling out cervical and/or endometrial pathology if haematometra is suspected. Patients may experience period-like pain, which can be reduced by analgesia.

In-patient operative hysteroscopy will be needed upon failure, to dilate the cervix. This is especially important as malignancies tend to be more advanced with failed saline sonohysterography. The technique is safe, with occasional vaso-vagal reaction and exacerbation of dormant pelvic infection being rare complications. It is easy to perform, relies on standard equipment and material available in most hospitals and does not require much training. It adds a small fraction to the duration of a standard scan. It guides the need for hysteroscopy, with significant cost savings.

The investigation can be part of one-stop bleeding and infertility clinics, where endometrial biopsy and out-patient hysteroscopy can be carried out and other aspects of patient care discussed and planned. It is likely to become the first line investigation for bleeding and its value could be enhanced further with future refinements.

Figure 2 a,b — added at proof

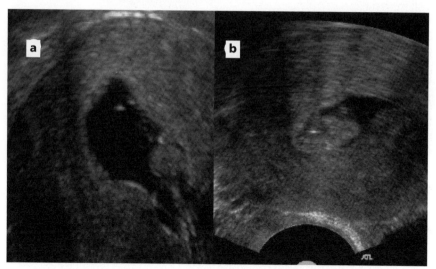

Fig. 2 Saline sonohysterography can distinguish between focal thickening (a) and endometrial polyp (b)

References

1 Chamberlain GVP. Gynaecology by Ten Teachers, 16th edn. London: Arnold 1995; 173–175

2 Mackenzie JZ, Bibby JG. Critical assessment of dilatation and curettage in 1209 women. Lancet 1978; ii: 566–569

3 Grimes DA. Diagnostic dilatation and curettage; a reappraisal. Am J Obstet Gynecol 1982; 142: 1–6

4 The Royal College of Obstetricians and Gynaecologists. In-patient Treatment – D&C in women age 40 or less. RCOG guidelines No. 3. London: RCOG Press, 1994

5 Widrich T, Bradley LD, Mitchinson AR, Collins RL. Comparison of saline infusion sonography with office hysteroscopy for the evaluation of the endometrium. Am J Obstet Gynecol 1996; 174: 1327–1334

6 Weeks AD, Duffy SRG. Abnormal uterine bleeding; Diagnosis and medical management. Prog Obstet Gynaecol 1996; 12: 309–326

7 Lumsden MA, Norman J, Critchley H. Menstrual Problems for the MRCOG. London: RCOG Press, 1997; 21–39

8 Clark TJ, Bakour SH, Gupta JK, Khan KS. Evaluation of outpatient hysteroscopy and ultrasonography in the diagnosis of endometrial disease. Obstet Gynecol 2002; 99: 1001–1007

9 Clifford K, Regan L. Recurrent pregnancy loss. Prog Obstet Gynaecol 1994; 11: 97–110

10 Pinion SB. The future of hysteroscopic surgery. Prog Obstet Gynaecol 1994; 11: 245–260

11 Asherman JG. Amenorrhoea traumatica (atretica). J Obstet Gynecol Br Emp 1948; 55: 23

12 Ayida G, Chamberlain P, Barlow D, Kennedy S. Uterine cavity assessment prior to *in vitro* fertilisation: comparison of transvaginal scanning, saline contrast hysterosonography and hysteroscopy. Ultrasound Obstet Gynecol 1997; 10: 59–62

13 Cullinan JA, Fleischer AC, Kepple DM, Arnold AL. Sonohysterography: a technique for endometrial evaluation. Radiographics 1995; 15: 501–504

14 Goldstein SR. Saline infusion sonohysterography. Clin Obstet Gynaecol 1996; 39: 248–258

15 Laifer-Narin SL, Ragavendra N, Lu DS, Sayre J, Perrella RR, Grant EG. Transvaginal saline hysterosonography: characteristics distinguishing malignant and various benign conditions. AJR Am J Roentgenol 1999; 172: 1513–1520

16 De Crespigny L, Kuhn R, McGinnes D. Saline infusion sonohysterosalpingography: an under-utilised technique. Aust NZ J Obstet Gynaecol 1997; 37: 206–209

17 Bronz L, Suter T, Ruscca T. The value of transvaginal sonography with and without saline instillation in the diagnosis of uterine pathology in pre- and postmenopausal women with abnormal bleeding or suspect sonographic findings. Ultrasound Obstet Gynaecol 1997; 9: 53–58

18 Okaro E, Condous G, Bourne T. The use of ultrasound in the management of gynaecological conditions. Prog Obstet Gynaecol 2002; 15: 273–297

19 Bonilla-Musoles F, Simon C, Serra V, Sampio M, Pellicer A. An assessment of hystersalpingosonography as a diagnostic tool for uterine cavity defects and tubal patency. J Clin Ultrasound 1992; 20: 175–181

20 Gaucherand P, Piacenza JM, Salle B, Rudigoz RC. Sonohysterography of the uterine cavity; Preliminary investigations. J Clin Ultrasound 1995; 23: 339–348

21 Lindheim SR, Sauer MV. Upper genital tract screening with hysterosonography in patients receiving donated oocytes. Int J Gynecol Obstet 1998; 60: 47–50

22 Senoh D, Tanaka H, Akiyama M, Yanagihara T, Hata T. Saline infusion contrast intrauterine sonographic assessment of the endometrium with high-frequency, real-time miniature transducer in normal menstrual cycle: a preliminary report. Hum Reprod 1999; 14: 2600–2603

23 Keltz MD, Olive DL, Kim AH, Arici A. Sonohysterography for screening in recurrent pregnancy loss. Fertil Steril 1997; 67: 670–674

24 Cicinelli E, Romano F, Anastasio PS, Blasi N, Parisi C. Sonohysterography versus hysteroscopy in the diagnosis of endouterine polyps. Gynecol Obstet Invest 1994; 38: 226–271

25 Epstein E, Ramirez A, Skoog L, Valentin L. Transvaginal sonography, saline contrast sonohysterography and hysteroscopy for the investigation of women with postmenopausal bleeding and endometrium > 5 mm. Ultrasound Obstet Gynecol 2001; 18: 157–162

26 Gull B, Karlsson B, Wikland M, Milson I, Granberg S. Factors influencing the presence of uterine cavity fluid in a random sample of asymptomatic postmenopausal women. Acta Obstet Gynecol Scand 1998; 77: 751–757

27 Breckenbridge JW, Kurtz AB, Ritchie WGM, Machat EL. Postmenopausal uterine fluid collection: an indicator of carcinoma. AJR Am J Roentgenol 1982; 139: 529–534

28 Synder JT, Anasti J. A comparison of two saline infusion sonography catheters. Obstet Gynaecol 2000; 95: 31S

29 Baldwin MT, Dudiak KM, Gorman B, Marks CA. Focal intracavitary masses recognized with the hyperechoic line sign at endovaginal US and characterised with hysterosonography. Radiographics 1999; 19: 927–935

30 Parsons AK, Lense JJ. Sonohysterography for endometrial abnormalities: preliminary results. J Clin Ultrasound 1993; 21: 87–95

31 Buttery BW. Ultrasonic hysterography: a new technique. Lancet 1973; 2: 595–596

32 Campbell S, Bourne TH, Tan SL, Collins WP. Hysterosalpingo contrast sonography (HyCoSy) and its future role within the investigation of infertility in Europe. Ultrasound Obstet Gynecol 1994; 4: 245–253

33 Schlief R, Deichert U. Hysterosalpingo-contrast sonography of the uterus and fallopian tubes: results of a clinical trial of a new contrast medium in 120 patients. Radiology 1991; 178: 213–215

34 Goldstein SR, Monteagudo A, Popiolek D, Mayberry P, Timor-Tritsch I. Evaluation of endometrial polyps. Am J Obstet Gynecol 2002; 186: 669–674

35 Bourne TH, Lawton F, Leather A, Granberg S, Campbell S, Collins WP. Use of intracavitary saline instillation and transvaginal ultrasonography to detect tamoxifen-associated endometrial polyps. Ultrasound Obstet Gynecol 1994; 4: 73–75

36 Lahti E, Blanco G, Kauppila A, Apaja-Sarkkinen M, Taskinen P J, Laatikainen T. Endometrial changes in postmenopausal breast cancer patients receiving tamoxifen. Obstet Gynecol 1993; 81: 660–664

37 Timmerman D, Deprest J, Bourne T, Berghe IVD, Collins WP, Vergote I. A randomised trial on the use of ultrasonography or office hysteroscopy for endometrial assessment in postmenopausal patients with breast cancer who were treated with tamoxifen. Am J Obstet Gynecol 1998; 179: 62–70

38 Donnez J, Gillerot S, Bourgonion D, Clerckx F, Nisolle M. Neodynium:Yag laser hysteroscopy in large submuous fibroids. Fertil Steril 1990; 54: 999–1003

39 Goldstein SR. Use of ultrasonohysterography for triage of perimenopausal patients with unexplained uterine bleeding. Am J Obstet Gynecol 1994; 170: 565–570

40 Baskett TF, O'Connor H, Magos AL. A comprehensive one-stop menstrual problem clinic for the diagnosis and management of abnormal uterine bleeding. Br J Obstet Gynaecol 1996; 103: 76–77

41 Lindheim SR, Kavic S, Shulman SV, Sauer MV. Operative hysteroscopy in the office setting. J Am Assoc Gynecol Laparosc 2000; 7: 65–69

42 Gupta JK, Chien PF, Volt D, Clark TJ, Khan KS. Ultrasonographic endometrial thickness for diagnosing endometrial pathology in women with postmenopausal bleeding: a meta-analysis. Act Obstet Gynecol Scand 2002; 81: 799–816

43 Goldstein SR, Nachtigall M, Snyder JR, Nachtigall L. Endometrial assessment by vaginal ultrasonography before endometrial sampling in patients with postmenopausal bleeding. Am J Obstet Gynecol 1990; 163: 119–123

44 Granberg S, Wickland M, Karlsson B, Norstrom A, Friberg LG. Endometrial thickness as measured by endovaginal ultrasonography for identifying endometrial abnormality. Am J Obstet Gynecol 1991; 164: 47–52

45 Smith-Bindman R, Kerlikowske K, Feldstein VA et al. Endovaginal ultrasound to exclude endometrial cancer and other endometrial abnormalities, JAMA 1998; 280: 1510–1517

46 Dubinsky TJ, Stoechlein K, Abu-Ghazzeh, Parvey HR, Maklad N. Prediction of benign and malignant endometrial disease; Hysterosonographic-pathologic correlation. Radiology 1999; 210: 393–397

47 Karlsson B, Granberg S, Wickland M et al. Transvaginal ultrasonography of the endometrium in women with postmenopausal bleeding: a Nordic multicentre study. Am J Obstet Gynecol 1995; 172: 1488–1494

48 Sheikh M, Sawhney S, Khurana A, Al-Yatama M. Alteration of sonographic texture of the endometrium in postmenopausal bleeding: a guide to further management. Acta Obstet Gynecol Scand 2000; 79: 1006–1010

49 Bernard JP, Lecuru F, Darles C, Robin F, De Bievre P, Taurelle R. Saline contrast sonohysterography as first-line investigation for women with uterine bleeding. Ultrasound Obstet Gynecol 1997; 10: 121–125

50 Fujiwaki R, Hata T, Hata K, Kitao M. Intrauterine assessment of embryonic development. Am J Obstet Gynecol 1995; 173: 1770–1774

51 Hata T. Intrauterine sonography for the assessment of embryonic development. Med Imag Int 1996; 6: 11–15

52 Hata T, Fujiwaki R, Senoh D, Hata K. Intrauterine sonographic assessments of embryonal liver length. Hum Reprod 1996; 11: 1278–1281

Nicholas J. Raine-Fenning

Three-dimensional ultrasound and reproductive medicine

Conventional ultrasound provides two-dimensional views of three-dimensional structures that an experienced ultrasonographer has to examine dynamically in order to create their own three-dimensional impression of the object of interest.[1] In contrast, three-dimensional ultrasound allows the simultaneous assessment of individual sectional planes, which may be examined in turn to maximise the information available.[2,3] It provides the examiner with more spatial information as well as several different viewing modalities to maximise diagnostic capability dependent upon the particular field of interest.[4] Uniquely, three-dimensional ultrasound allows demonstration of the coronal plane perpendicular to the transducer face facilitating the identification of surface irregularities which can then be accounted for during volume measurement.[5]

The following review briefly discusses the advantages of three-dimensional ultrasound, in terms of its spatial awareness and associated measurement parameters, and their application within the field of reproductive medicine and represents an extension of a review recently published in the *British Medical Ultrasound Society Bulletin*.

THREE-DIMENSIONAL DATA ANALYSIS

Three-dimensional imaging is invariably associated with photographic-like images of the developing fetus. However, to appreciate the real benefits of three-dimensional ultrasound one has to consider what it offers in terms of new measurement parameters.

The most obvious parameter considered is that of volume. Whilst volume may be estimated from measurements made with conventional two-dimensional ultrasound, such measurements use various formulae based

Nicholas J. Raine-Fenning MBChB MRCOG PhD
Clinical Lecturer, Academic Division of Reproductive Medicine, School of Human Development, D Floor, East Block, Queen's Medical Centre, Nottingham NG7 2UH, UK
(E-mail: nick.fenning@nottingham.ac.uk)

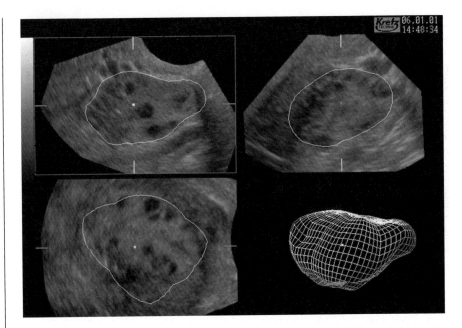

Fig. 1 The VOCAL technique of volume calculation. Virtual Organ Computer-aided AnaLysis (VOCAL) allows the dataset to be rotated through 180° about a central axis defined by the application of two callipers. The number of planes available for volume calculation is determined by a rotation step that may de adjusted according to the complexity of the organ being studied. Here, the 30° rotation step has been used and the ovarian cortex outlined in the coronal or C plane using the manual mode. The resultant three-dimensional ovarian model is shown in the lower right of the image.

upon certain geometric assumptions.[6] Volume estimation based on three-dimensional ultrasound still involves a degree of geometric assumption, as data are reconstructed based upon their most probable position within a Cartesian grid system, but utilises much more information. There are two basic methods employed to calculate volume from a three-dimensional dataset: the conventional 'full planar' or 'contour' method and the more recently introduced 'rotational' method possible through the VOCAL-imaging program (Virtual Organ Computer-aided AnaLysis™) which also generates a three-dimensional model of the object of interest (Fig. 1). Volume calculation by either of these techniques has proven highly reliable and valid both *in vitro* and *in vivo*.[7-14] Both techniques involve the manual delineation of the object of interest in the multiplanar display that shows the three perpendicular planes characteristic of three-dimensional ultrasound (Fig. 2).

VOCAL also facilitates the assessment of blood flow in a novel manner through the quantification of the power Doppler signal both within the defined volume of interest and also within the surrounding tissue through the application of a shell parallel to the originally defined surface contour (Fig. 3). Three 'indices of vascularity' are calculated: (i) the **vascularisation index** (VI) reflects the ratio of power Doppler information within the total dataset relative to both colour and grey information; (ii) the **flow index** (FI) represents the mean power Doppler signal intensity; and (iii) the **vascularisation flow index**

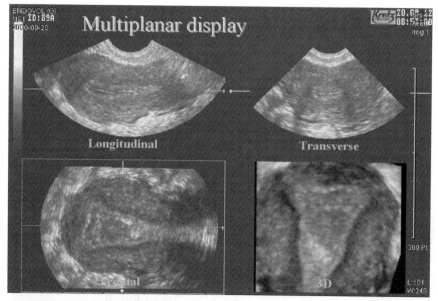

Fig. 2 The multiplanar display. A typical multiplanar display of a three-dimensional ultrasound dataset of the uterus is shown with the three mutually related orthogonal planes at 90° to one another. The upper left image represents the longitudinal plane (the A plane), the upper right image the transverse plane (the B plane) and the lower left image the coronal plane (the C plane). Volume calculation can be conducted in any plane using the remaining two as reference points. The lower right image shows a rendered three-dimensionak view of the uterus and endometrial cavity with its surrounding and relative hypochoeic junctional zone.

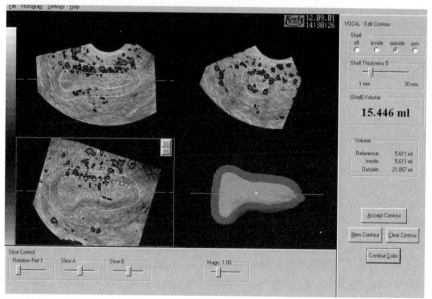

Fig. 3 Three-dimensional power Doppler angiography of the uterine blood supply. A three-dimensional dataset containing power Doppler information has been acquired from the uterus. VOCAL has then been used to define the myometrial-endometrial border and to apply a shell 5 mm outside of that contour to define the sub-endometrium, which can be clearly seen to be more vascular than the endometrium itself. The power Doppler information within the endometrium or sub-endometrial shell may then be quantified using various mathematical algorithms.

represents a combination of the two.[15] The exact relationship of these indices to true flow and vascularity *in vivo* remains to be established, but they have been shown to vary both within an individual and between different subjects suggesting they could have a valuable role in identifying and categorising differences between patient groups. Importantly, the indices may be calculated in a reproducible manner between observers[16] following the three-dimensional acquisition of power Doppler data which itself has also been shown to be reliable.[17]

CLINICAL APPLICATIONS

Three-dimensional ultrasound has been used to redefine the changes that occur within the female pelvis during the normal menstrual cycle, to investigate women with subfertility and suspected pelvic pathology, to predict ovarian reserve and endometrial receptivity in women undergoing assisted reproduction treatment and to examine women with problems in the early stages of pregnancy.

Normal physiology

Three-dimensional ultrasound has been used to quantify volume and vascular changes within the ovary and uterus that occur during the menstrual cycle and to examine the effect of age on these parameters.

Lee *et al.*[18] used three-dimensional ultrasound to examine the change in the ratio between uterine and endometrial volume that occurs during the menstrual cycle. The mean endometrial volume was 1.23 cm³ in relation to a mean uterine volume of 48.93 cm³ and the change in ratio between these two parameters was found to correlate well with the day of menstrual cycle with endometrial growth occurring during the follicular phase, plateauing in the peri-ovulatory period before decreasing in the late luteal phase. In our own study of 27 healthy female volunteers, we noted a similar significant increase in both endometrial volume and thickness during the follicular phase ($P < 0.001$) with a subsequent plateau in growth from around the time of ovulation until the next menstrual period. These changes in endometrial thickness and volume were highly correlated ($R^2 = 0.767$;: $P < 0.001$). Sub-group analysis revealed significant differences in endometrial morphometry between different patient groups and whilst endometrial thickness was consistent across the study population, parity was associated with a significantly greater endometrial volume than nulliparity (4.159 versus 2.234 cm³; $P < 0.05$).

We have also studied changes in endometrial and sub-endometrial blood flow using three-dimensional power Doppler angiography in the same 27 women and found a characteristic pattern not previously described with ultrasound.[19] The three-dimensional 'indices of vascularity' within both the endometrium and sub-endometrium increased during the proliferative phase peaking around 3 days prior to ovulation ($P < 0.001$) before decreasing to a nadir 5 days post-ovulation ($P < 0.001$). Thereafter, the degree of vascularity gradually increased during the transition from early to mid-secretory phase. This is contrary to what we had expected which, in keeping with the velocity information derived from pulsed wave Doppler studies of both uterine and spiral artery blood flow, was a peak in endometrial blood flow during the peri-implantation window. However, similar serial changes have been reported in women following the instillation of radio-labelled ^{133}Xe into the uterine cavity[20] and a decrease in uterine artery blood flow noted in ewes,[21] sows,[22] and cows in association with the reversal in oestrogen to progesterone ratio that occurs during the luteal phase of the cycle following oestrous.[23,24] These results warrant further investigation and confirmation but are clearly exciting and serve to demonstrate the different information obtainable with power and pulsed wave Doppler.

Much less is known about ovarian and follicular blood flow during the normal menstrual cycle. Jarvela et al.[25] examined the ovaries of 30 women at a single time point during the late follicular phase of the menstrual cycle prior to IVF treatment. A dominant follicle was identified in 80% of cycles and as expected the volume of this ovary was higher (9.9 ± 4.0 cm^3 versus 6.8 ± 2.8 cm^3; $P < 0.001$) and mean greyness lower (43.3 ± 5.0 versus 47.2 ± 4.0; $P < 0.001$) than that of the contralateral non-dominant ovary. Peri-follicular vascularity, assessed through the application of a 2-mm shell, was significantly higher than that of the total ovary for both the VI (9.0 ± 5.9 versus 5.5 ± 2.5; $P < 0.003$) and VFI (4.2 ± 2.8 versus 2.5 ± 1.3; $P < 0.046$) highlighting both the importance of flow to folliculogenesis and the degree of angiogenesis that occurs in this region even prior to the formation of the corpus luteum.

Pan et al.[26] noted a progressive reduction in ovarian vascularity with age in their study of 100 consecutive women attending for routine cervical cytology. Of the study group, 58 women were defined as being pre-menopausal, based on menstruation occurring within the last 3 months and 22 women were adjudged to be postmenopausal having not menstruated within the last 12 months with the remaining 20 women considered perimenopausal as they had menstruated 3–12 months earlier. The vascularisation index, flow index and vascularisation flow index in the postmenopausal group were all approximately half that seen than in the women considered peri-menopausal (VI, 0.53 ± 1.75 versus 1.11 ± 0.93; FI, 5.18 ± 5.31 versus 12.00 ± 3.86; and VFI, 0.09 ± 0.32 versus 0.18 ± 0.15, respectively) and highest in the pre-menopausal women (VI, 6.95 ± 8.35; FI, 15.98 ± 7.59; VFI, 1.25 ± 1.59). The change in serum oestradiol paralleled these results. This may reflect a reduction in ovarian reserve and function or simply indicate that ovarian blood flow is dependent upon adequate oestrogen levels. The latter is supported by a subsequent study by the same group which showed an improvement in ovarian blood flow in postmenopausal women in response to continuous-combined hormone replacement therapy (HRT).[27] Compared to 15 control patients not using HRT, a significant increase in the three-dimensional indices of vascularity was observed in 20 women receiving a 3-month course of 0.625 mg conjugated equine oestrogen in combination with 5 mg of medroxyprogesterone acetate daily (VFI, 0.13 ± 0.11 versus 0.59 ± 0.49; FI, 30.47 ± 12.06 versus 38.41 ± 10.21; VI, 0.31 ± 0.27 versus 1.12 ± 0.95).

Investigation of subfertility

Three-dimensional ultrasound has been used to diagnose uterine anomalies, assess tubal patency and to examine a spectrum of intrauterine and ovarian pathologies.

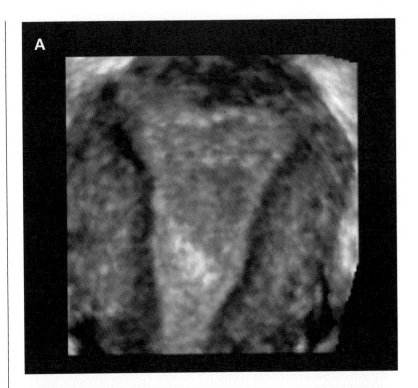

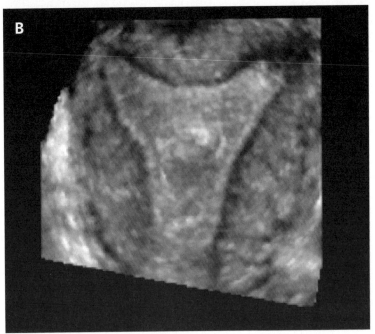

Fig. 4 Uterine anomalies. (A) A three-dimensional reconstruction of a normal uterus with its characteristic pyramidal appearance and horizontal fundal contour. This contour is mildly concave in the arcuate uterus (B) and exaggerated in the septum of the sub-septate uterus (C).

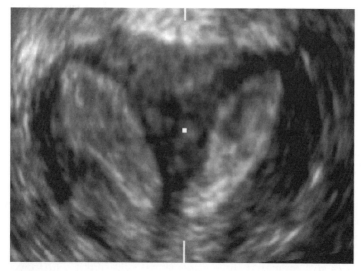

Fig. 4C

Uterine anomalies

Congenital uterine anomalies are associated with an increased risk of repeated first and second trimester miscarriage and preterm delivery.[28] A meta-analysis of published retrospective data indicated a marked improvement after hysteroscopic septoplasty, which itself has minimal postoperative sequelae.[29] Accurate and reliable diagnosis is important, therefore, as it allows the identification of patients at risk of these complications and timely surgical intervention. This is undoubtedly the area where three-dimensional ultrasound has contributed the most and has become the investigation of choice in units where available. This reflects its ability to demonstrate both the endometrial cavity and the myometrium simultaneously in the coronal plane as shown by an early study of 61 patients with a history of recurrent miscarriage or infertility (Fig. 4).[30] Hysterosalpingography had shown the presence of a normal uterus in 44 (72.1%) patients, an arcuate uterus in nine (14.8%) and a major fusion defect in three cases (4.9%). Whilst two-dimensional ultrasound was associated with five false-positive diagnoses of arcuate uteri and three of major uterine anomalies, three-dimensional ultrasound agreed with hysterosalpingography in all of these cases. Shortly afterwards, other groups began to report similarly favourable results suggesting three-dimensional ultrasound offers a 100% specificity for the exclusion of uterine anomalies and is able to differentiate between the different anomalies.[31,32]

Three-dimensional ultrasound has since been used to determine the prevalence of uterine anomalies in various patient groups and to characterise outcome on the basis of the anomaly. As many as 24% of women with recurrent pregnancy loss may have uterine anomalies,[33] which is roughly 4 times that seen in low-risk women where the prevalence is in the order of 5–6%.[34,35] In terms of the type of anomaly, a similar distribution is seen between different groups with arcuate uteri being the most common, followed by subseptate then bicornuate uteri with the more complex anomalies such as uterus didelphys and single uterine horns the least prevalent. Women with a subseptate uterus have a significantly higher proportion of first-trimester loss and women with an arcuate uterus a significantly greater proportion of second-trimester loss ($P < 0.01$) and preterm labour ($P < 0.01$) compared to women with a normal uterus.[33] Another important finding derived from these three-dimensional studies has been that outcome is related not only to the degree of defect but also to the remaining cavity length which is significantly shorter in both arcuate and subseptate uteri in women with recurrent miscarriage.[35] The measurement techniques and classifications reported allow comparison between the studies, as a degree of standardisation has been used based upon measurement of fundal distortion from the mid-point of an imaginary horizontal line joining the upper aspects of the cornuae to the upper aspect of the uterine cavity. This has been shown to be reliable between observers examining stored three-dimensional datasets.[36]

Intra-uterine pathology

La Torre *et al.*[37] compared three-dimensional ultrasound with conventional imaging with and without saline contrast in 23 patients in whom subsequent hysteroscopy had revealed the presence of 16 endometrial polyps. Standard two-dimensional ultrasound demonstrated a relatively poor specificity of only 69.5% suggesting the presence of polyps in 23 patients. This was improved to 94.1% when two-dimensional ultrasound was used in conjunction with saline infusion as only 17 patients were then thought to have polyps. Three-dimensional ultrasound performed almost as well diagnosing the presence of polyps in 18 patients with a specificity of 88.8% and subsequently correctly identified all 16 polyps when used in conjunction with saline infusion (Fig. 5). A similar improvement in specificity with three-dimensional ultrasound has been shown by Sylvestre *et al.*[38] in their study of 209 subfertile patients thought to have an intra-uterine lesion on transvaginal two-dimensional ultrasound or hysterosalpingography. Using saline infusion sonography with two-dimensional and then three-dimensional ultrasound, 92 patients were subsequently identified as having a variety of intra-uterine lesions suggesting a sensitivity and specificity of 97% and 11% for two-dimensional ultrasound, 87% and 45% for three-dimensional ultrasound and 98% and 100% for two-dimensional saline infusion sonography. Of 59 patients that had undergone hysteroscopy, the sensitivity and positive predictive value of saline infusion sonography were 98% and 95% when performed in combination with two-dimensional ultrasound and 100% and 92% with three-dimensional ultrasound, respectively. The study clearly demonstrates how simple contrast media potentially increase the specificity of two-dimensional ultrasound as 55% (116 of 209) of patients were found to have normal cavities following the infusion of saline. This was largely due to the correct localisation of leiomyomas as intramural rather than submucosal (54/101). This is extremely important in the clinical setting, as whilst three-dimensional ultrasound improves further on two-dimensional imaging it is not currently available in all units and its use, therefore, has significant implications in terms of cost and training. Saline infusion on the other hand may be undertaken easily using various dedicated systems or modifications of readily available cheaper catheters such as a paediatric feeding tube.

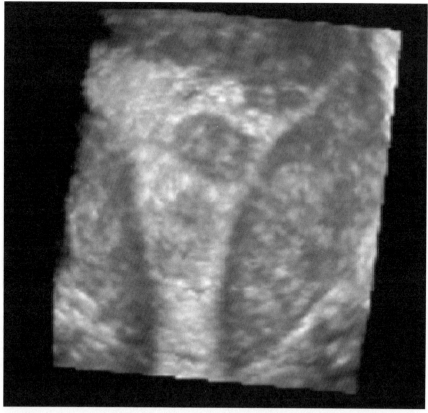

Fig. 5 Endometrial polyps. The coronal view may be used to locate the position of intrauterine pathology and confirm the presence of individual smaller polyps often confused as large single fibroids with conventional imaging that are suitable for routine polypectomy rather then hysteroscopic resection. Two polyps are readily evident in this three-dimensional reconstruction when conventional imaging had suggested the presence of a single large polyp or sub-mucosal fibroid (Fig. 3).

Polycystic ovaries

Several groups have used three-dimensional ultrasound to demonstrate ovarian volume and vascularity are increased in polycystic ovarian syndrome.[39–42] Three-dimensional ultrasound also allows for the measurement of stromal volume through the calculation and subtraction of total follicular volume from total ovarian volume (Fig. 6). Using this technique, Kyei-Mensah et al.[43] showed stromal volume was positively correlated with serum androstenedione concentrations ($P < 0.01$) in 26 women with clinical evidence of polycystic ovaries. However, using a similar approach, Nardo et al.[44] were unable to demonstrate any relationship between serum FSH, LH or testosterone and ovarian stromal volume in 23 infertile women with clomiphene citrate-resistant polycystic ovary syndrome at the same stage of the menstrual cycle.

Endometriosis

Wu et al.[45] used three-dimensional power Doppler angiography to examine the effect of surgery on ovarian blood flow in 22 women undergoing assisted

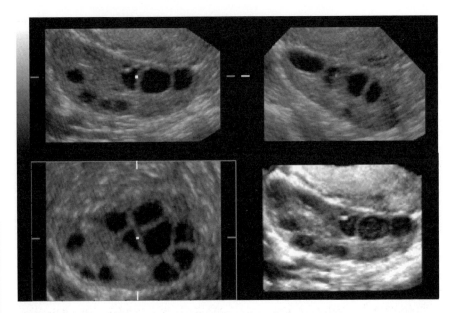

Fig. 6 Polycystic ovaries. Three-dimensional ultrasound facilitates objective assessment of the ovarian stroma, through measurement of its mean grey signal intensity, its vascularity and its volume, which may be calculated by subtracting total follicular volume from total ovarian volume using the multiplanar view shown here. The three-dimensional reconstruction in the lower right image shows the follicles arranged peripherally around an echodense stroma.

reproduction treatment following the laparoscopic removal of large endometriomas. Ovarian blood flow within the study group was compared to that of 26 women with tubal factor infertility and no known ovarian pathology on the day of human chorionic gonadotrophin. Whilst ovarian volume was spared, all three indices of vascularity were significantly decreased in the endometriosis group. This is clearly an interesting area and one of concern that requires further study.

Ovarian torsion

Yaman et al.[46] reported a case of unilateral ovarian torsion in a pregnant patient with bilateral hyperstimulated ovaries 2 weeks following embryo transfer. Three-dimensional power Doppler angiography demonstrated a significant improvement in ovarian vascularity within 1 h of laparoscopic treatment (VI, 3.81 versus 0.24; FI, 42.80 versus 21.99; VFI, 1.63 versus 0.05, respectively) whereas conventional assessment with pulsed-wave Doppler showed no significant difference in the impedance to blood flow within the ovarian vessels (RI, 5.1 versus 5.2). A single case, admittedly, but once again one that suggests more information is obtainable with three-dimensional ultrasound than with conventional ultrasound thereby allowing differentiation between patient groups not currently possible.

Intra-uterine contraceptive devices

Bonilla-Musoles et al.[47] compared the ability of two-dimensional and three-dimensional ultrasound to correctly identify and locate intra-uterine contraceptive devices in 66 asymptomatic women. Hysteroscopy, performed in 14 cases where there was a discrepancy between the methods, confirmed the three-dimensional findings in all cases. In contrast, two-dimensional ultrasound was unable to correctly identify the type of intra-uterine device in six cases (9.1%) or to identify the position of the device in two cases (3.0%). Lee et al.[48] also used three-dimensional ultrasound to examine 96 women at a mean interval of 22 days following the insertion of a TCu380A intra-uterine device. Complete and simultaneous imaging of all parts of the device, stem and arms, was possible in 95% of cases. Volume rendering was required to identify 30 devices, but the multiplanar display was sufficient in 64% of cases. Inappropriately located intra-uterine devices may result in pain but more importantly have a reduced efficacy and a prospective randomised trial comparing two- and three-dimensional ultrasound would be worthwhile, therefore.

Fibroids

Fleischer et al.[49] used three-dimensional colour Doppler ultrasound to track fibroid size and vascularity in 20 patients with a total of 31 fibroids following embolisation. The reduction in size and vascularity was asynchronous, a marked decrease in vascularity occurring within 1 day of embolisation whilst the greatest volume change occurred at 3 months. The absolute reduction in size did appear to depend upon the initial degree of vascularity with a greater decrease in patients with hypervascular fibroids than those with isovascular or hypovascular fibroids as defined by their vascular appearance relative to that of the myometrium. The same group also retrospectively compared three-dimensional colour Doppler ultrasound with selective uterine artery arteriography in 15 of these patients.[50] A mean reduction in vascularity of 44% (19% to 78%) was noted and there was agreement between the two forms of assessment in the majority of cases (13 of 15 patients; 87%). In the 2 cases (13%) of disagreement, three-dimensional imaging suggested collateral flow not seen at arteriography. Aside from providing quantifiable information, colour Doppler was also subjectively felt to improve the delineation of the size, location and extent of myometrial involvement. Three-dimensional colour Doppler ultrasound may offer a predictive tool, therefore, to identify women most likely to obtain benefit from this procedure but in the absence of an appropriately blinded and randomised study this should be interpreted with caution.

Tubal patency

The combination of contrast media and three-dimensional ultrasound has also been used to assess tubal patency. Kiyokawa et al.[51] found three-dimensional saline sonohysterosalpingography was able to demonstrate the entire contour of the uterine cavity in 96% of cases compared to only 64% cases with conventional X-ray hysterosalpingography and was associated with a positive predictive value and specificity of predicting tubal patency of 100% in 25 unselected infertile patients. Sladkevicius et al.[52] found three-dimensional power Doppler imaging demonstrated free spill almost twice as often as conventional imaging (114 versus 58 tubes, respectively) when used during hysterosalpingo-contrast sonography. Sankpal et al.[53] reported less promising results with the same technique when they re-assessed tubal patency in 15 women who had normal X-ray HSG examinations within the previous year. An important distinction was their use of saline rather than a positive contrast agent but it may be that the technique has a distinct learning curve and numbers were small.

Assisted reproduction treatment

Ultrasound is used to monitor the response to controlled ovarian stimulation and to guide the transvaginal collection of oocytes and subsequent trans-cervical transfer of embryos to the uterus. Three-dimensional ultrasound may be used in all of these areas but has largely been applied as a predictor of ovarian response or 'ovarian reserve' and as a determinant of endometrial receptivity.

Three-dimensional markers of 'ovarian reserve'

Of the ultrasound markers suggested as predictive of ovarian response, the three that have been specifically addressed by three-dimensional ultrasound studies are antral follicle counts, ovarian volume and ovarian blood flow.

Pellicer et al.[54] were amongst the first to use three-dimensional ultrasound as an adjunct to conventional markers of ovarian reserve when they examined ovarian volume and the number of 'selectable follicles' measuring 2–5 mm in a small group of low responders on day three of the menstrual cycle. Both the number of selectable follicles and the total number of antral follicles were significantly decreased in the 'low responder' group who also demonstrated significantly higher serum FSH levels despite having values within the normal range. Ovarian volume measurements, however, were similar between the two groups. Pohl et al.[55] also used three-dimensional ultrasound to quantify the number of follicles of varying diameter in 113 patients following 'down-regulation' but prior to ovarian stimulation. Patients with a higher number of follicles measuring 5–10 mm were younger ($P < 0.01$), had a significantly higher number of oocytes retrieved ($P < 0.0001$) and were more likely to conceive ($P < 0.05$). Kupesic et al.[56] also suggested that the antral follicle count is a better predictor than three-dimensional measures of ovarian volume and blood flow. A minimal ovarian volume may be important however. Schild et al.[57] noted a pregnancy rate of only 6.7% (1 of 15) in patients with a minimum unilateral ovarian volume of $<= 3$ cm^3, which represented a single SD below the mean, versus 21.9% (30 of 137) in patients with an initial minimum ovarian volume above 3 cm^3. This difference was not significant, however, and cancellation rates due to poor ovarian response or failed fertilisation were similar in both groups.

There is no doubt that antral follicle counts, when used in categorical classifications, are an important predictor of 'ovarian reserve' and may be measured with a high level of agreement both between and within observers.[58] Three-dimensional ultrasound, however, does not appear to offer any significant advantage over two-dimensional imaging even at higher follicle counts when interobserver reliability is reduced. Ovarian volume has a limited predictive ability that does not appear to supersede that of antral follicle counts. This has allowed researchers to turn their focus to the ovarian blood flow and use three-dimensional ultrasound to examine the effect of ovarian vascularity on the response of the ovary to controlled ovarian stimulation.

Jarvela et al.[59] used three-dimensional power Doppler angiography after pituitary 'down-regulation' and during gonadotrophin stimulation to compare ovarian vascularity in 33 women with normal ovarian reserve, as judged by antral follicle counts, to 12 women who had demonstrated a previous poor response. The number of oocytes retrieved correlated with the antral follicle count (R = 0.458;, $P < 0.01$) and ovarian volume (R = 0.388; $P < 0.05$) but not with ovarian vascularity. All three indices of vascularity were shown to increase significantly during gonadotrophin stimulation in the group with normal ovarian reserve only, but this was related to the antral follicle count re-iterating the importance of this marker as an independent variable. Kupesic et al.[60] similarly showed the number of oocytes retrieved and subsequent conception rate to be greater in patients with a greater ovarian volume and a greater ovarian stromal vascularity but not independently of a higher number of antral follicles.

Three-dimensional markers of 'endometrial receptivity'

Schild et al.[61] measured endometrial thickness and volume in a total of 47 IVF cycles on the day of oocyte retrieval. There were no significant differences between the group of fifteen patients that conceived (31.9%) and the remaining 32 non-pregnant women in terms of the mean endometrial thickness (10.8 ± 2.3 mm versus 11.8 ± 3.4 mm) or volume (4.9 ± 2.2 cm^3 versus 5.8 ± 3.4 cm^3), respectively. Yaman et al.[62] reported similar findings with no differences in endometrium volume (4.16 ± 1.97 cm^3 versus 4.53 ± 1.79 cm^3) or endometrium thickness (11 ± 2 mm versus 11 ± 2 mm) in 21 pregnant and 44 non-pregnant women on the day of hCG administration. However, whilst there was no absolute endometrial thickness required for pregnancy, a minimal endometrial volume above 2.5 cm^3 favoured pregnancy. Raga et al.[63] described a cut-off point of 2 cm^3 on the day of embryo transfer and observed no pregnancies at endometrial volumes below 1 cm^3. Even if there is a lower limit in endometrial volume below which pregnancy will not occur, conventional measurement of endometrial thickness is already known to have a similar negative predictive value with conception less likely in patients with an endometrium measuring less than 5 mm in diameter.

Kupesic et al.[64] reported more predictive information could be derived at the time of embryo transfer when three-dimensional power Doppler was used to quantify endometrial vascularity. Of 89 patients studied, successful conception cycles were associated with a significantly higher endometrial flow index (13.2 ± 2.2 versus 11.9 ± 2.4; $P < 0.05$). Wu et al.[65] also found three-dimensional power Doppler angiography to be an important determinant of 'endometrial receptivity' but on the day of hCG administration in 54 patients undergoing their first IVF cycle. The subendometrial vascularisation flow index (VFI) proved the best predictor of conception being superior to the vascularisation index (VI), flow index (FI) and endometrial volume in the receiver operating characteristics curve analysis. Interestingly, three-dimensional ultrasound may also be used to examine endometrial vascularity and determine 'endometrial receptivity' prior to ovarian stimulation. Schild et al.[66] reported significantly lower indices of vascularity at down-regulation in 15 patients that subsequently conceived (20%) than in 60 non-conception cycles ($P < 0.05$) with the flow index the strongest predictive factor of IVF success ($P < 0.05$). Endometrial measurements were once again not correlated with outcome. This may reflect a more profound pituitary suppression, but is more likely to reflect a group of patients more responsive to exogenous hormonal therapy.

Procedures

Feichtinger[67] reported the transvaginal needle-guided aspiration of 10 follicles from a single patient using three-dimensional ultrasound. The use of three-dimensional imaging was associated with a mean delay of 5.00 ± 1.22 s during the interactive volume calculation whilst the needle tip was located but the procedure proved successful with oocytes recovered from all follicles. It is difficult to see how three-dimensional imaging can significantly improve oocyte retrieval, which is usually a straightforward procedure; however, further randomised work is warranted particularly in complex patients and possibly in patients undergoing assisted reproduction and *in vitro* maturation where oocytes are retrieved from smaller 'immature' follicles.

Poehl *et al.*[68] used the spatial appearance of intrafollicular cumulus-like structures with the number and maturity of information provided by the multiplanar display to correlate the oocytes retrieved from 50 women undergoing IVF treatment. All follicles measuring 16 mm or more were carefully examined for the presence of cumuli in all three perpendicular planes or in a reconstructed three-dimensional composite image. A total of 296 mature oocytes were eventually retrieved from 318 follicles and 218 of these fertilised successfully. In all, 262 cumuli had been visualised within these follicles and this correlated well with the number of retrieved oocytes ($r^2 = 0.83$; $P < 0.0001$), oocyte maturity ($r^2 = 0.78$; $p < 0.0001$) and fertilisation rate ($r^2 = 0.65$; $P < 0.0001$). Serum oestradiol also correlated well with the number of follicles and fertilised oocytes.

Early pregnancy

Miscarriage

Gestational sac volume has been proposed as representative of the competence of the early uteroplacental unit and, therefore, a potential predictor of pregnancy outcome.[69] In one of the first reported applications of three-dimensional ultrasound, Steiner *et al.*[69] studied 38 pregnancies at 5–11 weeks' gestation and found gestational sac volume measurements to significantly correlated with gestational age ($r = 0.74$; $P < 0.001$) and more than two standard deviations below the mean in three of five embryonic or anembryonic pregnancy failures. However, Acharya and Morgan[70] have recently shown a clear relationship between gestational sac volume and sac diameter also exists in patients with embryonic pregnancy failure and that measurements are unable to predict eventual outcome during conservative management. Babinszki *et al.*[71] did find a relationship between gestational sac and yolk sac volume and adverse outcome in a group of 49 patients who had conceived following treatment for subfertility, but crown rump length performed equally as well.

Currently, therefore, one may conclude that whilst there is a distinct relationship between gestational age and three-dimensional measurements of

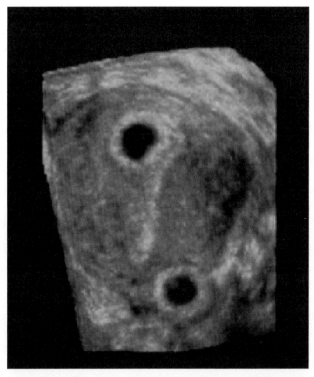

Fig. 7 Ectopic pregnancy. The spatial orientation of three-dimensional ultrasound and its ability to demonstrate the coronal plane of the uterus in its natural position may help in the diagnosis and exclusion of ectopic pregnancy. This is particularly true in cases of heterotropic pregnancy where an intrauterine pregnancy is associated with an ectopic twin gestation. This image shows a normally sited intrauterine pregnancy in the upper uterine cavity together with a left-sided cervical ectopic gestation in the lower part of the image.

gestational and yolk sac volume, these parameters do not appear to improve upon the predictive value of current tests in determining the eventual outcome in either viable or non-viable intrauterine pregnancies.

Pregnancy of unknown location

The improved spatial orientation afforded by three-dimensional ultrasound has been used to evaluate endometrial shape in cases of pregnancy of unknown location in an attempt to improve the sensitivity and specificity of ultrasound. Rempen et al.[72] described the persistence of a distinct symmetry with regard to the median longitudinal axis of the uterus in the coronal plane in 90% of extra-uterine pregnancies which was lost in intra-uterine pregnancies. Su et al.[73] reported a case of an anembryonic cervical pregnancy diagnosed at 10 weeks associated with a large arteriovenous malformation managed conservatively with selective uterine artery embolisation. Three-dimensional power Doppler ultrasonography proved useful in the initial diagnosis and subsequent monitoring of the response to treatment. These studies suggest a potential role for three-dimensional ultrasound; however, in the absence of properly blinded data, it is impossible to predict whether it will improve upon conventional ultrasound. The spatial orientation and additional information afforded by the coronal plane do lend themselves to assessment of the endometrial cavity as illustrated so elegantly by the three-dimensional studies on uterine anomalies so one should be optimistic in this regard. We have successfully used three-dimensional imaging in several cases of pregnancy of unknown location and particularly so in twin pregnancies following assisted reproduction treatment and embryo transfer where heterotropic pregnancy is so much more likely (Fig. 7).

CONCLUSIONS

Three-dimensional ultrasound offers several advantages over conventional imaging in reproductive medicine. The spatial orientation and additional information derivable from individual sectional planes has significantly enhanced our knowledge of uterine anomalies and contributed to our understanding of how these affect pregnancy outcome and may offer insight into the location of pregnancies of unknown location. Quantitative three-dimensional analysis of volume and vascularity has proven less informative, however, and whilst individual studies suggest a potential role for such measurements, these do not appear to out-perform current assessments.

Three-dimensional ultrasound largely remains an exciting research tool with the converted applying it in different forms and areas of interest and in doing so unearthing significant new information about normal physiology and pathophysiological change that direct further work. Our role is to continue to test it prospectively and against current forms of assessment but to remain realistic and to examine how it may be most appropriately applied in the clinical setting.

References

1 Linney AD, Deng J. Three-dimensional morphometry in ultrasound. Proc Inst Mech Eng [H] 1999; 213: 235–245

2 King DL, King Jr DL, Shao MY. Three-dimensional spatial registration and interactive display of position and orientation of real-time ultrasound images. J Ultrasound Med 1990; 9: 525–532

3 Brunner M, Obruca A, Bauer P, Feichtinger W. Clinical application of volume estimation based on three-dimensional ultrasonography. Ultrasound Obstet Gynecol 1995; 6: 358–361

4 Riccabona M, Pretorius DH, Nelson TR, Johnson D, Budorick NE. Three-dimensional ultrasound: display modalities in obstetrics. J Clin Ultrasound 1997; 25: 157–167

5 Maymon R, Herman A, Ariely S, Dreazen E, Buckovsky I, Weinraub Z. Three-dimensional vaginal sonography in obstetrics and gynaecology. Hum Reprod Update 2000; 6: 475–484

6 Gilja OH, Hausken T, Berstad A, Odegaard S. Measurements of organ volume by ultrasonography. Proc Inst Mech Eng [H] 1999; 213: 247–259

7 Kyei-Mensah A, Maconochie N, Zaidi J, Pittrof R, Campbell S, Tan SL. Transvaginal three-dimensional ultrasound: reproducibility of ovarian and endometrial volume measurements. Fertil Steril 1996; 66: 718–722

8 Raine-Fenning NJ, Campbell BK, Collier J, Brincat MB, Johnson IR. The reproducibility of endometrial volume acquisition and measurement with the VOCAL-imaging program. Ultrasound Obstet Gynecol 2002; 19: 69–75

9 Farrell T, Leslie JR, Chien PF, Agustsson P. The reliability and validity of three

dimensional ultrasound volumetric measurements using an *in vitro* balloon and *in vivo* uterine model. Br J Obstet Gynaecol 2001; 108: 573–582

10 Riccabona M, Nelson TR, Pretorius DH. Three-dimensional ultrasound: accuracy of distance and volume measurements. Ultrasound Obstet Gynecol 1996; 7: 429–434

11 Raine-Fenning NJ, Clewes JS, Kendall NR, Bunkheila AK, Campbell BK, Johnson IR. The interobserver reliability and validity of volume calculation from three-dimensional ultrasound datasets in the *in vitro* setting. Ultrasound Obstet Gynecol 2003; 21: 283–291

12 Riccabona M, Nelson TR, Pretorius DH, Davidson TE. *In vivo* three-dimensional sonographic measurement of organ volume: validation in the urinary bladder. J Ultrasound Med 1996; 15: 627–632

13 Kyei-Mensah A, Zaidi J, Pittrof R, Shaker A, Campbell S, Tan SL. Transvaginal three-dimensional ultrasound: accuracy of follicular volume measurements. Fertil Steril 1996; 65: 371–376

14 Amer A, Hammadeh ME, Kolkailah M, Ghandour AA. Three-dimensional versus two-dimensional ultrasound measurement of follicular volume: are they comparable? Arch Gynecol Obstet 2003; 268: 155–157

15 Pairleitner H, Steiner H, Hasenoehrl G, Staudach A. Three-dimensional power Doppler sonography: imaging and quantifying blood flow and vascularization. Ultrasound Obstet Gynecol 1999; 14: 139–143

16 Raine-Fenning NJ, Campbell BK, Clewes JS, Kendall NR, Johnson IR. The reliability of the semi-quantification of ovarian, endometrial and sub-endometrial perfusion using three-dimensional power Doppler angiography and shell-imaging. Ultrasound Obstet Gynecol 2003; 22: 633–639

17 Jarvela IY, Sladkevicius P, Tekay AH, Campbell S, Nargund G. Intraobserver and interobserver variability of ovarian volume, gray-scale and color flow indices obtained using transvaginal three-dimensional power Doppler ultrasonography. Ultrasound Obstet Gynecol 2003; 21: 277–282

18 Lee A, Sator M, Kratochwil A, Deutinger J, Vytiska-Binsdorfer E, Bernaschek G. Endometrial volume change during spontaneous menstrual cycles: volumetry by transvaginal three-dimensional ultrasound. Fertil Steril 1997; 68: 831–835

19 Raine-Fenning NJ, Campbell BK, Kendall NR, Clewes JS, Johnson IR. Quantifying the changes in endometrial vascularity throughout the normal menstrual cycle with three-dimensional power Doppler angiography. Hum Reprod 2004; 19: 330–338

20 Fraser IS, McCarron G, Hutton B, Macey D. Endometrial blood flow measured by xenon 133 clearance in women with normal menstrual cycles and dysfunctional uterine bleeding. Am J Obstet Gynecol 1987; 156: 158–166

21 Greiss Jr FC, Anderson SG. Uterine vascular changes during the ovarian cycle. Am J Obstet Gynecol 1969; 103: 629–640

22 Ford SP, Christenson RK. Blood flow to uteri of sows during the estrous cycle and early pregnancy: local effect of the conceptus on the uterine blood supply. Biol Reprod 1979; 21: 617–624

23 Waite LR, Ford SP, Young DF, Conley AJ. Use of ultrasonic Doppler waveforms to estimate changes in uterine artery blood flow and vessel compliance. J Anim Sci 1990; 68: 2450–2458

24 Ford SP, Chenault JR, Echternkamp SE. Uterine blood flow of cows during the oestrous cycle and early pregnancy: effect of the conceptus on the uterine blood supply. J Reprod Fertil 1979; 56: 53–62

25 Jarvela IY, Sladkevicius P, Kelly S, Ojha K, Nargund G, Campbell S. Three-dimensional sonographic and power Doppler characterization of ovaries in late follicular phase. Ultrasound Obstet Gynecol 2002; 20: 281–285

26 Pan HA, Cheng YC, Li CH, Wu MH, Chang FM. Ovarian stroma flow intensity decreases by age: a three-dimensional power Doppler ultrasonographic study. Ultrasound Med Biol 2002; 28: 425–430

27 Pan HA, Li CH, Cheng YC, Wu MH, Chang FM. Quantification of ovarian stromal Doppler signals in postmenopausal women receiving hormone replacement therapy. Menopause 2003; 10: 366–372

28 Kupesic S. Clinical implications of sonographic detection of uterine anomalies for reproductive outcome. Ultrasound Obstet Gynecol 2001; 18: 387–400

29 Homer HA, Li TC, Cooke ID. The septate uterus: a review of management and reproductive outcome. Fertil Steril 2000; 73: 1–14

30 Jurkovic D, Geipel A, Gruboeck K, Jauniaux E, Natucci M, Campbell S. Three-dimensional ultrasound for the assessment of uterine anatomy and detection of congenital anomalies: a comparison with hysterosalpingography and two-dimensional sonography. Ultrasound Obstet Gynecol 1995; 5: 233–237

31 Raga F, Bonilla-Musoles F, Blanes J, Osborne NG. Congenital Mullerian anomalies: diagnostic accuracy of three-dimensional ultrasound. Fertil Steril 1996; 65: 523–528

32 Wu MH, Hsu CC, Huang KE. Detection of congenital Mullerian duct anomalies using three-dimensional ultrasound. J Clin Ultrasound 1997; 25: 487–492

33 Woelfer B, Salim R, Banerjee S, Elson J, Regan L, Jurkovic D. Reproductive outcomes in women with congenital uterine anomalies detected by three-dimensional ultrasound screening. Obstet Gynecol 2001; 98: 1099–1103

34 Jurkovic D, Gruboeck K, Tailor A, Nicolaides KH. Ultrasound screening for congenital uterine anomalies. Br J Obstet Gynaecol 1997; 104: 1320–1321

35 Salim R, Regan L, Woelfer B, Backos M, Jurkovic D. A comparative study of the morphology of congenital uterine anomalies in women with and without a history of recurrent first trimester miscarriage. Hum Reprod 2003; 18: 162–166

36 Salim R, Woelfer B, Backos M, Regan L, Jurkovic D. Reproducibility of three-dimensional ultrasound diagnosis of congenital uterine anomalies. Ultrasound Obstet Gynecol 2003; 21: 578–582

37 La Torre R, De Felice C, De Angelis C, Coacci F, Mastrone M, Cosmi EV. Transvaginal sonographic evaluation of endometrial polyps: a comparison with two dimensional and three dimensional contrast sonography. Clin Exp Obstet Gynecol 1999; 26: 171–173

38 Sylvestre C, Child TJ, Tulandi T, Tan SL. A prospective study to evaluate the efficacy of two- and three-dimensional sonohysterography in women with intrauterine lesions. Fertil Steril 2003; 79: 1222–1225

39 Jarvela IY, Mason HD, Sladkevicius P et al. Characterization of normal and polycystic ovaries using three-dimensional power Doppler ultrasonography. J Assist Reprod Genet 2002; 19: 582–590

40 Wu MH, Tang HH, Hsu CC, Wang ST, Huang KE. The role of three-dimensional ultrasonographic images in ovarian measurement. Fertil Steril 1998; 69): 1152–1155

41 Dolz M, Osborne NG, Blanes J et al. Polycystic ovarian syndrome: assessment with color Doppler angiography and three-dimensional ultrasonography. J Ultrasound Med 1999; 18: 303–313

42 Pan HA, Wu MH, Cheng YC, Li CH, Chang FM. Quantification of Doppler signal in polycystic ovary syndrome using three-dimensional power Doppler ultrasonography: a possible new marker for diagnosis. Hum Reprod 2002; 17: 201–206

43 Kyei-Mensah AA, LinTan S, Zaidi J, Jacobs HS. Relationship of ovarian stromal volume to serum androgen concentrations in patients with polycystic ovary syndrome. Hum Reprod 1998; 13: 1437–1441

44 Nardo LG, Buckett WM, White D, Digesu AG, Franks S, Khullar V. Three-dimensional assessment of ultrasound features in women with clomiphene citrate-resistant polycystic ovarian syndrome (PCOS): ovarian stromal volume does not correlate with biochemical indices. Hum Reprod 2002; 17: 1052–1055

45 Wu MH, Tsai SJ, Pan HA, Hsiao KY, Chang FM. Three-dimensional power Doppler imaging of ovarian stromal blood flow in women with endometriosis undergoing in vitro fertilization. Ultrasound Obstet Gynecol 2003; 21: 480–485

46 Yaman C, Ebner T, Jesacher K. Three-dimensional power Doppler in the diagnosis of ovarian torsion. Ultrasound Obstet Gynecol 2002; 20: 513–515

47 Bonilla-Musoles F, Raga F, Osborne NG, Blanes J. Control of intrauterine device insertion with three-dimensional ultrasound: is it the future? J Clin Ultrasound 1996; 24: 263–267

48 Lee A, Eppel W, Sam C, Kratochwil A, Deutinger J, Bernaschek G. Intrauterine device localization by three-dimensional transvaginal sonography. Ultrasound Obstet Gynecol 1997; 10: 289–292

49 Fleischer AC, Donnelly EF, Campbell MG, Mazer MJ, Grippo D, Lipsitz NL. Three-dimensional color Doppler sonography before and after fibroid embolization. J Ultrasound Med 2000; 19: 701–705

50 Muniz CJ, Fleischer AC, Donnelly EF, Mazer MJ. Three-dimensional color Doppler sonography and uterine artery arteriography of fibroids: assessment of changes in vascularity before and after embolization. J Ultrasound Med 2002; 21: 129–133

51 Kiyokawa K, Masuda H, Fuyuki T *et al.* Three-dimensional hysterosalpingo-contrast sonography (3D-HyCoSy) as an outpatient procedure to assess infertile women: a pilot study. Ultrasound Obstet Gynecol 2000; 16: 648–654

52 Sladkevicius P, Ojha K, Campbell S, Nargund G. Three-dimensional power Doppler imaging in the assessment of Fallopian tube patency. Ultrasound Obstet Gynecol 2000; 16: 644–647

53 Sankpal RS, Confino E, Matzel A, Cohen LS. Investigation of the uterine cavity and fallopian tubes using three-dimensional saline sonohysterosalpingography. Int J Gynaecol Obstet 2001; 73: 125–129

54 Pellicer A, Ardiles G, Neuspiller F, Remohi J, Simon C, Bonilla-Musoles F. Evaluation of the ovarian reserve in young low responders with normal basal levels of follicle-stimulating hormone using three-dimensional ultrasonography. Fertil Steril 1998; 70: 671–675

55 Pohl M, Hohlagschwandtner M, Obruca A, Poschalko G, Weigert M, Feichtinger W. Number and size of antral follicles as predictive factors *in vitro* fertilization and embryo transfer. J Assist Reprod Genet 2000; 17: 315–318

56 Kupesic S, Kurjak A. Predictors of IVF outcome by three-dimensional ultrasound. Hum Reprod 2002; 17: 950–955

57 Schild RL, Knobloch C, Dorn C, Fimmers R, van der Ven H, Hansmann M. The role of ovarian volume in an in vitro fertilization programme as assessed by 3D ultrasound. Arch Gynecol Obstet 2001; 265: 67–72

58 Scheffer GJ, Broekmans FJ, Bancsi LF, Habbema JD, Looman CW, Te Velde ER. Quantitative transvaginal two- and three-dimensional sonography of the ovaries: reproducibility of antral follicle counts. Ultrasound Obstet Gynecol 2002; 20: 270–275

59 Jarvela IY, Sladkevicius P, Kelly S, Ojha K, Campbell S, Nargund G. Quantification of ovarian power Doppler signal with three-dimensional ultrasonography to predict response during *in vitro* fertilization. Obstet Gynecol 2003; 102: 816–822

60 Kupesic S, Kurjak A, Bjelos D, Vujisic S. Three-dimensional ultrasonographic ovarian measurements and *in vitro* fertilization outcome are related to age. Fertil Steril 2003; 79: 190–197

61 Schild RL, Indefrei D, Eschweiler S, Van der Ven H, Fimmers R, Hansmann M. Three-dimensional endometrial volume calculation and pregnancy rate in an *in-vitro* fertilization programme. Hum Reprod 1999; 14: 1255–1258

62 Yaman C, Ebner T, Sommergruber M, Polz W, Tews G. Role of three-dimensional ultrasonographic measurement of endometrium volume as a predictor of pregnancy outcome in an IVF-ET program: a preliminary study. Fertil Steril 2000; 74: 797–801

63 Raga F, Bonilla-Musoles F, Casan EM, Klein O, Bonilla F. Assessment of endometrial volume by three-dimensional ultrasound prior to embryo transfer: clues to endometrial receptivity. Hum Reprod 1999; 14: 2851–2854

64 Kupesic S, Bekavac I, Bjelos D, Kurjak A. Assessment of endometrial receptivity by transvaginal color Doppler and three-dimensional power Doppler ultrasonography in patients undergoing *in vitro* fertilization procedures. J Ultrasound Med 2001; 20: 125–134

65 Wu HM, Chiang CH, Huang HY, Chao AS, Wang HS, Soong YK. Detection of the subendometrial vascularization flow index by three-dimensional ultrasound may be useful for predicting the pregnancy rate for patients undergoing *in vitro* fertilization-embryo transfer. Fertil Steril 2003; 79: 507–511

66 Schild RL, Holthaus S, d'Alquen J *et al.* Quantitative assessment of subendometrial blood flow by three-dimensional-ultrasound is an important predictive factor of implantation in an *in-vitro* fertilization programme. Hum Reprod 2000; 15: 89–94

67 Feichtinger W. Follicle aspiration with interactive three-dimensional digital imaging (Voluson): a step toward real-time puncturing under three-dimensional ultrasound control. Fertil Steril 1998; 70: 374–377

68 Poehl M, Hohlagschwandtner M, Doerner V, Dillinger B, Feichtinger W. Cumulus assessment by three-dimensional ultrasound for *in vitro* fertilization. Ultrasound Obstet Gynecol 2000; 16: 251–253

69 Steiner H, Gregg AR, Bogner G, Graf AH, Weiner CP, Staudach A. First trimester three-dimensional ultrasound volumetry of the gestational sac. Arch Gynecol Obstet 1994; 255: 165–170

70 Acharya G, Morgan H. Does gestational sac volume predict the outcome of missed miscarriage managed expectantly? J Clin Ultrasound 2002; 30: 526–531

71 Babinszki A, Nyari T, Jordan S, Nasseri A, Mukherjee T, Copperman AB. Three-dimensional measurement of gestational and yolk sac volumes as predictors of pregnancy outcome in the first trimester. Am J Perinatol 2001; 18: 203–211

72 Rempen A. The shape of the endometrium evaluated with three-dimensional ultrasound: an additional predictor of extrauterine pregnancy. Hum Reprod 1998; 13: 450–454

73 Su YN, Shih JC, Chiu WH, Lee CN, Cheng WF, Hsieh FJ. Cervical pregnancy: assessment with three-dimensional power Doppler imaging and successful management with selective uterine artery embolization. Ultrasound Obstet Gynecol 1999; 14: 284–287

Aarti Sharma Mohammed Yousef
Rianna Burrill William Atiomo

Recent developments in polycystic ovary syndrome

The polycystic ovary syndrome (PCOS) is one gynaecological condition where the knowledge base is rapidly evolving. Although traditional concepts of PCOS as a gynaecological/endocrine condition presenting with menstrual irregularities, anovulatory infertility, obesity, hirsutism and acne still prevail, there have been several recent developments in the literature on the agreed definition, pathophysiology, treatment and possible long-term health consequences. Some of the key developments include a new consensus definition, the identification of additional metabolic factors and genes which may be implicated in its pathophysiology, a plethora of publications on the possible beneficial effects of metformin on anovulatory infertility, an emphasis on the role of life-style modification in its management and concerns about possible long-term health risks of cardiovascular disease, endometrial, breast and ovarian cancer.

This chapter argues that the complexity of PCOS calls for a paradigm shift in future research directions to improve the understanding and management of these women taking into account the hypothesis-driven research which predominates the literature and which focuses on one gene or factor at a time is inappropriate in a syndrome as complex as PCOS. Fortunately, recent

Aarti Sharma MBBS MRCOG
Specialist Registrar in Obstetrics and Gynaecology, City Hospital, Nottingham, UK (correspondence to: Miss Aarti Sharma, c/o Mr Atiomo's Secretary, B Floor, East Block, Queen's Medical Centre, Clifton Boulevard, Nottingham NG7 2UH, UK)

Mohammed Yousef MBBCh MA MRCOG
Staff Grade Doctor in Obstetrics and Gynaecology, Queen's Medical Centre, Clifton Boulevard, Nottingham NG7 2UH, UK

Rianna Burrill BMedSci
Medical Student, University of Nottingham, Nottingham, UK

William Atiomo MBBS DM MA MRCOG
Clinical Senior Lecturer and Consultant Gynaecologist, Division of Obstetrics and Gynaecology, School of Human Development, University of Nottingham, B Floor, East Block, Queen's Medical Centre, Clifton Boulevard, Nottingham NG7 2UH, UK

advances in molecular biology and bioinformatics including cDNA microarrays and proteomics which now make it possible to analyse several thousand genes and proteins in one experiment will facilitate this paradigm shift to complexity, bioinformatics and mathematical modelling in PCOS-related research.

The chapter begins by reviewing recent developments in the definition, prevalence and pathophysiology of PCOS. The clinical features are then briefly reviewed followed by an exploration of recent developments in the management and possible long-term health consequences of PCOS. The chapter ends by briefly discussing the practical implications and benefits of a shift to 'complexity driven research in PCOS' but argues that even if this is adopted as a vital future evolution in PCOS research, there will still remain the challenge of making sense of all the data generated. The ultimate challenge of 'finding simplicity in complexity'.

DEFINITION

The main recent advance in the agreed definition of PCOS was agreed at the Rotterdam ESHRE/ASRM-sponsored PCOS consensus workshop.[1] Traditionally, there had been an on-going debate between gynaecologists in Europe and North America about how best to define PCOS. In the UK and Europe, most clinicians agreed that a the presence of polycystic ovaries on ultrasound was pivotal in its diagnosis and a diagnosis of PCOS was made if polycystic ovaries on ultrasound were found in combination with one or more of the clinical and biochemical features of androgen excess and chronic anovulation. However, in North America, the definition was based on an NIH consensus definition agreed in 1992,[2] which required that PCOS be diagnosed in women with chronic anovulation and evidence of androgen excess for which there is no other cause. Specifically, ovarian morphology was not thought to be essential in the diagnostic criteria. In an attempt to resolve the debate, the Rotterdam ESHRE/ASRM-sponsored PCOS consensus workshop group agreed that PCOS was a primarily condition of ovarian dysfunction whose cardinal features were hyperandrogenism and polycystic morphology on ultrasound. The workshop agreed that two of the following three criteria were required in order to diagnose the condition after exclusion of other causes of androgen excess. These three criteria were: (i) oligo- and/or anovulation; (ii) clinical and/or biochemical signs of hyperandrogenism; and (iii) polycystic ovary morphology on ultrasound scan, defined as the presence of 12 or more follicles in each ovary (with one ovary being sufficient for diagnosis) measuring 2–9 mm in diameter, and/or increased ovarian volume (> 10 ml).

This definition was, however, not to be applied to women on the oral contraceptive pill as it changes the ovarian morphology. It was also suggested that, in the presence of a dominant follicle (> 10 mm) or a corpus luteum, the scan was to be repeated in the next cycle.

Some unresolved practical issues still remain with this new definition. These include the variable quality of ultrasound scans which are often operator- and machine-dependent, and the omission of measures of insulin resistance in the diagnostic criteria, which is increasingly being recognised as being central to the pathophysiology of PCOS.

PREVALENCE

Using ultrasound scan criteria only, 20–33% of apparently healthy women in the child-bearing period have been found to have polycystic ovaries in population studies[3–6] whereas a prevalence of 4–10% in women of reproductive age is commonly quoted when the diagnosis is based on clinical, biochemical and ultrasound scan features.[5,7,8] However, 50–85% of 'these apparently healthy women' have symptoms or signs of the syndrome such as menstrual irregularity or hirsutism.

Recent studies in the literature on the prevalence of PCOS, again further heighten the need for a fundamental shift in research approach as previously discussed, particularly in view of reports showing that the phenotypic expression of PCOS appears to be dependent on racial origin. For example, Mexican American and south Asian women with PCOS[9] are more likely to suffer insulin resistance compared with Caucasians. South Asian women also have lower sex hormone binding globulin levels. European and Maori women with PCOS are more likely to present with hirsutism compared with other races[10] and the prevalence of PCO morphology has also been shown to be commoner in women with type 2 diabetes.[11]

Adopting the new consensus ESHRE/ASRM definition of PCOS as the gold standard over the next few years could potentially overcome this challenge; however, as the new ESHRE/ASRM consensus definition does not incorporate indices of insulin resistance, this will not be easy.

PATHOPHYSIOLOGY

Traditional concepts of PCOS as a primarily endocrine condition secondary to aberrations in the hypothalamo–pituitary–ovarian axis manifesting as high luteinising hormone/follicle stimulating hormone ratios, increased androgen production and high oestrone levels from peripheral conversion in adipose tissue of androgens are increasingly being challenged. New developments in research into the pathophysiology of PCOS have focused on the role of genetics, insulin resistance and the interrelationships between obesity and ghrelin (a gastric peptide with adipogenic activity).

Genetics

The familial pattern and identification of a possible male phenotype in PCOS makes it a condition that hypothetically is predominantly genetic in origin. Overall, studies on the genetics of PCOS do suggest that a gene or several genes may be associated with PCOS, based on the clustering of PCOS in families and studies of theca muscle and adipocytes from women with PCOS which have highlighted a unique molecular phenotype.

Results from some family studies suggest a possible autosomal dominant phenotype. However, the largest twin study on women with PCOS[12] found a high degree of discordance among twins with polycystic ovaries, which suggests a more complex pattern of inheritance than an autosomal dominant pattern of inheritance. Similarly, although some cytogenetic studies suggested that PCOS may be associated with a large deletion of chromosome 11[13] and X chromosome aneuploidies,[14] larger cytogenetic studies have failed to reveal any karyotypic abnormalities.[15]

Studies on candidate genes have focused on those involved in steroid hormone synthesis, genes involved in carbohydrate metabolism, genes involved in gonadotrophin action and the major histocompatibility region. These candidate genes include CYP11A, CYP17, CYP21, androgen receptor, SHBG gene, insulin receptor gene, insulin gene, insulin receptor substrate gene, capain 10, FSH β-subunit gene, dopamine receptor gene and follistatin.[16] Although there is no overwhelming evidence supporting linkage from many of these studies, the strongest evidence can be found in support of the region near the insulin receptor gene as it has been found in two different studies[17,18] where an association was demonstrated between a marker (D19S884 at 19p13.3) that is located 2 megabases centromeric from the insulin receptor.

A unique molecular phenotype of skeletal muscle and ovarian theca cells from women with PCOS also provides some evidence in support of a genetic aetiology. In one study, increased insulin receptor serine phosphorylation of skeletal muscle was found in 50% of a sample of women with PCOS.[19] Although it could be argued that epigenetic alterations could have occurred during the *in vitro* cultures of these cells, the results from microarray analysis of ovarian theca cells and skeletal muscle cultures from women with PCOS support the concept of a unique tissue molecular phenotype.[20] Larger and confirmatory studies are, however, awaited.

An overall appraisal of the evidence in support of a genetic basis for PCOS would, therefore, suggest that although there is some evidence that genetics underpins PCOS, the evidence is not overwhelming, and several genes or an interaction between several genes and environmental factors may be involved.

Insulin resistance

It is now clearly established that insulin resistance is present in obese and non-obese women with PCOS; however, the exact mechanisms of insulin resistance in PCOS remain elusive. Recent studies on mechanisms of insulin resistance in PCOS have focused on polymorphisms in genes regulating carbohydrate homeostasis as discussed above. However, none of these genes have been consistently shown to be related with PCOS.

One central paradox regarding insulin resistance in PCOS is the high responsiveness to insulin by the ovary, as opposed to the resistance of the whole body, and this model has been used to explain ovarian hyperandrogenaemia as it is thought to arise from a direct stimulatory effect of insulin on ovarian stromal cells. However, a recent study from China appears to contradict this hypothesis.[21] In a study of 44 women undergoing IVF treatment, of whom 11 had polycystic ovaries and 33 had normal ovulation, significant decreases in insulin-stimulated glucose incorporation into glycogen in cultured ovarian granulosa cells treated with troglitazone from women with PCOS were found compared with controls suggesting that ovarian cells are also insulin resistant. Although, admittedly, these were granulosa and not theca cells and they had been exposed to *in vitro* culture, it does raise the question of whether selective ovarian sensitivity does truly occur in PCOS.

Obesity and ghrelin

About 10–65% of women with PCOS are obese, and obesity in PCOS tends to be distributed around the abdomen (visceral fat). Generally, a significant correlation exists between obesity and infertility and obesity and miscarriage but the mechanisms have not been completely elucidated. There have recently been studies looking at the role of a complex interaction between obesity and reproductive function in the aetiology of PCOS mediated by ghrelin. Ghrelin is a novel gastric peptide which has orexigenic and adipogenic properties. Circulating ghrelin concentrations are influenced by nutritional status and, probably, regulate food intake and body weight. Ghrelin has been shown to modulate the secretory pattern of pituitary hormones, and it may exert direct effects on peripheral organs such as the gonads and endocrine pancreas. Four recent studies[22-25] have examined the role of ghrelin in women with PCOS and produced conflicting results. In one study, ghrelin levels were no different from controls; in another, ghrelin levels; were lower in obese women with PCOS compared with controls, and, in the third paper, women with PCOS had lower ghrelin levels compared with lean and obese controls. In the most recent study, however, circulating ghrelin levels were found to rise following anti-androgen treatment in women with PCOS, suggesting that androgens were an independent modulator of ghrelin levels. The complexity of the interrelationships between PCOS, androgens, ghrelin, obesity and infertility, however, remain to be unravelled.

CLINICAL FEATURES

Traditional concepts of our understanding of the clinical features of PCOS are largely unchanged; however, there have been some minor new developments. These developments include the failure to demonstrate a clear link between PCOS and recurrent miscarriage and a possible link between PCOS and epilepsy.

Presenting features in PCOS usually range from no symptoms to those of menstrual irregularities, hirsutism, obesity, acne, and infertility. It had been suggested in the past that miscarriage may be associated with PCOS. It was thought that this was due to the presence of high luteinising hormone and androgen levels in women with PCOS, as these hormones were associated with miscarriage. However, this link between PCOS and recurrent miscarriage has recently been questioned. In a recent cohort study looking at the prospective pregnancy outcome of 486 women who were antiphospholipid antibody negative and on no pharmacological treatment, similar live-birth rates were found amongst women with PCO (60.9%) compared with those with normal ovarian morphology (58.5%).[26]

Recent studies have also shown that epileptics may be more prone to PCOS. Although the link and mechanisms are debatable, it has been proposed that it may occur secondary to direct influences of epilepsy and anti-epileptic drugs on the endocrine control centres in the brain or to the effect of anti-epileptic drugs on insulin sensitivity.[27] However, in a recent study, the prevalence of polycystic ovaries and polycystic ovarian syndrome amongst epileptics was similar to that in general population.[28] Similarly, there is no reliable data showing a greater prevalence of PCO in women on valproate although previously there had been concerns raised about a possible link between PCOS and valproate use.[29]

LONG-TERM SEQUELAE OF PCOS

More recently, the potential longer term risks of PCOS have been a focus of research. Although it has been clearly established that PCOS predisposes to non-insulin dependent diabetes in later life,[30] significant controversy still exists as to the link between PCOS and cardiovascular mortality. This is because although there have been several studies showing that morbidity from cardiovascular disease is increased in women with PCOS, the only published study on mortality in PCOS did not confirm the link.[30]

Recent interest in the long-term risks of PCOS have also focused on its possible associations with endometrial, ovarian and breast cancer. An association between PCOS and endometrial carcinoma was first suggested in 1949.[31] The mechanism which is generally assumed to be responsible for any increased risk of endometrial carcinoma in women with PCOS relates to prolonged anovulation with consequent continued secretion of oestrogen unopposed by progesterone. However, in a recent appraisal of the evidence published in the *Lancet*, the evidence for an association between PCOS and endometrial cancer was inconclusive.[32]

Several lines of evidence also suggest that women with PCOS may also be at increased risk of having ovarian cancer. In a 1993 study,[33] a high frequency of hyperplastic and metaplastic changes were found on the surface epithelium or in the inclusion cysts in ovaries with contralateral polycystic ovarian disease, epithelial ovarian tumours and endometrial cancers compared to ovaries without hyperplastic or metaplastic changes. In another study linking clomiphene with ovarian cancer,[34] women with polycystic ovaries were found to have an adjusted relative risk of ovarian tumours of 4.1 compared with controls. Two large Danish studies also suggest that infertility on its own increases the risk of borderline and invasive ovarian tumours.[35,36] However, conflicting this link between PCOS and ovarian cancer is the study by Wild and colleagues on mortality in PCOS, where the standardised mortality ratio in women with PCOS was 0.34, suggesting a lower risk of ovarian cancer.

The association of PCOS with postmenopausal breast cancer has been evaluated in a large study and this did not show an increased incidence over controls. Therefore, women with PCOS do not require surveillance above that indicated in the Breast Screening Programme. On the other hand, a positive association has been shown between PCOS and a family history of breast cancer. In a cross-sectional study of 217 women with and without PCOS, the proportion of women with a positive family history of breast cancer was significantly greater in women with PCOS compared with controls.[37] Although these results have not yet been replicated, animal studies linking elevated testosterone, insulin, insulin-like growth factor 1, insulin-like growth factor 2, and abdominal obesity with breast cancer suggests that more research is called for in this area.

MANAGEMENT

Traditionally, treatment of PCOS has been mainly symptom oriented as no one cause could be attributed to the condition. However, with the recent identification of the central role of insulin resistance to the aetiology of PCOS, treatment is now aimed towards measures to improve insulin resistance as these have been shown to improve the regularity of menstrual cycles, ovulation, androgen levels and surrogate markers for longer term risk of diabetes and heart disease. Life-style modification and metformin which both improve insulin resistance have, therefore, been the focus of recent research.

Life-style modification

Life-style modification is very important in the treatment for PCOS, as weight loss and exercise show a striking improvement in ovulatory function and features of hyperandrogenism. Specifically, dietary modification, moderate exercise, cessation of smoking and moderate alcohol and caffeine intake are life-style modifications recommended in women with PCOS.[38] Studies investigating the effects of both reduced calorie diets (1000–1200 kcal/day) and very low calorie diets (VLCD: about 400 kcal/day) in obese women with PCOS have found significant weight loss, reductions in testosterone and an improvement in insulin sensitivity. There has been recent speculation about the effects of a high protein diet (Atkins) on weight loss and it would be interesting to determine if it is effective in women with PCOS. However, in the only published study comparing a high protein diet (30% protein) with a standard diet (15% protein) in women with PCOS (39), dietary composition had no effect on reproduction and a high-protein diet only conferred small improvements on lipids, glucose and the free androgen ratio. Larger, evaluative studies are required.

The effect of increased physical activity alone (no change in dietary intake) in obese women with PCOS was investigated by Randeva et al.[40] who reported a significant reduction in WHR, and plasma homocysteine concentrations (a cardiovascular risk marker) but no significant change in BMI amongst 12 obese women with PCOS who adhered to a 6-month exercise programme. Again, although no significant reduction in BMI was noted in 15 obese PCOS women offered diet and exercise counselling and support, improved ovulation, fertility and insulin sensitivity were found.[41] On the other hand, 25 (76%) of 33 obese women with PCOS lost at least 5% of their body weight when they were prescribed a hypocaloric diet and recommended to swim or do aerobics once or twice a week. Eighteen had a resumption of regular cycles and 15 experienced spontaneous ovulation; 10 spontaneous pregnancies occurred in patients who lost at least 5% of their weight.[42]

Although, to date, there have been no studies specifically considering the effects of smoking, alcohol and caffeine in PCOS, it is currently recommended that women with PCOS cease smoking and only consume moderate amounts of alcohol and caffeine.[38] These recommendations are made because all three have been shown to exacerbate the symptoms of PCOS. For example (although debates may exist), cigarette smoking has been linked to decreased fertility[43–46] and impaired insulin action.[47] Negative effects of alcohol on fertility[48,49] have also been reported. Finally, caffeine may influence fertility[50–52] and increase the risk of spontaneous abortion[51] though the research evidence is inconsistent.

Further research to determine whether advice on life-style modification outside a research setting (i.e. in day-to-day clinical practice) actually improves the symptoms of PCOS is required as preliminary data from a pilot study suggest that this may not be the case.[53]

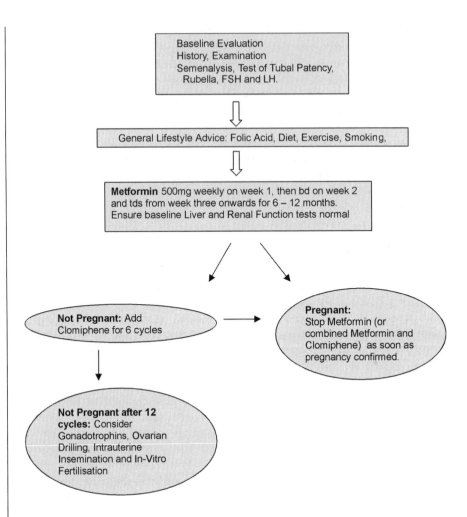

Fig. 1 Algorithm for the management of infertility in women with PCOS with metformin.

Metformin

There have been several studies evaluating the effectiveness of metformin in PCOS. In summary, these studies show that although there is clear evidence that metformin improves menstrual cyclicity and ovulation in PCOS, the effects on live-birth rates, hirsutism, acne and obesity are unclear (see Fig. 1). The most robust evidence on metformin use in PCOS comes from the findings of a recent systematic review.[54] In a meta-analysis of 13 randomised controlled trials, metformin was shown to be effective in achieving ovulation in women with PCOS (OR, 3.88; 95% CI 2.25–6.69) compared with placebo and for metformin and clomifene compared with clomifene alone (OR, 4.41; 95% CI 2.37–8.22). There was, however, no data on live-birth rates and no studies where metformin had been directly compared with clomifene as initial therapy for anovulatory PCOS.

Metformin can be offered to all women (obese and non-obese) with anovulatory infertility due to PCOS who have been trying to conceive for a year or more as a first-line drug or where clomiphene treatment has failed. There have been concerns expressed about the risk of hypoglycaemia in lean anovulatory women with PCOS on metformin treatment. However, the risk of hypoglycaemia with metformin treatment in PCOS is low, although the exact risks in lean women with PCOS is unclear. Theoretically, it would be extremely unlikely, particularly as insulin resistance is linked with anovulation in PCOS even in non-obese women. It is, however, recommended that all women going on metformin are advised to look out for signs of hypoglycaemia and stop treatment if this is suspected.

Strictly speaking, there is no agreed upper body mass index cut-off as is the case with clomifene; however, weight loss by exercise and diet modification should be advised as the first-line therapy, particularly as weight loss in obese patients with PCOS results in a striking improvement in ovulatory function and hyperandrogenism as previously discussed. Many pregnancy complications are linked to obesity, and it makes sense to advice women to lose weight as this reduces the occurrence of obesity-related pregnancy complications.[55]

Before prescribing metformin, renal and hepatic function should be checked as metformin can very rarely cause lactic acidosis in the presence of even mild renal impairment. Annual testing of renal and hepatic function is also indicated once on metformin therapy. An oral glucose tolerance test and fasting lipids should also ideally be checked as women with PCOS are at higher risk of being diabetes and having an atherogenic lipid profile. The oral glucose tolerance test should also be rechecked once pregnancy is confirmed.[56] The usual dose is 500 mg, three times daily. To minimise the mainly gastrointestinal side effects (mentioned below), it is commonly advised to take the tablets just before food and gradually increase the daily dose of metformin in increments of 500 mg weekly. Some prefer to prescribe it in a dose of 850 mg twice daily in order to improve compliance. A higher dose (850 mg tds) of metformin in obese women with PCOS does not appear to confer any further benefit.

The optimal period of metformin monotherapy for fertility is unknown. Some studies have shown a rapid return to spontaneous ovulation and normal menstrual rhythm within three months of the start of therapy.[57,58] Nestler et al.[58] suggested a 6-month trial where time is not of the essence. There is no correlation between length of trial and proportion ovulating with metformin alone.[54] It is, however, recommended that where metformin is used as stand-alone first-line therapy, it is continued for 6–12 months if regular ovulation is documented; however, if it has not been effective after 3–6 months' treatment, clomifene should be added for a further 6 months. Metformin should be stopped once pregnancy is confirmed as it is not licensed for use in pregnancy. Where pregnancy has not occurred, after a year of either metformin alone or metformin + clomifene combination therapy, then alternative treatments (laparoscopic ovarian drilling, gonadotrophins or in vitro fertilisation) should be considered.

There are currently no clear guidelines on the role of follicle tracking in women on metformin monotherapy as in theory the risks of multiple pregnancy and ovarian hyperstimulation are absent. Metformin is usually discontinued once pregnancy is confirmed although there is no evidence of animal or human fetal teratogenicity.

FUTURE RESEARCH CHALLENGES

There is still an absence of clear and consistent data about the effects of metformin on pregnancy rates, live-birth rates, hirsutism, obesity or in reducing the potential longer term health risks of PCOS. There is also a need for a better characterisation of PCOS given the complexity of its clinical presentation and unclear aetiology. Although there have been attempts to do this genetically given the familial associations in PCOS, there is still some uncertainty about the exact gene/genes involved. PCOS, however, probably arises from a complex interaction of genetic and environmental factors. Research approaches that integrate these variables are, therefore, more likely to improve our understanding of PCOS. Fortunately, recent developments in molecular biology make it possible to study an increased number of genes (mRNAs) and proteins expressed in human tissue using techniques such as microarrays and proteomics. Computational analysis and interpretation of derived biological data enable rapid assimilation, usable formats and algorithms for efficient management and interpretation of results.

These approaches to future research in PCOS will hopefully simplify our understanding of the aetiology, diagnosis and clinical management of the complex (or supercomplex) condition of PCOS. On the other hand, recent experience from cancer research where this strategy has been adopted has generated a further challenge of developing simple biologically relevant mathematical models from the complex datasets produced from experiments using microarrays.[59]

CONCLUSIONS

The key recent developments in PCOS include the following. A publication of a new ESHRE/ASRM consensus definition incorporating PCO morphology, chronic oligo/anovulation and hyperandrogenaemia. Advances in genetic studies searching for a genetic basis for PCOS including microarray analysis of ovarian theca cells demonstrating a unique molecular phenotype. Studies evaluating selective ovarian insulin resistance and the role of ghrelin, a gastric peptide, in PCOS. Studies evaluating possible long-term health risks of cardiovascular disease, endometrial, breast and ovarian cancer in PCOS. Studies demonstrating the positive impact of improved life-style advice through diet and exercise on PCOS and finally evidence of improved menstrual cyclicity and ovulation with metformin use.

There is a need for research into several unanswered questions in PCOS and for a paradigm shift to complexity driven research given the complexity of PCOS. This strategy acknowledges that in complex conditions such as PCOS, a complex interplay of genetic, epigenetic and environmental factors may influence its expression. Recent developments in molecular biology (such as microarrays) and computational biology which potentially enhanced this shift. However, the real challenge in adopting this new research approach is in making clinical sense of complex datasets produced – 'the challenge of finding simplicity in complexity'.

Useful website for further information on PCOS

<http://www.pcos.i8.com>

1 Rotterdam ESHRE/ASRM-Sponsored PCOS Consensus Workshop Group. Revised 2003 consensus on diagnostic criteria and long-term health risks related to polycystic ovary syndrome. Fertil Steril 2003; 81: 19–25

2 Zawadzki JK, Dunaif A. Diagnostic criteria for polycystic ovary syndrome: towards a rational approach. In: Dunaif A, Givens JR, Haseltine FP, Merriman GR. (eds) Polycystic Ovary Syndrome. Oxford; Blackwell, 1992; 377–384

3 Clayton, RN, Ogden V, Hodgkinson J et al. How common are polycystic ovaries in normal women and what is their significance for the fertility of the population? Clin Endocrinol 1992; 37: 127–134

4. Balen AH. The pathogenesis of polycystic ovarian syndrome: the enigma unravels. Lancet 1999; 354: 966–967

5 Polson DW, Adams J, Wadsworth J, Franks S. Polycystic ovaries – a common finding in normal women. Lancet 1998; i: 870–872

6 Farquhar CM, Birdsall MA, Manning P et al. The prevalence of polycystic ovaries on ultrasound scanning in a population of randomly selected women. Aust NZ J Obstet Gynaecol 1994; 34: 67–72

7 Hull MGR. Epidemiology of infertility and polycystic ovarian disease: endocrinological and demographic studies. Gynaecol Endocrinol 1987; 1: 233–245

8 Dunaif A. Insulin resistance and the polycystic ovarian syndrome: mechanisms and implications for pathogenesis. Endocrine Rev 1997; 18: 774–800

9 Wijeyaratne CN, Balen AH, Barth JH et al. Clinical manifestations and insulin resistance (IR) in polycystic ovary syndrome (PCOS) among South Asians and Caucasians: is there a difference? Clin Endocrinol 2002; 57: 343–350

10 Williamson K, Gunn AJ, Johnson N, Milsom SR. The impact of ethnicity on the presentation of polycystic ovarian syndrome. Aust NZ J Obstet Gynaecol 2001; 41: 202–206

11 Peppard HR, Marfori J, Iuorno MJ, Nestler JE. Prevalence of polycystic ovary syndrome among premenopausal women with type 2 diabetes. Diabetes Care 2001; 24: 1050–1052

12 Jahanfar S, Eden JA, Warren P, Seppala M, Nguyen TV. A twin study of polycystic ovary syndrome. Fertil Steril 1995; 63: 478–486

13 Meyer MF, Gerresheim F, Pfeiffer A, Epplen JT, Schatz H. Association of polycystic ovary syndrome with an interstitial deletion of the long arm of chromosome 11. Exp Clin Endocrinol Diabetes 2000; 108: 519–523

14 Rojanasakul A, Gustavson KH, Lithell H, Nillius SJ. Tetraploidy in two sisters with the polycystic ovary syndrome. Clin Genet 1985; 27: 167–174

15 Stenchever MA, Macintyre MN, Jarvis JA, Hempel JM. Cytogenetic evaluation of 41 patients with Stein-Leventhal syndrome. Obstet Gynecol 1968; 32: 794–801

16 Legro R, Strauss J. Molecular progress in infertility: polycystic ovary syndrome. Fertil Steril 2003; 78: 569–576

17 Urbanek M, Legro RS, Driscoll DA et al. Thirty-seven candidate genes for polycystic ovary syndrome: strongest evidence for linkage is with follistatin. Proc Natl Acad Sci USA 1999; 96: 8573–8578

18 Tucci S, Futterweit W, Conception ES et al. Evidence for association of polycystic ovary syndrome in Caucasian women with a marker at the insulin receptor gene locus. J Clin Endocrinol Metab 2001; 86: 446–449

19 Dunaif A, Xia J, Book CB, Schenker E, Tang Z. Excessive insulin receptor serine phosphorylation in cultured fibroblasts and in skeletal muscle. A potential mechanism for insulin resistance in the polycystic ovary syndrome. J Clin Invest 1995; 96: 801–810

20 Wood JR, Nelson VL, Ho C et al. The molecular phenotype of polycystic ovary syndrome (PCOS) theca cells and new candidate PCOS genes defined by microarray analysis. J Biol Chem 2003; 278: 26380–26390

21 Wu XK, Zhou SY, Liu JX, Pollanen P, Sallinen K, Makinen M, Erkkola R. Selective ovary resistance to insulin signalling in women with polycystic ovary syndrome. Fertil Steril 2003; 80: 954–965

22 Gambineri A, Pagotto U, Tschop M et al. Anti-androgen treatment increases circulating ghrelin levels in obese women with polycystic ovary syndrome. J Endocrinol Invest 2003; 26: 629–634

23 Orio Jr F, Lucidi P, Palomba S *et al*. Circulating ghrelin concentrations in the polycystic ovary syndrome. J Clin Endocrinol Metab 2003; 88: 942–945

24 Pagotto U, Gambineri A, Vicennati V, Heiman ML, Tschop M, Pasquali R. Plasma ghrelin, obesity, and the polycystic ovary syndrome: correlation with insulin resistance and androgen levels. J Clin Endocrinol Metab 2002; 87: 5625–5629

25 Schofl C, Horn R, Schill T, Schlosser HW, Muller MJ, Brabant G. Circulating ghrelin levels in patients with polycystic ovary syndrome. Clin Endocrinol Metab 2002; 87: 4607–4610

26 Rai R, Backos M, Rushworth F, Regan L. Polycystic ovaries and recurrent miscarriage – a reappraisal. Hum Reprod 2000; 15: 612–615

27 Bauer J, Isojarvi JI, Herzog AG *et al*. Reproductive dysfunction in women with epilepsy: recommendations for evaluation and management. J Neurol Neurosurg Psychiatry 2002; 73: 121–125

28 Polson DW. Polycystic ovary syndrome and epilepsy – a gynaecological perspective. Seizure 2003; 12: 397–402

29 Genton P, Bauer J, Duncan S *et al*. On the association between valproate and polycystic ovary syndrome. Epilepsia 2001; 42: 305–310

30 Wild S, Pierpoint T, Jacobs H, McKeigue P. Long-term consequences of polycystic ovary syndrome: results of a 31 year follow-up study. Fertility 2000; 3: 101–105

31 Speert H. Carcinoma of the endometrium in young women. Surg Gynaecol Obstet 1949; 88: 332–336

32 Hardiman P, Pillay OC, Atiomo W. Polycystic ovary syndrome and endometrial cancer. Lancet 2003; 361: 1810–1812

33 Resta L, Russo S, Colucci GA, Prat J. Morphologic precursors of ovarian epithelial tumors. Obstet Gynecol 1993; 82: 181–186

34 Rossing MA, Daling JR, Weiss NS, Moore DE, Self SG. Ovarian tumors in a cohort of infertile women. N Engl J Med 1994; 331: 771–776

35 Mosgaard BJ, Lidegaard O, Kjaer SK, Schou G, Anderson AN. Infertility, fertility drugs, and invasive ovarian cancer: a case-control study. Fertil Steril 1997; 67: 1005–1012

36 Mosgaard BJ, Lidegaard O, Kjaer SK, Schou G, Andersen AN. Ovarian stimulation and borderline ovarian tumors: a case-control study. Fertil Steril 1998; 70: 1049–1055

37 Atiomo W, El Mahdi E, Hardiman P. Familial associations in PCOS. Fertil Steril 2003; 80: 143–145

38 Norman RJ, Davies MJ, Lord J, Moran LJ. The role of lifestyle modification in polycystic ovary syndrome. Trends Endocrinol Metab 2002; 13: 251–257

39 Moran LJ, Noakes M, Clifton PM *et al*. Dietary composition in restoring reproductive and metabolic physiology in overweight women with polycystic ovary syndrome. J Clin Endocrinol Metab 2003; 88: 812–819

40 Randeva HS, Lewandowski KC, Drzewoski J *et al*. Exercise decreases plasma total homocysteine in overweight young women with polycystic ovary syndrome. J Clin Endocrinol Metab 2002; 87: 4496–4501

41 Huber-Buchholz MM, Carey DG, Norman RJ. Restoration of reproductive potential by lifestyle modification in obese polycystic ovary syndrome: role of insulin sensitivity and luteinizing hormone. J Clin Endocrinol Metab 1999; 84: 1470–1474

42 Crosignani PG, Colombo M, Vegetti W, Somigliana E, Gessati A, Ragni G. Overweight and obese anovulatory patients with polycystic ovary syndrome: parallel improvements in anthropometric indices, ovarian physiology and fertility rate induced by diet. Hum Reprod 2003; 18: 1928–1932

43 Florack EI, Zielhuis GA, Rolland R. Cigarette smoking, alcohol consumption, and caffeine intake and fecundability. Prevent Med 1994; 23: 175–180

44 Alderete E, Eskenazi B, Sholtz R. Effect of cigarette smoking and coffee drinking on time to conception [comment]. Epidemiology 1995; 6: 403–408

45 Barbieri RL. The initial fertility consultation: recommendations concerning cigarette smoking, body mass index, and alcohol and caffeine consumption. Am J Obstet Gynecol 2001; 185: 1168–1173

46 Munafo M, Murphy M, Whiteman D, Hey K. Does cigarette smoking increase time to conception? J Biosoc Sci 2002; 34: 65–73

47 Targher G, Alberiche M, Zenere MB *et al*. Cigarette smoking and insulin resistance in

patients with non-insulin-dependent diabetes mellitus. J Clin Endocrinol Metab 1997; 82: 3619–3624

48 Grodstein F, Goldman MB, Cramer DW. Infertility in women and moderate alcohol use [comment]. Am J Public Health 1994; 84: 1429–1432

49 Jensen TK, Hjollund NH, Henriksen TB *et al.* Does moderate alcohol consumption affect fertility? Follow up study among couples planning first pregnancy [comment]. BMJ 1998; 317: 505–510

50 Stanton CK, Gray RH. Effects of caffeine consumption on delayed conception [comment]. Am J Epidemiol 1995; 142: 1322–1329

51 Barbieri RL. The initial fertility consultation: recommendations concerning cigarette smoking, body mass index, and alcohol and caffeine consumption. Am J Obstet Gynecol 2001; 185: 1168–1173

52 Bolumar F, Olsen J, Rebagliato M, Bisanti L. Caffeine intake and delayed conception: a European multicenter study on infertility and subfecundity. European Study Group on Infertility Subfecundity. Am J Epidemiol 1997; 145: 324–334

53 Burrill R. Lifestyle Modification in PCOS. BMedSci Dissertation, University of Nottingham, 2004

54 Lord JM, Flight IHK, Norman RJ. Metformin in polycystic ovary syndrome: systematic review and meta-analysis. BMJ 2003; 327: 951–956

55 Clark AM, Thornley B, Tomlinson L *et al.* Weight loss in obese infertile women results in improvement in reproductive outcome for all forms of fertility treatment. Hum Reprod 1998; 13: 1502–1505

56 The Royal College of Obstetrics and Gynaecology Long-term consequences of polycystic ovary syndrome. Clinical Green Top Guideline No 33. London, RCOG Press, 2003

57 Pasquali R, Gambineri A, Biscott D *et al.* Effect of long-term treatment with metformin added to hypocaloric diet on body composition, fat distribution and androgen and insulin levels in abdominally obese women with and without the polycystic ovary syndrome. J Clin Endocrinol Metab 2000; 85: 2767–2774

58 Nestler JE, Jakubowicz DJ, Evans WS, Pasquali R Effects of metformin on spontaneous and clomiphene-induced ovulation in the in polycystic ovary syndrome. N Engl J Med 1998; 338: 1876–1880

59 Winegarden N. Microarrays in cancer: moving from hype to clinical reality. Lancet 2003; 362: 1428

James D. M. Nicopoullos
Jonathan W. A. Ramsay Carole Gilling-Smith

Assessment and management of azoospermia in the infertile couple

The investigation and treatment of subfertility is an integral part of a gynaecologist's workload. Infertility affects approximately one in seven couples in the UK and The Royal College of Obstetricians and Gynaecologists (RCOG) estimates that a typical health authority may see up to 230 new consultant referrals each year.[1] Since the first published study of the epidemiology of infertility in 1886 by Mathews Duncan (Fecundity, Fertility and Sterility), inconsistencies in the definition of infertility, approach to investigation and diagnostic criteria have led to considerable variations in the published prevalence of infertility and the relative contributions of particular aetiologies. Nevertheless, male factor infertility is consistently shown to be the commonest single diagnostic category.[2] The RCOG state that male factor infertility is responsible for up to 25% of all cases of infertility and may contribute in a further 25%.[3] Although the gynaecologist is invariably referred the female partner, it is essential that we are equipped to meet the needs of the subfertile 'couple' and deal with male-factor problems.

'Azoospermia', the complete absence of sperm in the ejaculate, is found in 1% of males[4] and the incidence in subfertile couples has been reported to be as high as 10–15%.[5] Recent NICE guidelines have drawn, once again, attention to the need for evidence-based management of infertile couples. The aim of this chapter is to review the aetiology, assessment and management of azoospermia, both in a general gynaecology clinic and assisted reproduction setting, and provide guidelines which will be helpful to both generalist and

James D. M. Nicopoullos MBBS BSc
Clinical Research Fellow, Assisted Conception Unit, Chelsea & Westminster Hospital, 369 Fulham Road, London SW10 9NH, UK (for correspondence, E-mail: james.nicopoullos@chelwest.nhs.uk)

Jonathan W. A. Ramsay MS FRCS
Assisted Conception Unit, Chelsea & Westminster Hospital, 369 Fulham Road, London SW10 9NH, UK

Carole Gilling-Smith MA PhD FRCOG
Assisted Conception Unit, Chelsea & Westminster Hospital, 369 Fulham Road, London SW10 9NH, UK

sub-specialist in order to counsel couples correctly on management options and chances of successful outcome.

HISTORICAL OVERVIEW

Whereas, 10 years ago, the use of donor sperm was the only option offering a realistic chance of parenting for the azoospermic or severely oligoastheno-teratospermic male, the development of micromanipulation techniques and the use of surgically retrieved sperm have revolutionised their management.

In vitro fertilisation (IVF) techniques were originally developed to tackle tubal-factor subfertility in women with normospermic partners. Despite initial hopes following the first pregnancy achieved using sperm aspirated from the epididymis of an azoospermic man,[6] they proved to be of limited use with a significantly reduced chance of fertilisation once the sperm count fell below < 5 x 10^6/ml.[7] However, with the advent of IVF, micromanipulation techniques, much practised previously in animal models, became feasible on human gametes. The initial techniques developed centred on the reduced ability of sperm in oligospermic men to penetrate the barrier to fertilisation represented by the zona pellucida: for example, 'zona drilling', in which the zona was punctured with acid Tyrode's solution;[8] partial zona dissection (PZD), where the zona was 'partially opened using mechanical force only';[9] and subzonal sperm injection (SUZI) into the perivitelline space.[10]

However, the success of PZD and SUZI in terms of fertilisation rate (FR < 20–25%) and pregnancy outcome remained moderate. It was not until the introduction of intracytoplasmic sperm injection (ICSI) by the work of Van Steirteghem and colleagues in Brussels that the management of male factor fertility moved significantly forward.[11] The results of a controlled comparison of SUZI and ICSI procedures on sibling oocytes showed a substantially higher FR with ICSI (4% versus 72%), and high FR and implantation rates (IR) with ICSI were reported in a series of 150 consecutive treatment cycles in couples previously not accepted for IVF or who had failed fertilisation with IVF.[11] A comparative study of conventional IVF versus ICSI for patients requiring microsurgical epididymal sperm aspiration (MESA) gave overall FR and pregnancy rates (PR) of 45% and 47%, respectively, for ICSI and 6.9% and 4.5%, respectively, for IVF.[12] The ability of ICSI to achieve high FR and PR, regardless of semen parameters[13] confirmed the role of ICSI in the management of azoospermic patients.

EVALUATION AND AETIOLOGY OF THE AZOOSPERMIC MAN

Once a diagnosis of azoospermia has been made and confirmed following repeat semen analyses and centrifugation of samples, the subsequent evaluation (Fig. 1) aims to identify any potential cause and decide into which of the two main classifications of azoospermia the patient falls (Table 1). This further evaluation should ideally occur in conjunction with an urologist with a special interest in male-factor subfertility. The correct classification of the azoospermic man into either obstructive azoospermia (OA) or non-obstructive azoospermia (NOA) is vital as the subsequent treatment options, genetic implications, counselling needs and chances of conception differ significantly

Table 1 Causes of azoospermia

Obstructive
    Infection
        Chlamydia
        Gonococcus
        Tuberculosis
        Filiriasis
        Bilharzias
    Surgery
        Childhood surgery (hernia, hydrocoele)
        Vasectomy
    Congenital bilateral absence of vas deferens
    Other respiratory associated conditions
        Young's syndrome
        Kartagener's syndrome
    Trauma
    Rare developmental abnormalities
        Ejaculatory duct obstruction
        Rete testis obstruction

Non-obstructive
    Genetic causes
        Y chromosome microdeletions
        Sex chromosomal anomalies (predominantly Kleinfelter's)
        Translocations
        Androgen insensitivity syndrome
        Noonan's syndrome
        Myotonic muscular dystrophy
        Sickle cell disease
    Crypto-orchidism
    Testicular trauma
    Testicular tumour
    Testicular torsion
    Viral orchitis (*e.g.* mumps)
    Varicocoele
    Toxins (chemotherapy/radiotherapy, *etc.*)

Miscellaneous
    Hypogonadotrophic hypogonadism
        Idiopathic
        Kallman's syndrome
        Prader Willi syndrome
        Lawrence-Moon-Biedle syndrome
        Familial cerebellar ataxia
        Trauma
        Tumour
    Retrograde ejaculation

between the two groups, and can only be confirmed with certainty on scrotal exploration and biopsy.

Obstructive azoospermia

Obstructive azoospermia (OA) is characterised by normal spermatogenesis. The testis will be of normal volume and examination will reveal normal virilisation. Therefore, the hypothalamic–pituitary–gonadal axis is unaffected and serum levels of follicle stimulating hormone (FSH) are normal (< 10 IU/l).

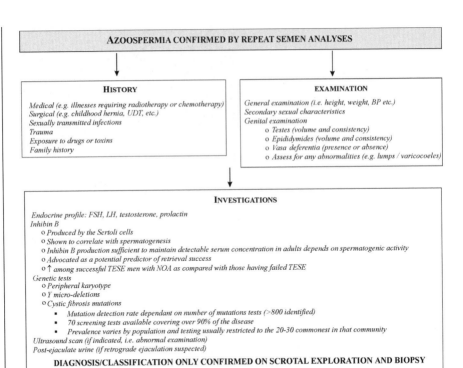

AZOOSPERMIA CONFIRMED BY REPEAT SEMEN ANALYSES

HISTORY

Medical (e.g. illnesses requiring radiotherapy or chemotherapy)
Surgical (e.g. childhood hernia, UDT, etc.)
Sexually transmitted infections
Trauma
Exposure to drugs or toxins
Family history

EXAMINATION

General examination (i.e. height, weight, BP etc.)
Secondary sexual characteristics
Genital examination
    o Testes (volume and consistency)
    o Epididymides (volume and consistency)
    o Vasa deferentia (presence or absence)
    o Assess for any abnormalities (e.g. lumps / varicocoeles)

INVESTIGATIONS

Endocrine profile: FSH, LH, testosterone, prolactin
Inhibin B
    o Produced by the Sertoli cells
    o Shown to correlate with spermatogenesis
    o Inhibin B production sufficient to maintain detectable serum concentration in adults depends on spermatogenic activity
    o Advocated as a potential predictor of retrieval success
    o ↑ among successful TESE men with NOA as compared with those having failed TESE
Genetic tests
    o Peripheral karyotype
    o Y micro-deletions
    o Cystic fibrosis mutations
        ▪ Mutation detection rate dependant on number of mutations tests (>800 identified)
        ▪ 70 screening tests available covering over 90% of the disease
        ▪ Prevalence varies by population and testing usually restricted to the 20-30 commonest in that community
Ultrasound scan (if indicated, i.e. abnormal examination)
Post-ejaculate urine (if retrograde ejaculation suspected)
DIAGNOSIS/CLASSIFICATION ONLY CONFIRMED ON SCROTAL EXPLORATION AND BIOPSY

Fig. 1 Evaluation of the azoospermic man.

Infection

The cause is often infective following chlamydial or gonococcal epididymitis. Less commonly in the industrialised world, infective agents such as filiriasis and tuberculosis are implicated.

Iatrogenic

Surgical obstruction can occur either at the time of childhood surgery (*e.g.* hernia repair, hydrocoele repair or orchidopexy) or intentionally at vasectomy. Up to 6% of men request reversal subsequent to vasectomy.[14] The success of reversal has been shown to be dependent on the skill and experience of the operator, time since vasectomy as well as the use of microsurgical techniques and type of reversal required. Patency and pregnancy rates have been quoted at 97% and 76% if performed within 3 years, 88% and 53% for 3–8 years, 79% and 44% for 9–14 years and 71% and 30% if more than 15 years after vasectomy.[15] Therefore, even with correct technique and done within 10 years of the original vasectomy, the procedure is not always successful. Furthermore, there is a significant discrepancy between patency and pregnancy rates, partly due to the 50–70% incidence of anti-sperm antibodies post-reversal[16,17] (as a consequence of the breach in the blood-testis barrier) and alterations in semen quality following the reversal.[18]

Congenital bilateral absence of the vas deferens (CBAVD)

CBAVD occurs in about 2% of obstructive azoospermics,[19] and in 1 in 1000 of the population. An increased frequency of cystic fibrosis gene mutations was reported for men diagnosed with CBAVD, and several series have observed that more than 50% carry a single mutation, and approximately 20% are compound heterozygotes.[20,21] Cystic fibrosis is a life-threatening autosomal recessive disorder with a carrier frequency of 1 in 25 in the UK, the mutation being carried on the short arm of chromosome 7 on the cystic fibrosis transmembrane conductance regulator (CFTR). More than 95% of males with cystic fibrosis are infertile secondary to obstructive azoospermia,[22] irrespective of the severity of their pancreatic or pulmonary disease and may present as an isolated finding or part of a specific genital phenotype. If such an abnormality is detected, it is imperative to test the female partner and counsel appropriately of the genetic risks. Even with a female partner negative for known mutations, there is still a 0.4% risk of an unknown mutation and, therefore, a 1 in 410 risk of an affected child. The pathology itself manifests as a consequence of fetal anomaly in the 7th week of gestation during Wolffian duct differentiation.

The CFTR protein may also be involved in the process of spermatogenesis and increased frequencies of CFTR mutations have been noted in populations of healthy infertile men with abnormal sperm parameters or non-obstructive azoospermia (16.7% versus 1.4–4% in normal controls).[23] There is also the separate entity of CBAVD associated with unilateral renal malformation that is not phenotypical of men with cystic fibrosis, as they have normal ureters and kidneys.

Young's syndrome

This syndrome was first described by Donald Young in 1970 and is characterised by chronic respiratory problems associated with obstructive azoospermia due to inspissated epididymal secretions. Examination reveals large, cystic epididymides and normal vasa. The OA may be progressive and may not be complete until years after puberty; therefore, patients may be able to conceive naturally in the early part of post-pubertal life. Aetiology is unknown but an association with childhood mercury poisoning has been suggested.[24]

Kartagener's syndrome

Immotile cilia syndrome (ICS) is a genetically heterogeneous disorder characterised by impaired motility of cilia and sperm tails (numerous genes involved in their construction implicated). Kartagener's syndrome is a rare (1 in 20,000) autosomal recessive subclassification of ICS, characterised by chronic sinusitis, dextrocardia and bronchiectasis. Homozygous men are almost always azoospermic secondary to globoz°spermia. The diagnosis is clinical, although may be confirmed by electron microscopy of cilia and sperm tails.[25]

Non-obstructive azoospermia

Non-obstructive azoospermia is characterised by impaired spermatogenesis, ranging from varying degrees of maturation arrest to Sertoli-cell only syndrome. Clinically, these men will usually have soft testis of decreased volume (< 15 ml); as a consequence of testicular dysfunction, a raised serum

FSH is probable. Common causes can be seen in Table 1, although the aetiology is unknown in about 50% of cases.[26]

Genetic

It has long been recognised that constitutional chromosomal abnormalities are more frequent in subfertile men than the general population. In an unselected group of 2372 infertile couples studied in Edinburgh, 2.1% of males had karyotypic abnormalities and over half of these were sex chromosomal.[27] One review has shown that 12% of azoospermic and severely oligospermic (< 10 x 10^6/ml) men have an abnormal karyotype.[28] A further review of the literature pooled data from six surveys of azoospermic men and five surveys of oligospermic men.[29] The cumulative data revealed an incidence of abnormality of 13.7% and 4.6% for the azoospermic and oligospermic populations, respectively. Klinefelter's syndrome (47XXY) or mosaicism (47XXY; 46XY) were the predominant abnormalities in the azoospermic men (10.8%). Unlike other causes of NOA, men with Kleinfelter often have small but firm atrophic testes, with long limbs as a consequence of late epiphyseal closure, scanty body hair and IQ levels 10–15 points lower than controls,[30] secondary to deficits in verbal ability. Other sex chromosomal anomalies and autosomal anomalies were found in 1.8% and 1.1%, respectively. Increased frequencies of reciprocal autosomal translocations have been reported in azoospermic men (0.9%),[29] and XY-autosome translocations have also been associated with aberrant spermatogenesis.[31]

Y-microdeletions

The association between deletions in the long arm of the Y chromosome and azoospermia was first suggested by Tiepolo and Zuffardi in 1976, who described 6 azoospermic men with a distal deletion of Yq11, proposing the presence of spermatogenesis-controlling factors at this site.[32] There followed extensive mapping of the Y chromosome into more than 100 sequence tagged sites (STS), which have been used to screen azoospermic and oligospermic men in an effort to further identify relevant genes and characterise microdeletions within these so-called 'azoospermia factor' (AZF) regions. Further analysis led to the identification of three non-overlapping regions along Yq (AZF a, b and c) in which the microdeletions were clustered.[33] A recent review of the literature encompassing nearly 5000 subfertile men screened for Y microdeletions shows an overall prevalence of 8%,[34] with the highest prevalence found in idiopathic NOA (16%). The authors confirmed a lack of clinical or histological genotype–phenotype pattern with no obvious relationship between the size of the microdeletion and the seminal pattern or testicular histology. Only when the entire Yq is deleted (AZFa–c) is the phenotype invariably azoospermic, and a total absence of sperm at testicular biopsy is always found when deletions extend into more than one region (*i.e.* AZFb–c or AZFa–c). *De novo* deletions of AZFc have been shown to occur at a frequency of 1 in 4000 newborn males.[35] There have been no reports that men with microdeletions have any other phenotypical abnormalities.

The genetic basis of NOA in a significant number of men makes genetic testing and referral for genetic counselling where appropriate essential.

Orchitis

Of adult cases of mumps, 25% are complicated by orchitis which develops as parotitis subsides. Inflammation and oedema (usually unilateral) lead to increasing pressure in the swollen testis produces ischaemia from blood vessel compression and necrosis of the seminiferous tubules.

Crypto-orchidism

In about 5% of newborn males, one or both testes may be undescended (0.8% by 1 year of age). If this is not corrected, ideally by 1 year of age, germ cell degeneration and dysplasia begins and is irreversible.

Miscellaneous

Hypogonadotrophic hypogonadism

Although 'non-obstructive' in nature (but with low serum FSH levels), hypothalamic disorders can be seen as a separate group of disorders causing azoospermia. This is most commonly as a consequence of defective GnRH secretion (Kallman's syndrome), associated with anosmia, cleft lip and palate, crypto-orchdism and colour blindness. Only one-third of cases will have a positive family history with X-linked, autosomal recessive and dominant variants.

Ejaculatory dysfunction

This group of disorders, that includes retrograde ejaculation, erectile dysfunction and anorgasmia, are strictly causes of 'aspermia' (absent ejaculate) and need to be considered as evaluation and treatment may mirror that for the azoospermic man. Retrograde ejaculation should be suspected in azoospermic men with a low volume semen sample, especially in the presence of a history of diabetes mellitus, multiple sclerosis, prostatectomy or bladder neck injury. The diagnosis is confirmed by evaluation of a post-ejaculate urine sample after alkalisation with ingestion of sodium bicarbonate.

MANAGEMENT OF THE AZOOSPERMIC MAN

The role of medical management of azoospermia is minimal. The primary outcome measure of the success of treatment of any infertile couple is live-birth rate (LBR); in the azoospermic men, this is predominantly achieved using assisted reproductive techniques in conjunction with surgical sperm retrieval.

Medical

Hypogonadotrophic hypogonadism (HH) and retrograde ejaculation are conditions that may be treated medically. HH can be reversed using either gonadotrophin injections (human chorionic gonadotrophin, 1000–2500 IU twice a week with human menopausal gonadotrophin, 150 IU twice a week) or pulsatile gonadotrophin-releasing hormone (5–20 mg every 120 min). A recent review suggested equal efficacy between the two (80–90% spermatogenesis but at levels below normal).[36] Maximal testicular size and spermatogenesis may take months or years to achieve. Alpha-agonists (*e.g.* phenylpropanaline 25 mg) may be used in urological practice initially for retrograde ejaculation with varying success.[36]

Surgical

Soon after ICSI with surgically retrieved sperm became accepted practice, a comparison of vasoepididymostomy and microsurgical epididymal sperm aspiration (MESA)/ICSI for treatment of epididymal obstruction secondary to vasectomy was reported.[37] In this study, patency rates of 85% at 6 months and pregnancy and delivery rates of 44% and 36% respectively at 1 year were

Table 2 Methods of sperm retrieval

	MESA	PESA	TESA	TESE
First reported	Temple-Smith *et al.* (1985)	Craft *et al.* (1995)	Craft and Tsirigiotis (1995)	Devroey *et al.* (1994)
Type of patient	Obstructive only	Obstructive only	Obstructive/ non-obstructive	Obstructive/ non-obstructive
Anaesthesia	Usually GA[a]	Usually LA	Usually LA	Usually GA[a]
Allows diagnosis	Yes	No	No	Yes
Allows reconstruction	Yes	No	No	–
Retrieval rates				
OA	Approaching 100%[38]	Approaching 100%	Approaching 100%[39]	Approaching 100%
NOA	–	–	11–13%[76,77]	Up to 50%[76,77]

IMPORTANT POINTS
Invasive
Open surgical procedure allowing scrotal exploration
Appropriate equipment and training required
Operating microscope required
Enables larger number of sperm to be aspirated for cryopreservation

Non-invasive
Blind aspiration procedure
Less likely to have sufficient sperm for cryopreservation

Non-invasive
Blind aspiration procedure
↓ Retrieval rates in NOA compared to TESE

Invasive
Open surgical procedure allowing scrotal exploration
Appropriate equipment and training required
Operating microscope required
↑ Retrieval rates in NOA compared to TESA[76,77]
More likely to retrieve sufficient sperm for cryopreservation
Repeatable with 89% success if sperm previously found[78]
No change in ICSI outcome with repeat retrievals[78]
↓ Retrieval at repeat with < 6 months interval between retrievals (80% versus 25%)[49]

[a]Can be attempted with LA spermatic cord block.

reported in their surgical cohort of patients, compared to a figure of 29% for delivery rate calculated by pooling data from previous reports for MESA/ICSI. In addition to the complications associated with assisted reproduction, the study showed that the cost per newborn was significantly higher for ICSI (US$51,024) as compared to that for vasectomy reversal (US$31,099). On this basis the authors concluded that MESA/ICSI should be reserved for cases not amenable to surgical reconstruction. This finding, although confirmed by others,[38] is now somewhat academic as current practice suggests the choice is not between surgical reversal or MESA/ICSI, but one is an adjunct to the other, with sperm retrieval vital at the time of attempted reversal in case of failure.

Sperm retrieval techniques

Obstructive azoospermia

In this group of patients, sperm retrieval is successful in almost 100% of cases.[39] Table 2 shows the types of retrieval available and their relative merits. If a simple sperm aspiration procedure (testicular [TESA] or percutaneous epididymal [PESA]) is as effective in terms of retrieval rates,[40] patient satisfaction,[41,42] and ICSI outcome[40] as an open MESA, and does not necessarily require the expertise of a urological surgeon, why can they not be performed routinely within an IVF unit by suitably trained gynaecologists or perhaps nursing staff? Although this is beginning to happen in some centres, we recommend the use of MESA (Fig. 2A) as the first-line method of retrieval in men with obstructive azoospermia in view of the opportunity it gives for diagnosis, reconstruction where appropriate, and retrieval of greater numbers of sperm for cryopreservation. Furthermore, the use of blind procedures such as PESA may result in more diffuse injury to epididymal tubules with subsequent scarring. This has been suggested to impair the efficacy of repeat procedures often required in view of the lower numbers of sperm retrieved.[43]

In men where MESA fails or where only immotile sperm are found, testicular sperm extraction (TESE), the method of choice in men with non-obstructive azoospermia, should be attempted.

Non-obstructive azoospermia

The focal 'patchy' nature of spermatogenesis in this group of patients makes an open TESE procedure the preferred method for retrieving sperm suitable for an ICSI procedure (Fig. 2B). As with MESA, TESE requires open surgery, with extraction of sperm by excisional biopsy followed by mincing of the testicular tissue and either milking the tubules microscopically with needles or digesting the tissue with enzymes. It also allows histopathological diagnosis and maximises the chances of sperm being available for cryopreservation.

The need to select the correct method of retrieval is highlighted by the lack of strong predictors for successful sperm recovery, apart from testicular histopathology.[40,44,45] An increase in the number of multiple and bilateral biopsies is needed, according to the severity of the diagnosis. One study demonstrated that in germ cell hypoplasia, maturation arrest and Sertoli-cell only syndrome, 97%, 83% and 50% of patients, respectively, had unilateral surgery and 72%, 60% and 40% had enough sperm for storage and treatment with one to three fragments of tissue.[45] Although FSH over 3 times the upper

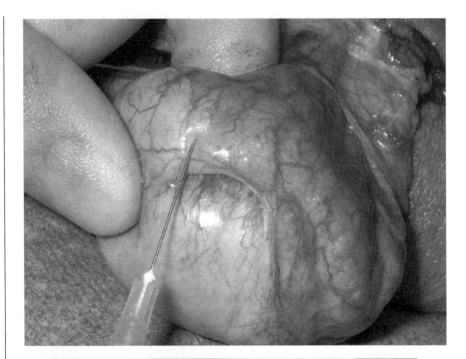

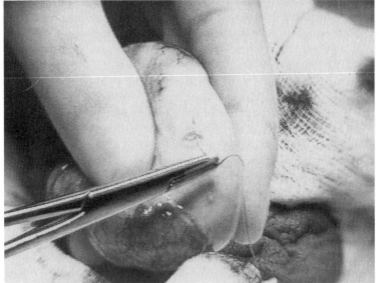

Fig. 2 (A) Microsurgical epidydmal sperm aspiration (MESA). (B) Testicular biopsy (testicular sperm extraction; TESE).

the limit of normal was classically used as an upper limit above which retrieval was not recommended, inhibin B is increasingly used as a better predictor of retrieval success.[46] As well as a marker of spermatogenesis (see Fig. 1), concentrations of inhibin B are significantly higher among successful TESE men with non-obstructive azoospermia as compared with those having failed TESE. One group has reported a value of > 40 pg/ml to be the best discriminator with a sensitivity of 90% and specificity of 100%.[46] Although inhibin B should be a part of the routine investigation of the azoospermic man, clinical decisions based on this assay alone should be avoided as successful retrieval with undetectable levels of inhibin B has been reported, and levels do not appear to significantly alter ICSI outcome should retrieval be successful.[47]

More recently, TESE procedures have been refined by the use of multiple testicular sampling[48] and microsurgical techniques[49] to maximise the chance of successful sperm recovery. It had been demonstrated that in almost half of the testes from which sperm cells were retrieved, spermatozoa were found in only some of the biopsies, and that performing only one biopsy would have missed 32% of the testes with sperm proven to be present.[48] Although multiple sampling has become common practice, consideration must be given to the physiological consequences of testicular sperm extraction, i.e. ultrasonographic abnormalities suggestive of resolving inflammation or haematoma in 82% of patients at 3 months, linear scars or calcification on scan at 6 months and evidence of devascularisation in two patients in one study[50] and a decrease in serum testosterone as long as 6 months after TESE in another.[51] This is partly compensated for by the use of microsurgical techniques where the ability to find sperm has been shown to increase from 45% to 63% with the use of an operating microscope, despite a 70-fold decrease in the volume of testicular tissue removed.[49] A prospective study comparing conventional TESE on one testis to microsurgical techniques on the contralateral testis found a significantly higher retrieval rate was (47% versus 30%) and both acute (15% versus 3%) and chronic complications (58% versus 30%) were significantly lower with microdissection TESE.[52]

ASSISTED REPRODUCTION

If we apply our current knowledge on ICSI outcome to clinical practice, we can formulate suitable management algorithms for the azoospermic man (Figs 3 and 4). It has consistently been shown that aetiology of azoospermia affects outcome with significantly impaired FR,[53–59] IR[58,59] and pregnancy outcome[53–57,59,60] using sperm from men with NOA compared to OA. This was confirmed by a meta-analysis that demonstrated an 18% decrease in fertilisation rate and 36% decrease in clinical pregnancy rate using sperm from men with NOA.[58] Furthermore, reports have compared ICSI outcome using ejaculated and surgically retrieved sperm, with significantly impaired pregnancy outcome using sperm from men with a non-obstructive but not an obstructive aetiology.[41,61,62] It is, therefore, sensible to discuss the two separately.

Obstructive azoospermia (Fig. 3)

Even when an obstructive diagnosis is strongly suspected, we always advise a definitive diagnostic scrotal exploration which: (i) confirms the classification of azoospermia; (ii) allows us to counsel patients correctly; and (iii) provides the opportunity for possible reconstruction. If live-birth rates are used to judge the outcome of assisted reproduction, meta-analysis of seven reports (as well as all of the individual papers) indicate that in OA a careful epididymal aspirate is

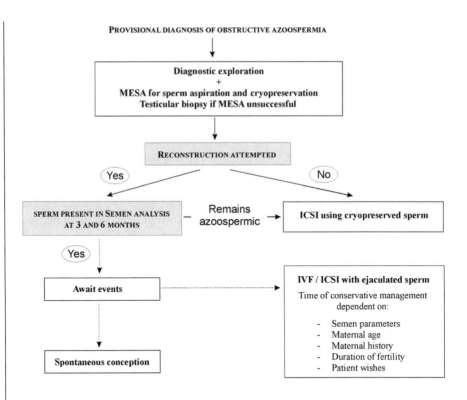

PROVISIONAL DIAGNOSIS OF OBSTRUCTIVE AZOOSPERMIA

Diagnostic exploration
+
MESA for sperm aspiration and cryopreservation
Testicular biopsy if MESA unsuccessful

RECONSTRUCTION ATTEMPTED

Yes   No

SPERM PRESENT IN SEMEN ANALYSIS AT 3 AND 6 MONTHS   — Remains azoospermic →   ICSI using cryopreserved sperm

Yes

Await events

IVF / ICSI with ejaculated sperm

Time of conservative management dependent on:

- Semen parameters
- Maternal age
- Maternal history
- Duration of fertility
- Patient wishes

Spontaneous conception

Fig. 3 Algorithm of the management of obstructive azoospermia.

as effective fresh as frozen-thawed.[63] It is thus sensible to plan epididymal aspiration (MESA) and storage from all patients who undergo scrotal exploration for use at a subsequent ICSI cycle. We have neither statistical nor scientific evidence to recommend the synchronous retrieval (SSR) of fresh epididymal gametes (*i.e.* sperm retrieval timed to coincide with oocyte retrieval of an ICSI cycle), except under specific circumstances where delay is inadvisable (*e.g.* advancing maternal age). Limiting the use of SSR in this way would minimise the risk of a cancelled cycle due to failed retrieval and eliminate the logistic difficulties we face when performing synchronous cycles. These logistic difficulties may be somewhat alleviated, however, by a recent report demonstrating that overnight incubation of both epididymal and testicular sperm following retrieval and ICSI at 24 h did not impair outcome.[64]

Where testicular aspiration is first-line management or if motile sperm is not retrieved at MESA necessitating testicular biopsy, how does this effect ICSI outcome in an obstructive azoospermic man? No differences in IR, clinical pregnancy rate (CPR) or live-birth rates (LBR) have been reported in any papers, and this is confirmed by a recent meta-analysis. We can, therefore, conclude that when a diagnosis of OA is made, epididymal aspiration remains the retrieval method of choice. However, when motile sperm are not found at epididymal aspiration in an obstructive azoospermic, the use of sperm retrieved from testicular tissue is an effective alternative.

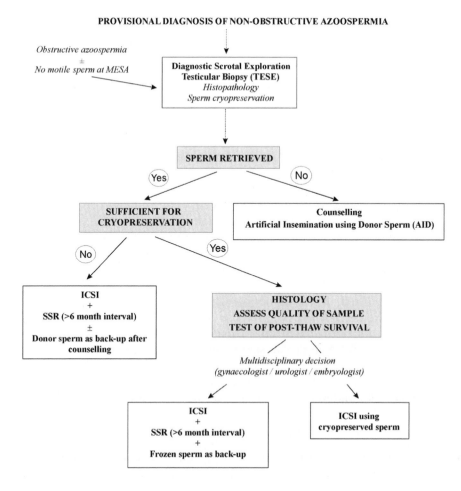

Fig. 4 Algorithm of assisted reproduction in the azoospermic man using testicular sperm.

Non-obstructive azoospermia (Fig. 4)

The situation with surgically retrieved testicular sperm in these cases is less clear. The lower retrieval rates when there is a non-obstructive cause of azoospermia always make a diagnostic testicular exploration and biopsy the correct option (TESE). The majority of reports have suggested no impairment in any outcome (FR, IR, CPR, LBR) between the use of fresh and frozen-thawed testicular sperm,[44,56,65–68] although the small numbers in some may have precluded them from achieving statistical significance. However, others have reported impaired FR,[63,69,70] IR,[69] and CPR[71] using frozen-thawed testicular sperm. To draw some conclusions from these reports, a meta-analysis (1476 cycles and 1377 transfers) comparing cycles using fresh or frozen-thawed sperm surgically retrieved from azoospermic men was carried out.[64] No difference in FR, CPR or OPR was noted when the testicular cycles were analysed separately, but implantation was significantly impaired using frozen-thawed sperm (RR, 1.75; 95% CI, 1.10–2.80; $P = 0.02$).

Therefore, if sufficient good-quality sperm are retrieved for cryopreservation at TESE, an ICSI cycle using the frozen-thawed sperm can be planned without statistically altering outcome. If sperm is retrieved, but is insufficient or inadequate for cryopreservation, SSR can be performed after discussing the use of donor-sperm as back-up should retrieval be unsuccessful. However, when looking at these testicular cycles our conclusions cannot unfortunately be this simple. We also need to take into account aetiology of azoospermia. The majority of studies reporting ICSI outcome use testicular sperm from a combination of men with obstructive and non-obstructive aetiologies without comparing the effect of cryopreservation by aetiology of infertility. The two papers that compared outcome with fresh and frozen-thawed testicular sperm from men with NOA only[45,66] showed no significant differences in either fertilisation or pregnancy outcome.

Despite this, it is difficult to conclude, as we have with epididymal sperm in men with OA, that the role of SSR is minimal. This is due to testicular retrieval in men with a non-obstructive aetiology commonly yielding few spermatozoa, often of poor motility and morphology, and the technical difficulty involved in the cryopreservation and thawing of such sperm. Therefore, the decision between the use of SSR (using donor or previously cryopreserved sperm as back up) or retrieval, followed by a planned cycle using frozen-thawed testicular sperm, should be made on an individual patient basis jointly by the clinical staff (urologist and gynaecologist) and embryologists. The option of a repeat retrieval (synchronous) is further validated by the findings of equal ICSI outcome using sperm from repeat TESE procedures.[50]

In view of the significantly impaired implantation rate using frozen-thawed testicular sperm found at meta-analysis,[63] there may also be a place for elective transfer of a higher number of embryos to achieve comparable pregnancy outcome in this situation. However, in our current drive to minimise high order multiple pregnancy, this would not be a recommendation we would support.

Assisted reproduction outcome

Although this review has given an overview of the management of the azoospermic couple, there still remains the question of ICSI outcome and what the patient should be told. The most recent UK data report live-birth rates of 25.7% per embryo transfer for ICSI (28.7% with maternal age under 38 years),[72] but pregnancy rates continue to vary considerably between units in the UK and outcome in an azoospermic man need to be considered accordingly. Therefore, couples with an obstructive aetiology should be counselled that the chances of successful ICSI outcome is likely to be similar to that achieved in their unit using ejaculated sperm. Couples with a non-obstructive aetiology should first be given a realistic estimate of their chances of successful retrieval, and then informed that even if sperm is found, ICSI outcome is likely to be significantly impaired. This is due to a reduction in sperm motility and morphology, as well as possible effects on the developmental competence of embryos derived from sperm retrieved in these cases. Higher sperm aneuploidy rates have been reported in these men[73] as well as a high incidence of mosaicism in embryos derived from TESE.[73] Although we have focused on the azoospermic man, we must not overlook the effect that maternal factors have on the outcome of assisted reproduction in such couples, with maternal age and ovarian reserve remaining significant determinants of success.[75,76]

CONCLUSIONS

The diagnosis, investigation, treatment and on-going research of azoospermia male factor infertility needs to remain an integrated multispecialty undertaking, ideally within an assisted reproductive setting, with dedicated gynaecological, urological and embryological staff supported by suitable counselling (both fertility and genetic) where needed. In our role as either gynaecologists or infertility specialists, it is vital that we ensure that this occurs and do not submit to the temptation of only focusing on the female partner.

References

1 The Royal College of Obstetricians and Gynaecologists. The Initial Investigation and Management of the Infertile Couple. Evidence-Based Clinical Guidelines No. 2. London: RCOG Press, 1998

2 Irvine DS. Epidemiology and aetiology of male infertility. Hum Reprod 1998: 13 (Suppl. 1): 33–44

3 Templeton A, Ashok P, Bhattacharya S et al. Male-factor infertility. In: Management of Infertility for the MRCOG and Beyond. London: RCOG Press, 2000; 23–46

4 Willott GM. Frequency of azoospermia. Forensic Sci Int 1982; 20: 9–10

5 Jarrow JP, Espeland MA, Lipschultz LI. Evaluation of the azoospermic patient. J Urol 1989; 142: 62–65

6 Temple-Smith PD, Southwick GJ, Yates CA, Trounson AO, de Kretzer DM. Human pregnancy by *in vitro* fertilisation using sperm aspirated from the epididymis. JIVFET 1985; 2: 119–122

7 Yovich JL, Stranger JD. The limitations of *in vitro* fertilisation from males with severe oligospermia and abnormal sperm morphology. JIVFET 1984; 1: 172–179

8 Gordon JW, Grunfield L, Garrisi GJ, Talansky BE, Richards C, Laufer N. Fertilisation of human oocytes by sperm from infertile males after zona pellucida drilling. Fertil Steril 1988; 50: 68

9 Cohen J, Malter H, Fehilly C et al. Implantation of embryos after partial opening of oocyte zona pellucida to facilitate sperm penetration. Lancet 1988; 2: 162

10 Ng SC, Bongso TA, Ratnam SS et al. Pregnancy after transfer of multiple sperm under the zona. Lancet 1988; 2: 290

11 Van Steirteghem AC, Nagy Z, Joris H et al. High fertilisation rates and implantation rates after intracytoplasmic sperm injection. Hum Reprod 1993; 8: 1061–1066

12 Silber SJ, Nagy ZP, Liu J, Godoy H, Devroey P, Van Steirteghem AC. Conventional *in-vitro* fertilisation versus intracytoplasmic sperm injection for patients requiring microsurgical sperm aspiration. Hum Reprod 1994; 9: 1705–1709

13 Nagy Z, Silber S, Liu J, Devroey P, Cecile J, Van Steirteghem A. The result of intracytoplasmic sperm injection is not related to any of the three basic sperm parameters. Hum Reprod 1995; 10: 1123–1129

14 Goldstein M. Vasectomy reversal. Comp Ther 1993: 19: 37

15 Belker AM, Thomas AJ, Fuchs EF, Konnak JW, Sharlip ID. Results of 1469 microsurgical vasectomy reversals by the Vasovasostomy Study Group. J Urol 1991; 145: 505–511

16 Li TS. Sperm immunology, infertility, and fertility control. Obstet Gynecol 1974; 44: 607–623

17 Linnet L. Clinical immunology of vasectomy and vasovasostomy. Urology 1983; 22: 101–114

18 Urry RL, Bennion Heaton J, Moore M, Muddleton RG. A fifteen year study of alterations in semen quality occurring after vasectomy reversal. Fertil Steril 1990; 53: 341–345

19 Donat R, McNeill AS, Fitzpatrick DR *et al*. The incidence of cystic fibrosis gene mutation in patients with congenital bilateral absence of the vas deferens in Scotland. Br J Urol 1997; 79: 74–77

20 Chillon M, Casals T, Mercier B. Mutation in the cystic fibrosis gene in patients with congenital absence of vas deferens. N Engl J Med 1995; 32: 1475–1480

21 Phillipson GTM, Petrucco OM, Matthews CD. Congenital bilateral absence of the vas deferens, cystic fibrosis mutation analysis and intracytoplasmic sperm mutation. Hum Reprod 2000; 15: 431–435

22 Welsh MJ, Tsui LC, Boat TF, Beaudet AL. Cystic fibrosis. In: Scriver CR, Beaudet AL, Sly WS, Valle D. (eds) The Metabolic and Molecular Basis of Inherited Disease, 7th edn. New York: McGraw-Hill, 1995; 3943–3954

23 Van der Veen K, Messer L, van der Veen H *et al*. Cystic fibrosis mutation screening in healthy men with reduced sperm quality. Hum Reprod 1996; 11: 513–517

24 Hendry WF, Ahern RP, Cole PJ. Was Young's syndrome caused by exposure to mercury in childhood. BMJ 1993; 307: 18–25

25 Afzelius BA. A human syndrome caused by immobile cilia. Science 1976; 193: 317–319

26 Jequier AM, Holmes SC. Primary testicular disease presenting as azoospermia or oligospermia and factors influencing disease. Br J Urol 1993; 71: 731–735

27 Chandley AC. The chromosomal basis of human infertility. Br Med Bull 1979; 35: 181–186

28 De Breekeleer M, Dao TN. Cytogenetic studies in male infertility: a review. Hum Reprod 1992; 6: 245–250

29 Van Assche E, Bonduelle M, Tournaye H *et al*. Cytogenetics of infertile men. Hum Reprod 1996; 11 (Suppl 4): 1–24

30 Rovet J, Netley C, Bailey J *et al*. Intelligence and achievement in children with extra X aneuploidy: a longitudinal perspective. Am J Med Genet 1995; 60: 356–363

31 Johnson MD. Genetic risks of intracytoplasmic sperm injection in the treatment of male infertility: recommendations for genetic counselling and screening. Fertil Steril 1998; 70: 397–411

32 Tiepolo L, Zuffardi O. Localisation of factors controlling human spermatogenesis in the non-fluorescent portion of the Y chromosome long arm. Hum Genet 1976; 38: 119–124

33 Vogt PH, Edelmann A, Kirsch S *et al*. Human Y chromosome azoospermia factors (AZF) mapped to different subregions in Yq11. Hum Mol Genet 1996; 5: 933–943

34 Forresta C, Moro E, Ferlin A. Y chromosome microdeletions and alterations in spermatogenesis. Endocrine Rev 2001; 22: 226–239

35 Reijo R, Alagappan RK, Patrizio P, Page DC. Severe oligospermia resulting from deletions of azoospermia factor gene on Y chromosome. Lancet 1996; 347: 1290–1293

36 Kamischke A, Nieschlag E. Analysis of medical treatment of male infertility. Hum Reprod 1999; 14 (Suppl 1): 1–23

37 Kolettis PN, Thomas AJ. Vasoepididymostomy for vasectomy reversal: a critical assessment in the era of intracytoplasmic sperm retrieval. J Urol 1997; 158: 467–470

38 Fuchs EF, Burt RA. Vasectomy reversal performed 15 years or more after vasectomy: correlation of pregnancy outcome with partner age and with pregnancy results of in vitro fertilisation with intracytoplasmic sperm injection. Fertil Steril 2000; 77: 519

39 Tounaye H, Verhayen G, Nagy P *et al*. Are there any predictive factors for successful testicular sperm recovery in azoospermic patients. Hum Reprod 1997; 12: 80–86

40 Tournaye H, Clasen K, Aytoz A, Nagy Z, Van Steirteghem A, Devroey P. Fine needle aspiration versus open biopsy for testicular sperm recovery: a controlled study in azoospermic patients with normal spermatogenesis. Hum Reprod 1998; 13: 901–904

41 Wood S, Thomas K, Sephton V, Cowan C, Lewis-Jones DI, Kingsland CR. Patient satisfaction with surgical sperm retrieval. Hum Fertil 2000; 3: Abstract 146

42 Gorgy A, Meniru GI, Bates S, Craft IL Percutaneous epididymal sperm aspiration and testicular sperm aspiration for intracytoplasmic sperm injection under local anaesthesia. Assist Reprod Rev 1998; 8: 79–93

43 Pasqualotto FF, Rossi-Ferragut LM, Rocha CC, Iconelli A, Ortiz V, Borges E. The efficacy of repeat percutaneous epididymal sperm aspiration procedures. J Urol 2003; 169:

1779–1781

44 Amer M, El Haggar S, Moustafa T, El-Naser T, Zohdy W. Testicular sperm extraction: impact of testicular histology on outcome, number of biopsies to be performed and optimal time for repetition. Hum Reprod 1999; 14: 3030–3034

45 Sousa M, Cremades N, Silva J et al. Predictive value of testicular histology in secretory azoospermic subgroups and clinical outcome after microinjection of fresh and frozen-thawed sperm and spermatids. Hum Reprod 2002; 17: 1800–1810

46 Ballesca JL, Balasch B, Calafell JM et al. Serum inhibin B determination is predictive of successful testicular sperm extraction in men with non-obstructive azoospermia. Hum Reprod 2000; 15: 1734–1738

47 Bailly M, Guthauser B, Bergere M et al. Effects of low concentrations of inhibin B on the outcomes of testicular sperm extraction and intracytoplasmic sperm injection. Fertil Steril 2003; 79: 905–908

48 Hauser R, Botchan A, Amit A et al. Multiple testicular sampling in non-obstructive azoospermia – is it necessary? Hum Reprod 1998; 13: 3181–3085

49 Schlegel PS. Testicular sperm extraction: microdissection improves sperm yield with minimal tissue excision. Hum Reprod 1999; 14: 131–135

50 Schlegel PN, Su L. Physiological consequences of testicular sperm extraction. Hum Reprod 1997; 12: 1688–1692

51 Manning M, Junemann K, Alken P. Decrease in testosterone blood concentrations after testicular sperm extraction for intracytoplasmic sperm injection in azoospermic men. Lancet 1998; 352: 37

52 Amer M, Ateyah A, Hany R, Zohdy W. Prospective comparative study between microsurgical and conventional testicular sperm extraction in non-obstructive azoospermia: follow-up by serial ultrasound examinations. Hum Reprod 2000; 15: 653–656

53 Kahraman S, Ozgur S, Alatas C et al. High implantation rates with testicular sperm extraction and intracytoplasmic sperm injection in obstructive and non-obstructive azoospermia. Hum Reprod 1996; 11: 673–676

54 Mansour RT, Kamal A, Fahmy I, Tawab N, Serour GI, Aboulghar MA. Intracytoplasmic sperm injection in obstructive and non-obstructive azoospermia. Hum Reprod 1997; 12: 1974–1979

55 Fahmy I, ,Mansour R, Aboulghar M et al. Intracytoplasmic sperm injection using surgically retrieved epididymal and testicular spermatozoa in cases of obstructive and non-obstructive azoospermia. Int J Androl 1997; 20: 37–44

56 Palermo GD, Sclegel PN, Hariprashad JJ et al. Fertilisation and pregnancy outcome with intracytoplasmic sperm injection for azoospermic men. Hum Reprod 1999; 14: 741–748

57 De Croo I, Van der Elst J, Everaert K, De Sutter P, Dhont M. Fertilisation, pregnancy, and embryo implantation rates after ICSI in cases of obstructive and non-obstructive azoospermia. Hum Reprod 2000; 15: 1381–1388

58 Nicopoullos JDM, Gilling-Smith C, Almeida PA, Ramsay JWA. Does the aetiology of azoospermia affect the outcome of intracytoplasmic sperm injection? Reproduction 2003; Abstract Series 30 P82: 86

59 Vernaeve V, Tournaye H, Osmanagaoglu K et al. Intracytoplasmic sperm injection with testicular spermatozoa is less successful in men with non-obstructive azoospermia than in men with obstructive azoospermia. Fertil Steril 2003; 79: 529–533

60 Pasqualotto FF, Rossi-Ferragut LM, Rocha CC, Iconelli A, Borges E. Outcome of in vitro fertilisation and intracytoplasmic injection of epididymal and testicular sperm obtained from patients with obstructive and non-obstructive azoospermia. J Urol 2002; 67: 1753–1756

61 Ghazzawi IM, Sarraf MG, Taher MR, Khalifa FA. Comparison of the fertilising ability of spermatozoa from ejaculates, epididymal aspirates and testicular biopsies using intracytoplasmic sperm injection. Hum Reprod 1998; 13: 348–352

62 Ubaldi F, Nagy ZP, Rienzi L et al. Reproductive capacity of spermatozoa from men with testicular failure. Hum Reprod 1999; 14: 2796–2800

63 Nicopoullos JDM, Gilling-Smith C, Almeida PA, Ramsay JWA. Fresh or frozen sperm in azoospermic men, a meta-analysis? Hum Reprod 2003; 18 (Suppl 1): o-064 18

64 Wood S, Sephton V, Searle T et al. Effect on clinical outcome of the interval between collection of epididymal and testicular spermatozoa and intracytoplasmic sperm

injection in obstructive azoospermia. J Androl 2003; 24: 67–72

65 Gil-Salom M, Romero J, Minguez Y et al. Pregnancies after intracytoplasmic sperm injection with cryopreserved testicular spermatozoa. Hum Reprod 1996; 11: 1309–1313

66 Friedler S, Raziel A, Soffer Y, Strassburger D, Komarovsky D, Ron-El R. Testicular sperm retrieval by percutaneous fine needle sperm aspiration compared with testicular sperm extraction by open biopsy in men with non-obstructive azoospermia. Hum Reprod 1997; 12: 1488–1493

67 Habermann H, Seo R, Cielsak J, Niederberger N, Prins GS, Ross R. In vitro fertilisation outcomes after intracytoplasmic sperm injection with fresh or frozen-thawed testicular spermatozoa. Fertil Steril 2002; 73: 955–960

68 Windt ML, Coetzee K, Kruger TF, Menkweld R, Van der Merwe JP. Intracytoplasmic sperm injection with testicular spermatozoa in men with azoospermia. J Assist Reprod Genet 2002; 19: 53–59

69 De Croo I, Van der Elst J, Everaert K, De Sutter P, Dhont M. Fertilisation, pregnancy, and embryo implantation rates after ICSI with fresh or frozen-thawed testicular sperm. Hum Reprod 1998; 13: 1893–1897

70 Wood S, Thomas K, Schnauffer K, Troup S, Kingsland C, Lewis-Jones I. Reproductive potential of fresh and cryopreserved epididymal and testicular spermatozoa in consecutive intracytoplasmic sperm injection cycles in the same patients. Fertil Steril 2002; 77: 1162–1166

71 Christodoulou K, Jerkovic S, Geyer J et al. The effect of TESA cryopreservation on the outcome of ICSI cycles. BFS/ACE abstracts, 2002

72 Human Fertilisation and Embryology Authority. The Patients' Guide to IVF Clinics. London: HFEA, 2002

73 Palermo GD, Colombero LT, Hariprashad JJ, Sclegel P, Rosenwaks Z. Chromosome analysis of epididymal and testicular sperm in azoospermic patients undergoing ICSI. Hum Reprod 2002; 17: 570–575

74 Silber S, Escudero T, Lenahan K, Abdelhadi I, Kilani Z, Munne S. Chromosomal abnormalities in embryos derived from testicular sperm extraction. Fertil Steril 2003; 79: 30–38.

75 Silber S, Nagy Z, Devroey P, Camus M, Van Steirteghem AC. The effect of female age and ovarian reserve on pregnancy rate in male infertility: treatment of azoospermia with sperm retrieval and intracytoplasmic sperm injection. Hum Reprod 1997; 12: 2693–2700

76 Nicopoullos JDM, Gilling-Smith C, Almeida PA, Ramsay JWA. Maternal age rather than time since vasectomy remains the principal determinant of ICSI success in men with azoospermia post vasectomy. Reproduction 2003, Abstract Series 30; 030: 23

77 Friedler S, Raziel A, Soffer Y, Strassburger D, Komarovsky D, Ron-El R. Testicular sperm retrieval by percutaneous fine needle sperm aspiration compared with testicular sperm extraction by open biopsy in men with non-obstructive azoospermia. Hum Reprod 1997; 12: 1488–1493

78 Rosenlund B, Kvist U, Ploen L, Rozell BL, Sjoblom P, Hillenslo T. A comparison between open and percutaneous needle biopsies in men with azoospermia. Hum Reprod 1998; 13: 1266–1271

79 Friedler S, Raziel A, Schachter M, Strassburger D, Bern O, Ron-El R. Outcome of first and repeated testicular sperm extraction and ICSI in patients with non-obstructive azoospermia. Hum Reprod 2002; 17: 2356–2361

N. Hammadieh O. Olufowobi M. Afnan K. Sharif

Factors affecting the outcome of *in vitro* fertilisation treatment

Infertility (the inability to conceive after 1 year of regular unprotected intercourse) is a common problem affecting 1 in 7 couples.[1] Although the incidence of infertility has not changed over the past few decades,[2] our ability to help infertile couples achieve a pregnancy has significantly increased. This is mainly due to the introduction of assisted reproductive techniques (ART), most notably *in vitro* fertilisation treatment (IVF), and it has been estimated that about 48% of infertile couples will require ART to have a realistic chance of achieving a pregnancy.[3]

Since the birth of Louise Brown (the world's first IVF baby) in 1978,[4] numerous and significant advances have taken place in the science and practice of IVF, resulting in increased success rates. For example, in the UK, the clinical pregnancy rate and live-birth rate per cycle started have increased from 18.0% and 14.0% in 1991 to 23.4% and 19.6% in 1999, respectively.[5] However, despite the apparent uniformity of the techniques used in different IVF centres, the success rates vary widely, sometimes by up to 10-fold.[6] Understanding the factors affecting the outcome of IVF is important for many reasons. First, techniques more likely to lead to success would be used. Second, some factors

Nahed Hammadieh MD MRCOG
Subspeciality Trainee in Reproductive Medicine, Cardiff Assisted Reproduction Unit, University Hospital of Wales, Heath Park, Cardiff CF14 4XW, UK
(for correspondence, E-mail: hammadiehn@cf.ac.uk)

Olufemi Olufowobi MRCOG
Clinical Research Fellow in Reproductive Medicine, Assisted Conception Unit, Birmingham Women's Hospital, Metchley Park Road, Birmingham B15 2TG, UK

Masoud Afnan FRCOG
Consultant Obstetrician and Gynaecologist, Assisted Conception Unit, Birmingham Women's Hospital, Metchley Park Road, Birmingham B15 2TG, UK

Khaldoun Sharif FRCOG MFFP MD
Consultant Obstetrician and Gynaecologist, Assisted Conception Unit, Birmingham Women's Hospital, Metchley Park Road, Birmingham B15 2TG, UK

could be altered (surgically, medically, or by changing life-style) before the IVF treatment, thus maximising the chances of success. Other factors may not be amenable to change (*e.g.* age), but understanding them would allow for a more realistic prognosis to be given. Finally, when comparing published results from different centres, accounting for these factors would allow for a more valid comparison.[7] Understanding these factors is equally important for the reproductive medicine specialists who perform the IVF and for the generalist gynaecologists who make most of the referrals. In addition, it is important for the infertile couple, particularly in this day and age of increased patient involvement in the medical decision-making process.

For the purpose of this review, we searched the Cochrane database (CD lib 2000), Medline (1966–2002) and manually searched bibliographies of selected published articles. Search terms included IVF, age, follicle stimulating hormone (FSH), inhibins, ovarian volume, cause of infertility, duration of infertility, secondary infertility, cumulative pregnancy rate, embryo transfer (ET), pregnancy rate (PR), live-birth rate, obesity, smoking, ethnicity, ovarian stimulation, intracytoplasmic sperm injection (ICSI) and embryo cryopreservation were used as text words. [MeSH (medical subject headings), AND, OR] were used to improve the search quality. On line and manual search on related areas in infertility journals (*Human Reproduction* and *Fertility & Sterility*) were carried out. For completeness, the reference lists of all papers have been checked to widen the search.

PATIENT CHARACTERISTICS AND ITS EFFECT

Age

A woman's ability to become pregnant declines with age, both naturally and with treatment.[8,9] The Human Fertilisation and Embryology Authority (HFEA) is a regulatory body established in the UK in 1990, and keeps a formal register of all treatments involving the use of gametes outside the body or donated gametes. The HFEA database has been used by Templeton *et al.*[9] to examine the relationship between age and IVF outcome. The analysis was based on 36,961 fresh IVF cycles. The statistical analysis took into consideration confounding factors such as number of embryos transferred, embryo quality, cause of infertility and duration of infertility. The authors showed that the live-birth rates per cycle started declined from 16.1% for a woman aged 30 years to 1.9% for a woman aged 45 years (Fig. 1).

In a similar study, Kooij *et al.*[10] found that a woman's age was strongly related to the implantation rate (number of gestational sacs with fetal heart seen on ultrasound at 6 weeks' gestation, divided by number of embryos replaced). They reported a reduction in implantation of approximately 7% per year in the older (> 37 years) age groups. It was suggested that the age-related decrease in the implantation rate was most likely caused by a decrease in embryo viability (capacity of the embryo to implant and develop). In addition, IVF cycle cancellation was higher in the older women due to poor ovarian response. Mardesic *et al.*[11] found in their study a 3-fold increase in cancellation rates in older women compared to younger ones (50% in women 38–40 years old versus 17.7% in women less than 30 years).

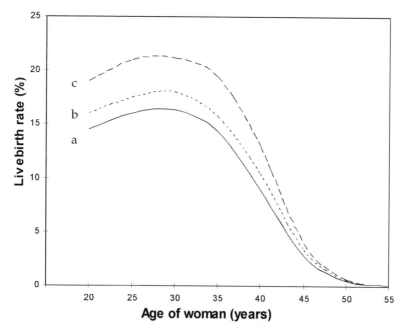

Fig. 1 Effect of age of woman on live-birth rate (a) per treatment cycle started, (b) per egg collection and (c) per embryo transfer. (a) Reproduced with permission from Elsevier (*The Lancet* 1996; 348: 1402–1406).

This adverse effect of older age is mainly related to the age of oocyte, as it can be overcome to a large extent by the use of eggs donated from younger women.[12]

Ovarian reserve

It is well known that women of similar age can respond differently to IVF. This has given rise to the concept of chronological age versus ovarian age. The ovarian age reflects the ability of the ovary to release oocytes with good potential for pregnancy, which is termed ovarian reserve. Its assessment is useful in predicting response and success in IVF cycles.[13–15] Women with decreased ovarian reserve respond poorly to controlled ovarian hyperstimulation and have poor clinical outcome in IVF treatment cycles.[13–15] Ovarian reserve can be tested for in different ways – basal FSH concentration, inhibin level, ovarian volume and morphology, and anti-mullerian hormone.

High basal FSH level
Basal (b) FSH is the concentration of FSH in the early follicular phase (menstrual days 2–5). With increasing age, elevated bFSH reflects the pituitary response to diminishing ovarian reserve. Women with raised bFSH levels have a high cancellation rate, fewer numbers of oocytes collected together with an impaired implantation rate as well as poorer IVF success rates. Sharif *et al.*[13] measured bFSH in 344 women before undergoing their first IVF cycles and found it better than age in predicting cancellation rate and number of oocytes collected.

Serum inhibin levels

Inhibins (A and B) are heterodimeric molecules and members of the transforming growth factor family of peptides. Inhibin A is produced primarily during the late follicular phase by the corpus luteum, and inhibin B is produced by granulosa cells. Inhibins predict the sensitivity to ovarian stimulation, the number of eggs harvested and the IVF outcome.[14] Seifer et al.[14] showed in a matched control study that day 3 serum inhibin-B level > 45 pg/ml is an additional prognostic factor for predicting the ovarian response and outcome after ovulation induction in IVF cycles. The cancellation and clinical pregnancy rates per cycle started in women with inhibin-B level > 45 pg/ml were 5% and 26%, respectively. For women with low inhibin-B level (level < 45 pg/ml), cancellation and clinical pregnancy rates were 19% and 7%. The differences between the two groups were statistically significant.

Ovarian volume

Ovarian volume or size decreases with increasing age. Women with small ovaries (ovarian volume > 1 SD below the mean) have a poor response to ovarian stimulation and a higher cancellation rate compared with women who have ovaries larger than the mean (cancellation rate 20% versus 5%).[15] Lass *et al.*[15] suggested that assessment of ovarian volume should form an integral part of infertility evaluation.

Anti-mullerian hormone

Anti-mullerian hormone (AMH) is a glycoprotein hormone that belongs to the transforming growth factor-β superfamily. It is mainly expressed in pre-antral and early follicles and thus its secretion might reflect the activity of pre-antral and early follicles. This makes it a promising parameter in the evaluation of ovarian follicle reserve. AMH level on menstrual cycle day 3 decreases progressively with age. Von Rooij *et al.*[16] recently analysed serum AMH of 119 patients who underwent IVF treatment for the first time. The authors found that the serum AMH levels correlated with the number of antral follicles assessed by ultrasound on day 3 of a spontaneous cycle and the number of oocytes retrieved. The correlation was statistically significant. Inclusion of inhibin B and bFSH concentrations to AMH in a multivariate model improved the prediction of ovarian response.

In current clinical practice, bFSH is the most widely used test for assessing ovarian reserve. As with all hormonal tests, the cut-off values depend on the specific assay used, which could be different in different laboratories.

Cause of infertility

The live-birth rates by diagnosis category following IVF vary little according to the recent American Society for Reproductive Medicine/Society for Assisted Reproductive Technology (ASRM/SART) report,[12] and the HFEA database analysis by Templeton *et al.*[9] According to the SART data, the live birth rates by diagnostic category were: male factor 27.1%, endometriosis 25.8%, ovulatory dysfunction 22.5%, tubal factors 25.3%, unexplained infertility 25.4%). Most were near the overall national success rate of 24.9%. The higher success rates in the male factor group may be explained by the increased number of intracytoplasmic sperm injection (ICSI) cycles for more severe cases of male infertility (accounting for 40% of all IVF cycles). The better success rate of ICSI may be attributed to the fact that many ICSI couples do not have additional compromising female factors such as tubal disease.

Hydrosalpinx

IVF patients with hydrosalpinges have poor prognosis. Many recent reports including a meta-analysis[18] confirmed that the presence of a hydrosalpinx during IVF-embryo transfer had negative consequences on the pregnancy rate, the implantation rate, the rate of early pregnancy loss, and the live delivery rate per embryo transfer. Strandell et al.[18] demonstrated in their randomised Scandinavian multicentre trial that there was a significant improvement in implantation and delivery rates in patients with ultrasound visible hydrosalpinges patients who had salpingectomies for the damaged tubes compared with the control group (25.6% versus 22.5% and 40.0% versus 17.5%, respectively). The differences in outcomes were statistically significant.

The fluid of hydrosalpinges may constitute a mechanical barrier to implantation by causing the embryo to float and thus making attachment to the endometrium difficult. It has also been suggested that the fluid is nutritionally deficient to support the developing embryo leading to early demise. Others have proposed that the fluid is toxic thereby compromising the developmental potential of the embryo. Thus the precise mechanism(s) by which the fluid of the hydrosalpinx inhibits implantation and predisposes to miscarriage and hence poor IVF outcomes in such women is not clear but appears to be multifactorial; nonetheless, improved outcomes have been reported following salpingectomy.[18]

Male factor

The poor success rates of couples with male factor infertility undergoing IVF treatment is well recognised and relates essentially to poor fertilisation rates. However, the use of ICSI treatment for severe male factor infertility has dramatically improved the outcome for these couples.[19] Severe male factor fertility is defined as severe abnormality of 1 or moderate abnormality of 2 or more of the 3 the main parameters of seminal fluid analysis (sperm count < 5 x 10^6/ml, sperm rapid progressive motility < 10% and morphology < 5% each constitute severely abnormal parameters).[20]

Endometriosis

The effect of endometriosis on ART results is unclear. Azim et al.[21] showed that the fertilisation rate, pregnancy rate (PR) per transfer, and birth rate were significantly lower in patients with severe endometriosis (stages III and IV) compared with tubal infertility. On the other hand, the HFEA database[5] and SART register[11] did not show lower pregnancy rate in patients with endometriosis, but it did not take into account the stage of endometriosis.

Leiomyomas (fibroids)

These are a common gynaecological problem occurring in about 30% of women over the age of 30 years. The cause/effect of fibroids and infertility remains controversial in most series. Ramzy et al.[22] reported that fibroids not causing deformity of the uterine cavity and < 7 cm in mean diameter, did not affect the implantation or miscarriage rates in ART. On the other hand, Eldar-Geva et al.[23] in their study classified fibroids according to their location. They found that fibroids had a negative impact on implantation and pregnancy rates even when there was no deformity of the uterine cavity.

It seems that patients with submucosal or large intramural leiomyoma (7 cm diameter), especially if associated with uterine cavity deformity, should be advised to have myomectomy prior to IVF treatment.

Duration of infertility

Increasing duration of infertility is associated with a decrease in the probability of spontaneous pregnancy in untreated infertile couples. Analysis of the HEFA database demonstrated the decrease in live-birth rate with increasing duration of infertility in ART despite adjustment for age.[9] After age adjustment, the data showed that there was a significant decrease in pregnancy rate with increasing duration of infertility (15.3% for 1–3 years, 14% for 4–6 years, 12.9% for 7–9 years, 12.4% for 10–12 years and 8.6% for > 12 years of infertility).

History of previous pregnancy

Secondary infertility is a good prognostic factor in untreated infertile couples especially if the pregnancy ended in a live birth. Similarly, previous pregnancy substantially increases the likelihood of success after IVF, especially when the previous pregnancy resulted from previous IVF treatment and ended in a live birth.[9]

A large study by Croucher et al.[24] demonstrated a significant increase in pregnancy rate in women experiencing a clinical or biochemical pregnancy in a first cycle compared to those whose first cycle yielded a negative result.

Table 1 Outcome of a second cycle after a pregnancy in the first IVF cycle

First cycle outcome	Delivered in first IVF	Miscarried in first IVF	Ectopic in first IVF
No. of patients having a second cycle	166	111	26[a]
No. of pregnancies (%)	56 (32.5)	35 (31.5)	6[a] (23.1)
Live births (%)[b]	42 (75)	23 (65.7)	3 (50.0)
Miscarriages (%)[b]	7 (12.5)	9 (25.7)	2 (33.3)
Ectopic pregnancies (%)[b]	2 (3.6)	1 (2.9)	1 (16.7)
Lost of follow-up (%)[b]	4 (7.1)	1 (2.9)	
Biochemical pregnancies (%)[c]	2 (1.2)	6 (5.4)	1 (3.8)
Others	1 termination	1 termination	

IVF, in vitro fertilisation.
[a]Includes pregnancies defined as on-going because a fetal heart was detected at 10, 12 or 20 weeks' gestation but whose final outcome is unknown.
[b]The percentage values are from the number of pregnancies.
[c]The percentage values are from the number of cycles.
There were no statistical differences between the groups.
Reproduced by permission of Oxford University Press/Human Reproduction.

Thus, the outcome in the next cycle in terms of biochemical pregnancy, miscarriage, ectopic pregnancy and successful live-birth rates is much dependent on the outcome of the first cycle (Table 1).

Rank of IVF attempts

Because the chance of conception with a single IVF treatment is still low, couples are often interested in understanding not only their chances of getting pregnant per cycle, but also their expected chances of getting pregnant after a specified number of IVF cycles. Meldrum et al.[25] in a multicentre trial assessed pregnancy and delivery rates following repeated IVF treatment. The delivery rate for cycles 1, 2, 3, 4 and > 4 were 27%, 27.4%, 23.4%, 16.1% and 15.4%, respectively. In this study, previous cycles were included from other centres. There was significant decrease in delivery rate at cycle rank four or more. A similar pattern was also found in an analysis of the HFEA database.[9] The live-birth rates were 14%, 11.4% and 8.9% after the first, third and fifth attempts of IVF cycle, respectively.

Obesity

The evidence for the impact of obesity on pregnancy rates after IVF is conflicting. Clark et al.[26] suggested fecundity in obese women is reduced compared to normal weight women in both spontaneous and assisted conceptions. These authors employed a weight-loss programme in a prospective study to evaluate the effect of weight loss on the reproductive outcome for all forms of fertility treatment in infertile obese, body mass index (BMI) 30 kg/m². The authors observed that weight loss resulted in significant improvement in reproductive outcome for all fertility treatments. On the other hand, Lashen et al.[27] reported no significant difference on IVF embryo transfer outcome between obese patients whose BMI was > 27.9 kg/m² and a control group with BMI of 20–24 kg/m². All potentially confounding factors were corrected for in both groups. Furthermore, the findings by Wass et al.[28] revealed that BMI appeared not to have an affect on the pregnancy rate (PR), but that an android body fat distribution in females impaired the pregnancy rate in IVF patients. The authors defined upper-body fatness as a waist:hip ratio (WHR) > 0.80. Women with WHR > 0.80 had a PR of 15.9% when compared with 29.9% in women with WHR between 0.70–0.79 (OR, 0.42; 95% CI, 0.2–0.9; P = 0.03]. The underlying mechanism is still not clear but this might relate to the androgen levels. The excessive androgen levels in women with high WHR could have a negative effect on oocyte development resulting in poor quality embryos.

Smoking

The negative effects of cigarette smoking on general health are well known, but smoking may also affect fertility. The biological plausibility of the effect of smoking on ovarian function has been noted in observational studies where smokers were shown to have an earlier menopause by 1–1.5 years. Cigarette smoking is associated with a prolonged and dose-dependent adverse effect on ovarian function and oocyte quality. Furthermore, smoking could affect tubal or cervical function either directly or indirectly, and could be toxic to sperm.[29] A meta-analysis by Feichtinger et al.[29] showed that the pregnancy rate amongst women smokers were significantly lower than non-smokers after their IVF attempts (14% versus 21%, respectively). Therefore, women should be advised to quit smoking before assisted reproduction treatments.

Ethnicity

Lashen et al.[30] showed that there is no significant difference in clinical pregnancy (16% versus 17%) and implantation rate (13% versus 17%) between Asian women from the Indian sub-continent and white Caucasian women undergoing IVF treatment in a UK centre. Both groups were similar in terms of age, day 3 bFSH and indication for IVF.

CLINIC CHARACTERISTICS AND ITS EFFECT

Whilst it is hard to change the couple's characteristics, patients can choose which clinic they attend, and clinics can vary significantly in their IVF success rates. For example, in the UK the success rates for IVF and ICSI treatments vary from one centre to another, ranging from 3.8% to 36.4% per cycle started.[6] It is possible that these differences are genuine, i.e. because some clinics are better than others in their clinical and embryology practices. On the other hand, patient selection could be responsible for at least a part of such large differences.[7] Some clinics are known to decline to treat patients with poor prognostic factors such as abnormal basal FSH, older women, etc. Another explanation could be the differences in reporting cycles which do not get to egg collection (the cancelled cycles). It is well known that success rates in ART are reported differently. This may be per number of cycles started, oocyte retrievals or embryo transfers.[7]

Stimulation protocol

Although the world's first IVF baby had resulted from a natural unstimulated cycle,[4] controlled ovarian hyperstimulation is now used in most IVF centres. It leads to the creation of numerous embryos, which could be available for transfer or cryopreservation, thus increasing the chance of pregnancy.[31]

Gonadotrophin releasing hormone (GnRH) agonists

GnRH agonists are synthetic analogues of native GnRH. They exhibit higher receptor affinity and prolonged action. On initial administration, there is increased FSH and LH production for about a week, the so-called 'flare-up effect'. Their chronic administration (after 2–3 weeks) leads to receptor down-regulation and pituitary desensitisation. The resultant hypogonadotrophic state leads to ovarian quiescence, which is a reversible process.

The use of GnRH agonist in down-regulation protocols has been shown to improves the IVF outcome, by allowing as many follicles as possible to reach maturity thereby increasing the number of oocytes collected and reducing the cancellation rate. GnRH agonists are effective in preventing premature LH surge and consequently spontaneous ovulation.[31] This makes cycle monitoring much easier.

GnRH agonists protocols

GnRH agonists are used in IVF in two distinctly different ways – the long protocol, and the short or flare protocol. A major distinction between these regimens is based on the duration of use before the initiation of gonadotrophin therapy. In the long protocol, GnRH agonists are administered until the pituitary is completely desensitised, at which point ovarian stimulation is initiated with gonadotrophins while the administration of the agonist is continued. The agonist may be started in the early follicular, mid-luteal and late luteal phase.

The short, or flare, protocol consists of combined administration of agonists and gonadotrophins from the beginning of the cycle, usually day 1 or 2 of the follicular phase.

In a meta-analysis by Hughes et al.,[32] there were no significant differences between the long and short protocols in terms of clinical pregnancy and cancellation rates. However, Cramer et al.,[33] in a prospective observational study of women undergoing IVF treatment, reported that patients who received the short protocol had 11% fewer oocytes retrieved and a 35% reduction in the clinical pregnancy rate (CPR) compared with those who received a long protocol. The authors suggested that the difference in CPR could be due to the decreased number of oocytes retrieved or higher E2 or LH levels in patients who had the short protocol.

GnRH antagonists

The GnRH antagonist acts by competitively binding to gonadotrophic cells receptors. This competitive blockade leads to an immediate arrest of gonadotrophin secretion, without initial flare-up. This has the advantage of shorter duration treatment. However, a systematic review by Al-Inany and Aboulghar[34] in which five randomised control trials were analysed showed that the clinical pregnancy rate per woman randomised was significantly lower in the antagonist group. A fixed regimen of GnRH antagonists (a fixed dose and starting day) was used in these studies, and the authors suggested that future research should investigate the results of using variable regimens, individually tailored to the woman's response.

Gonadotrophin stimulation regimens

Step-up stimulation regimen – In the step-up regimen, the stimulation starts usually with a relatively small dose (75 IU FSH); thereafter, the dose is maintained or increased according to patient response which is monitored by ultrasound assessment of the growth of the follicles and, in some units, oestradiol level. Van Hooff et al.[35] reported that increasing the stimulation dose did not improve the outcome in poor responders.

Fixed stimulation regimen – Many centres use the patient's age, bFSH and previous IVF cycle outcome to determine a fixed stimulation dose. In the fixed dose or standard regimen, the same dose is used throughout the stimulation period. The fixed dose regimen varies from unit to unit. The Assisted

Conception Unit in Birmingham (UK) uses the following regimen. First, the patient has her bFSH measured, and those with abnormally high values (> 11 IU/l), indicating poor ovarian reserve, get 450 IU gonadotrophins daily for ovarian stimulation. In patients with normal bFSH (90% of patient population), the dose is determined by the age. Patients who are ≤ 30 years receive 150 IU daily, patients who are 31–35 years old receive 225 IU, patients who are 36–39 years old receive 300 IU, and those who are 40 years old or over receive 450 IU. All polycystic ovarian syndrome (PCOS) patients are given reduced dose (75 IU less daily), as they are potentially at high risk of developing ovarian hyperstimulation syndrome (OHSS).

Step-down stimulation regimen – In the step-down regimen, the starting dose is usually high and according to the patient's response the dose is reduced or maintained.[36] The objective of this protocol is to reach the threshold for maximal FSH stimulation and thereafter reduce the dose, thereby mimicking the FSH secretion pattern in natural cycle. The theoretical benefit is that the more matured follicles will continue their growth, but there will be fewer new and small follicles recruited later in the cycle, thereby reducing the risk of OHSS.

Types of gonadotrophin

The strategy of stimulating the ovaries with exogenous gonadotrophins to induce multiple follicular development in women undergoing ART is now well established. The role of FSH in this process is essential, whereas LH plays a relatively minor role. Until recently, the main source of FSH was urine of postmenopausal women. This human menopausal gonadotrophin (hMG) consists of FSH, LH and urinary proteins. Advances in purification techniques using monoclonal antibodies has enabled the extraction of FSH from urine to produce highly purified FSH free of contaminant proteins and LH. This was an attempt to improve the efficacy of FSH. The improved efficacy was demonstrated in the meta-analysis by Daya et al.,[37] who reported that in IVF cycles the use of FSH was associated with a significantly higher number of oocytes retrieved and clinical pregnancy rates compared to the hMG group.

Further advance continues to be made in this area to improve IVF outcome. Recent developments in biotechnology have led to production of recombinant gonadotrophins for ovulation induction in IVF programmes. The theoretical advantages of this product over urine derived-gonadotrophins include batch-to-batch consistency, purity of the product, which reduces the risks of side effects, and that production is independent of urine collection. There have been many studies comparing recombinant FSH (rFSH) with highly purified urinary FSH (uFSH). The evidence is conflicting. Daya and Gunby,[38] in a systematic review of all randomised trials to date comparing rFSH with uFSH for controlled ovarian hyperstimulation, found that treatment with rFSH resulted in significantly higher clinical pregnancy rates compared with uFSH. The overall common odds ratio (OR) in favour of rFSH was 1.2 (95% CI, 1.42; $P = 0.03$). Even when the cost was taken into account, using the actual market costs of the FSH preparations, the conclusion was that the cost effectiveness of rFSH is better than uFSH,[39] that is the cost per pregnancy is lower when the recombinant preparation is used.

Patient monitoring

Controlled ovarian hyperstimulation (COH) in IVF cycles involves serial transvaginal ultrasound scans (TVS) to monitor follicular development and serum hormonal assessments. The purpose is to monitor follicle development/growth, predict a premature luteinising hormone surge, the optimum time for hCG administration, early prediction for severe ovarian hyperstimulation syndrome and to improve the stimulation response in poor responders. With the use of GnRH agonists (or antagonists) during ovarian stimulation in IVF cycle, there is no longer a need for LH monitoring. Many IVF centres are still using oestradiol (E2) levels for controlled ovarian hyperstimulation monitoring, although TVS alone has shown to be adequate and is successfully used in monitoring IVF cycles without any negative effect on the outcome.[40]

The frequency of monitoring during an IVF stimulation cycle varies amongst different centres, with little evidence as to which one is best.

Number of embryos transferred

Multiple pregnancy is associated with increased pregnancy complications such as hyperemesis gravidarum, pregnancy induced hypertension, anaemia, low birth weight, premature delivery, congenital malformations and increased admission into special care baby unit with an attendant overall cost of care. Therefore, it is imperative for any assisted conception programme to aim at maximising the chance of a healthy singleton delivery at term, and minimise the risk of multiple pregnancies. The need to reduce the rates of multiple pregnancies is the motive of the HFEA recent embryo transfer policy, that is reducing the number of embryos normally transferred from three to two. The UK HFEA's recommendations for good clinical practice advised that it should be the usual practice to transfer a maximum of two embryos during IVF treatment cycle. The decision continues to generate concerns for patients who genuinely believe the policy may be associated with a reduction in the success of IVF. However, the HFEA data[5] have been very re-assuring in showing that reducing the number of embryos transferred in the majority of cases reduced the risk of multiple birth (particularly triplets) without reducing the chance of singleton births (Table 2).

A similar finding has been reported in a randomised control trial for a cohort of patients who were less than 37 years old, on their first IVF attempt, and had at least three good quality embryos. The pregnancy rates were similar when either two or three embryos were transferred as long as the embryos were of good quality (42.5% versus 48.5%).[41] The most convincing data in

Table 2 Two and three embryo transfers for fresh stimulated IVF cycles

No. of embryos transferred	No of cycles	Live birth rate per stated cycles	Multiple birth rate
2	6838	28.6%	26.4%
3	7102	25.8%	34.9%

Reproduced with permission from the Human Fertilisation and Embryology Authority.

strong support of the two embryo transfer policy as a means of reducing multiple gestation and its inherent complications are from the HEFA database in which Templeton et al.[42] demonstrated that when there are at least four embryos to select from, the woman's chance of birth is not diminished by transferring only two embryos.

Furthermore, there has been a recent call to reduce this further to one embryo of good quality, especially for selected patients who are at high risk of multiple pregnancies. This is the basis of a new strategy on trial in Scandinavian countries where they are implementing a one embryo transfer policy in selected cases.

Embryo transfer technique

Despite the huge improvements in IVF technology over the last few years, the majority of transferred embryos fail to result in pregnancy. This failure may be due to poor embryo quality, poor uterine receptivity or to embryo transfer technique.

Most embryo transfers proceed smoothly and do not require particular manipulation. Unfortunately, there are occasions when embryo transfer may be technically difficult. Often the difficulty relates to stenosed external cervical os, very narrow endocervical canal and acute anteversion or retroversion of the uterus. These may make passage of the embryo catheter into and through the endocervical canal difficult. It has been shown that difficult transfers might negatively affect the IVF success rate.[43] Unfortunately, in the absence of objective criteria for defining a difficult transfer, this parameter remains an uncertain prognostic indicator of pregnancy outcome.

Some authors have advocated the use of transabdominal ultrasound guidance to facilitate embryo transfer in IVF treatment. The rationale for using this technique is to track the catheter tip for proper placement of the embryos at the thickest part of the endometrium, avoiding contact with the fundus. Coroleu et al.[44] found in a randomised control trial that the pregnancy rate was significantly higher among the ultrasound-guided embryo transfer group (50%) compared with the 'clinical touch' (transfer without the aid of ultrasound guidance) group (33.7%). There was also a significant increase in the implantation rate (25.3% versus 18.1%). Both groups were adjusted for age, cause of infertility and characteristics of the IVF cycle.

Interestingly, outcomes can vary greatly among individual practitioners performing ET. Hearns-Stokes et al.,[45] in a retrospective analysis of 393 clinical pregnancies from 850 embryo transfers, reported significant differences in pregnancy rates after embryo transfer performed by different providers. The observed differences could not be explained by the number of high-grade embryos transferred, the number of transfers performed, or the age of the patient. Also experience alone did not fully account for the observed differences in pregnancy rates amongst providers. Other authors have failed show this difference.[46]

Other important variables which have been demonstrated to affect pregnancy rates following ET are the presence of uterine contractions during ET, usually stimulated by touching the uterine fundus, difficult transfer, transmyometrial transfer or use of a tenaculum. This stimulation of uterine contractility may lead to the relocation or the expulsion of the transferred embryos, thereby reducing the success of treatment. The type of catheter may affect the outcome, the 'soft' catheter is more favoured as this is less traumatic and less likely to induce uterine contractions.[47]

Embryo cryopreservation programmes

Cryopreservation of embryos and subsequent frozen embryo transfer is a well-established treatment in most IVF programmes, substantially contributing to cumulative pregnancy rates.[31] The main aim of embryo cryopreservation is to increase the chances of achieving a live birth from a single controlled ovarian hyperstimulation cycle. In addition, it will of course offer a chance for a sibling pregnancy if the patient has been successful from the fresh cycle. The value of embryo cryopreservation can be seen in other respects as well:

1. It may reduce the risks of multiple pregnancies by limiting the number of embryos the patients want to replace in a fresh cycle.

2. It decreases the potential risk of ovarian hyperstimulation syndrome by permitting the elective freezing of all embryos for replacement in a subsequent cycle.

3. It may also reduce the cost of further treatment to the patient as additional transfer cycles are produced without having to repeat the more expensive fresh controlled ovarian hyperstimulation cycle.

4. It reduces the risks associated with a fresh cycle, that is risks associated with ovulation induction drugs and oocyte retrieval.

The average clinical pregnancy and live-birth rates in frozen embryo replacement cycles in the UK are 15% and 12.2%, respectively.[5] Wang and colleagues[31] in a large review study (897 cycles) observed that the contribution from embryo cryopreservation programmes to IVF outcome is substantial as it increased the PR of women who had frozen-thawed embryo transfer by 11%. However, only 55% of the women had embryos good enough to freeze.

Factors known to affect the pregnancy rate in fresh IVF treatment cycles, such as age of patients and number of embryos transferred, have the same effect in frozen-thawed embryo replacement cycles. However, the major factors affecting outcome of the cryopreservation programme are the number of oocytes retrieved in the initial stimulation cycle, the number of embryos available for cryopreservation and the pregnancy outcome of the fresh cycle.[31]

It has been shown that the outcome of the previous cycle has a prognostic value on the outcome of subsequent cycles.[9] This suggestion was corroborated by Karlstrom et al.[48] who found that for women who became pregnant following fresh embryo transfer a pregnancy rate of 29% was obtained in the subsequent frozen cycle. The pregnancy rate of those who did not conceive in the fresh cycle was lower, at 21%. Furthermore, Kowalik and colleagues[49] compared the clinical outcome after cryopreservation of 690 embryos obtained from intracytoplasmic sperm injection (239 embryos) and IVF (451 embryos). The authors observed similar embryo survival rates between the two groups (73.3% and 70.5%, respectively) irrespective of the stage at cryopreservation.

Also there was no significant difference in the pregnancy rates per transfer (32.3% and 31.8%). However, there was a difference in the clinical miscarriage rates (23.8% and 16.7%) between the ICSI and IVF groups, respectively.

ICSI TREATMENT

The introduction of ICSI in 1991 by Palermo[50] has revolutionised treatment of male factor infertility, almost irrespective of the severity of the condition. The good success rates of ICSI in male factor infertility appear unaffected by the semen characteristics and sperm quality even when epididymal or testicular spermatozoa are used.[51] As the only requirement for ICSI is the presence of at least one living spermatozoa per oocyte, few spermatozoa are required for treatment. Percutaneous epididymal sperm aspiration (PESA), microsurgical epididymal sperm aspiration (MESA), testicular sperm aspiration (TESA) and testicular sperm extraction (TESE) are surgical sperm retrieval methods that are used world-wide to collect sperm from azoospermic men who would otherwise have required donor sperm treatment before the advent of ICSI. Ubaldi et al.[52] found that no differences were observed with regard to embryo quality and clinical pregnancy rates in three groups of patients when ejaculated spermatozoa, epididymal or testicular spermatozoa were used.

The high success rate of ICSI treatment has compelled many authors to advocate a wider scope for its indications, that is ICSI for treatment of non-male factor infertility. Khamsi et al.,[53] in a prospective randomised controlled study, reported that in IVF patients with non-male factor infertility, ICSI increases the fertilisation rate and formation of good quality embryos. It also avoids the problem of total fertilisation failure in almost all cases. However, a recent Cochrane Systematic Review[54] did not support this notion of improved success of ICSI in non-male factor infertility. The Cochrane Systemic Review included eight randomised control trials comparing ICSI with conventional IVF and showed that for couples with normal semen fluid analysis there was no difference in fertilisation rates or pregnancy rates for the different groups.

CONCLUSIONS

The major factors that affect pregnancy and live birth rates in IVF are: (i) the age of the woman, the rates declining after the age of 30 years; (ii) increasing duration of infertility is associated with poor outcomes; and (iii) previous pregnancy, most importantly previous live birth, is a good prognostic factor. Low basal FSH, high inhibin B level, AMH and good ovarian volume are measures of ovarian reserve and useful predictors of successful ovarian stimulation and IVF outcome. Broadly speaking, the aetiology of a woman's infertility has a minimal effect on IVF outcome. However, the presence of hydrosalpinx significantly impairs the implantation and pregnancy rates in ART. Large intramural or submucosal fibroids, especially if distorting the uterine cavity, should be removed as they are associated with decreased implantation rates, increased miscarriage rate and consequently lower live-birth rate. Weight loss and cessation of smoking appear to have a positive impact on the outcome of IVF, whilst more research is needed to evaluate the effect of race on IVF outcome.

At the beginning of treatment, couples should be informed of the chances for conceiving spontaneously as compared to chances with ART. The chances of a couple conceiving can be estimated from the prognostic factors discussed above, that is success should be individualised. This is more meaningful and useful than giving general figures for the clinic as a whole.

As well as giving the chances for an individual cycle, it is also important to give an idea of the cumulative conception rates, both with repeated cycles and with frozen embryo transfers.

A correlate of pregnancy rate is the risk of multiple pregnancy. The higher the chance of a pregnancy in ART, the higher the risk of multiple pregnancies.

KEY POINTS FOR CLINICAL PRACTICE

- IVF is an effective treatment for many causes of infertility. Couples should be counselled properly about their chances of getting pregnant before starting treatment.
- Age is the best predictor of pregnancy.
- Basal FSH levels and inhibin B are the best readily available predictors of ovarian reserve in clinical practice.
- Obesity is associated with infertility and poor reproductive outcome. Weight loss is advisable prior to any assisted reproductive programmes and may increase the chances of successful conception.
- Smoking has been implicated in women with poor oocyte quality and is associated with a reduction in success rate in women undergoing assisted reproduction cycles.
- Smoking is detrimental both to sperm quality and function.
- Factors such as leiomyomata, hydrosalpinges and endometriosis, which have been implicated in poor IVF outcome, should be appropriately managed prior to embarking on IVF treatment.
- Every attempt should be made to avoid multiple pregnancies with IVF treatment, particularly triplet pregnancies.
- ICSI is an appropriate and effective treatment for severe male factor infertility.
- Embryo cryopreservation should be discussed with and offered to all couples undergoing IVF treatment. This will provide the opportunity to cryopreserve good quality embryos that can be used for future treatment.
- All assisted conception units must have quality control procedures and regularly evaluate their results to permit the maintenance of acceptable standards and early recognition of factors that may compromise IVF outcome.

References

1 Hull MG, Glazener CM, Kelly NJ *et al.* Population study of causes, treatment, and outcome of infertility. BMJ 1985; 291: 1693–1697
2 Templeton A, Fraser G, Thompson B. Infertility, epidemiology and referral practice. Hum Reprod 1991; 6: 1391–1394
3 School of Public Health, University of Leeds. Centre for Health Economics, University of York, Research Unit, Royal College of Physicians. Effective Health Care. Bulletin 1992 (2): 11
4 Steptoe PC, Edwards RG. Birth after re-implantation of a human embryo. Lancet 1978; 2: 366
5 Human Fertilisation and Embryology Authority. Ninth Annual Report and Accounts. London: The Stationary Office, 2000; 11–19

6 Human Fertilisation and Embryology Authority. The Patients' Guide to IVF Clinics. London: HFEA, 2000

7 Sharif K, Afnan M. The IVF league tables: time for a reality check. Hum Reprod 2003; 18: 483–485

8 Menken J, Trussel J, Larsen U. Age and infertility. Science 1986; 233: 1389–1394

9 Templeton AA, Morris JK, Parslow W. Factors that effect outcome of *in vitro* fertilisation treatment. Lancet 1996; 348: 1402–1406

10 Van Kooij RJ, Looman CWN, Habbema JDF, Dorland M, Velde ER. Age-dependent decrease in embryo implantation rate after *in vitro* fertilisation. Fertil Steril 1996; 66: 769–775

11 Mardesic T, Muller P, Zetova L, Mikova M. Factors affecting the results of in vitro fertilization-I. The effect of age. Ceska Gynekol 1994; 59: 259–261

12 Society For Assisted Reproductive Technology and the American Society for Reproductive Medicine. 1998 Assisted Reproductive Technology Success Rates, Fourth annual report

13 Sharif K, Elgendy M, Lashen H, Afnan M. Age and basal follicle stimulating hormone as predictors of *in vitro* fertilisation outcome. Br J Obstet Gynaecol 1998; 105: 107–112

14 Seifer DB, Lambert-Messerlian G, Hogan WJ, Gardiner AC, Blazar AS, Berke A. Day 3 serum inhibin-B is predictive of assisted reproductive technologies outcome. Fertil Steril 1997; 67: 110–114

15 Lass A, Skull J, McVeigh E, Margara R, Winston RM. Measurement of ovarian volume by transvaginal sonography before ovulation induction with human menopausal gonadotrophin for *in vitro* fertilisation can predict poor response. Hum Reprod 1997; 12: 294–297

16 Van Rooij JA, Broekmans FJ, te Velde ER *et al*. Serum anti-mullerian hormone levels: a novel measure of ovarian reserve. Hum Reprod 2002; 17: 3065–3071

17 Camus E, Poncelet C, Goffint F *et al*. Pregnancy rates after *in vitro* fertilisation in cases of tubal infertility with and without hydrosalpinx: a meta-analysis of published comparative studies. Hum Reprod 1999; 14: 1243–1249

18 Strandell A, Lindhard A, Waldenstrom U, Thorburn J, Janson PO, Hamberger L. Hydrosalpinx and IVF outcome: a prospective, randomized multicentre trial in Scandinavia on salpingectomy prior to IVF. Hum Reprod 1999; 14: 2762–2769

19 Van Steirteghem AC, Nagy Z, Staessen C *et al*. High fertilisation and implantation rates after intracytoplasmic sperm injection. Hum Reprod 1993; 8: 1061–1066

20 World Health Organization. Laboratory Manual for the Examination of Human Semen and Sperm–Cervical Mucus Interaction, 4th edn. Cambridge: Cambridge University Press, 1999; 10, 14–17

21 Azim F, Lessing B, Geva E *et al*. Patients with stage III and VI endometriosis have a poor outcome of *in vitro* fertilisation-embryo transfer than patients with tubal infertility. Fertil Steril 1999; 72: 1107–1109

22 Ramzy AM, Sattar M, Amin Y, Mansour RT, Serour GI, Aboulghar MA. Uterine myomata and outcome of assisted reproduction. Hum Reprod 1998; 13: 198–202

23 Eldar-Geva T, Meagher S, Healy DL, Maclachlan V, Breheny S, Wood C. Effect of intramural, subserosal, and submucosal uterine fibroids on the outcome of assisted reproductive technology treatment. Fertil Steril 1998; 70: 687–691

24 Croucher CA, Lass A, Margara R, Winston RM. Predictive value of the results of a first *in vitro* fertilisation cycle on the outcome of subsequent cycles. Hum Reprod 1998; 13: 403–408

25 Meldrum DR, Silverberg KM, Bustillo M, Stokes L. Success rate with repeated cycles of *in vitro* fertilisation-embryo transfer. Fertil Steril 1998; 69: 1005–1009

26 Clark AM, Thornley B, Tomlinson L, Galletley C, Norman RJ. Weight loss in obese infertile women results in improvement in reproductive outcome for all forms of fertility treatment. Hum Reprod 1998; 13: 1502–1505

27 Lashen H, Ledger W, Bernal AL, Barlow D. Extremes of body mass do not adversely affect the outcome of superovulation and *in vitro* fertilization. Hum Reprod 1999; 14: 712–715

28 Wass P, Waldenstrom U, Rossner S, Hellberg D. An android body fat distribution in females impairs the pregnancy rate of *in vitro* fertilization-embryo transfer. Hum Reprod 1997; 12: 2057–2060

29 Feichtinger W, Papalambrou K, Poehl M, Krischker U, Neumann K. Smoking and *in vitro* fertilization: a meta-analysis. J Assist Reprod Genet 1997; 14: 596–599

30 Lashen H, Afnan M, Sharif K. A controlled comparison of ovarian response to controlled stimulation in first generation Asian women compared with white Caucasian undergoing *in vitro* fertilisation. Br J Obstet Gynaecol 1999; 106: 407–409

31 Wang XJ, Ledger W, Payne D, Jeffery R, Mathew CD. The contribution of embryo cryopreservation to *in vitro* fertilisation/gamete intra-fallopian transfer: 8 years experience. Hum Reprod 1994; 9: 103–109

32 Hughes EG, Federkow DM, Daya S, Sagle M, Van de Koppel P, Cllins JA. The routine use of gonadotrophin-releasing hormone agonists prior to *in vitro* fertilisation and gamete intrafallopian transfer: a meta-analysis of randomised control trials. Fertil Steril 1992; 58: 888–896

33 Cramer DW, Poers RD, Oskowitz PS *et al*. Gonadotrophin-releasing hormone agonist use in assisted reproduction cycles: the influence of long and short regimens on pregnancy rates. Fertil Steril 1999; 72: 83–89

34 Al-Inany H, Aboulghar M. Gonadotrophin-releasing hormone antagonists for assisted conception. Cochrane Database of Systematic Reviews, 2002 (issue 3)

35 Van Hooff MH, Alberda AT, Huisman GJ, Zellmaker GH, Leerentveld RA. Doubling the human menopausal gonadotrophin dose in the course of an *in vitro* fertilisation treatment cycle in low responders: a randomised study. Hum Reprod 1993; 8: 369–373

36 Fauser BCJM, Donderwinkle P, Schoot DC. The step down principle in gonadotrophin treatment and the role of GnRH analogues. Baillière's Clin Obstet Gynaecol 1993; 7: 309–330

37 Daya S, Gunby J, Hughes EG, Collins JA, Sagle MA. Follicle-stimulating hormone versus human menopausal gonadotrophin for in vitro fertilisation cycles: a meta-analysis. Fertil Steril 1995; 64: 347–354

38 Daya S, Gunby J. Recombinant versus urinary follicle stimulating hormone for ovarian stimulation in assisted reproduction. Hum Reprod 1999; 14: 2207–2215

39 Balasch J, Barri PN. Reflections on the cost-effectiveness of recombinant FSH in assisted reproduction. J Assist Reprod Genet 2001; 18: 45–55

40 Roset J, Verhoeff A, Van Heusden AM, Zellmaker GH. Minimal monitoring of ovarian hyperstimulation: a useful simplification of the clinical phase of *in vitro* fertilisation treatment. Fertil Steril 1995; 64: 552–556

41 Staessen C, Janssenswillen C, Van den Abbeel E, Devroev P, Vansterteghem AC. Avoidance of triplet pregnancy by elective transfer of two good quality embryos. Hum Reprod 1993; 8: 1650–1653

42 Templeton AA, Morris JK. Reducing the risk of multiple births by transfer of two embryos after *in vitro* fertilisation. N Engl J Med 1998; 339: 573–577

43 Nabi A, Awonuga A, Birch H, Barlow S, Stewart B. Multiple attempts at embryo transfer: does this affect *in vitro* fertilisation outcome? Hum Reprod 1997; 12: 1188–1190

44 Coroleu B, Carreras O, Veiga A *et al*. Embryo transfer under ultrasound guidance improves pregnancy rate after *in vitro* fertilisation. Hum Reprod 2000; 15: 616–620

45 Hearns-Stokes RM, Miller BT, Scott L, Creuss D, Chakraborty KP, Segars HJ. Pregnancy rates after embryo transfer depend on the provider at embryo transfer. Fertil Steril 2000; 74: 80–86

46 Visser DS, Fourie FL, Kruger HF. Multiple attempts at embryo transfer: effects on pregnancy outcome in an *in vitro* fertilisation and embryo transfer program. J Assist Reprod Genet 1993; 15: 107–112

47 Schoolcraft WB, Surrey ES, Gardner DK. Embryo transfer: technique and variables affecting success. Fertil Steril 2001; 76: 863–870

48 Karlstrom PO, Bergh T, Forsberg AS, Sandkvist U, Wikland M. Prognostic factors for the success rate of embryo freezing. Hum Reprod 1997; 12: 1263–1266

49 Kowalik A, Palermo GD, Barmat L, Veek L, Rimarachin J, Rosenwaks Z. Comparison of clinical outcome after cryopreservation of embryos obtained from intracytoplasmic sperm injection and in vitro fertilisation. Hum Reprod 1998; 13: 2848–2851

50 Palermo G, Joris H, Devroey P, Van Steirteghem AC. Pregnancies after intracytoplasmic sperm injection of a single spermatozoon into an oocyte. Lancet 1992; 340: 17–18

51 Mansour R, Aboulghar MA, Serour GI, Amin Y, Ramzi AM. The effect of sperm

parameters on the outcome of intracytoplasmic sperm injection. Fertil Steril 1995; 64: 982–986

52 Ubaldi F, Liu J, Nagy Z *et al*. Indications for and results of intracytoplasmic sperm injection (ICSI). Int J Androl 1995; 18 (Suppl 2): 88–90

53 Khamsi F, Yavas Y, Roberge S, Wong JC, Lacanna IC, Endman M. Intracytoplasmic sperm injection increased fertilisation and good-quality embryo formation in patients with non-male factor indications for *in vitro* fertilisation: a prospective randomized study. Fertil Steril 2001; 75: 342–347

54 Van Rumste MM, Evers JL, Farquhar CM, Blake DA. Intra-cytoplasmic sperm injection versus partial zona dissection, subzonal insemination and conventional techniques for oocyte insemination during in vitro fertilisation (Cochrane Review). The Cochrane Library, 1999

Horace M. Fletcher Joseph Frederick

Abdominal myomectomy revisited

Leiomyomata uterii (uterine fibroids) are benign tumours of the smooth muscle of the uterus. These tumours are extremely common with prevalence rates varying from 20–50% of women depending on the age, ethnicity, parity, and method used to assess their presence. In one series, they were said to be present in 77% of postmortem specimens where detailed examination of the uterus was done looking for these fibroids. In that series, over 50% of the women were said to be asymptomatic.[1]

In Jamaica, the incidence is high, as 90% of the women seen are of African ancestry and these tumours are said to be especially prevalent in such women. At the University Hospital of the West Indies, about 30% of the women admitted to the gynaecological ward are for the treatment of uterine fibroids. This is the most common reason for major surgery in our institution.

These tumours seem to grow under the influence of the hormone oestrogen and are most often seen after the menarche. The typical patient is nulliparous or of low parity and the main complaints are menorrhagia, symptoms of anaemia, dysmenorrhoea, pressure symptoms, abdominal distension and infertility. Infertility appears to be an incidental finding rather than a consequence of the fibroids, except in the case of submucous fibroids.[2,3] Rare complications include degeneration, torsion, prolapse of a submucous fibroid, ureteric obstruction and malignant transformation. As a result of these problems many women will present to their doctor for treatment and an assessment of the patient is needed as well as counselling prior to any definitive treatment.

Horace M. Fletcher BSc MB BS DM(O&G) FRCOG FACOG
Senior Lecturer and Consultant, Department of Obstetrics and Gynaecology, University of the West Indies, Mona, Kingston 7, Jamaica (for correspondence, E-mail: hfletchr@cwjamaica.com)

Joseph Frederick MB BS DM(O&G) FRCOG FACOG
Professor and Consultant, Department of Obstetrics and Gynaecology, University of the West Indies, Mona, Kingston 7, Jamaica

NO TREATMENT NEEDED

Not all fibroids require treatment and in some women treatment may be more hazardous than to leave the fibroids alone. No treatment is needed in asymptomatic women with small fibroids especially those found after pelvic examination which are less than 12-week size or those found as incidental findings at ultrasonography. Asymptomatic women who have reproductive desires and are fertile are best left alone. In these women, it is believed that surgical treatment is potentially hazardous because of the risk of tubal occlusion from adhesion formation. Perimenopausal women are sometimes not treated if the symptoms are minor, as the fibroids tend to shrink after the menopause with the loss of oestrogen stimulation. However, with the recent push for hormonal replacement in all menopausal women, it is probably time to re-think this recommendation. Surgical removal of fibroids during pregnancy is not recommended, with treatment confined to the use of analgesia for pain from red degeneration. The removal of fibroids at the time of Caesarean section has long been contra-indicated although recent reports have suggested both hysterectomy and even myomectomy in experienced hands is possible and safe.[4] Finally, women too ill to undergo surgery safely despite symptoms are better off in delaying treatment until well enough to do so.

HYSTERECTOMY

This is the treatment of choice for most women who have completed their reproductive life. This is usually recommended because of the high recurrence rate after myomectomy of 27% over 10 years with the need for re-operation.[5] The procedure can be done vaginally if the fibroids are small less than 12-week size (vaginal hysterectomy for fibroids larger than this has been reported but is best left to the experienced). Laparoscopic hysterectomy is also possible in small fibroids and this can be done totally abdominally with morcellation of the fibroids to remove them or as a laparoscopic-assisted vaginal hysterectomy. The usual method of removal is by abdominal hysterectomy by laparotomy. This can be done as a total abdominal hysterectomy or as a subtotal abdominal hysterectomy which is an old procedure that has found a new resurgence due to recent studies demonstrating better bladder function in women with this procedure compared to those with total hysterectomy. Hysterectomy is, however, not the method of choice in women who wish to conserve their uterus for reproductive or social reasons and should be avoided in these women due to the psychological impact of the procedure.

CONSERVATIVE PROCEDURES

Conservative procedures include medical procedures to treat the complications such as iron replacement in anaemic patients. Medical treatment of fibroids includes depot-medroxy progesterone acetate (DMPA) to reduce bleeding and gonadotrophin releasing hormone (GnRH) agonists to reduce bleeding and to shrink the fibroids. Conservative procedures also include surgical procedures such as endometrial ablation in women with menorrhagia who are too ill to undergo laparotomy. Myolysis is a relatively new method where the fibroids are coagulated with a bipolar needle during laparoscopy.[6]

A new procedure of selective embolisation of the blood supply to solitary myomata has shown some promise as a conservative procedure. This procedure is believed to be beneficial even in patients with multiple fibroids as embolisation of the blood supply appears to affect the fibroids more than the normal myometrium. However, where the blood supply is severely compromised there is a risk of uterine infection and bowel necrosis[7] or endometrial atrophy with amenorrhea and infertility.[8]

The main conservative surgical procedure is myomectomy. This can be done as hysteroscopic myomectomy of submucous fibroids, laparoscopic myomectomy of subserous fibroids and myomectomy by laparotomy for any type of fibroid.

Medical treatment prior to myomectomy

DMPA and other progestogens such as norethisterone have been used to reduce the menorrhagia associated with uterine fibroids. The effect is temporary and there is no impact on the size or growth of the fibroids. They may, however, be useful adjuncts to surgery.[9,10]

GnRH agonists were introduced and showed much promise initially. They reduce the size and growth of fibroids albeit only temporarily. All studies have shown that there is no benefit to give this treatment for more than 3 months and that all the fibroids regrow within 12 months of treatment.[11] The main benefits are improvement of the patients' well-being prior to surgery with reduction in anaemia and reduction in fibroid size thereby reducing the need for non-cosmetic subumbilical incisions. The ease of myomectomy post-GnRH treatment is controversial with some reports claiming that the procedure is easier because the fibroids are smaller and others reporting that the removal is more difficult because of an indistinguishable capsule.[12] There is, however, potential for its use prior to minimal invasive procedures such as laparoscopic and hysteroscopic myomectomy because of the reduction in tumour size.

Pre-operative counselling

All patients scheduled for myomectomy should have extensive counselling regarding the efficacy of the procedure the complications and the possibility of hysterectomy depending on what obtains at surgery. Patients should be told that the procedure may not relieve symptoms and also that the fibroids can regrow. Patients who are nulliparous and those with fertility desires should be told that complications such as haemorrhage and adhesion formation can cause tubal occlusion with iathrogenic infertility. The possibility of a hysterectomy should be discussed as intra-operative events may make this the better option for the patient. Patients who refuse to give consent to possible hysterectomy should not be operated on.

Myomectomy

Recommendations by the American College of Obstetricians and Gynecologists are that hysterectomy is indicated in women with 'large' asymptomatic myomata with a uterine size of equal to or greater than 12 weeks' gestation (or weight 280 g) determined by physical examination.[13] This is surely not a recommendation that we follow in Jamaica since fibroids we see tend to be gigantic. Most of our patients present late and also tend to have rapid growth of the fibroids. We do not use size as a determination as to whether or not we do myomectomy and we have been successfully able to remove up to 81 fibroids from a single uterus.[14]

Small fibroids can be successfully removed during laparoscopy or hysteroscopy in carefully selected patients. Laparoscopy is useful for subserous or intramural fibroids. This is usually a long and tedious process with closure of the cavity a challenging, and sometimes difficult, undertaking. Hysteroscopy is useful for submucous fibroids the main risk being perforation of the uterus. These procedures are not usually possible in our patients due to the size and number of fibroids we encounter and also due to the inevitable presence of the fibroids in the three layers of the uterus.

Myomectomy by laparotomy is the method of choice in most patients. In this procedure, an abdominal incision is made over the uterus and the fibroids removed individually by shelling them out of their capsule. The inevitable complications are bleeding which is sometimes tremendous and adhesion formation postoperatively with infertility or bowel obstruction. Adhesion formation can be reduced by careful operative technique limiting the number of incisions and by using oxidised regenerated cellulose absorbable barrier (Interceed®: Johnson and Johnson, Summerville, NJ, USA) to reduce contact between damaged tissues.[15,16]

The procedure

Most fibroids can be removed through a low transverse incision (Pfannenstiel incision). To decide if this is possible, one should evaluate the uterus pre-operatively. If the uterus is larger than a size equivalent to 20 weeks' gestation and is immobile, if there have been previous difficult surgery or pelvic sepsis with adhesions, other pelvic pathology such as ovarian tumours, then a sub-umbilical midline incision is the better choice.

One method used commonly in our institution during the Pfannenstiel incision is to place the transverse incision into the rectus sheath about 5 cm above the transverse incision into the skin. This usually makes it much easier to manipulate large fibroids and allows proper placement of the myoma screw. This also allows for an excellent cosmetic result in the skin as the resulting scar is low in the line of the pubic region (Fig. 1).

When the abdominal cavity is opened, the uterus should be mobilised and removed from the abdominal cavity prior to any incision being made. Grasping the fundus or a fibroid and pulling it through the incision can usually remove the uterus. In cases where this is not possible, the removal can be achieved with the aid of a myoma screw placed as far posteriorly as is possible. With the myoma screw in the right hand, the left hand is placed behind the uterus and serves the purposes of retraction of the abdominal wall and internal organs such as bowel, away from the point of entry of the myoma screw and also to feel for inadvertent exit of the instrument. The aim is to place the myoma screw into a large fibroid and to avoid injury to the fallopian tubes ovaries or bowel. When it is properly inserted, with steady traction antero-inferiorly the uterus can usually be easily

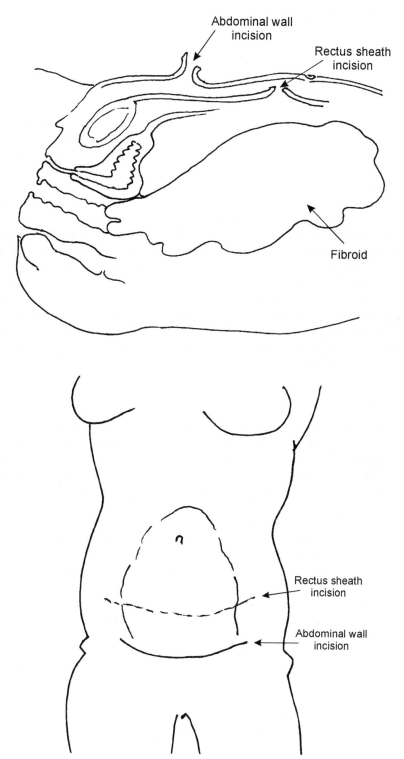

Fig. 1 Rectus incision made about 5 cm higher than skin incision making it easier to place the myoma screw near the fundus of the enlarged uterus.

delivered through the incision. Great care should be taken during this procedure to avoid damage to the vessels in the broad ligament as these are sometimes congested and easily torn. Once the uterus is delivered, an assessment is made of the tubes, ovaries and the uterus. The presence of severe endometriosis of pelvic inflammatory disease should not prevent the surgeon from doing a myomectomy in patients who wish to retain their uterus. However if in the judgement of the surgeon the patient's symptoms are best relieved by a hysterectomy, this should be performed. Assessment of the uterus entails careful evaluation of the anatomy to see exactly where the main fibroids are located. Fibroids located adjacent to the intramural part of the fallopian tubes are difficult to remove because of the risk of tubal occlusion. Fibroids located low down on the uterus anteriorly or posteriorly are also a problem because of the risk of damage to the bladder or other pelvic structures. Pedunculated fibroids adherent to other structures also present a problem and require careful removal to avoid organ damage and ensure haemostasis. The surgeon should carefully plan his incisions aiming to remove as many fibroids as possible with as few incisions as possible. Transverse, inverted U, or wedge-shaped incisions done around the largest fibroids are best. They can be done anteriorly, posteriorly or both. Most of the fibroids can be removed through these major incisions; however, if this is not possible, the smaller supplementary incisions can be made over fibroids out of reach of the primary incision.

Prevention of bleeding has always been a challenge to the surgeon. The use of Bonney's clamp and Rubin's tourniquet were for many years the mainstay of prevention of this complication. These older methods have, however, been replaced in most centres by better procedures such as the use of vaso-occlusive injections (*e.g.* vasopressin). The use of the tourniquet and the clamp, to a lesser extent, caused trauma to the broad ligament and also proved to be inefficient resulting in some bleeding still as well as iatrogenic adhesions in the peri-ovarian area. In both methods, the occlusion does not include the infundibulopelvic ligament with the ovarian blood supply, which forms one arm of the anastamosis in the broad ligament. Occluding only one arm was, therefore, not enough to achieve good haemostasis. Some authors have advocated occlusion of the infundibulopelvic ligament with ring forceps or intestinal clamps but these result in a reduction in the blood supply to the ovaries with unknown effects on their subsequent function. These mechanical methods of occlusion also required that the occlusion be released every 20 min with the inevitable outcome of bleeding.

The use of vasopressin has been described for prevention of bleeding at myomectomy by laparoscopy and laparotomy. It has been used intramurally as well as perivascularly. It has been clearly shown to be better than both placebo[14] and tourniquet[17] in reducing blood loss and reducing the need for blood transfusion. The method described by Frederick *et al.*[14] requires injection of the diluted vasopressin solution (1 ml 20 U vasopressin with 19 ml normal saline) perivascularly into the broad ligament at the junction of the anastamosis of the ovarian and uterine blood supply (Fig. 2). This is done under direct vision to avoid inadvertent intravascular injection of the solution. Some solution is also injected beneath the peritoneum, along the proposed incision lines. This results in an immediate blanching of the uterus, with no effect on the ovaries or fallopian tubes.

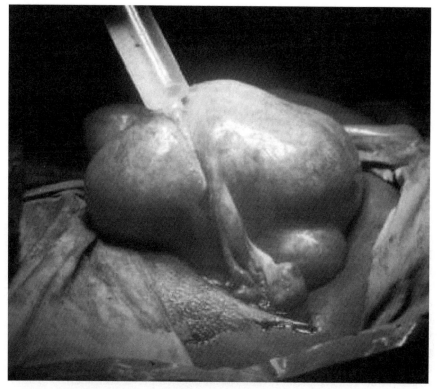

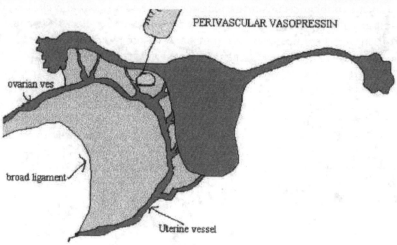

Fig. 2 Perivascular vasopressin injection into the broad ligament.

The myomectomy is then performed with as few incisions as possible and with gentle tissue handling. Obvious bleeding points are occasionally seen and these are clamped directly and ligated. The reduction in blood loss gives us the confidence to patiently dissect out all fibroids, and results in less need for blood transfusion. Theoretically, we believe that the reduced blood loss should result in less postoperative morbidity but this was not proven by the two studies.

Subserous/pedunculated fibroids

These are usually the easiest fibroid to remove. An elliptical incision around the base of the fibroid is made and the stalk and fibroid removed. The incision can be made with a scalpel or better with cutting diathermy to reduce bleeding even further. With broad-base stalks be careful not to make the incision too wide as the defect left will be difficult to close.

Intramural fibroids

The incision is made over the fibroid deep enough to enter the false capsule. The fibroid is then grasped with a tenaculum or the myoma screw and with traction on the fibroid and counter traction with a moistened towel used to bluntly push off the myometrium. The fibroid can be removed with minimal damage to deeper tissue such as the endometrium.

Sub-mucous fibroids

These are removed by opening the endometrial cavity and palpating for fibroids. This is not always needed as bimanual palpation of the uterus can confirm the absence of these fibroids. This bimanual palpation is invaluable at all stages of the procedure to detect small intramural fibroids as well. When the intra-cavitary fibroids are encountered, one can sometimes remove them through a single incision over the fibroid. Others can be removed by avulsion, if small and pedunculated. Opening the cavity is also of value in allowing drainage of blood through the vagina instead of into the peritoneal cavity where it may cause a paralytic ileus or an infected pelvic collection.

Closure of the incisions made requires good haemostasis and closure of all dead space where there is the potential for blood to collect. Haematomata result in persistent postoperative pyrexia. It is sometimes of value to trim off excess myometrial tissue to ensure that there is reduced chance of leaving behind dead space. Myometrial incisions are best closed with a strong suture such as 1/0 poly-glycolic acid (Vicryl: Ethicon, Edinburgh, UK). The serosa is then approximated with a subcuticular suture and closed with 3/0 poly-glycolic acid sutures. These suture materials are better than the traditional catgut sutures as there is less tissue reaction and less adhesion formation.

The incisions are then covered with a layer of an adhesion barrier (Interceed®) which is only placed when all bleeding has been controlled. The adhesion barrier (Interceed®) can be sutured in place or spread over the incisions and the uterus carefully replaced into the abdominal cavity without suturing.

Repeat myomectomy

In our setting, where many patients develop fibroids in their late 20s early 30s, it is common for us to see recurrence of fibroids prior to the completion of the patient's reproductive life. In some of these patients, recurrent myomectomy is a valid option that we undertake and this is done if the patient has a recurrence of symptoms such as menorrhagia, severe pain or an abdominal mass. The procedure is similar to that described for the primary myomectomy except for the fact that, in these patients, the likelihood of adhesions is more common and the risks and complication also greater.

These patients are, therefore, carefully counselled and a bowel preparation done pre-operatively. The bladder is also drained throughout the operation by Foley catheterisation.

The patients are evaluated in a similar fashion and if the uterus is large (> 20 weeks) and relatively immobile we opt for the use of a sub-umbilical mid-line incision as opposed to a low-transverse incision. Adhesions to bowel and bladder are very common and careful dissection is needed to avoid damage to these structures. In dissecting dense adhesions, it is best to leave a part of the uterine peritoneum behind than to inadvertently make a hole into large bowel. Haemostasis is achieved with vasopressin and adhesions are prevented with adhesion prevention barriers. In a series of 57 patients, Frederick et al.[18] found that the success of performing a repeat myomectomy was high with only one patient having transformation of the operation to hysterectomy, but complications such as blood loss and pyrexia were high and fertility rates low at 15% compared to the 50% usually described for the primary procedure.[19,20]

Myomectomy in pregnancy

This has for many years been an absolute contra-indication. However, in the more recent literature, it appears that this is not always necessarily the case. The main principles of myomectomy during pregnancy are that: (i) this should be a procedure undertaken by an experienced surgeon; (ii) it should be done only with the full consent and knowledge of the patient; and (iii) it should be avoided unless the baby is being delivered at the same time (Caesarean myomectomy). Reports of myomectomy and the pregnancy continuing are rare and only done in dire circumstances where the symptoms are extreme and the patient fully aware of the risk of losing the pregnancy as well as her uterus.

Caesarean myomectomy is a more feasible undertaking. It is, however, important to remember that the baby must be delivered prior to attempting myomectomy and also that if the bleeding from the Caesarean section is heavy, then the myomectomy should probably best be done as an interval procedure.[4]

CONCLUSIONS

Uterine fibroids are very common and in many patients no treatment is needed. Medical treatment of fibroids is inadequate when used alone. The use of surgical treatment is mandatory in many women to relieve symptoms. The safety of surgical techniques has been enhanced by adjuncts to surgery such as pretreatment with GnRh agonists, intra-operative adhesion prevention and haemostatic agents such as vasopressin. Probably a combination of all these techniques will result in optimal treatment until newer methods are found to prevent fibroids and to treat them medically.

References

1 Cramer S, Patel A. Frequency of uterine fibroids. Am J Clin Pathol 1990; 94: 435–438
2 Pritts E. Fibroids and infertility. Obstet Gynecol Surv 2001; 56: 483–491
3 Poncelet C, Benifla J, Darai E, Madelenat P. Myoma and infertility: analysis of the literature. Gynecol Obstet Fertil 2001; 29: 413–421

4 Brown D,. Fletcher H, Myrie M, Reid M. Caesarean myomectomy a safe procedure. A retrospective case controlled study. J Obstet Gynaecol 1999; 19: 139–141

5 Candiani G, Fedele L, Parazinni F, Villa L. Risk of recurrence after myomectomy. Br J Obstet Gynaecol 1991; 98: 385–389

6 Donnez J, Squifflet J, Polet R, Nisolle M. Laparoscopic myolysis. Hum Reprod Update 2000; 6: 609–613

7 Al-Fozan H, Tulandi T. Factors affecting early surgical intervention after uterine artery embolization. Obstet Gynecol Surv 2002; 57: 810–815

8 Tropeano G, Litwicka K, Di Stasi C, Romano D, Mancuso S. Permanent amenorrhea associated with endometrial atrophy after uterine artery embolization for symptomatic uterine fibroids. Fertil Steril 2003; 79: 132–135

9 Lumbiganon P, Rugpao S, Phandu-Fung S, Laopaiboon M, Vudhikamraksa N, Werawatakui Y. Protective effect of depot-medroxyprogesterone acetate on surgically treated leiomyomas: a multicentre case control study. Br J Obstet Gynaecol 1996; 103: 909–914

10 Sheth S, Das S. Preoperative management of anaemia to avoid blood transfusion. Int J Obstet Gynecol 2002; 77: 245–247

11 Healy D, Vollenhoven B. The role of GnRH agonists in the treatment of uterine fibroids. Br J Obstet Gynaecol 1992; 99 (Suppl 7): 23–26

12 Benagiano G, Morini A, Primero F. Fibroids: overview of current and future treatment options. Br J Obstet Gynaecol 1992; 99: 18–22

13 Reiter R, Wagner P, Gambone J. Routine hysterectomy for large asymptomatic uterine leiomyomata: a reappraisal. Obstet Gynecol 1992; 79: 481–484

14 Frederick J, Fletcher H, Hardie M Simeon D, Mullings A. Intramyometrial vasopressin as haemostatic agent during myomectomy. Br J Obstet Gynaecol 1994; 101: 435–437

15 Mais V, Ajossa S, Piras B, Guerro S, Marongiu D, Melis G. Prevention of *de-novo* adhesion formation after laparoscopic myomectomy. A randomised trial to evaluate the effectiveness of an oxidized regenerated cellulose adhesion barrier in infertile women. Hum Reprod 1995; 10: 3133–3135

16 Sawada T, Nishizawa H, Nishio E, Kadowaki M. Postoperative adhesion prevention with an oxidized regenerated cellulose adhesion barrier in infertile women. J Reprod Med 2000; 45: 387

17 Fletcher H, Frederick J, Hardie M, Simeon D. A randomized comparison of vasopressin and tourniquet as hemostatic agents during myomectomy. Obstet Gynecol 1996; 87: 1014–1018

18 Frederick J, Hardie M, Reid M, Fletcher H, Wynter S, Frederick C. Operative morbidity and reproductive outcome in secondary myomectomy: a prospective cohort study. Hum Reprod 2002; 17: 2967–2971

19 Berkeley A, De Cherney A, Polan M. Abdominal myomectomy and subsequent fertility. Surg Gynecol Obstet 1983; 156: 319–322

20 Kably Ambe A, Anaya Coeto H, Garza Rios P. Abdominal myomectomy and subsequent fertility. Ginocol Obstet Mex 1990; 58: 274–276

Geoffrey Trew

Postoperative adhesions and their avoidance

Should adhesion reduction agents be used in all operations? This is an important question which needs urgent debate. Considering the mounting experience and evidence we have of adhesions and their impact and in the face of new developments in anti-adhesion agents, we are now moving to a time when not to use an adhesion reduction agent during therapeutic intraperitoneal surgery could be considered potentially negligent!

ADHESIONS – THE IMPACT

Adhesions are an almost inevitable consequence of abdominal and pelvic surgery, with almost 95% of patients following laparotomy being shown to have adhesions at subsequent surgery.1

They are an everyday problem in clinical and surgical practice, a major cause of morbidity and expense, an occasional cause of mortality and a leading and debilitating cause of chronic pain for patients – estimated as the most common pathology associated with chronic pain.[2,3] Of small bowel obstructions, 74% are adhesion-related[4] and it is estimated that 20–40% of secondary infertility in women is as a result of adhesions.[5,6] Adhesions also pose an important complicating factor for surgeons and patients undergoing future surgery. Adhesions from previous surgery significantly increase subsequent operating time by a median 18 min[7] and even in the hands of experienced colorectal surgeons there is a 19% risk of inadvertent enterotomy.[8] Many clinicians feel that the prevention of adhesions is one of the biggest unmet needs in surgery; but, because of the historic inability to prevent adhesion formation after surgery, it has been said that there is a sense of 'fatalism' that has affected the surgical community

Geoffrey Trew
Consultant in Reproductive Medicine and Surgery, Hammersmith and Queen Charlotte's Hospital and Honorary Senior Lecturer, Imperial College, London, UK (E-mail: g.trew@imperial.ac.uk)

Most health surgeons lack full awareness of the magnitude and consequences of adhesions. There are several reasons for this: (i) adhesive complications can occur unpredictably, sometimes several years after a procedure, and are frequently treated by physicians or specialists other than the initial surgeon; (ii) the aetiology of adhesion formation remains incompletely understood; and (iii) there is a nearly century-long track record of failure or limited applicability of traditional adhesion prevention modalities until the recent introduction of newer agents.

Lack of awareness of the clinical significance and frequency of adhesion formation has been cited as the greatest impediment to reducing adhesion formation[9] and, until recently, the extent of burden of adhesion-related disease was unclear. Surgeons have been known to claim that 'adhesions are not a problem for (my) patients' or that they 'don't get any adhesions after surgery'.[9] Thus, many have not always appreciated the need to act to try to reduce adhesions.

EPIDEMIOLOGY OF ADHESION-RELATED RE-ADMISSIONS

Adhesive intestinal obstruction has been shown to be responsible for 3.5% of all laparotomies;[10] in the UK, it accounted for 0.9% of all admissions and 3.3% of 4502 major laparotomies in a 24-year (1964–1988) study of 28,297 adult surgical admissions,[1,11] but largely the epidemiology of adhesions was unclear.

The Surgical and Clinical Research (SCAR) group has undertaken most work in this area. Their initial work followed-up adhesion-related hospital re-admissions in Scotland for 10 years in a cohort of patients undergoing open abdominal or pelvic surgery.[12] They found that up to one in three patients were re-admitted at least twice for adhesion-related problems or operations potentially complicated by them during this period and the re-admissions continued steadily through the 10 years. This research also indicated that patients undergoing open surgical procedures on the colon and rectum in general surgery[13] and fallopian tubes and ovaries in gynaecological surgery[14] were at most risk of adhesion-related re-admissions. An assessment of the prevalence of adhesions demonstrated that adhesion-related admissions were as common in 1994 as hospital admissions for appendicectomies, hip replacements and coronary bypass grafts. Recently, this group has examined more current epidemiology and reported that 40% of laparoscopic gynaecology cases have at least a comparable risk of adhesion-related re-admission to similar surgery by laparotomy.[15]

Although it is not possible to identify which adhesions will create complications, logic and clinical observation[11] indicate that those involving key organs and tissues (e.g. the small intestine or the uterus and adnexa) are the most likely to be symptomatic. In the treatment of adhesion-related small bowel obstruction, outcomes following conservative treatment have been shown to be worse if adhesions are a result of previous appendectomy or tubal or ovarian surgery.[16]

PATHOPHYSIOLOGY

Adhesions are basically abnormal attachments between tissues and organs[17] and may be congenital or acquired.[18,19] The development of acquired adhesions

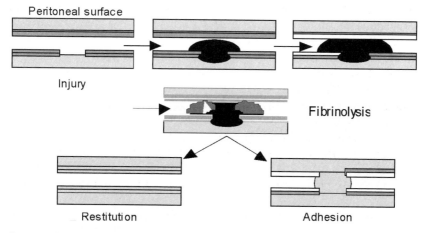

Peritoneal surface

Injury

Fibrinolysis

Restitution   Adhesion

Fig. 1 Pathogenesis of adhesions.[22]

is a generalised phenomenon in response to trauma to the peritoneum, the surface of which is extremely delicate as its cells are very loosely interconnected. The trauma may be inflammatory or surgical, and may include: exposure to infection or to intestinal contents; ischaemia; irritation from foreign materials (such as sutures, gauze particles, or glove dusting powder); desiccation; or overheating by lamps or irrigation fluid.[2] Adhesion formation is a surface event associated with peritoneal wound healing.

Abrasion and other trauma lead to disruption of the mesothelium and fibrin is then deposited at the damaged surfaces by bleeding and post-traumatic inflammation. This fibrin mass enlarges, reaching another tissue surface and forming a bridge between the surfaces.

Adhesion formation generally requires the contact of two traumatised mesothelial surfaces,[20,21] or of one surface and the omentum. Locally generated fibrinolytic factors are released which may degrade all or part of this fibrin bridge but surgery infection and hypoxia dramatically diminish fibrinolytic activity – in this case, fibroblasts and other cells may migrate across the bridge remnants transforming it into an adhesion (Fig. 1).

The most important events determining whether the pathway taken is adhesion formation or re-epithelialisation are, therefore, the apposition of two damaged surfaces and the extent of fibrinolysis.

While the severity and extent of adhesions may change over weeks and months, the incidence of an adhesion (*i.e.* whether it develops at all) is decided in the 5–7 days after peritoneal trauma takes place and the development of the adhesions commences very early during surgery. Since many of the traumas listed above are a routine part of surgery, it is not surprising that the formation of postsurgical adhesions is almost universal.[1]

STEPS TO REDUCE ADHESIONS

In the knowledge of the factors influencing the development of adhesions during surgery, there are basic steps that should be taken to help reduce adhesion development (Table 1). The fundamental step in adhesion avoidance

Table 1 Basic steps to reduce adhesion development

- Careful surgical technique
- Excellent haemostasis
- Minimise tissue handling by careful technique, magnification and microsurgery, if appropriate
- Reduce infection risk
- Avoid gastrointestinal contamination
- Reduce drying of tissues including using irrigation/lubrication
- Limit use of cautery
- Limit use of sutures and choice of fine non-reactive suture
- Avoid foreign bodies such as materials with loose fibres
- Use of starch-free gloves

is careful surgical technique.[23] Tissue should be handled as little as possible and there is a need for meticulous haemostasis. Infection should be kept to a minimum by avoiding spillage of intestinal contents and appropriate use of prophylactic antibiotics. Desiccation should be kept to a minimum by the use of minimal access techniques and the use of irrigation fluids during the course of open surgery. Abdominal packs should be used sparingly as these cause significant desiccation and peritoneal abrasions. Where packing is required the packs should be soaked in an irrigation fluid such as Hartmann's solution. Excessive diathermy should be avoided and monofilament sutures should be used where possible. Careful technique to avoid large avascular pedicles can also be beneficial. Talc or starch containing gloves should never be used.

However, any type of surgery (however good the surgeon!) and any site of surgery can cause postoperative adhesion formation; while steps as listed above should be taken during all surgery, a fundamental paradox is that the method used to separate adhesions – surgery – is the one that induces them.

The most important factor in bringing about a reduction in the consequences of adhesion-related disease is education. Surgeons need to be constantly aware of the potential adhesive complications of any procedure and the need to reduce them.

ADHESION REDUCTION AGENTS

In recent years, there have been considerable steps toward the development of effective anti-adhesions agents and there is a clear place for agents that are safe, simple to use, clinically effective and affordable. A number of adjuvants have been developed to help to further reduce adhesion complications – both pharmacological agents and physical barriers.

Pharmacological agents

The processes of adhesion formation present various theoretical opportunities for pharmacological intervention. However, these are limited by the ability to deliver drugs to the site and to keep them there long enough to be effective.[24] Surgical sites are often cut off from normal blood supply and, therefore, systemic administration is ineffective, while the rapid absorption through the peritoneal membrane quickly removes most agents delivered intraperitoneally. Moreover, many processes involved in adhesion formation are also part of normal wound healing, so any pharmacological agent needs to reduce fibrin deposition yet still allow for re-epithelialisation.

A number of anti-inflammatory drugs including NSAIDs such as ibuprofen, and corticosteroids have been investigated but shown doubtful clinical efficacy. While NSAIDs have been shown to reduce adhesion reformation in animals, it is thought perhaps that their lack of clinical effectiveness may result from inadequate drug delivery.[25]

There are a number of experimental areas of drug investigation involving naturally occurring fibrinolytic enzymes including tissue plasminogen activator (tPA) and phospholipids (phosphatidylcholine). However, the dose of fibrinolytics required to reduce fibrinogenesis is too close to the anticoagulatory dose, thereby increasing the risk of impaired wound healing and haemorrhage. Work continues to research a range of agents that could potentially impact on the basic pathways of adhesion formation but there potential impact on helping to reduce adhesions in a surgical setting is some way off as the work is still largely experimental.

Physical separators

Barriers are currently the most useful adjuncts to reduce adhesion formation. The key need of any barrier is that it effectively separates all the traumatised peritoneal surfaces during the critical period of adhesion development in the 5–7 days after surgery. This separation can broadly be achieved by use of solid mechanical barriers (films and gels) to keep tissue surfaces physically separated during the healing process, or by the use of fluids for hydroflotation.

Solid mechanical barriers

Solid mechanical barriers have been used for some time initially in the form of omental or peritoneal grafting and more recently inert barriers have been introduced to be used at the site of trauma, for instance over a suture line for procedures such as myomectomy. Preclude® (expanded polytetrafluoroethylene, PTFE: Gore-tex) has been available for some time but has the fundamental disadvantage that it must be sutured in place and then removed at a second-look laparoscopy which substantially limits its applicability in peritoneal surgery. Subsequently, absorbable barriers have introduced.

Interceed® (oxidised regenerated cellulose) was introduced in 1990 and there is a substantial literature on its use. It has been shown to reduce adhesion formation whilst not affecting wound healing.[26] It can be used at most intraperitoneal locations and in laparoscopic surgery. It is, however, relatively difficult to handle and laparoscopic application is challenging. Moreover, its efficacy is reduced by the presence of blood so meticulous haemostasis must be achieved before it can be applied – in the presence of blood it turns black and is rendered ineffective. Recent work with Interceed has indicated that its effect on reducing adhesions is translated in infertile patients to improved pregnancy outcomes.[27] While this was a study in a limited number of patients, the use of Interceed resulted in significant increase in the pregnancy rate compared to surgical controls. While Interceed has limited applicability in routine surgery, these results are important as for the first time they provide evidence that an impact of an anti-adhesion agent on the secondary marker of adhesion reduction translates to a positive increase in clinical outcomes – in this case pregnancy.

Seprafilm® (hyaluronic acid/carboxymethylcellulose) is another barrier film[28,29] which is placed over a suture line. It also persists during the period of re-epithelialisation and is spontaneously absorbed. It does not conform to the shape of the pelvic organs as well as Interceed and is more useful as a barrier placed between the bowel or omentum and the anterior abdominal wall at the time of wound closure where it can prevent adherence and potentially reducing the risk of enterotomy at subsequent laparotomy. Recent work, however, while demonstrating its general safety in colorectal surgery has indicated that use at the site of an anastomosis is to be avoided due to increased anastamotic leaks.[30,31] To effect adequate coverage in colorectal surgery, a mean of 4.5 sheets/patient was also used which is expensive.[30,31]

Gel barriers

A fundamental limitation of site-specific barriers is the requirement of the surgeon to predict where clinically significant adhesions are likely to form. Additionally, they are generally difficult to use in laparoscopic surgery. In the knowledge of these limitations, gel barriers have also been developed. Hyaluronic acid has been used in a number of such preparations. It is a naturally occurring polysaccharide component of connective tissue which is fairly readily absorbed from the peritoneal cavity. The intraperitoneal residence time can be increased by cross-linking. In the physical barrier Seprafilm®, it is cross-linked with carboxymethylcellulose. Two gel formulations have been developed. In Hyalobarrier Gel™, hyaluronic acid is cross-linked to hyaluronic acid. This agent is, however, not widely available or used. More widely available and well used is Intergel®, where the hyaluronic acid is cross-linked with ferric chloride. Initial experience with Intergel was favourable.[32,33] In a laparotomy study followed by second-look laparoscopy, administration of 300 ml of Intergel into the peritoneal cavity at the end of surgery was shown to reduce adhesions at both surgical and non-surgical sites, including those anatomical locations where gravity alone would be likely to reduce the chance of distribution.[32,33] It was easier to apply at both open surgery or laparoscopy and seemed promising although expensive. It was, however, withdrawn from the market early in 2003 due to problems with late-onset postoperative pain.

The most recent gel barrier coating system developed is SprayGel™, which was approved for use in laparoscopic and open surgery in Europe at the end of 2001. This consists of two water-based synthetic polyethylene glycol (PEG) solutions – one clear and one coloured with methylene blue to make it easy to see where it has been used. When sprayed together, these two solutions react with each other at the target tissue, where they mix to form a hydrogel film that provides a physical barrier. This barrier remains in place for up to 7 days, and then is absorbed and cleared through the kidneys.

In preliminary clinical trials, use of SprayGel resulted in a statistically significant decrease in incidence, severity and extent of post-surgical adhesion formation found at second look laparoscopy compared with findings at initial surgery.[34,35] A larger scale pivotal study has been set up in the US but has recently been halted due to lack of efficacy in the treatment arm compared to control – considered to be a study design issue.

The use of SprayGel is limited by the complex set-up of the equipment, the skill and time required to evenly spray and coat tissues. It is also site-specific limiting efficacy to the sites it is administered and it is expensive.

Macromolecular solutions

A further strategy in adhesion reduction has been the intraperitoneal instillation of macromolecular solutions. The investigation of such solutions was led by Hyskon® (32% dextran 70). Dextran is an α-1,6-linked dextrose polymer, originally used (at 6%) as a plasma expander, which absorbed systemically but metabolised very slowly. In clinical practice, it can produce undesirable local and systemic side effects due to its osmotic and anaphylactic properties.[36] It is indicated for use as an aid to hysteroscopy and not as an anti-adhesion agent; clinical trials did not find Hyskon to be an effective adhesion reduction device.[37]

Hydroflotation

Hydroflotation has long been suggested as a technique which may be efficacious both at the site of application and elsewhere in the pelvis. This involves the instillation of a fluid into the peritoneal cavity at the end of the procedure to provide a physical, fluid barrier preventing apposition of damaged peritoneal surfaces. Saline, lactated Ringer's solution or Hartmann's solution have all been (and still are) widely used. However, these crystalloids are rapidly absorbed and do not work to reduce adhesions.[38] These solutions are absorbed from the peritoneal cavity at the rate of 30–60 ml/h, so that by 24 h after surgery, little, if any, crystalloid solution would be left in the pelvis.[39,40]

More recently, Adept® (4% icodextrin solution) has been approved for adhesion reduction. Icodextrin was originally developed as a peritoneal dialysate and has been marketed and used as such for a number of years in 7.5% solution. There is now more than 26,000 patient years of safety data with 7.5% solution and Adept has been used as an anti-adhesion solution in over 30,000 patients undergoing routine surgery. Adept has a sufficiently long intraperitoneal residence to provide hydroflotation during the crucial period of adhesion formation (Fig. 2).[41]

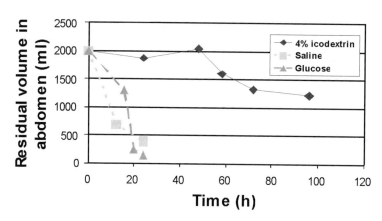

Fig. 2 Icodextrin hydroflotation mechanism.[41]

It looks and handles like normal saline or Hartmann's solution, is isosmolar and does not potentiate infection. As well as being easy to use, requiring no change to routine surgical practice or any special training, it is inexpensive. Preclinical studies confirmed that when used as an intra-operative wash and postoperative instillate Adept significantly reduced the incidence, severity and extent of postoperative adhesions.[42] No differences have been demonstrated between Adept and lactated Ringer's solution in the healing and strength of midline incisions and bowel anastamoses.[43]

Initial clinical studies are encouraging. A multicentre US study in patients undergoing laparoscopic gynaecological surgery, powered to confirm safety, has shown a net 30% improvement in adhesion reduction in patients treated with 4% icodextrin compared with a net 16% increase in adhesions in patients in whom Ringer's lactated solution was used.[44] Two major clinical trials in laparoscopic gynaecological surgery are on-going powered to demonstrate efficacy – a US study on patients undergoing adhesiolysis and a European study focusing on formation of *de novo* adhesions. The results of these will hopefully confirm the clinical efficacy of Adept.

In the meantime, a patient registry (ARIEL) allowing surgeons to record and report experiences of use of Adept in routine gynaecological and general surgery is on-going.[45,46] Feedback on almost 2000 patients has been received at time of writing and shows that Adept is well received by surgeons and well tolerated by patients. It is easy to use in both open and laparoscopic surgery with a good safety profile.

Icodextrin is also a satisfactory vehicle for drug administration and is approved in the UK and other European countries as a pharmacological agent for the administration of intraperitoneal drug therapy. Heparin has been successfully added by some surgeons who previously had used heparinised Hartmann's solution for irrigation purposes. Antibiotics have also been added. An interesting area of future research would be to consider the addition of pharmacological agents such as tPA to icodextrin. tPA has been shown to significantly reduce adhesion formation in the rabbit model without affecting haemostasis, bowel anastomosis or wound strength.[47] Its use has not been reported in human studies.

ECONOMIC BURDEN

As well as an important clinical burden associated with adhesions, the economic burden to the healthcare system is substantial. The SCAR data from 1994 showed 4199 admissions for surgery due to adhesions – 2096 were for surgery and 2103 were treated non-operatively.[12] Analysis of the published average length of stay for general (5.4 days) and gynaecological surgery (3.4 days) showed that at 1994 prices, treatment costs in that one year alone were £6.1 million, equivalent to a cost of more than £72 million if extrapolated to the whole UK.[48] This represented 2% of expenditure on the hospital and community services sector in Scotland in that year – a conservative estimate bearing in mind the nature of the SCAR study and that the burden of adhesions is on-going.

An attributable-risk, cost-of-illness study was recently carried out in the US.[49] A hospital discharge database was used to identify all abdominal adhesion procedures performed in 1994 and the costs were calculated from Medicare records. The results were compared with data from 1988. Adhesiolysis accounted for 303,836 hospital admissions in 1994 and $1.3 billion in hospitalisation and surgeon costs.

Modelling cost effectiveness

Postoperative adhesions clearly have an important impact on successful clinical outcomes of surgery and pose an important cost burden. In considering the implementation of an anti-adhesion strategy, as well as knowing the clinical efficacy of an adhesion-reduction agent, there is a need to know if adopting use of a particular agent will be cost effective.

Epidemiological data from the SCAR study in open lower abdominal surgery[13] has been used to model the cumulative costs over time of adhesion-related ('directly' or 'possibly related') re-admissions, with or without surgery.[50]

Adhesion-related re-admissions usually present as SBO[51] and cost data from an audit of adhesion-related SBO (re-admissions without surgery £1,606.15 – mean hospital stay 7 days and with surgery £4,677.41 – mean hospital stay 16 days)[52] can be applied to the SCAR incidence data over the 10 years of the study. This model can be used to compare the 'control' costs for 100 lower abdominal patients where no adhesion-reduction strategy is implemented with the costs of treating 100 patients with an adhesion-reduction agent. For the purposes of the model, we have hypothetically priced these at either £50 or £200 per patient treatment. The level of clinical efficacy required to reduce the costs of adhesion-related re-admissions so that the costs of using an adhesion-reduction agent will be repaid at various time periods after use in surgery can then been estimated. Applying this model to a low cost adhesion-reduction agent (hypothetically priced at £50 per patient), it is estimated that a 32.6% reduction in re-admissions will be required to payback the £50 cost of the product within the first year, and only a 16.0% reduction in re-admissions will be required to payback the £50 spent after 3 years. Thereafter, for each patient, cost savings will occur (Fig. 3).

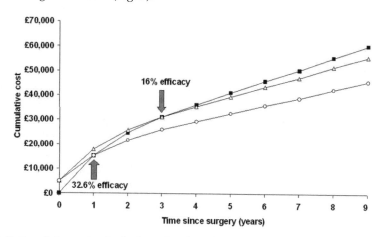

Fig. 3 Cumulative costs of adhesion-related re-admissions since surgery for 100 patients without treatment (control, filled squares) or with an adhesion-reduction product priced at £50 per treatment patient. Modelled on year one efficacy, required payback cost of treatment alone after one (open circles) or three (open triangles) years.

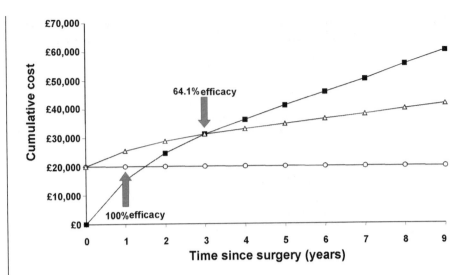

Fig. 4 Cumulative costs of adhesion-related re-admissions since surgery for 100 patients without treatment (control, filled squares) or with an adhesion-reduction product priced at £200 per treatment patient. Modelled on efficacy required to payback cost of treatment after one (open circles) or three (open triangles) years.

An adhesion-reduction agent hypothetically costing £200 per patient will not return the initial costs per patient within the first year even if it results in a 100% reduction in re-admissions, but the product would return the initial costs if a reduction in adhesion-related re-admissions of 64.1% could be demonstrated after 3 years (Fig. 4).

It is clear from this that in considering the choice of adhesion-reduction strategy, the cost of the product versus the clinical impact of the agent needs to be carefully considered. The price at which any agent used will be cost neutral is not very high – and this has important considerations in relation to selecting agents for use.

MEDICOLEGAL CONSIDERATIONS

Postoperative adhesions are an important cause of morbidity and represent a significant burden to the health service. The use of careful surgical technique and limited use of physical barriers has been the mainstay adopted to date amongst the few surgeons who recognise the problems of adhesions. However, with rising evidence of the impact of postoperative adhesions on successful surgical outcome, as surgeons we need to be cognoscente of the potential for medicolegal interest,[53,54] if we do not actively consider an anti-adhesion strategy at least in what mounting evidence suggests is 'high-risk' surgery (Table 2).

Adhesions remain an almost inevitable consequence of surgery — the major cause of small bowel obstruction, and significant causes of both female infertility and chronic pelvic pain. Even if adhesions are 'silent' posing no issues for patients, the risks of complications at re-operative surgery are considerable.

Table 2 'High-risk' surgery

Gynaecology	Ovarian cystectomy
	Tubal surgery
	Surgery for endometriosis
	Myomectomy
General surgery	Abdominal wall adhesiolysis
	Small bowel resection
	Formation and closure of ileostomy
	Hartmann's procedure
	Anterior resection ± stoma
	Lower anterior resection
	Abdominoperineal excision
	Colectomy
	Colostomy closure/formation

When consenting our patients for surgery, do we then tell them of any of these risks or potential strategies that could be implemented to reduce them? In a recent UK survey of trainee surgeons, only 14% of trainees routinely warned patients of the risk of adhesion formation.[55] The International Adhesions Society have also been undertaking work to review this with patients.[56] In only 10.4% of cases were adhesions mentioned as part of the informed consent process and in 14.4% adhesions were discussed but not part of the consent.

In patients undergoing specific adhesiolysis operations, 54% of patients reported being given some kind of information about adhesions before surgery and only 46% were given information on anti-adhesion agents. However, in procedures not involving adhesiolysis only 10% of patients reported receiving any adhesion information and only in 6% of cases was information given on anti-adhesion agents.

Perhaps it is time for us to consider whether this is acceptable practice?

Considering laparoscopic surgery, tissue damage to underlying structures has been shown to be the commonest cause of successful surgical negligence suits[57] and it is estimated that there is a risk of bowel injury in 10–25% of laparoscopic adhesiolysis cases[58] and a 19% risk of inadvertent enterotomy during re-operative laparotomy.[8] Moreover, in a study of misadventure data following laparoscopic surgery, while injury to the common bile duct was the most frequent, perforation of the small bowel or colon was the second most common injury and two-thirds of injuries were initially missed and not recognised until after conclusion of the surgical procedure.[59] Risk of damage was greater when there were difficulties visualising structures – which can be a common issue with adhesions.

In an analysis of medicolegal claims,[53] the most common reasons cited were:
1. Failure to diagnose adhesion-related problems.
2. Delay in diagnosis.
3. Bowel damage at adhesiolysis – laparoscopy > laparotomy.
4. Infertility or risk of infertility.
5. Starch granuloma (use of starch-powdered gloves).
6. Failure to take precautions to prevent adhesions.

In the period 1994–1999, the UK Medical Defence Union received 77 adhesion-related claims and there were out-of-court settlements in 14 cases in 11 years ranging from £7,960 to £124,261 – an average £50,765 per case.[53] And that was up until 1999!

Since 1999, evidence on the epidemiological and economic burden of adhesions and their risk to patients has expanded considerably,[8,12-15,22,52,58] and it is clear from recent work by SCAR2[15] that there has been little change in the epidemiology of adhesions even with advances in our surgical techniques: in some instances, surprisingly, laparoscopic surgery appears to be as adhesiogenic as open surgery – if not more so.[15]

Since 1999, there have been important advances in both scientific evidence and our practical knowledge of using anti-adhesion agents. Not all of them are difficult or costly to use and there is promising evidence of efficacy not only in reduction of adhesions but in subsequent outcomes and considerable work is on-going.

This author suggests that the time has come when we as operating surgeons need to discuss adhesions with our patients and actively seek to use an anti-adhesion agent, at least in what we know are adhesiogenic procedures (Table 2). Not to do so may lead us to be considered negligent.

If we were the patient what might we reasonably expect?

Until recently, English courts have generally adopted the standard of accepted medical practice based on the 'Bolam test' of negligence – that practitioners are not negligent if they act in accordance with practice accepted by a responsible body of medical opinion. However, recent judgements in both English and Australian courts suggest that judges are moving away from accepting what 'reasonable doctors' might do to supporting what 'reasonable patients' might expect. This is something we as surgeons need to seriously consider in light of increased evidence of the risks of postoperative adhesions and the availability of approved anti-adhesion agents. It is also something we need to ensure hospital management and budget holders are alerted to.

References

1 Menzies D, Ellis H. Intestinal obstruction from adhesions - how big is the problem? Ann R Coll Surg Engl 1990; 72: 60–63
2 Holmdahl L, Risberg B, Beck DE et al. Pathogenesis and prevention – panel discussion and summary. Eur J Surg 1997; 163: 54–62
3 Rapkin AJ. Adhesions and pelvic pain: a retrospective study. Obstet Gynecol 1986; 68: 13–15
4 Menzies D. Postoperative adhesions: their treatment and relevance in clinical practice. Ann R Coll Surg Engl 1993; 75: 147–153
5 Hershlag A, Diamond MP, DeCherney AH. Adhesiolysis. Clin Obstet Gynaecol 1991; 34: 395–402
6 Mishell DR, Davajan V. Evaluation of the infertile couple. In: Mishell DR, Davajan V, Lobo RA. (eds) Infertility Contraception & Reproductive Endocrinology, 3rd edn. Massachusetts: Blackwell, chapter 26
7 Coleman MG, McLain AD, Moran BJ. Impact of previous surgery on time taken for incision and division of adhesions during laparotomy. Dis Colon Rectum 2000; 43: 1297–1299

8 Van Der Krabben AA, Dijkstra FR, Nieuwenhuijzen M *et al.* Morbidity and mortality of inadvertent enterotomy during adhesiotomy. Br J Surg 2000; 87: 467–471

9 Diamond MP. Prevention of adhesions. In: Sciarra J. (ed) Gynecology and Obstetrics. Philadelphia: Harper & Row, 1988; 211–222

10 Holmdahl L, Risberg B. Adhesions: prevention and complications in general surgery. Eur J Surg 1997; 163: 169–174

11 Menzies D. Peritoneal adhesions. Incidence, cause and prevention. Ann Surg 1992; 24: 29–45

12 Ellis H, Moran BJ, Thompson JN *et al.* Adhesion-related hospital readmissions after abdominal and pelvic surgery: a retrospective cohort study. Lancet 1999; 353: 1476–1480

13 Parker MC, Ellis H, Moran BJ *et al.* Postoperative adhesions: ten-year follow-up of 12,584 patients undergoing lower abdominal surgery. Dis Colon Rectum 2001; 44: 822–830

14 Lower AM, Hawthorn RJS, Ellis H *et al.* The impact of adhesions on hospital readmissions over ten years after 8489 open gynaecological operations: an assessment from the Surgical and Clinical Adhesions Research Study. Br J Obstet Gynaecol 2000; 107: 855–862

15 Lower AM, Hawthorn RJS, Clark D *et al.* Adhesion-related readmissions following gynaecological laparoscopy or gynaecological laparotomy in Scotland. An epidemiological study of 24,046 patients. Hum Reprod 2003; 18: 53–54

16 Meagher AP, Moller C, Hoffmann DC. Non-operative treatment of small bowel obstruction following appendicectomy or operation on the ovary or tube. Br J Surg 1993; 80: 1310–1311

17 Wiseman D. Polymers for the prevention of surgical adhesions. In: Domb AJ. (ed) Polymeric Site-specific Pharmacotherapy. New York: John Wiley, 1994; 370–421

18 Ellis H. The causes and prevention of intestinal adhesions. Br J Surg 1982; 69: 241–243

19 Ellis H. Prevention and treatment of adhesions. Infect Surg 1983; November: 803–807

20 Haney AF, Doty E. The formation of coalescing peritoneal adhesions requires injury to both contacting peritoneal surfaces. Fertil Steril 1994; 61: 767–775

21 Lamont PM, Menzies D, Ellis H. Intra-abdominal adhesion formation between two adjacent deperitonealised surfaces. Surg Res Commun 1992; 13: 127–130

22 Holmdahl L. Making and covering surgical footprints. Lancet 1999; 353: 1456–1457

23 Monk BJ, Berman ML, Monitz FJ. Adhesions after extensive gynaecological surgery: clinical significance, etiology and prevention. Am J Obstet Gynecol 1994; 170: 1396–1403

24 Risberg B. Adhesions: preventive strategies. Eur J Surg 1997; 163 (Suppl 577): 32–39

25 diZerega GS. Contemporary adhesion prevention. Fertil Steril 1994; 61: 219–235

26 Interceed (TC7) Adhesion Barrier Study Group. Prevention of postsurgical adhesions by Interceed, an absorbable adhesion barrier: a prospective randomised multicentre clinical study. Fertil Steril 1989; 51: 933–938

27 Sawada T, Nishizawa H, Nishio E, Kadowaki M. Postoperative adhesion prevention with an oxidized regenerated cellulose adhesion barrier in infertile women. J Reprod Med 2000; 45: 387–389

28 Diamond MP and the Seprafilm Study Group. Reduction of adhesions after uterine myomectomy by Seprafilm membrane (HAL-F): a blinded, prospective, randomised, multicentre clinical study. Fertil Steril 1996; 66: 904–910

29 Becker JM, Dayton MT, Fazio VW *et al.* Prevention of postoperative abdominal adhesions by a sodium hyaluronate-based bioresorbable membrane: a prospective, randomized, double-blind multicenter study. J Am Coll Surg 1996; 183: 297–306

30 van Goor H on behalf of the Adhesions Study Group Steering Committee. First results of a prospective randomised multicentre controlled study of the safety of Seprafilm adhesion barrier in abdominopelvic surgery. PAX VIth International Symposium on Peritoneum, Amsterdam, 2003

31 Beck DE, Cohen Z, Fleshman JW, Kaufman HS, vanGoor H, Wolff BG. Prospective, randomized, multicentre, controlled study of the safety of Seprafilm adhesion barrier in abdominopelvic surgery. Dis Colon Rectum 2003; In press

32 Johns DB, Keyport GM, Hoehler F, diZerega GS Intergel Adhesions Prevention Study Group. Reduction of postsurgical adhesions with Intergel adhesion prevention solution: a multicenter study of safety and efficacy after conservative gynecologic surgery. Fertil Steril 2001; 76: 595–604

33 Lundroff P, van Geldorp H, Tronstad SE *et al*. Reduction of post-surgical adhesions with ferric hyaluronate gel: a European Study. Hum Reprod 2001; 16: 1982–1988

34 Mettler L, Audebert A, Lehmann-Willenbrock E *et al*. A prospective clinical trial of SprayGel as a barrier to adhesion formation: interim analysis. In: Bruhat M, Silva Carvalho JL, Campo R *et al*. (eds) Proceedings of the 10th Congress of the European Society for Gynaecological Endoscopy. Bologna, Italy: Monduzzi, 2001; 223–228

35 Johns DA, Ferland R. Initial feasibility study of a sprayable hydrogel adhesion barrier system in patients undergoing laparoscopic ovarian surgery. Fertil Steril 2002; 77: S21–S22

36 Gauwerky JFH, Heinrich D, Kubli F. Complications of intraperitoneal dextran application for prevention of adhesions. Biol Res Pregnancy 1986; 7: 93–97

37 Rosenberg SM, Board JA. High molecular weight dextran in human infertility surgery. Am J Obstet Gynecol 1984; 148: 380–385

38 Wiseman DM, Trout JR, Diamond MP. The rates of adhesion development and the effects of crystalloid solutions on adhesion development in pelvic surgery. Fertil Steril 1998; 70: 702–711

39 Shear L, Swartz C, Shinaberger J *et al*. Kinetics of peritoneal fluid absorption in adult man. N Engl J Med 1965; 272: 123–127

40 Hart R, Magos A. Laparoscopically instilled fluid: the rate of absorption and the effects on patient discomfort and fluid balance. Gynaecol Endosc 1996; 5: 287–291

41 Hosie K, Gilbert JA, Kerr D *et al*. Fluid dynamics in man of an intraperitoneal drug delivery solution: 4% icodextrin. Drug Delivery 2001; 8: 9–12

42 Verco SJS, Peers EM, Brown CB *et al*. Development of a novel glucose polymer solution (icodextrin) for adhesion prevention: pre-clinical studies. Hum Reprod 2000; 15: 1764–1772

43 Rodgers KE, Verco SJS, diZerega GS. Effects of intraperitoneal 4% icodextrin solution on the healing of bowel anastomoses and laparotomy incisions in rabbits. Colorect Dis 2003; 5: 324–330

44 diZerega GA, Verco SJS, Young P *et al*. A randomized, controlled pilot study of the safety and efficacy of 4% icodextrin solution (Adept®) in the reduction of adhesions following laparoscopic gynaecological surgery. Hum Reprod 2002; 17: 1031–1038

45 Sutton C, Menzies DM, Pouly JL *et al*. European experience with icodextrin 4% solution in routine surgical practice. 1st European Endoscopic Surgery Week, Glasgow, 15–18 June 2003

46 Menzies D, Parker MC, Sutton C *et al*. European experience with icodextrin 4% solution in routine surgical practice. European Council of Coloproctology 9th Biennial Congress, Athens, May 31–June 4 2003

47 Menzies D, Ellis H. The role of plasminogen activator in adhesion prevention. Surg Gynecol Obstet 1991; 172: 362–366

48 Parker MC on behalf of the SCAR Study Steering Group. The economic and practical implications of adhesive small bowel disease. ASCRS and Tripartite Meeting Symposium: Adhesive Small Bowel Obstruction Following Colon and Rectal Surgery: Can we do better? May 3 1999, Abstract

49 Fox Ray N, Denton WG, Tharner M, Henderson SC, Perry S. Abdominal adhesiolysis: inpatient care and expenditure in the United States in 1994. Ann Coll Surg 1998; 186: 1–9

50 Wilson MS, Menzies D, Knight AD, Crowe AM. Demonstrating the clinical and cost effectiveness of adhesion reduction strategies. Colorect Dis 2002; 4: 355–360

51 Ellis H. The magnitude of adhesion-related problems. Ann Chir Gynaecol 1998; 87: 9–11

52 Menzies D, Parker M, Hoare R, Knight AD. Small bowel obstruction due to postoperative adhesions: treatment patterns and associated costs in 110 hospital admissions. Ann R Coll Surg Engl 2001; 83: 40–46

53 Ellis H. Medico-legal consequences of postoperative intra-abdominal adhesions. J R Soc Med 2001; 94: 331–332

54 Skene L, Smallwood R. Informed consent: lessons from Australia. BMJ 2002; 324: 39–41

55 Nash G, Pullen A. Are current surgical trainees preventing future adhesions complications? Adhesions News & Views 2002; 2: 12

56 Wiseman D. Adhesions and informed consent: patients' awareness of adhesions prior to surgery. VIth International Symposium on Peritoneum (PAX), Amsterdam 2003. PAX Abstracts pp 21: VIII(4)

57 Pownall M. Tissue damage is commonest cause of surgical negligence suits. BMJ 1999; 318: 692

58 Swank DJ, Swank-Borderwijk SCG, Hop WCJ *et al*. Laparoscopic adhesiolysis in patients with chronic abdominal pain: a blinded controlled multi-centre trail. Lancet 2003; 361: 1247–1251

59 Ferriman A. Laparoscopic surgery: two-thirds of injuries initially missed. BMJ 2000; 321: 784

60 Bolam vs Freirn Barnet Hospital Management Committee [1957] 1 WLR 582; [1957]2 All ER 118 (QBD)

61 Skene L, Smallwood R. Informed consent: lessons from Australia. BMJ 2002; 324: 39–41

Olanrewaju O. Sorinola Roksana Begum

Ureteric injuries during gynaecological surgery

From a historical viewpoint, since the earliest recorded ureteric injury repairs of Berard in 1841 and Simon in 1869,[1] the subject of ureteric injury and repair has stimulated the concern of pelvic surgeons. The importance of the ureters in the management of gynaecological disease has always been recognised, as gynaecological disease can involve the ureters directly or can cause the course of the ureters to deviate. The anatomical proximity of the female urinary and genital tracts makes injury to the ureters a constant threat during gynaecological surgery. It is one of the most serious complications of a major gynaecological procedure with incidence varying from 0.4–2.5% as reported in different studies for benign conditions,[2-4] but it can be as high as 30% in operations for malignancies.[5] About 75% of ureteric injuries occur during an abdominal gynaecological procedure with incidence of 0.5–1% for abdominal hysterectomy compared with 0.1% for vaginal hysterectomy. This difference is primarily due to the fact that an abdominal hysterectomy is often done in patients with extensive disease adjacent to the ureters, which places them at greater risk; in vaginal hysterectomy, unless there is complete procidentia, there is usually no distortion of the anatomy of the lower ureter.

Ureteric trauma can easily be missed, particularly when unilateral and a high index of suspicion is necessary for early diagnosis. Only one-third of the cases are diagnosed intra-operatively. Delay in making a diagnosis can be disastrous leading to severe morbidity and even loss of renal function. Therefore, ureteric injuries are far more serious and troublesome than injury to the bladder or the rectum, the other two important sites of potential surgical

Olanrewaju O. Sorinola MBBS MRCOG MMedSci
Consultant Obstetrician and Gynaecologist and Honorary Senior Lecturer University of Warwick,
Warwick Hospital, Lakin Road, Warwick CV34 5BW, UK
(for correspondence, E-mail: lanre.sorinola@swh.nhs.uk)

Roksana Begum MBBS MRCOG
Staff Grade, Warwick Hospital, Lakin Road, Warwick CV34 5BW, UK

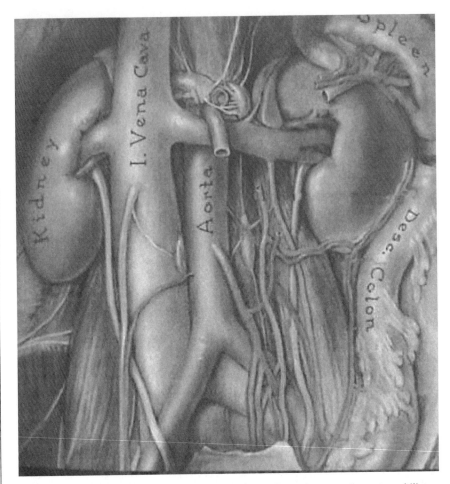

Fig. 1 The right ureter lying on the psoas muscle and crossing over the external iliac vessels to enter the pelvis.

trauma during pelvic surgery. Although ureteric injuries can occur with colorectal surgery for cancer and inflammatory bowel disease, with appendicectomy, with iliac endarterectomy, and with procedures done by urological surgeons, about 75% of injuries result from gynaecological operations.[1] Injuries to the urinary tract (especially the ureter) during operations represent the most common reason for medicolegal action against gynaecological surgeons.

ANATOMICAL CONSIDERATIONS

All gynaecologists should be familiar with the anatomical features of the ureter and the sites where it is susceptible to injuries. The ureter is composed of three anatomical layers: (i) the transitional epithelium lining the lumen; (ii) the smooth muscle comprising of longitudinal, circular and spiral fibres providing regular and efficient peristaltic waves; and (iii) the adventitial sheath containing and protecting the blood vessels.

Each ureter is about 25-30 cm in length and traverses retroperitoneally from renal pelvis to the bladder. Anatomically, the two major components, abdominal and pelvic ureters, are almost equal in length, 12–15 cm each. The abdominal portions lie on the anterior surface of the psoas muscle, descending posterolaterally as they cross over the iliac vessels to the pelvic inlet (Fig. 1). They are crossed anteriorly by the ovarian vessels as they approach the pelvis. The right ureter is located to the right of the lower part of the inferior vena cava and enters the pelvis by crossing over the external iliac artery. The left ureter lies posterior to the left colic vessels and passes posterior to the sigmoid mesocolon and enters the pelvis by crossing over the common iliac artery.

Within the pelvis, each ureter lies in loose areolar tissue on the lateral wall close to the internal iliac artery in front of the sacroiliac joint. In normal pelvis, the ureter can usually be visualised throughout its course beneath the peritoneum along the lateral wall of the true pelvis until it disappears beneath the uterine vessels (Fig. 2) and into the tunnel through the cardinal ligament before entering the bladder. Ureteral peristalsis can be seen through the peritoneum on the pelvic sidewall and can be stimulated by simply stroking it longitudinally along its course. The ureter passes beneath the uterine artery about 1.5 cm lateral to the cervix at the level of the internal os. It passes medially over the anterior vaginal fornix before entering the wall of the

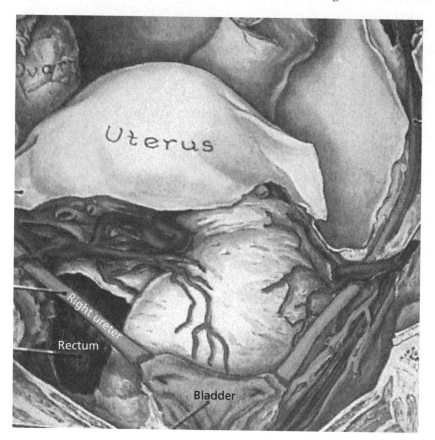

Fig. 2 The ureters passing beneath the uterine vessels.

bladder, just above the trigone. This angulation is often referred to as the 'knee of the ureter' and the lowest 1–2 cm can sometimes be palpable bimanually through the vagina.

The ureter has blood supply from multiple sources, which gives it preferential healing capabilities following injury. The upper segment of the ureter has a freely anastomosing arterial network with branches from renal and ovarian arteries. The middle segment derives its blood supply directly from aortic branches and the common iliac artery, while the pelvic ureter has branches from the uterine, vaginal, middle haemorrhoidal, vesical, and hypogastric arteries. Care must be taken during dissection to prevent injury to the blood supply. As the blood supply to the upper and middle portions of the ureter is from its medial side, ureteric exploration is best done from the lateral margin; whereas the blood supply to the pelvic ureter is principally from the lateral side, therefore dissection should be along its medial side.

Anatomical locations of ureteric injury

Unilateral ureteric injury is more common with bilateral injury occurring in only 5–10% of cases. The earliest anatomical descriptions of the ureter emphasised that the left ureter was often closer to the cervix than the right and some studies have also shown a predominance of left-sided injuries.[6–8] However, as shown by the classic study of Sampson,[9] the proximity of the ureter to either side of the cervix can vary considerably with the position of the uterus in the pelvis, even in the absence of pathology and injury to either ureter is just as common.

The ureter is vulnerable to injury at the following sites in the pelvis:
1. *At the pelvic brim during ligation of the infundibulopelvic ligament as the ureters lie beneath the insertion of the ligament.*
2. *At the base of the broad ligament, where the ureter passes beneath the uterine artery (Fig. 2).*
3. *Beyond the uterine vessels as the ureter passes through its tunnel in the cardinal ligament at the level of the internal cervical os.*
4. *At the anterolateral fornix of the vagina as the ureter enters the bladder (i.e. the intramural portion near the insertion into the trigone).*
5. *Along the course of the ureter on the lateral pelvic sidewall just above the uterosacral ligament.*
6. *Lateral pelvic sidewall over the iliac vessels during lymph node dissection.*

Authors vary as to whether the commonest site of injury is at the pelvic brim in the area of the infundibulopelvic ligament[6] or in the distal ureter during ligation of the uterine arteries.[1,3,7,10,11] The consensus is that distal ureter injury is commoner but, as already discussed above, the ureter can be injured at any of the listed locations.

TYPES AND CAUSE OF INJURY

Intra-operative injury to the ureter may result from:
1. Ligation with suture.
2. Crushing from misapplication of a clamp.

Table 1 Gynaecological procedures associated with ureteric injury

Abdominal	Vaginal	Laparoscopic
Hysterectomy	Hysterectomy	Division of adhesions
Wertheim's hysterectomy	Anterior colporrhaphy	Transection of uterosacral ligaments
Oophorectomy	Cervical biopsy	Colposuspension
Uterine suspension	Vesicovaginal fistula repair	Treatment of endometriosis
Burch colposuspension		Sterilisation (especially electrocoagulation)
Vesicovaginal fistula repair		

3. Transection (partial or complete).
4. Angulation with secondary obstruction (partial or complete).
5. Ischaemia – risk of injury from diathermy applied to bleeding points. There is also a risk of avascular necrosis if the peri-ureteric tissues carrying the blood supply are stripped or diathermised.
6. Resection of a segment of the ureter, usually intentional during an extensive operation for a malignant disease.
7. Electrical, thermal, or laser energy, or from the linear stapler during laparoscopic surgery.

Combinations of the above injuries can occur during a procedure. Table 1 lists the different gynaecological procedures associated with ureteric injury.

Factors predisposing to ureteric injury

In most patients, no identifiable risk factors are found. However, any condition disrupting the normal anatomy of the ureter increases the likelihood of injury, *e.g.* large ovarian masses, fibroids (including broad ligament fibroids), endometriosis, and pelvic inflammatory disease. Other risk factors are previous pelvic surgery, history of pelvic irradiation, and, less commonly, congenital abnormalities such as ureteric duplication, mega-ureter, and ectopic ureter or kidney. About 1% of women have duplications of the ureter, usually unilateral. The surgeon should keep in mind the possibility of ureteric duplication on one or both sides of the pelvis. If one ureter is identified on one pelvic sidewall, it cannot be assumed that it is the only one present.

Two large retrospective studies[11,12] reviewed the incidence of ureteric injuries and its associated risk factors. Significantly, pelvic malignancies were present in 44% of the cases with ureteric injury. The authors concluded that this was most likely due to dense adhesions, large masses displacing the ureter, and anatomical changes distorting the course of the ureter. However, it is noteworthy that half of all the ureteric injuries had no identifiable risk factors and occurs in the so called 'simple' hysterectomy.[11]

PREVENTION OF URETERIC INJURY

The most important aspect of ureteric injury is primary prevention (*i.e.* prevention of the injury before it occurs). Provided the gynaecological surgeon understands the anatomy of the ureter and how the ureter is involved in gynaecological disease and gynaecological surgery, prevention of ureteric injuries should not be a difficult task in most operations. Primary prevention of ureteric injury begins pre-operatively with a careful evaluation of the patient's gynaecological disease and recognition of the risk to the ureter with the surgical procedure planned.[13] Second, by using the skills described in the following sections, most ureteric injuries can be prevented. However, even the most skilful gynaecological surgeon will injure the ureter inadvertently, but on rare occasions.

Abdominopelvic surgery

An important axiom in all surgical procedures is that an adequate incision must be made so that proper exposure can be accomplished. Exposure of important structures in the pelvis should not be limited by a limited incision. Primary prevention includes first and foremost the surgeon's cognisance of the risk of ureteric injury throughout the entire pelvic dissection. A sound knowledge of abdominal and pelvic anatomy is the most important factor in reducing the incidence of ureteric injury especially in those areas where the ureter is most susceptible to injury.

Simple measures such as: (i) tracing of the ureters if at any doubt before clamping tissues (*e.g.* by opening the peritoneum lateral to the infundibulopelvic ligament and identifying the ureter on the medial leaf of the peritoneum); (ii) adequate mobilisation of the bladder during hysterectomy; (iii) avoidance of blind clamping for haemostasis; and (iv) the use of the intrafascial technique for hysterectomy in benign pelvic disease can prevent injuries in many cases.[14]

A simple manoeuvre that facilitates the identification of the ureter involves the following steps:

1. Divide the round ligament near the lateral pelvic side wall, then open the lateral peritoneum 10-15 cm in a cephalad direction.

2. Place an index finger on the external iliac artery, which can easily be identified from its superficial, consistent anatomical position and pulsating characteristic.

3. By moving the finger upward (cephalad), the first structure to be exposed, crossing and in contact with the iliac artery, will be the ureter.

4. As the index finger is placed on the ureter, the infundibulopelvic ligament should be behind the middle phalanx and can be safely clamped with the ureter clearly visualised. Remember the distance between the infundibulo-pelvic ligament clamps and the ureter may be only 1 cm or less.

5. The ureter is then followed towards the cardinal ligament, where it passes under the uterine artery. It is gently pushed laterally and downward, moving it away from the cervix and with traction on the uterus to expose the uterine artery, the ureter is protected when the uterine arteries are ligated.

Another axiom in surgery is that important structures in the operative field that are at risk of injury should always be dissected sufficiently to allow their

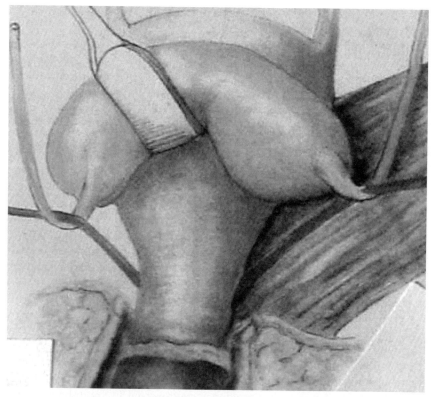

Fig. 3 The need to develop adequate vesico-uterine space during vaginal hysterectomy due to the closeness of the ureters.

identification and retraction out of harm's way throughout the operation. Although dissection or mobilisation of the ureters may not be always be indicated, the ureters should be clearly identified in the pelvis particularly in areas where it is most susceptible to injury. However, endometriosis and/or pelvic inflammatory disease may disfigure the region where the ureter crosses the uterine artery at the midplane of the pelvis, while large broad ligament or cervical leiomyomas may obscure the operative field, making the dissection extremely difficult. The gynaecological surgeon has to be mindful of these areas during surgery.

Vaginal surgery

The key in vaginal hysterectomy is to develop an adequate vesico-uterine space to protect the ureters from injury by surgical clamps and sutures (Fig. 3). This is achieved by downward traction on the cervix and counter traction upward beneath the bladder. The ureters can be palpated by applying gentle traction on the cervix, combined with upward traction on the upper vagina exposing the entry point of the ureter into the trigone. It is crucial to clamp, cut, and ligate only small bites of paracervical and parametrial tissue adjacent to the uterus thereby ensuring that the ureters stay safely away from the operative field. In posterior culdoplasty, sutures placed in the uterosacral ligaments to support the vaginal apex after the uterus is removed can kink or obstruct the ureters if not done carefully.

The key in anterior colporrhaphy is not to start too laterally or to insert sutures too deeply to prevent needle injury to the ureters while plicating the bladder. During anterior colporrhaphy the distance between the ureter and the surgeon's needle in the upper third of the vagina is only about 0.9 cm, as shown by Hofmeister[15] using fluoroscopic imaging.

Laparoscopic surgery

Primary prevention of ureteric injury with operative laparoscopy involves many of the principles mentioned earlier. If the ureter cannot be visualised, retroperitoneal dissection to locate the ureter will help to decrease the incidence of injury and help to make the diagnosis promptly if an injury occurs. Electrocoagulation of bleeding points around the uterosacral ligaments is especially risky and might better be done with sutures or clips. In laparoscopic-assisted hysterectomy, a stapler is applied across the uterine artery and the cardinal ligaments. Sometimes the width and length of the stapler makes safe application difficult and these pedicles are better ligated vaginally.

Other preventive measures

Ureteric stent

Some surgeons perform pre-operative ureteric stent placement if a difficult surgery is anticipated. The benefit of the procedure is controversial. In a retrospective study by Kuno et al.,[16] prophylactic ureteric catheterisation was not found to statistically affect the rate of injury in their cases. Bothwell et al.[17] found a 1% risk of iatrogenic injury to the ureter and mentioned that catheters do not prevent the incidence of ureteric injury; however, catheters may aid in intra-operative detection of ureteric injury. Lighted ureteric stents has become very popular in advanced laparoscopic surgery.[18] These allow visualisation of the ureter, but are of limited value in the presence of masses and dense adhesions.

Imaging

Pre-operative imaging using an IVP or contrast-enhanced computed tomo-graphy if distorted anatomy is anticipated or previous urinary tract compromise is suspected has been advocated by some surgeons. Piscitelli et al.[19] retrospectively reviewed 493 cases of hysterectomy for benign disease, 299 (60%) of whom received a pre-operative IVP routinely; 77 patients (27%) had abnormal findings. The IVP findings commonly associated with abnormality were uterine size of 12 weeks or greater or an adnexal mass of 4 cm or larger. One can argue that these findings can be elicited on pelvic examination, helping to direct which patients should undergo pre-operative imaging rather than as a routine. Endometriosis, pelvic inflammatory disease, uterovaginal prolapse and previous intra-abdominal surgery were not associated with an increased prevalence of abnormal IVP findings. The incidence of ureteric injuries in the IVP group and the non-IVP group was not significant in their study. Though there is no proof that a pre-operative IVP reduces the risk of ureteric injury, many surgeons feel that pre-operative knowledge of the lower urinary tract anatomy helps to avoid such injuries. However, this has to be balanced against the cost of pre-operative IVP and the fact that a normal pre-operative IVP does not dispel the surgeon's responsibility to dissect and identify the ureters in all pelvic operations.

DIAGNOSIS

It is important to keep in mind the timeless statement of Higgins that has benefited so many pelvic surgeons: 'the venial sin is injury to the ureter; the moral sin is failure of recognition'. Secondary prevention involves recognition of the ureteric injury during the operation so that immediate repair can take place and reduce serious postoperative morbidity and loss of kidney function. Unfortunately, only one-third of ureteric injuries are still recognised intra-operatively.

INTRA-OPERATIVE

Any suspicion of ureteric injury during operation should be clarified and dealt with intra-operatively. The surgeon must promptly identify the ureter and evaluate the nature and severity of the injury. Proximal ureter may be dilated if it is obstructed distally. Dye test with intravenous phenazopyridine HCl (pyridium), indigo carmine or methylene blue (about 5 ml) can be used to demonstrate urinary extravasation more clearly (within 3–5 min) and identify the location of the ureteric injury. Presence of peristalsis does not always guarantee full viability, as avascular necrosis may be evident later. Other surgeons advocate the use of fluorescein or Wood's lamp if devascularisation is suspected.[2]

Some surgeons perform intra-operative cystoscopy after a high-risk urogynaecological or pelvic reconstructive surgery. There is no consensus whether cystoscopy should be performed after all gynaecological surgery. In a review article by Gilmour et al.,[20] the incidence of ureteric injury was found to be higher in eight studies where routine intra-operative cystoscopy with or without dye test was performed. Up to 90% of unsuspected ureteric injuries were identified intra-operatively and repaired successfully in these studies. While there is no doubt that cystoscopy along with dye test is justified whenever there is any concern of ureteric damage, cystoscopy has the disadvantages of increased operating time with extra training and skills required. Also, routine cystoscopy does not guarantee recognition of all of ureteric injuries as non-obstructive, partially obstructive or late injuries secondary to ischaemia and avascular necrosis can be missed.

Recently, some authors have been exploring the diagnostic potential of peri-operative ultrasound using a laparoscopic ultrasound probe.[21] In a small animal and human study involving six animal and four human ureters, they found that if ureteric diameter in peri-operative ultrasonography exceeds 3.0 mm or if no peristaltic activity is visible during 5 min of follow-up, or if a clear echodense caudally progressing contraction segments are absent, ureteric complication should be suspected. However, this was quite a small study, plus the need for a laparoscopic USS probe and the small variations of ureteric diameters makes the clinical application of this study doubtful for now.

Table 2 Symptoms and signs of ureteric injury

Symptoms	Time of presentation
Loin or flank pain	0–21 days
Fever	0–21 days
Adynamic ileus/peritonitis	0–7 days
Fistulas	0–30 days
Lower abdominal/pelvic mass	20–40 days
Anuria (if bilateral)	< 24 h
Asymptomatic	Incidental finding

Postoperative

Approximately two-thirds of the cases are diagnosed postoperatively. The clinical presentations are listed in Table 2.

Ureteric trauma can easily be missed, particularly in the case of unilateral injury.[4] If the contralateral kidney is healthy, it will compensate for the loss with only a transient rise in serum creatinine. Eventually, the affected kidney will lose its function. The patients may complain of loin pain due to hydronephrosis. Pyrexia is common. A urinary fistula may arise at any time during the first 4 weeks after the operation communicating with any nearby structure (ureterovaginal/uretero-uterine) or with the skin (ureterocutaneous).

If the urine is unable to escape, it will accumulate as a localised urinoma, which can present as abdominal distension, swinging pyrexia, or urinary ascites with ileus or peritonitis. Anuria develops in cases of bilateral ureteric obstruction (5–10% cases are bilateral). It is, however, important to remember that unilateral ureteric injury can be asymptomatic. Early postoperative diagnosis of ureteric injury typically takes place 7–10 days after surgery. However, the non-specific presentation sometimes means a delay in diagnosis, Dowling *et al.*[22] reported a mean delay of 10–21 days in almost two-thirds of cases.

Table 3 Investigations of ureteric injury

White cell count
Urea and electrolytes
Intravenous pyelogram (IVP)
     Hydronephrosis
     Delayed function
     Non-visualisation
     Extravasation
     Urinoma
     Stricture
Retrograde/antegrade ureterogram/nephrostogram (Fig. 4)
     Extravasation
     Fistula
     Obstruction
Ultrasound of abdomen and pelvis (Fig. 5)
CT scanning (with or without contrast)
Fistulogram/double dye test
Cystoscopy
Fluid analysis from drains, ascitic collection

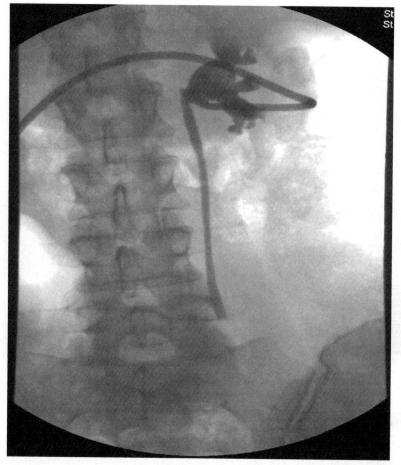

Fig. 4 Nephrostogram (PA view) showing dye in the nephrostomy tube and the right ureter down to the pelvic brim (at the level of the sacroiliac joint, junction of the middle and distal third of the ureter) but not beyond.

Investigations

The main diagnostic investigations are summarised in Table 3. Postoperatively, there is usually leukocytosis, there may be a slight rise in creatinine level in unilateral obstruction, but uraemia is seen more in bilateral obstruction. IVP is the mainstay of diagnoses postoperatively, which may show hydronephrosis, hydroureter, delayed function or extravasation. It may be normal in as many as 7% of cases.[2] Nephrostogram (Fig. 4) or retrograde ureterogram may provide further useful information. Transabdominal ultrasound or CT scanning may show hydronephrosis, urinoma or ascites. The ureter affected by the injury can also be identified by cystoscopy. As a rule, the ureteric orifice will not spurt urine on the affected side. With fistula, a double dye test is done with methylene blue in the bladder and phenazopyridine HCl (Pyridium) intravenously. An orange-stained swab in the vagina confirms the fistula is ureterovaginal, while a blue-stained swab confirms a vesicovaginal fistula. Biochemical analysis of the fluid will confirm the presence of urine in cases of urinoma or ureterocutaneous fistulas.

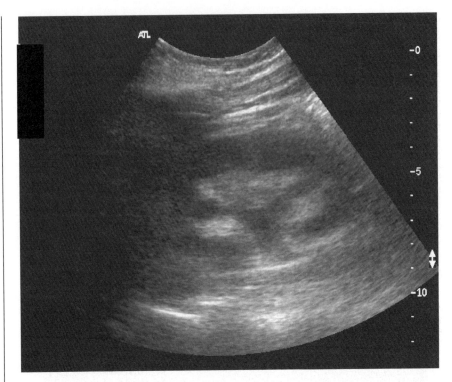

Fig. 5 Abdominal USS showing moderate right renal hydronephrosis.

MANAGEMENT

The aims of treatment are preservation of renal function and restoration of anatomical continuity. The approach to ureteric repair depends on the cause, location/extent of injury, and the time at which it is recognised. If the injury goes unrecognised, the following are the possible sequelae:

1. Spontaneous resolution and healing when injury is minimal.
2. Hydronephrosis (Fig. 5) and gradual loss of renal function in complete obstruction.
3. Urinoma/urinary ascites ± infection in ureteric transection or necrosis with urinary extravasation.
4. Fistula formation: ureterovaginal/uretero-uterine or ureterocutaneous
5. Stenosis at the site of injury or of the fistula tract with insidious loss of renal function.

Intra-operative period

Minor injury diagnosed intra-operatively is best managed by suturing, deligation or ureteric stent placements. The stents stay in place for 3–6 weeks, and are then removed by flexible cystoscopy (Fig. 6) followed by an IVP to confirm ureteric patency. In case of crush injury with minimal trauma, a stent only can be used. Due to risk of devascularisation, when the trauma is more extensive, the area involved is better excised and anastomosis or re-implantation of the ureter is

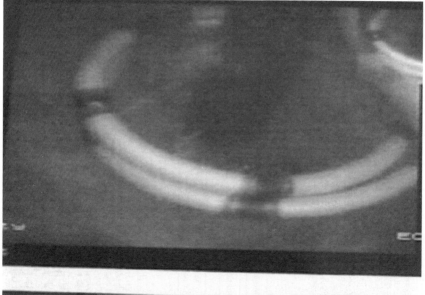

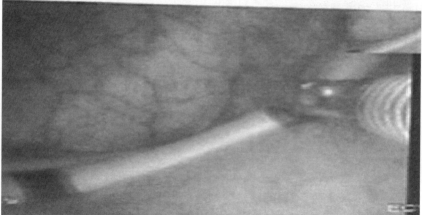

Fig. 6 A double J ureteric stent being removed by flexible cystoscopy.

performed. Major injuries diagnosed intra-operatively are managed according to the algorithm in Figure 7 with over 90% cure rate.

Postoperative period

The management strategy remains slightly controversial when ureteric injury is found in the postoperative period. The two decisions required are early versus late intervention and conservative/minimally invasive approach against an open repair.[23] Minor injuries can be managed by antegrade or retrograde stent placement which was successfully achieved in about one-third of cases in different studies.[14,24] Successful endoscopic management using stenting ± balloon dilatation requires minimal loss of ureteric segment (less than 2 cm for strictures), some continuity of the ureteric wall and early intervention (*i.e.* within 4 weeks) after the injury to achieve a cure rate of 88%.

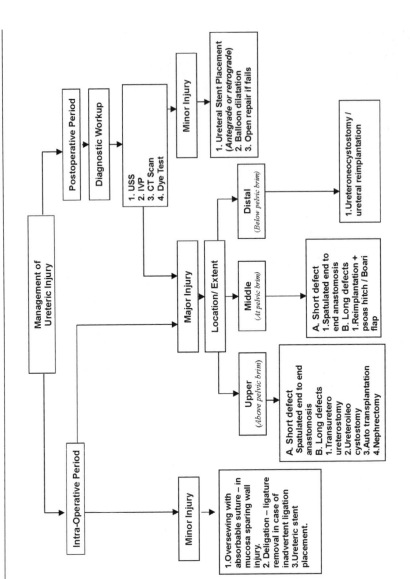

Fig. 7 Schematic flow chart of the management of ureteric injuries.

Table 4 Principles of ureteric repair

Meticulous ureteric dissection preserving ureteric sheath with its blood supply

Tension-free anastomosis by ureteric mobilisation

Use minimum amount of fine absorbable suture to attain a watertight closure

Use peritoneum or omentum to surround the anastomosis especially if the peri-ureteric tissue is rigid and fibrotic, as better healing of the repair site is achieved

Drain the anastomotic site with a closed suction drain to prevent urine accumulation

Stent the anastomotic site with a ureteric catheter

Consider a proximal diversion – diversion of the urinary stream with percutaneous nephrostomy is usually necessary if the defect is large, the ureter has been completely transected or the ureter lies in a bed of inflammation[25]

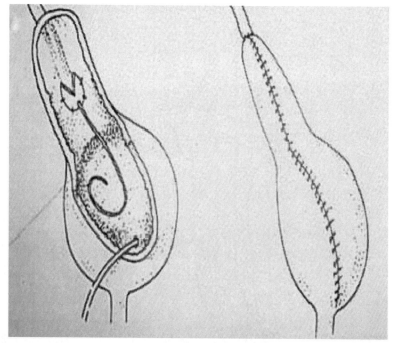

Fig. 8 Boari flap procedure – picture on left shows a flap being made from the bladder while the one on the right shows the flap sutured to end of the shortened ureter.

Major injuries

The principles guiding ureteric repair are detailed in Table 4. For most major injuries, a nephrostomy tube is commonly inserted while awaiting definitive surgery in order to preserve renal function.

In case of injury to the distal part (*i.e.* within 5 cm of the ureterovesical junction), ureteric re-implantation into the bladder is performed. The submucosal tunnel technique of ureteroneocystostomy has been found to be useful to prevent vesico-ureteric reflux, with lower risk of pyelonephritis and renal insufficiency secondary to chronic reflux and infection. However, some surgeons prefer refluxing-type ureteric anastomosis due to technical simplicity, shorter operating time, decreased risk of distal ureteric stricture and the ability to gain an additional 2–3 cm of ureteric length that would have been lost in the ureteric tunnel.[26] This coupled with the fact that the pressure system in the adult female urinary system is less than in the male makes urinary reflux less common in the adult female and submucosal tunnelling less of an issue.

Injury to the ureter in the middle part is best managed by spatulated end-to-end anastomosis to reduce the risk of stricture. For longer defects, to prevent tension at the anastomotic site, ureteroneocystostomy is performed with a Psoas hitch or a Boari flap. In the Psoas hitch technique, the principle is to mobilise the bladder and fix it to the Psoas tendon of the affected side. This bridges the gap in the ureteric length and also keeps tension off the anastomosis. In the Boari flap technique, a broad-based flap is dissected off the bladder to reach the injured ureter to be re-implanted, without tension (Fig. 8).

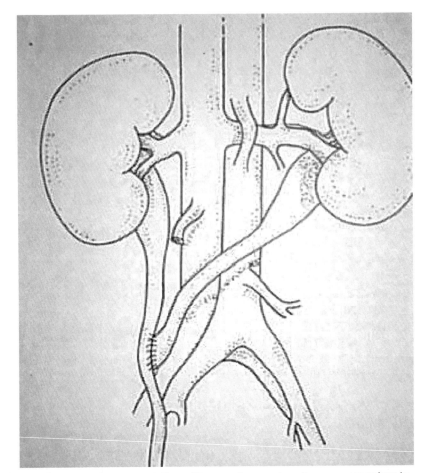

Fig. 9 Diagrammatic representation of transuretero-ureterostomy – a procedure in which a damaged ureter is anastomosed to the contralateral ureter.

In case of injuries to the upper part of the ureter (above the pelvic brim), where primary anastomosis is not possible, transuretero-ureterostomy is performed (Fig. 9). In some cases, other procedures like interposition of a length of isoperistaltic ileum or autotransplantation of the kidney into the pelvis may be necessary. Nephrectomy may be appropriate when the other renal function is normal. Patients will need regular clinical and radiological follow-up postoperatively as there is a risk of developing ureteric stricture following repair even after a year.[27]

A number of factors affect the healing of the ureter after injury and repair.[1] The ureter should always be handled gently, preferably with non-crushing clamps and forceps. Clear dissection of the ureter from its bed should be limited to that required for the operation. Unnecessary dissection should be avoided but should always be sufficient to accomplish repair without tension on the suture line. The ureter is capable of closing its own defect by regenerating its own components. Several factors will encourage uro-epithelial growth. If careful mucosa-to-mucosa approximation is done, if urinary leakage is minimal, and if there is no tension on the suture line, the defect can be bridged by new growth of transitional epithelium in less than 2 weeks. The growth of new smooth muscle across the gap will complete the repair. Resumption of peristaltic activity across the repair site is usually seen in about a month.

Fistulas and repair

Following unrecognised ureteric injury, a fistulous tract may develop between the ureter and uterus/vagina or skin. Occasionally, a fistula may stop draining spontaneously; however, this does not mean that fistula has healed. Most likely, it is due to scar formation and stenosis of the fistulous tract. It is usually necessary to relieve the obstruction to preserve renal function. In cases of ureterovaginal or uretero-uterine fistulas, stent placement with continuous bladder drainage for up to 6 weeks may be sufficient to allow healing.[28] When minimal invasive treatment fails, open repair is necessary after an interval when the local inflammation has subsided. Open repair may involve re-implantation or ureteric re-anastomosis depending on the site of injury as indicated in Figure 7. The same principles apply.

MEDICOLEGAL CONSIDERATIONS

The first step in risk management and prevention of litigation is at the initial consultation for operation. The necessity and risks associated with the procedure to be performed should be discussed in detail with the patient and properly documented in the case notes and the GP letter.

Medicolegal sequelae are increasingly becoming a major area of concern. Brudenell[29] reported a number of cases in which the legal view was of negligence on the part of the gynaecologist involved and damages in excess of £100,000 were awarded. The main issues that came out from the cases were as follows:

1. Following a straightforward hysterectomy for menorrhagia, despite following a correct procedure by pushing the bladder down so that the top of the vagina could be visualised all round, the gynaecologist was still found negligent in causing a ureteric injury. The legal view was that of misjudgement on the part of the surgeon, for not making a proper visual assessment of the position of the bladder, which would have ascertained that ureters were in a position of safety.

2. At a difficult hysterectomy due to an enlarged uterus with multiple large vascular fibroids, the ureter was injured, resulting in a ureterovaginal fistula 4 weeks later. The legal view was that there was lack of planning on the part of the consultant as he allowed his registrar to do the case and poor decision making on his part, as he did not take over the case when there was persistent bleeding. Large vascular fibroids did not constitute a sufficient explanation for the damage to the ureter.

3. Again following a 'simple' abdominal hysterectomy for menorrhagia, the ureter was ligated in its lower part, diagnosis made after 1 week, and ureter re-implanted into the bladder. The view was that obstruction would not have occurred but for error amounting to negligence on the part of the surgeon.

The legal view increasingly appears to be that most, if not all, ureteric injuries are due to negligence on the part of the gynaecologist involved. However, occasionally ureteric injury might be defensible according to Lord Denning's[30] proposal in the Court of Appeal that: 'in a professional man, an error of judgement is not necessarily negligent'. Gynaecologists should remember the view expressed by Lezen and Stotler:[31] 'that many ureteric injuries occur during difficult open dissection and may not be preventable even by the most experienced and skilled surgeons'.

To prevent litigation, any difficulty encountered during the operation including identification and visualisation of the ureters should be carefully documented in the notes. When removal of the cervix is difficult, subtotal hysterectomy may be appropriate for the patient to avoid risk of damage to the ureter.

Any suspicion of ureteric damage intra-operatively should be properly investigated and managed with expert urological assistance. Postoperatively, early investigation and diagnosis is very important as it is easier to repair and also patient morbidity is reduced. Postoperatively, patients should have follow-up with both urology and gynaecology consultants. They should be advised to report immediately in case of any symptoms in the future.

KEY POINTS FOR CLINICAL PRACTICE

- For every surgical procedure, associated benefits and risks should be discussed in details with the patient and documented properly in the notes.

- Gynaecological surgeons must have a thorough knowledge of the anatomy of the ureter and be aware of the sites where it is liable to be injured.

- Pre-operative intravenous urography or stent placement has not been shown to decrease the incidence of ureteric injuries.

- Since only one-third of the injuries are recognised intra-operatively, a high index of suspicion and early investigations are necessary for diagnosis.

- Early diagnoses and management will reduce postoperative morbidity and save renal loss.

- Timing of repair should be individualised; current studies suggest that there is no difference in outcome in early or late repair.

References

1 Thompson JD. Operative injuries to the ureter: prevention, recognition, and management. In: Thompson JD, Rock JA (eds) Te Linde's Operative Gynaecology, 8th edn. Philadelphia: Lippincott-Raven, 1997; 40: 1135–1173

2 Drake MJ, Noble JG. Ureteric trauma in gynecologic surgery. Int Urogynecol 1998; 9: 108–117

3 Brandt FT, Akbuquerque CDC, Lorenzato FR. Transperitoneal unstented ureteral reimplantation for injuries postgynecological surgery. World J Urol 2001; 19: 216–219

4 Chan JK, Morrow J, Manetta A. Prevention of ureteral injuries in gynecologic surgery. Am J Obstet Gynecol 2003; 188: 1273–1277

5 Liapis A, Bakas P, Sykiotis K, Creatsas G. Urinoma as a complication of iatrogenic ureteric injuries in gynecological surgery. Eur J Obstet Gynaecol Reprod Biol 2000; 91: 83–85

6 Meiro D, Moriel EZ, Zilberman M, Farkas A. Evaluation and treatment of iatrogenic ureteral injuries during obstetric and gynecologic operations for non-malignant conditions. J Am Coll Surg 1994; 178: 144–148

7 Mattingly RF, Borkowf HI. Acute operative injury to the lower urinary tract. Clin Obstet Gynecol 1978; 5: 123–149

8 Blandy JP, Badenoch DF, Fowler CG et al. Early repair of iatrogenic injury to the ureter or bladder after gynaecological surgery. J Urol 1991; 146: 761

9   Sampson JA. The relation between carcinoma cervicis uteri and the ureters and its significance in the more radical operations for that disease. John Hopkins Med Bull 1904; 156: 72

10 Reucken RK, Jansen AA, Bornman MS *et al*. Trauma of the ureter. S Afr J Surg 1991; 29: 154

11 Goodno JA, Powers TW, Harris VD. Ureteral injury in gynaecologic surgery: a ten-year review in a community hospital. Am J Obstet Gynecol 1995; 172: 1817–1822

12 Liapis A, Bakas P, Giannopoulos V, Creatsas G. Ureteral injuries during gynaecological surgery. Int Urogynecol J 2001; 12: 391–394

13 Smith JC. How to avoid litigation: the urologist's view. Br J Urol 1997; 80 (Suppl. 1): 33–34

14 Sakellariou P, Protopapas AG, Voulgaris Z *et al*. Management of ureteric injuries during gynaecological operations: 10 years' experience. Eur J Obstet Gynaecol Reprod Biol 2002; 101: 179–184

15 Hofmeister FJ. Pelvic anatomy of the ureter in relation to surgery performed through the vagina. Clin Obstet Gynecol 1982; 25: 821

16 Kuno K, Menzin A, Kauder HH, Sison C, Gal D. Prophylactic ureteral catheterization in gynecologic surgery. Urology 1998; 52: 1004–1008

17 Bothwell WN, Bleicher RJ, Dent TL. Prophylactic ureteral catheterization in colon surgery. Dis Colon Rectum 1994; 37: 330–334

18 Low RK, Moran ME. Laparoscopic use of the ureteral illuminator. Urology 1993; 42: 455–457

19 Piscitelli JT, Simel DL, Addison A. Who should have intravenous pyelograms before hysterectomy for benign disease? Obstet Gynecol 1987; 69: 541–545

20 Gilmour DT, Dwyer PL, Carey MP. Lower urinary tract injury during gynaecologic surgery and its detection by intraoperative cystoscopy. Obstet Gynecol 1999; 94: 883–889

21 Helin-Martikainen HL, Kirkinen P, Heino A. Ultrasonography of the ureter after surgical trauma. Surg Endosc 1998; 12: 1141–1144

22 Dowling RA, Coriere JN, Sandler CM. Iatrogenic ureteral injury. J Urol 1986; 135: 912–915

23 Aslan P, Brooks A, Drummond M, Woo H. Incidence and management of gynaecological related ureteric injuries. Aust NZ J Obstet Gynaecol 1999; 39: 178–181

24 Elabd S, Ghoniem G, Elsharaby M *et al*. Use of endoscopy in the management of postoperative ureterovaginal fistula. Int Urogynecol J 1997; 8: 185–190

25 Utrie JW. Bladder and ureteral injury: prevention and management. Clin Obstet Gynaecol 1998; 41: 755–763

26 Ahn M, Loughlin KR. Psoas hitch ureteral reimplantation in adults – analysis of a modified technique and timing of repair. Urology 2001; 58: 184–187

27 Meretyk S, Albala DM, Clayman RV, Denstedt JD, Kavoussi LR. Endoureterotomy for treatment of ureteral strictures. J Urol 1992; 147: 1502–1506

28 Chang R, Marshall FF, Mitchell S. Percutaneous management of benign ureteral strictures and fistulas. J Urol 1987; 137: 1126–1131

29 Brudenell M. Medico-legal aspects of ureteric damage during abdominal hysterectomy. Br J Obstet Gynaecol 1996; 103: 1180–1183

30 Denning in Whitehouse vs Jordan. Court of appeal judgement case No. All ER650;1980

31 Lezen MA, Stotler ML. Surgical ureteral injuries. Urology 1991; 38: 497–506

Alaa El-Ghobashy Simon Herrington

20

Cervical cancer: epidemiology and molecular characterisation

World-wide, cervical carcinoma is the second most frequent cancer in women after breast carcinoma and, therefore, presents a serious global problem.[1] However, invasive cancer of the cervix is considered to be a preventable condition, since it is associated with a long pre-invasive stage (cervical intra-epithelial neoplasia, CIN) making it amenable to screening and treatment. Despite clinical screening programmes becoming more effective, cervical cytology still has significant limitations since cytomorphological criteria are unable to predict progression to invasive cancer in an individual with a precancerous lesion.

Cervical carcinoma has epidemiological characteristics similar to those of a sexually transmitted infectious disease and, hence, a number of infectious agents have been implicated in its pathogenesis.[2] In more than 95% of cases, considerable evidence has now been gathered to implicate human papillomavirus (HPV) infection in the subsequent development of CIN and cancer.[3,4] The precise role of a cancer-associated virus is often difficult to understand because of the delay (latent phase) of many years between the initial viral infection and the development of cancer.[5]

RISK FACTORS FOR THE DEVELOPMENT OF CERVICAL NEOPLASIA

It remains unclear which factors, in addition to HPV, are important for the development of cervical carcinoma.[6] Numerous studies of the epidemiology of cervical cancer have shown strong associations with several risk factors, including smoking, oral contraceptive usage and certain nutritional

Alaa El-Ghobashy MBChB MSc MRCOG
Specialist Registrar in Obstetrics and Gynaecology, University Hospital of North Staffordshire, West Midlands, UK

Simon Herrington FRCP DPhil FRCPath
Professor of Pathology, University of St Andrews, Bute Medical School, Westburn Lane, St Andrews, Fife KY16 9TS, UK (for correspondence, E-mail: csh2@st-andrews.ac.uk)

Table 1 Risk factors for the development of cervical cancer

Sexual factors
Parity
Circumcision
Smoking
Oral contraceptives
Dietary factors
Socio-economic status
Oncogenes and tumour suppressor genes
Immunological factors
Chromosomal aberrations
Infectious agents
    Chlamydia trachomatis
    Herpes viruses
    Human immunodeficiency virus (HIV)
    Human papilloma virus (HPV)

deficiencies.[7,8] Furthermore, a number of recent studies have highlighted the need for considering male factors, since the sexual behaviour of the male appears to play an important role in determining the risk of cervical cancer in female partners (Table 1).

Sexual factors

Cervical cancer is virtually unknown in virgins and nuns and the disease is statistically more frequent in married than in unmarried women. Sexual intercourse has been implicated as a major prerequisite for the development of invasive cervical cancer. Other variables include age at first intercourse, the frequency and the number of sexual partners. Women with cervical cancer are more likely to have commenced sexual activity during adolescence[9,10] and the number of sexual partners is an important factor associated with the development of the disease.[11] Although it is difficult to obtain precise figures, several investigators have shown that increasing the number of sexual partners has the effect of increasing the risk of developing CIN and invasive disease.[12,13] Investigators reported that the risk associated with 10 or more partners is nearly 3 times higher than that associated with one partner or none.[14,15]

Recently, a UK national case-control study of cervical cancer reported a strong relation between both squamous cell and adenocarcinoma and the lifetime number of sexual partners.[16]

Parity

The role of parity in the development of cervical cancer has not yet been fully clarified. Early reports suggested that women with cervical cancer had more children than controls.[16] This association between high parity and squamous cell carcinoma of the cervix disappeared when allowance was made for the correlation between high parity and an early age at marriage. Cervical trauma and/or hormonal and nutritional changes during pregnancy and labour might play a role in cervical carcinogenesis.[17,18]

Other studies failed to report any relationship between parity and the risk of developing cervical intra-epithelial disease and cancer in high and low parity populations.[19,20]

Circumcision

Male circumcision was thought to protect women from the development of cervical cancer. However, investigations taking ethnic differences into account failed to prove an association between male circumcision and a reduced risk of the disease in women.[21]

In one study, the incidence of cervical cancer was compared in Hindu and Muslim women in India. A higher incidence was found in the former group. It was suggested that the difference was due to Muslim men, unlike Hindu men, being circumcised.[22]

A recent report revealed that only 5.5% of circumcised men harbour HPV in comparison with 19.6% of uncircumcised men. Monogamous women whose partners were circumcised had a lower risk of cervical cancer.[23]

Smoking

In 1977, Winkelstein[24] proposed that cigarette smoking was a causative factor in the development of cervical cancer. In a review by Green et al.,[16] long duration of smoking (20 or more years) was associated with a 2-fold increase in the risk of squamous cell rather than adenocarcinoma. A study from Venezuela which compared female sex workers who smoked with those who did not. The results showed that the incidence of pre-invasive and invasive cervical lesions increased with the increase in the number of cigarettes smoked per day and the total duration of smoking.[25]

The causal nature of the relation between smoking and cervical cancer remains uncertain as it involves other confounding factors (e.g. sexual, dietary, etc.). In some studies, the relative risk remained high after some of these confounding factors were eliminated.[26] In others, the significant correlation vanished after multifactorial analyses adjusted for behavioural factors, suggesting that smoking is a risk marker, but not a causal factor.[27]

Smoking damages DNA in cervical epithelium by the production of DNA adducts. Polycyclic hydrocarbon DNA adducts, which may lead to induction of mutations, are more frequent in biopsies from smokers than in those from non-smokers. An in vitro study demonstrated that cigarette smoke condensate leads to malignant transformation of HPV-16 immortalised human endocervical cells. High levels of smoke-derived nicotine and cotinine present in the cervical mucus of smokers may act alone or in association with HPV in the development of the disease.[28]

A recent meta-analysis of cigarette smoking and cervical cancer supports this association. The authors proposed a multifactorial hypothesis involving HPV interaction with tar, from smoking, as the aetiology of cancer.[29]

Oral contraceptives

The relationship between oral contraceptives and the development of cervical cancer has been investigated in previous studies. The International Agency for

Research in Cancer (IARC) multicentre study concluded that the use of oral contraceptives increases the cervical cancer risk up to 4-fold after 5 or more years among HPV DNA positive women.[30]

It is not clear whether oral contraceptives act as co-carcinogens in association with transmissible agents or whether they provide exogenous stimuli to potentially hazardous endogenous hormonal influences.

A recent study identified a significant association between the use of oral contraceptives and adenocarcinomas but only a weak association with squamous cell carcinomas. When other factors such as HPV infection, sexual history and cytological screening were taken into account, the association between oral contraceptives and invasive adenocarcinomas, squamous cell carcinoma *in situ* and invasive squamous cell carcinoma disappeared. However, a positive association remained between current use of oral contraceptives and cervical adenocarcinoma *in situ*.[31]

The Oxford Family Planning Association contraceptive study followed a cohort of 17,000 women for 22 years. Ever-users of oral contraceptives were found to have an elevated odds ratio (OR) for all types of cervical neoplasia (OR, 1.40; 95% CI, 1.00–1.96). The reported odds were high for invasive carcinoma (OR, 4.44), intermediate for carcinoma *in situ* (OR, 1.73) and low for CIN (OR, 1.07). The authors suggested a possible effect of oral contraceptive use in the later stages of cervical carcinogenesis, and a lesser effect during the preneoplastic phases.[32]

As oral contraceptives seem to increase the risk of cervical cancer moderately, particularly in HPV positive women, it has been questioned whether oral contraceptives might act as a promoter for HPV-induced carcinogenesis.[33] However, a recent systematic review of 19 epidemiological studies of the risk of HPV infection and oral contraceptives failed to find any evidence for a strong positive or negative association between oral contraceptives and HPV positivity, a major prerequisite for cervical carcinogenesis.[34]

A recent review reported that oral contraceptive users start having sexual intercourse at an earlier age, have more sexual partners and rarely use barrier methods of contraception. All the latter factors act as promoters for HPV-induced carcinogenesis.[35]

Dietary factors

It has been proposed that there is a link between certain dietary factors and the development of cervical carcinoma. Vitamin C and dietary folate have been associated with a reduced risk of cervical neoplasia.[36–38] Vitamin E also has an apparently protective effect against the development of cervical cancer. In addition to certain dietary factors that provide a probable protective effect, there are certain micronutrient deficiencies – such as those of riboflavin, ascorbic acid and zinc – that are associated with cervical cancer.[37,39]

Several case-controlled studies have been performed to investigate the effects of micronutrients on CIN and cervical cancer development. In one particular study, it was shown that food rich in total vitamin A, in particular high retinol food, might play a protective role against cervical cancer.[40,41] Nevertheless, a recent review showed limited evidence for the role of dietary factor in HPV carcinogenesis.[42]

Socio-economic status

Socio-economic factors have been linked with cervical cancer.[43] Women of low social classes tend to have lower screening attendance rates than those of high classes, both in industrialised and non-industrialised countries. Socio-economic differences in screening practices tend to decrease when participation is promoted and social support is offered.[44]

Poor personal hygiene and medical care, poor living conditions, unstable marriages and early age at first intercourse are factors associated with both low socio-economic conditions and cervical cancer.[45]

A recent meta-analysis reported an increased incidence, of nearly 100%, between high and low social class categories for the development of invasive cervical cancer; however, the risk was only 60% for pre-invasive lesions. This risk was observed in all countries but it was stronger in low/middle income countries and in North America than in Europe.[46]

Another meta-analysis of the efficacy of patient letter reminders in cervical cancer screening showed that this method is less effective in lower socio-economic groups who had a lower response rate.[47]

Oncogenes and tumour suppressor genes

Integration of HPV DNA into host cervical cells is essential for the development of cervical cancer. This leads to disruption of the E2 gene and up-regulation of E6 and E7 proteins with subsequent inactivation of p53 and retinoblastoma (Rb) tumour suppressor proteins. p53 gene changes have been detected in CIN 3 and invasive cervical cancers associated with HPV.[48,49]

There is a common p53 polymorphism that results in either a proline or an arginine at position 72 of the protein. The arginine form of p53 is more susceptible to degradation by the HPV E6 oncoprotein than the proline form.[50,51] The arginine/proline polymorphism at codon 72, exon 4 of the p53 gene has been associated with a 7-fold increased risk of cervical cancer (OR, 7.4; 95% CI, 2.1–29.4).[52–54]

There is debate regarding the significance of the association between p53 polymorphism and cervical neoplasia and whether it reflects an association with the neoplastic process independently of HPV infection.[55–57]

Recently, co-overexpression of p53 and bcl2 proteins has been associated with HPV in 105 cases of cervical cancer, suggesting that high-risk HPV infection might modulate the expression of these apoptosis-related proteins.[58]

Immunological factors

Host factors are critical in regulating tumour growth, and cytokines that modulate immunological control may be of particular importance. The type 1 cytokines, interleukin 2 (IL-2) and interferon-γ (IFN-γ), are immunostimulatory and are thus capable of limiting tumour growth. The type 2 cytokines, IL-4 and IL-10, are immuno-inhibitory and are thus capable of stimulating tumour growth.[59,60]

In one study, the levels of IL-10 and IL-12 in the blood of women with intra-epithelial lesions were measured. It was found that the relative ratios of both of these cytokines were significantly lowered in individuals with intra-epithelial lesions compared with normal individuals.[61] This suggests that the cytokine network involving these particular cytokines is disrupted by HPV infection.

Reduced production of IL-2 was noticed in a group of patients with high-grade CIN. In contrast, IL-4 and IL-10 production was elevated in the same group compared with that in the group with low-grade disease or with that in healthy control subjects. The highest production of IL-4 and IL-10 was detected in patients with HPV infection that had extended beyond the genital tract.[59] The authors suggested a shift from type 1 to type 2 cytokine production in individuals who had extensive HPV infection, further emphasising the point that immune dysregulation occurs in CIN patients and might be linked with disease progression.

It has been shown that immunosuppressed women infected with HIV are at increased risk of developing CIN compared with HIV-infected women who are not immunosuppressed.[62]

Human leukocyte antigens (HLA) are important in the regulation of the immune response to foreign antigens. Certain HLA genotypes have been associated with an increased risk of cervical neoplasia. This might be due to the reduced ability of these genotypes to clear HPV infection. Lie et al.[63] demonstrated that Norwegian women carrying the HLA DQB 1*0301 allele had an increased risk of developing CIN 3 after infection with HPV 16. However, no increase in the frequency of disease recurrence was observed among women carrying this allele.[63] In addition, Odunsi et al.[64] showed that increased susceptibility to HPV 16, 18, 31 and 33 infections in a Caucasian population in the UK was associated with MHC II haplotypes 0401/0301 and 1101/0301, whereas the haplotype 0101/0501 was protective.

Chromosomal aberrations

Chromosomal imbalance or aneuploidy is now considered to be an established marker of cancers including cancer of the cervix.[65,66] It is known that more than 20% of women are infected with HPV but only very few develop clinically relevant dysplastic lesions or even cancer. During an acute HPV infection, expression of viral genes, including the E6 and E7 oncogenes, is restricted to differentiated epithelial cells which have lost the ability to replicate and are, therefore, at no increased risk for acquiring functional mutations upon genotoxic damage. However, high-grade cervical dysplasia develops by dysregulated expression of viral oncogenes in replicating epithelial stem cells. The E6–E7, and to a lesser extent E5, gene products affect the control of the cell cycle and mitotic spindle pole formation through complex interactions with various cellular protein complexes. This induces chromosomal instability, telomerase activation and eventually cell immortalisation.[67,68]

Many different molecular cytogenetic techniques, including comparative genomic hybridisation (CGH), spectral karyotyping (SKY) and fluorescence in situ hybridisation (FISH), have been developed to investigate chromosomes in neoplastic and invasive lesions of the cervix.[69]

Chromosomal aberrations can lead to mutational inactivation or loss of tumour suppressor genes (TSGs), activation and amplification of oncogenes. Oncogene amplification is not a major mechanism in cervical carcinogenesis. However, cytogenetic and loss of heterozygosity (LOH) results from CIN and invasive cancer revealed alterations at specific chromosomal regions, pointing to the localisation of TSGs. Genetic alterations at chromosomes 3p, 6p, 11q were frequently found earlier in cervical cancer. Primary invasive carcinoma showed additional allelic losses at chromosome arms 6q, 17p and 18q. Putative senescence genes relevant for HPV-induced carcinogenesis are located on chromosomes 2, 4 and 10. Genes for telomerase suppression are presumably located on chromosomes 3, 4 and 6.[70]

Kirchhoff et al.[71] showed that chromosomal aberrations were detected in both pre-invasive and invasive cervical cancers, although the total number of aberrations was much higher in the latter category. The most consistent chromosomal gain was mapped to chromosome arm 3q in 35% of pre-invasive cases and in 72% of invasive cases. Chromosome aberrations were detected in 13/17 pre-invasive cases with a total of 61 involved chromosome arms. However, in the invasive cases, frequent gains occurred on 1q (45%), 8q (41%), 15q (41%), 5p (34%), and Xq (34%), and frequent losses were mapped to chromosome arms 3p (52%), 11q (48%), 13q (38%), 6q (38%), and 4p (34%).[71]

Infectious agents

Infection with a variety of transmissible agents might play a role in the development of cervical cancer. The most important risk factors are *Chlamydia trachomatis*, herpes viruses and human papillomaviruses.

Chlamydia trachomatis

C. trachomatis has been isolated from the endocervix in 8.2% of women with CIN and 18.2% of women with invasive cancer in comparison with 1% of controls.[72] One sero-epidemiological study demonstrated an association between serum antibodies to *C. trachomatis* and increased risk for cervical squamous cell carcinoma.[73] In a study of women from Brazil and The Philippines, the authors examined *C. trachomatis* infection as a cause of invasive cervical cancer (ICC) among women with human papillomavirus (HPV) infection. *C. trachomatis* seropositivity was associated with sexual behaviour but not with HPV infection. *C. trachomatis* increased the risk of squamous cervical cancer among HPV-positive women (OR, 2.1; 95% CI, 1.1–4.0). Results were similar in both countries. There was a suggestion of increasing squamous cancer risk with increasing *C. trachomatis* antibody titres. The authors concluded that *C. trachomatis* infection could be a possible factor, together with HPV, in the aetiology of squamous cervical cancer, and its effect might be mediated by chronic cervical inflammation.[74]

Serum antibodies to chlamydial heat shock protein 60-1 were found to be associated with an increased risk of cervical cancer. This suggests that persistent *C. trachomatis* infection may contribute to cervical neoplasia.[75]

Herpes viruses

In animals and in humans, herpes viruses have been associated with a variety of pathological conditions. The herpes viruses include cytomegalovirus (CMV), Epstein-Barr virus (EBV), varicela-zoster virus (VZV) and herpes simplex viruses 1 and 2 (HSV-1, HSV-2). All of these viruses except VZV induce malignant transformation in tissue culture and correlate with several malignant disorders in humans. It has been suggested that herpes viruses may also act as causative agents in cervical neoplasia.[76] A multicentre case-control study, investigating the correlation between HSV-2 and HPV in invasive cervical cancer, revealed that HSV-2 seropositivity was higher among patients with cervical squamous-cell carcinoma (44.4%) or adeno- or adenosquamous-cell carcinoma (43.8%) than among control subjects (25.6%). Moreover, among the HPV DNA-positive women, HSV-2 seropositivity was associated with a high risk of squamous-cell carcinoma (OR, 2.19; 95% CI, 1.41–3.40) and adeno- or adenosquamous carcinoma (OR, 3.37; 95% CI, 1.47–7.74) after adjustment for potential confounders. A similar association between HSV-2 seropositivity and squamous-cell carcinoma risk was observed after further controlling for markers of sexual behaviour (OR, 1.96; 95% CI, 1.24–3.09).[77]

Human immunodeficiency virus (HIV)

HIV-positive women are more likely to be infected with oncogenic HPV types and to have CIN lesions and invasive cervical cancer. Although the magnitude of the increased risk of cervical cancer in HIV-positive women is not clear, it is evident that it will remain elevated even in the anti-retroviral therapy era. Full screening for CIN remains necessary in HIV-positive patients.[78]

Meta-analysis from studies between 1986 and 1998 revealed that there is strong association between HIV and HPV and cervical cancer. HIV positive women had higher odds for the disease (OR, 8.8; 95% CI, 6.3–12.5) than HIV negative women (OR, 5; 95% CI, 3.7–6.8). These data suggest an interaction between both types of infection that leads to immunomodulation and subsequently neoplasia.[79]

Human papillomaviruses (HPVs)

Papillomaviruses are epitheliotropic viruses that belong to the Papovaviridae family. Infection across species is uncommon, with the exception of bovine papillomaviruses (BPV) which can induce fibropapillomas.[80] A recent meta-analysis investigated different types of HPV in cervical cancer. The prevalence of HPV type 16 was 46–63% of all cases of squamous cell carcinomas followed by HPV 18 (10–14%), HPV 45 (2–8%), HPV 31 (2–7%) and HPV 33 (3–5%) in all countries except Asia, where HPV 58 and HPV 52 were identified with high frequency. In adenocarcinoma, the prevalence of HPV was significantly lower than squamous carcinoma (76.4% and 87.3%, respectively). HPV 18 was predominant in adenocarcinoma followed by HPV 16.[81]

The clinical implications of human papillomavirus infection in cervical carcinogenesis were discussed in an earlier issue of *Progress in Obstetrics and Gynaecology*.[82]

BIOLOGICAL MARKERS OF CERVICAL NEOPLASIA

Early detection and treatment of cervical precancerous lesions has the potential to improve patient outcome. A possible approach to the understanding of the mechanisms by which cervical carcinoma arises is to study protein expression of putative markers in cervical neoplasia of various histological risk.[83,84] One way of achieving this goal is through the detection of cell cycle control proteins, the expression of which is modulated by HPV infection.[85,86]

Proliferation markers

pKi-67 is a large nuclear protein that is expressed in proliferating cells. The Ki-67 nuclear antigen is present in S, G_2, and M phase, but is absent in G_0 and during DNA-damage-induced cell cycle arrest. Immunostaining with monoclonal antibody Ki-67 provides a reliable means of rapidly evaluating the growth fraction of normal and neoplastic human cell populations.[87]

Most cervical squamous intra-epithelial lesions are readily diagnosed based on histological features. However, the interobserver variation in the diagnosis of these lesions is well known. Furthermore, atrophic squamous epithelium, diathermy artefacts after cervical loop excision, and squamous metaplasia can be confused with high-grade CIN. Ki-67 (MIB-1) has been shown to be helpful in these equivocal cases.[88,89] In normal squamous mucosa, staining for Ki-67 is usually limited to the parabasal cells. An atrophic epithelium and diathermy artefact exhibits little or no staining. In contrast, nuclear staining, throughout the full thickness of the epithelium, is seen in CIN III. A low degree of scattered basal and parabasal staining is usually detected in metaplasia.[88,90]

Proliferating cell nuclear antigen (PCNA) has also been used as a marker of cell proliferation, although its practical value is limited owing to a lower specificity for replicating cells and fixation-dependent immunostaining.[91] Meanwhile, previous studies have shown that PCNA can be useful for evaluating proliferative activity in CIN and cervical carcinoma, and may be used to distinguish CIN III from CIN I–II and evaluate the malignant potential of tumour tissues.[92,93]

Cyclins

Cyclins were first described in marine invertebrates as proteins whose accumulation and degradation oscillated during the cell cycle.[94] Regulation of the cell cycle depends on the sequential activation and inactivation of cyclin-dependent kinases (cdks), through the periodic synthesis and destruction of cyclins. Nine cdks (referred to as cdk 1–9) have been identified in mammalian cells. Moreover, at least 16 mammalian cyclins have been identified: A, B1, B2, C, D1, D2, D3, E, F, G1, G2, H, I, K, T1, and T2. All cyclins contain a common region known as the cyclin box, which is a domain used to bind and activate cdks. However, not all cyclins and cdks function in regulating the cell cycle. Other functions identified include regulation of transcription, DNA repair, differentiation and apoptosis.[95]

In cancers, increased cyclin expression may result from translocation, gene amplification or mutation. The levels of cyclins D1 and E, for example, are frequently increased in cancers.[96]

In cervical squamous lesions, cyclin D1 expression is abrogated by high-risk but not low-risk HPV infection, whilst cyclin A and E expression is up-regulated by both groups of viruses.[97] Moreover, cyclin B expression is up-regulated in high-grade squamous intraepithelial lesions (CIN II, CIN III) but not in low-grade lesions (CIN I, condylomata).

Recent work has revealed increased expression of cyclin A (Fig. 1A) and cyclin B, and to a lesser extent cyclin E, in glandular cervical neoplasia. Furthermore, immunohistochemical detection of cyclins, particularly cyclin B may be of value in the diagnostic assessment of these lesions.[98]

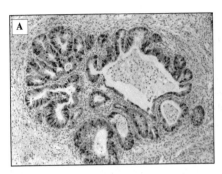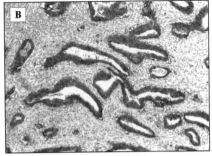

Fig. 1 Cyclin A expression in cervical glandular intra-epithelial neoplasia (A), and p16^INK4a expression in cervical adenocarcinoma (B).

A recent workshop under the auspices of The Royal College of Obstetricians and Gynaecologists reported that cell-cycle control proteins show significant promise as markers of oncogenic HPV infection.[99]

Cyclin-dependent kinase (CDK) inhibitors

Cyclin-dependent kinase inhibitors (CDKIs) play an important role in regulation of the cell cycle.[100] CDKIs compete with cyclin-dependent kinases at their binding sites with cyclins in the G_1 phase of the cell cycle. This blocks the kinase activity of CDK(s) and subsequently prevents phosphorylation of the Rb gene family and transition to S phase.[101]

Inactivation of CDKIs is implicated in the aetiology of various malignant tumours (*e.g.* breast, pancreatic and bladder carcinomas, *etc.*).[102]

Two groups of CDKI have been identified: the p21 and the p16 family of inhibitors.[103] P21 is known as a universal inhibitor as it interacts with a number of cyclin/CDK complexes. In addition, p21 binds to the proliferating cell nuclear antigen (PCNA) to inhibit DNA replication.[104] Unlike p21, the p16 protein specifically targets CDK4 and CDK6 preventing them from complexing with D-type cyclins.[85,105]

Strong p16 overexpression is observed in cervical squamous intra-epithelial lesions (CIN) and squamous cell carcinomas that are associated with high-risk HPV types,[106] indicating that the suppressor function of p16 can be overcome in the presence of viral oncoproteins, particularly E7.

Recently, p16 has been found to be a useful diagnostic marker for cervical neoplastic squamous and glandular lesions. It has also been shown that p16 is preferentially expressed in CIN 2–3 and CIN 1 infected with high-risk HPV types.[107,108]

In addition, p16 may be useful in the distinction between cervical glandular intra-epithelial neoplasia (CGIN) and benign mimics. Cases of CGIN and cervical adenocarcinoma almost invariably show strong diffuse positive staining for p16 (Fig. 1B), while most benign mimics are negative or show focal positivity.[89,109]

The role of p21 in the aetiology of cervical carcinomas has not been well analysed. Lu *et al.*[110] found enhanced expression of this cell-cycle inhibitor in most cervical adenocarcinomas relative to normal glands.

Markers of apoptosis

Bcl2 is a proto-oncogene that is located on chromosome 18 and encodes a 25-kDa protein. This extends cell survival by blocking apoptosis.[111] Immunohistochemical expression of *bcl2* was observed in cervical tubo-endometrioid metaplasia but not in CGIN. Positive staining has also been found in a proportion of cervical adenocarcinomas suggesting that it may have a role in the evolution of these tumours through inhibition of apoptosis.[112]

One of the proteins that oppose the action of the *bcl2* protein is bax. This protein promotes apoptosis and inhibits the anti-apoptotic activity of *bcl2*. Several reports of malignant human tumours have shown a significant association between positive bax expression alone and more favourable prognosis.[113,114] However, other studies showed no significant role for bax expression in cervical cancer.[114,115]

Mutations of p53, a tumour suppressor gene, are the most frequent mutations encountered in human tumours.[116] In cervical cancer, the presence of the p53 protein varies among different studies from a few percent to 62%.[115,117] Accumulation of p53 is often the result of stabilisation of p53 protein caused by mutations of the p53 gene. However, p53 mutation is uncommon in cervical neoplasia. Rather, p53 function is abrogated by the action of HPV E6 protein, which binds to and inactivates p53. Up-regulation of p53 protein expression in this context most likely represents over-expression of wild-type protein. The p53 protein up-regulates bax but down-regulates *bcl2* thereby tilting the *bcl2*/bax equilibrium towards bax causing induction of the cell death.[118] Data from cervical cancer cell lines revealed an inverse relationship between the levels of p53 and *bcl2*. These findings suggest that the relative level of p53 may modulate the ratio of *bcl2*/bax, and that loss of p53 expression in conjunction with an increased *bcl2*/bax ratio may lead to prolonged cell survival without tumour progression.[119]

Heat shock protein 27 (hsp27) is a molecular chaperone that may be constitutively present in cells, and is thought to protect cells from various stresses, such as supra-optimal temperature, anoxia or chemical agents. The expression of hsp27 has been shown to correlate with resistance to stress. Moreover, species' thresholds for hsp27 expression correlate with levels of stress that they naturally undergo.[120] Recent data have shown that, at a cut-off value of 40% for hsp27 expression, neoplastic cervical lesions could be identified from benign mimics with a sensitivity of 67.2% and specificity of 70% and with a positive predictive value of 82%.[121]

Minichromosome maintenance proteins

Minichromosome maintenance proteins (MCMs) play essential roles in eukaryotic DNA replication. These proteins are down-regulated in cells undergoing differentiation or quiescence and, thus, serve as specific markers for proliferating cells.[122] Several reports have indicated the usefulness of MCM proteins as markers of cancer cells in histopathological diagnosis. However, their mode of expression and pathophysiological significance in cancer cells remain to be clarified. Immunohistochemical studies of surgical material from the uterine cervix have shown that MCMs are ubiquitously expressed in cancer cells. Furthermore, the positive rate and level of MCM expression appeared to

Table 2 Useful molecular markers in cervical cancer diagnosis

Molecular marker	Differential diagnosis
Cyclin B	TEM versus CGIN
Ki-67	CIN versus metaplasia and atrophy
	Cervical adenocarcinoma versus benign glandular lesions
p16^{INK4a}	CIN versus metaplasia and atrophy CGIN versus TEM
p53	Cervical adenocarcinoma versus benign glandular lesions
Bcl2	TEM versus CGIN
CEA	Cervical adenocarcinoma versus benign glandular lesions
	Cervical versus endometrial adenocarcinoma
Chromogranin A	Neuro-endocrine carcinoma
Synaptophysin	Neuro-endocrine carcinoma
Vimentin	Cervical versus endometrial adenocarcinoma

CEA, Carcino-embryonic antigen; CIN, cervical intra-epithelial neoplasia; CGIN, cervical glandular intra-epithelial neoplasia; TEM, tubo-endometrioid metaplasia.

be higher in cancer cells than in normal proliferating cells of the uterine cervix and dysplastic cells, suggesting that they may be useful diagnostic markers.[123]

Other markers of diagnostic utility

Close morphological examination usually allows a confident distinction between different cervical lesions. However, in doubtful cases, other biological markers might also be of value (Table 2).

Carcino-embryonic antigen (CEA)

Neoplastic cervical lesions can be difficult to differentiate from benign mimics. This problem is more significant in small cervical biopsies and in some cases of minimal deviation adenocarcinoma. CEA may help in these circumstances.[124,125] Positive staining is seen in cervical adenocarcinoma and CGIN, whereas normal glands are negative. CEA is not a highly sensitive or specific marker. It may be expressed, in a focal pattern, in some cases of well-differentiated adenocarcinoma. Cervical squamous mucosa and benign glandular lesions with squamous metaplasia may also exhibit positive staining. Furthermore, endocervical glands with radiation-induced atypia show focal cytoplasmic staining for CEA.[126] Combined panels of antibodies (*e.g.* Ki-67, p53 and CEA,[127] or Bcl2, p16 and Ki67[128]) may be useful in discriminating benign and malignant lesions.

Vimentin (VIM)

Histological examination of adenocarcinoma present in an endometrial biopsy or endocervical curettage specimens represents a challenge to pathologists. The combination of CEA and VIM may be helpful in differentiating these lesions. VIM is an intermediate filament, which is characteristic, although not unique, to mesenchymal tumours. CEA is expressed by most cases of cervical adenocarcinoma. In contrast, endometrial adenocarcinomas are negative.[129,130] VIM is expressed in the majority of endometrial adenocarcinomas but only by a small percentage of cervical adenocarcinomas.[131-133] A recent study has suggested that the combination of VIM and oestrogen receptor (ER) scores may identify the endometrial origin of the tumour with 95% accuracy.[134]

Chromogranin A and synaptophysin

Cervical neuro-endocrine tumours vary from well-differentiated carcinoid tumours to poorly differentiated small and large cell tumours. It is crucial to distinguish between these tumours and other cervical carcinomas since this affects patient management. Chromogranin A and synaptophysin are two commonly used markers that stain neuro-endocrine tumours, with synaptophysin being of high sensitivity.[135,136]

KEY POINTS FOR CLINICAL PRACTICE

- Cervical cancer is the second most frequent cancer, world-wide, in women after breast carcinoma.

- Cervical cytology has limited ability to predict progression to invasive cancer in an individual with an intra-epithelial lesion.

- Human papillomavirus is thought to be necessary, but not sufficient, for the development of cervical neoplasia.

- Early detection and treatment of cervical intra-epithelial lesions has the potential to improve the outcome of patients.

- Cell-cycle control protein expression is modulated by HPV infection.

- Close morphological examination allows confident diagnosis of cervical lesions in most instances. In doubtful cases, biological markers are helpful in establishing the diagnosis.

- Cell-cycle control proteins show significant promise as markers of oncogenic HPV infection and possibly neoplastic potential

References

1 Parkin DM, Pisani P, Ferlay J. Estimates of the worldwide incidence of 25 major cancers in 1990. Int J Cancer 1999; 80: 827–841
2 Arends MJ, Buckley CH, Wells M. Aetiology, pathogenesis, and pathology of cervical neoplasia. J Clin Pathol 1998; 51: 96–103
3 Stoler MH, Rhodes CR, Whitbeck A, Wolinsky SM, Chow LT, Broker TR. Human papillomavirus type 16 and 18 gene expression in cervical neoplasias. Hum Pathol 1992; 23: 117–128
4 Schiffman MH, Brinton LA. The epidemiology of cervical carcinogenesis. Cancer 1995; 76: 1888–1901
5 Park TW, Fujiwara H, Wright TC. Molecular biology of cervical cancer and its precursors. Cancer 1995; 76: 1902–1913
6 Murthy NS, Sehgal A, Satyanarayana L et al. Risk factors related to biological behaviour of precancerous lesions of the uterine cervix. Br J Cancer 1990; 61: 732–736
7 Brinton LA. Epidemiology of Cervical Cancer – Overview. Lyons: IARC 1992; 3–23
8 Birley HD. Human papillomaviruses, cervical cancer and the developing world. Ann Trop Med Parasitol 1995; 89: 453–463
9 Cuzick J, Sasieni P, Singer A. Risk factors for invasive cervix cancer in young women. Eur J Cancer 1996; 32A: 836–841
10 Biswas LN, Manna B, Maiti PK, Sengupta S. Sexual risk factors for cervical cancer

among rural Indian women: a case-control study. Int J Epidemiol 1997; 26: 491–495

11 Brinton LA, Herrero R, Reeves WC, de Britton RC, Gaitan E, Tenorio F. Risk factors for cervical cancer by histology. Gynecol Oncol 1993; 51: 301–306

12 Skrabanek P. Cervical cancer in nuns and prostitutes: a plea for scientific continence. J Clin Epidemiol 1988; 41: 577–582

13 Critchlow CW, Wolner-Hanssen P, Eschenbach DA et al. Determinants of cervical ectopia and of cervicitis: age, oral contraception, specific cervical infection, smoking, and douching. Am J Obstet Gynecol 1995; 173: 534–543

14 Kataja V, Syrjanen S, Yliskoski M et al. Risk factors associated with cervical human papillomavirus infections: a case-control study. Am J Epidemiol 1993; 138: 735–745

15 Koutsky L. Epidemiology of genital human papillomavirus infection. Am J Med 1997; 102: 3–8

16 Green J, Berrington de Gonzalez A et al. Risk factors for adenocarcinoma and squamous cell carcinoma of the cervix in women aged 20–44 years: the UK National Case-Control Study of Cervical Cancer. Br J Cancer 2003; 89: 2078–2086

17 Brinton LA, Reeves WC, Brenes MM et al. Parity as a risk factor for cervical cancer. Am J Epidemiol 1989; 130: 486–496

18 Gopalkrishna V, Murthy NS, Sharma JK et al. Increased human papillomavirus infection with the increasing number of pregnancies in Indian women. J Infect Dis 1995; 171: 254–255

19 Ferrera A, Velema JP, Figueroa M et al. Co-factors related to the causal relationship between human papillomavirus and invasive cervical cancer in Honduras. Int J Epidemiol 2000; 29: 817–825

20 Deacon JM, Evans CD, Yule R et al. Sexual behaviour and smoking as determinants of cervical HPV infection and of CIN3 among those infected: a case-control study nested within the Manchester cohort. Br J Cancer 2000; 83: 1565–1572

21 Anderson LM, May DS. Has the use of cervical, breast, and colorectal cancer screening increased in the United States? Am J Public Health 1995; 85: 840–842

22 Jayant K. Additive effect of two risk factors in the aetiology of cancer of the cervix uteri. Br J Cancer 1987; 56: 685–686

23 Castellsague X, Bosch FX, Munoz N et al. Male circumcision, penile human papillomavirus infection, and cervical cancer in female partners. N Engl J Med 2002; 346: 1105–1112

24 Winkelstein Jr W. Smoking and cancer of the uterine cervix: hypothesis. Am J Epidemiol 1977; 106: 257–259

25 Nunez JT, Delgado M, Pino G, Giron H, Bolet B. Smoking as a risk factor for preinvasive and invasive cervical lesions in female sex workers in Venezuela. Int J Gynaecol Obstet 2002; 79: 57–60

26 Kanetsky PA, Gammon MD, Mandelblatt J et al. Cigarette smoking and cervical dysplasia among non-Hispanic black women. Cancer Detect Prev 1998; 22: 109–119

27 Sikstrom B, Hellberg D, Nilsson S, Mardh PA. Smoking, alcohol, sexual behaviour and drug use in women with cervical human papillomavirus infection. Arch Gynecol Obstet 1995;, 256: 131–137

28 Yang X, Jin G, Nakao Y, Rahimtula M, Pater MM, Pater A. Malignant transformation of HPV 16-immortalized human endocervical cells by cigarette smoke condensate and characterization of multistage carcinogenesis. Int J Cancer 1996; 65: 338–344

29 Haverkos HW, Soon G, Steckley SL, Pickworth W. Cigarette smoking and cervical cancer: Part I: a meta-analysis. Biomed Pharmacother 2003; 57: 67–77

30 Moreno V, Bosch FX, Munoz N et al. Effect of oral contraceptives on risk of cervical cancer in women with human papillomavirus infection: the IARC multicentric case-control study. Lancet 2002; 359: 1085–1092

31 Lacey Jr JV, Brinton LA, Abbas FM et al. Oral contraceptives as risk factors for cervical adenocarcinomas and squamous cell carcinomas. Cancer Epidemiol Biomarkers Prev 1999; 8: 1079–1085

32 Zondervan KT, Carpenter LM, Painter R, Vessey MP. Oral contraceptives and cervical cancer – further findings from the Oxford Family Planning Association contraceptive study. Br J Cancer 1996; 73: 1291–1297

33 La Vecchia C, Tavani A, Franceschi S, Parazzini F. Oral contraceptives and cancer. A review of the evidence. Drug Safety 1996; 14: 260–272

34 Green J, Berrington de Gonzalez A, Smith JS *et al*. Human papillomavirus infection and use of oral contraceptives. Br J Cancer 2003; 88: 1713–1720

35 Deligeoroglou E, Michailidis E, Creatsas G. Oral contraceptives and reproductive system cancer. Ann NY Acad Sci 2003; 997: 199–208

36 VanEenwyk J, Davis FG, Colman N. Folate, vitamin C, and cervical intraepithelial neoplasia. Cancer Epidemiol Biomarkers Prev 1992; 1: 119–124

37 Potischman N. Nutritional epidemiology of cervical neoplasia. J Nutr 1993; 123: 424–429

38 Mackerras D, Irwig L, Simpson JM *et al*. Randomized double-blind trial of beta-carotene and vitamin C in women with minor cervical abnormalities. Br J Cancer 1999; 79: 1448–1453

39 Guo WD, Hsing AW, Li JY, Chen JS, Chow WH, Blot WJ. Correlation of cervical cancer mortality with reproductive and dietary factors, and serum markers in China. Int J Epidemiol 1994; 23: 1127–1132

40 Kanetsky PA, Gammon MD, Mandelblatt J *et al*. Dietary intake and blood levels of lycopene: association with cervical dysplasia among non-Hispanic, black women. Nutr Cancer 1998; 31: 31–40

41 Shannon J, Thomas DB, Ray RM *et al*. Dietary risk factors for invasive and in-situ cervical carcinomas in Bangkok, Thailand. Cancer Causes Control 2002; 13: 691–699

42 Castellsague X, Bosch FX, Munoz N. Environmental co-factors in HPV carcinogenesis. Virus Res 2002; 89: 191–199

43 Kawachi I, Kennedy BP, Gupta V, Prothrow-Stith D. Women's status and the health of women and men: a view from the States. Soc Sci Med 1999; 48: 21–32

44 Segnan N. Socioeconomic Status and Cancer Screening. Lyons: IARC Sci Publ, 1997; 369–376

45 Hildesheim A, Gravitt P, Schiffman MH *et al*. Determinants of genital human papillomavirus infection in low-income women in Washington, DC. Sex Transm Dis 1993; 20: 279–285

46 Parikh S, Brennan P, Boffetta P. Meta-analysis of social inequality and the risk of cervical cancer. Int J Cancer 2003; 105: 687–691

47 Tseng DS, Cox E, Plane MB, Hla KM. Efficacy of patient letter reminders on cervical cancer screening: a meta-analysis. J Gen Intern Med 2001; 16: 563–568

48 Wong YF, Chung TK, Cheung TH *et al*. p53 polymorphism and human papillomavirus infection in Hong Kong women with cervical cancer. Gynecol Obstet Invest 2000; 50: 60–63

49 do Horto dos Santos Oliveira L, Rodrigues Ede V, de Salles Lopes AP, Fernandez Ade P, Cavalcanti SM. HPV 16 detection in cervical lesions, physical state of viral DNA and changes in p53 gene. Sao Paulo Med J 2003; 121: 67–71

50 Yamashita T, Yaginuma Y, Saitoh Y *et al*. Codon 72 polymorphism of p53 as a risk factor for patients with human papillomavirus-associated squamous intraepithelial lesions and invasive cancer of the uterine cervix. Carcinogenesis 1999; 20: 1733–1736

51 Madeleine MM, Shera K, Schwartz SM *et al*. The p53 Arg72Pro polymorphism, human papillomavirus, and invasive squamous cell cervical cancer. Cancer Epidemiol Biomarkers Prev 2000; 9: 225–227

52 Storey A, Thomas M, Kalita A *et al*. Role of a p53 polymorphism in the development of human papillomavirus-associated cancer. Nature 1998; 393: 229–234

53 Rosenthal AN, Ryan A, Al-Jehani RM, Storey A, Harwood CA, Jacobs IJ. p53 codon 72 polymorphism and risk of cervical cancer in UK. Lancet 1998; 352: 871–872

54 Makni H, Franco EL, Kaiano J *et al*. P53 polymorphism in codon 72 and risk of human papillomavirus-induced cervical cancer: effect of inter-laboratory variation. Int J Cancer 2000; 87: 528–533

55 Giannoudis A, Graham DA, Southern SA, Herrington CS. p53 codon 72 ARG/PRO polymorphism is not related to HPV type or lesion grade in low- and high-grade squamous intra-epithelial lesions and invasive squamous carcinoma of the cervix. Int J Cancer 1999; 83: 66–69

56 Andersson S, Rylander E, Strand A, Sallstrom J, Wilander E. The significance of p53 codon 72 polymorphism for the development of cervical adenocarcinomas. Br J Cancer 2001; 85: 1153–1156

57 Rezza G, Giuliani M, Garbuglia AR *et al*. Lack of association between p53 codon-72 polymorphism and squamous intraepithelial lesions in women with, or at risk for,

human immunodeficiency virus and/or human papillomavirus infections. Cancer Epidemiol Biomarkers Prev 2001; 10: 565–566

58 Grace VM, Shalini JV, Lekha TT, Devaraj SN, Devaraj H. Co-overexpression of p53 and bcl-2 proteins in HPV-induced squamous cell carcinoma of the uterine cervix. Gynecol Oncol 2003; 91: 51–58

59 Clerici M, Merola M, Ferrario E et al. Cytokine production patterns in cervical intraepithelial neoplasia: association with human papillomavirus infection. J Natl Cancer Inst 1997; 89: 245–250

60 Tjiong MY, van der Vange N, ten Kate FJ et al. Increased IL-6 and IL-8 levels in cervicovaginal secretions of patients with cervical cancer. Gynecol Oncol 1999; 73: 285–291

61 Jacobs N, Giannini SL, Doyen J et al. Inverse modulation of IL-10 and IL-12 in the blood of women with preneoplastic lesions of the uterine cervix. Clin Exp Immunol 1998; 111: 219–224

62 Smith JR, Kitchen VS, Botcherby M et al. Is HIV infection associated with an increase in the prevalence of cervical neoplasia? Br J Obstet Gynaecol 1993; 100: 149–153

63 Lie AK, Skarsvag S, Haugen OA et al. Association between the HLA DQB1*0301 gene and human papillomavirus infection in high-grade cervical intraepithelial neoplasia. Int J Gynecol Pathol 1999; 18: 206–210

64 Odunsi K, Terry G, Ho L, Bell J, Cuzick J, Ganesan TS. Susceptibility to human papillomavirus-associated cervical intra-epithelial neoplasia is determined by specific HLA DR-DQ alleles. Int J Cancer 1996; 67: 595–602

65 Southern SA, Herrington CS: Interphase karyotypic analysis of chromosomes 11, 17 and X in invasive squamous-cell carcinoma of the cervix: morphological correlation with HPV infection. Int J Cancer 1997; 70: 502–507

66 Graham DA, Southern SA, McDicken IW, Herrington CS. Interphase cytogenetic evidence for distinct genetic pathways in the development of squamous neoplasia of the uterine cervix. Lab Invest 1998; 78: 289—296

67 von Knebel Doeberitz M. New markers for cervical dysplasia to visualise the genomic chaos created by aberrant oncogenic papillomavirus infections. Eur J Cancer 2002; 38: 2229–2242

68 Fehrmann F, Laimins LA. Human papillomaviruses: targeting differentiating epithelial cells for malignant transformation. Oncogene 2003; 22: 5201–5207

69 Harris CP, Lu XY, Narayan G, Singh B, Murty VV, Rao PH. Comprehensive molecular cytogenetic characterization of cervical cancer cell lines. Genes Chromosomes Cancer 2003; 36: 233–241

70 Kaufmann AM, Backsch C, Schneider A, Durst M. HPV induced cervical carcinogenesis: molecular basis and vaccine development. Zentralbl Gynakol 2002; 124: 511–524

71 Kirchhoff M, Rose H, Petersen BL et al. Comparative genomic hybridization reveals a recurrent pattern of chromosomal aberrations in severe dysplasia/carcinoma in situ of the cervix and in advanced-stage cervical carcinoma. Genes Chromosomes Cancer 1999; 24: 144–150

72 Hare MJ, Taylor-Robinson D, Cooper P. Evidence for an association between Chlamydia trachomatis and cervical intraepithelial neoplasia. Br J Obstet Gynaecol 1982; 89: 489–492

73 Koskela P, Anttila T, Bjorge T et al. Chlamydia trachomatis infection as a risk factor for invasive cervical cancer. Int J Cancer 2000;, 85: 35–39

74 Smith JS, Munoz N, Herrero R et al. Evidence for Chlamydia trachomatis as a human papillomavirus cofactor in the etiology of invasive cervical cancer in Brazil and the Philippines. J Infect Dis 2002; 185: 324–331

75 Paavonen J, Karunakaran KP, Noguchi Y et al. Serum antibody response to the heat shock protein 60 of Chlamydia trachomatis in women with developing cervical cancer. Am J Obstet Gynecol 2003; 189: 1287–1292

76 Boyle DC, Smith JR. Infection and cervical intraepithelial neoplasia. Int J Gynecol Cancer 1999; 9: 177–186

77 Smith JS, Herrero R, Bosetti C et al. Herpes simplex virus-2 as a human papillomavirus cofactor in the etiology of invasive cervical cancer. J Natl Cancer Inst 2002; 94: 1604–1613

78 de Sanjose S, Palefsky J. Cervical and anal HPV infections in HIV positive women and men. Virus Res 2002; 89: 201–211

79 Mandelblatt JS, Kanetsky P, Eggert L, Gold K. Is HIV infection a cofactor for cervical squamous cell neoplasia? Cancer Epidemiol Biomarkers Prev 1999; 8: 97–106

80 Koller LD, Olson C. Attempted transmission of warts from man, cattle, and horses and of deer fibroma, to selected hosts. J Invest Dermatol 1972; 58: 366–368

81 Clifford GM, Smith JS, Plummer M, Munoz N, Franceschi S. Human papillomavirus types in invasive cervical cancer worldwide: a meta-analysis. Br J Cancer 2003; 88: 63–73

82 Papadopoulos A, Devaja O, Cason J, Raju K. (eds) The Clinical Implications of Human Papillomavirus Infection in Cervical Carcinogenesis and Emerging Therapies. London: Churchill Livingstone, 2000; 281–293

83 Duska LR, Flynn CF, Chen A, Whall-Strojwas D, Goodman A. Clinical evaluation of atypical glandular cells of undetermined significance on cervical cytology. Obstet Gynecol 1998; 91: 278–282

84 Azodi M, Chambers SK, Rutherford TJ, Kohorn EI, Schwartz PE, Chambers JT. Adenocarcinoma in situ of the cervix: management and outcome. Gynecol Oncol 1999; 73: 348–353

85 Serrano M, Hannon GJ, Beach D. A new regulatory motif in cell-cycle control causing specific inhibition of cyclin D/CDK4. Nature 1993; 366: 704–707

86 Khleif SN, DeGregori J, Yee CL et al. Inhibition of cyclin D-CDK4/CDK6 activity is associated with an E2F-mediated induction of cyclin kinase inhibitor activity. Proc Natl Acad Sci USA 1996; 93: 4350–4354

87 Gerdes J, Lemke H, Baisch H, Wacker HH, Schwab U, Stein H. Cell cycle analysis of a cell proliferation-associated human nuclear antigen defined by the monoclonal antibody Ki-67. J Immunol 1984; 133: 1710–1715

88 Mittal K, Mesia A, Demopoulos RI. MIB-1 expression is useful in distinguishing dysplasia from atrophy in elderly women. Int J Gynecol Pathol 1999; 18: 122–124

89 Keating JT, Cviko A, Riethdorf S et al. Ki-67, cyclin E, and p16^{INK4} are complimentary surrogate biomarkers for human papilloma virus-related cervical neoplasia. Am J Surg Pathol 2001; 25: 884–891

90 Pirog EC, Baergen RN, Soslow RA et al. Diagnostic accuracy of cervical low-grade squamous intraepithelial lesions is improved with MIB-1 immunostaining. Am J Surg Pathol 2002; 26: 70–75

91 Busmanis I. Biomarkers in carcinoma of the cervix: emphasis on tissue-related factors and their potential prognostic factors. Ann Acad Med Singapore 1998; 27: 671–675

92 Xue Y, Feng Y, Zhu G, Zhang X. Proliferative activity in cervical intraepithelial neoplasia and cervical carcinoma. Chin Med J (Engl) 1999; 112: 373–375

93 Herbsleb M, Knudsen UB, Orntoft TF et al. Telomerase activity, MIB-1, PCNA, HPV 16 and p53 as diagnostic markers for cervical intraepithelial neoplasia. Apmis 2001; 109: 607–617

94 Rosenthal ET, Hunt T, Ruderman JV. Selective translation of mRNA controls the pattern of protein synthesis during early development of the surf clam, Spisula solidissima. Cell 1980; 20: 487–494

95 Johnson DG, Walker CL. Cyclins and cell cycle checkpoints. Annu Rev Pharmacol Toxicol 1999; 39: 295–312

96 Chao Y, Shih YL, Chiu JH et al. Overexpression of cyclin A but not Skp 2 correlates with the tumor relapse of human hepatocellular carcinoma. Cancer Res 1998; 58: 985–990

97 Southern SA, Herrington CS. Differential cell cycle regulation by low- and high-risk human papillomaviruses in low-grade squamous intraepithelial lesions of the cervix. Cancer Res 1998; 58: 2941–2945

98 El-Ghobashy A, Shaaban A, Herod J, Innes J, Prime W, Herrington CS. Overexpression of cyclin A and cyclin B as markers of neoplastic glandular lesions of the cervix. Gynecol Oncol 2004; 92: 628–634

99 Royal College of Obstetricians and Gynaecologists. Study Group Recommendations – Lower Genital Tract Neoplasia. London: RCOG Press, 2003

100 Harper JW, Elledge SJ. Cdk inhibitors in development and cancer. Curr Opin Genet Dev 1996; 6: 56–64

101 Xiong Y. Why are there so many CDK inhibitors? Biochim Biophys Acta 1996; 1288: 1–5

102 Ruas M, Peters G. The p16^{INK4a}/CDKN2A tumor suppressor and its relatives. Biochim Biophys Acta 1998; 1378: F115–F177

103 Pavletich NP. Mechanisms of cyclin-dependent kinase regulation: structures of Cdks, their cyclin activators, and Cip and INK4 inhibitors. J Mol Biol 1999; 287: 821–828

104 Waga S, Hannon GJ, Beach D, Stillman B. The p21 inhibitor of cyclin-dependent kinases controls DNA replication by interaction with PCNA. Nature 1994; 369: 574–578

105 Hirai H, Roussel MF, Kato JY, Ashmun RA, Sherr CJ. Novel INK4 proteins, p19 and p18, are specific inhibitors of the cyclin D-dependent kinases CDK4 and CDK6. Mol Cell Biol 1995; 15: 2672–2681

106 Sano T, Oyama T, Kashiwabara K, Fukuda T, Nakajima T. Expression status of p16 protein is associated with human papillomavirus oncogenic potential in cervical and genital lesions. Am J Pathol 1998; 153: 1741–1748

107 Jenkins D, Klaes R, Brenner A. p16[ink4a] immunohistochemistry improves interobserver agreement in the diagnosis of cervical intraepithelial neoplasia. J Pathol 2001; 195: 2A

108 Klaes R, Benner A, Friedrich T et al.: p16[INK4a] immunohistochemistry improves interobserver agreement in the diagnosis of cervical intraepithelial neoplasia. Am J Surg Pathol 2002; 26: 1389–1399

109 El-Ghobashy A, Shaaban A, Innes J, Prime W, Herrington CS. Quantitative analysis of cyclin dependent kinase inhibitors, p16 and p21, distinguishes neoplastic cervical glandular abnormalities. Unpublished data

110 Lu X, Toki T, Konishi I, Nikaido T, Fujii S. Expression of p21WAF1/CIP1 in adenocarcinoma of the uterine cervix: a possible immunohistochemical marker of a favorable prognosis. Cancer 1998; 82: 2409–2417

111 Hockenbery DM, Zutter M, Hickey W, Nahm M, Korsmeyer SJ. BCL2 protein is topographically restricted in tissues characterized by apoptotic cell death. Proc Natl Acad Sci USA 1991; 88: 6961–6965

112 McCluggage G, McBride H, Maxwell P, Bharucha H: Immunohistochemical detection of p53 and bcl-2 proteins in neoplastic and non-neoplastic endocervical glandular lesions. Int J Gynecol Pathol 1997; 16: 22–27

113 Xie X, Clausen OP, De Angelis P, Boysen M. Bax expression has prognostic significance that is enhanced when combined with AgNOR counts in glottic carcinomas. Br J Cancer 1998; 78: 100–105

114 Tjalma WA, Weyler JJ, Bogers JJ et al. The importance of biological factors (bcl-2, bax, p53, PCNA, MI, HPV and angiogenesis) in invasive cervical cancer. Eur J Obstet Gynecol Reprod Biol 2001; 97: 223–230

115 Crawford RA, Caldwell C, Iles RK, Lowe D, Shepherd JH, Chard T. Prognostic significance of the bcl-2 apoptotic family of proteins in primary and recurrent cervical cancer. Br J Cancer 1998; 78: 210–214

116 Vogelstein B, Kinzler KW. p53 function and dysfunction. Cell 1992; 70: 523–526

117 Benjamin I, Saigo P, Finstad C et al. Expression and mutational analysis of P53 in stage IB and IIA cervical cancers. Am J Obstet Gynecol 1996; 175: 1266–1271

118 Haldar S, Negrini M, Monne M, Sabbioni S, Croce CM. Down-regulation of bcl-2 by p53 in breast cancer cells. Cancer Res 1994; 54: 2095–2097

119 Liang XH, Mungal S, Ayscue A et al. Bcl-2 protooncogene expression in cervical carcinoma cell lines containing inactive p53. J Cell Biochem 1995;, 57: 509–521

120 Feder ME, Hofmann GE. Heat-shock proteins, molecular chaperones, and the stress response: evolutionary and ecological physiology. Annu Rev Physiol 1999; 61: 243–282

121 El-Ghobashy A, Shaaban A, Innes J, Prime W, Herrington CS. Upregulation of heat shock protein 27 in metaplastic and neoplastic lesions of the endocervix. International J Gynecol Cancer 2004; In press

122 Freeman A, Morris LS, Mills AD et al. Minichromosome maintenance proteins as biological markers of dysplasia and malignancy. Clin Cancer Res 1999; 5: 2121–2132

123 Ishimi Y, Okayasu I, Kato C et al. Enhanced expression of Mcm proteins in cancer cells derived from uterine cervix. Eur J Biochem 2003; 270: 1089–1101

124 Michael H, Grawe L, Kraus FT. Minimal deviation endocervical adenocarcinoma: clinical and histologic features, immunohistochemical staining for carcinoembryonic antigen, and differentiation from confusing benign lesions. Int J Gynecol Pathol 1984; 3: 261–276

125 Gilks CB, Young RH, Aguirre P, DeLellis RA, Scully RE. Adenoma malignum (minimal deviation adenocarcinoma) of the uterine cervix. A clinicopathological and immunohistochemical analysis of 26 cases. Am J Surg Pathol 1989; 13: 717–729

126 Lesack D, Wahab I, Gilks CB. Radiation-induced atypia of endocervical epithelium: a histological, immunohistochemical and cytometric study. Int J Gynecol Pathol 1996; 15: 242–247

127 Cina SJ, Richardson MS, Austin RM, Kurman RJ. Immunohistochemical staining for Ki-67 antigen, carcinoembryonic antigen, and p53 in the differential diagnosis of glandular lesions of the cervix. Mod Pathol 1997; 10: 176–180

128 Cameron RI, Maxwell P, Jenkins D, McCluggage WG. Immunohistochemical staining with MIB1, bcl2 and p16 assists in the distinction of cervical glandular intraepithelial neoplasia from tubo-endometrial metaplasia, endometriosis and microglandular hyperplasia. Histopathology 2002; 41: 313–321

129 Wahlstrom T, Lindgren J, Korhonen M, Seppala M. Distinction between endocervical and endometrial adenocarcinoma with immunoperoxidase staining of carcinoembryonic antigen in routine histological tissue specimens. Lancet 1979; 2: 1159–1160

130 Cohen C, Shulman G, Budgeon LR. Endocervical and endometrial adenocarcinoma: an immunoperoxidase and histochemical study. Am J Surg Pathol 1982; 6: 151–157

131 Dabbs DJ, Geisinger KR, Norris HT. Intermediate filaments in endometrial and endocervical carcinomas. The diagnostic utility of vimentin patterns. Am J Surg Pathol 1986; 10: 568–576

132 Dabbs DJ, Sturtz K, Zaino RJ. The immunohistochemical discrimination of endometrioid adenocarcinomas. Hum Pathol 1996; 27: 172–177

133 Zhu L, Li B. [Clinical pathological analysis and immunohistochemical expression of primary cervical adenocarcinoma in 98 cases]. Zhonghua Bing Li Xue Za Zhi 1999; 28: 252–255

134 Kamoi S, Al-Juboury MI, Akin MR, Silverberg SG. Immunohistochemical staining in the distinction between primary endometrial and endocervical adenocarcinomas: another viewpoint. Int J Gynecol Pathol 2002; 21: 217–223

135 Albores-Saavedra J, Gersell D, Gilks CB et al. Terminology of endocrine tumors of the uterine cervix: results of a workshop sponsored by the College of American Pathologists and the National Cancer Institute. Arch Pathol Lab Med 1997; 121: 34–39

136 Conner MG, Richter H, Moran CA, Hameed A, Albores-Saavedra J. Small cell carcinoma of the cervix: a clinicopathologic and immunohistochemical study of 23 cases. Ann Diagn Pathol 2002; 6: 345–348

Frank Lawton

How can we improve the prognosis of endometrial cancer?

A superficial glance at the overall survival figures for patents with endometrial cancer may lead the casual observer to conclude that the question in the title is only one of academic interest. The observer might conclude that a 5-year survival of around 75% is considerably better than that for many other cancers and, in addition, is achieved relatively easily by means of simple hysterectomy and bilateral salpingo-oophorectomy plus, possibly, postoperative radiotherapy. Furthermore, with such a good prognosis, the observer might rightly draw to the attention of interested parties that to show that innovative therapies have a positive therapeutic impact, randomised studies with huge numbers would be needed to demonstrate even a small percentage improvement in survival. This disease is 'benign' in comparison with all other major gynaecological cancers. Despite this, there would appear to be major interest in this disease as evidenced by the large number of factors mooted to be of prognostic significance (Table 1). This may be due to the fact that a disease which claims the lives of one in four patients within 5 years of diagnosis cannot be described as benign and that the status quo only encourages therapeutic complacency. Whilst it is true that for patients with pure adenocarcinoma confined to the endometrium the outlook may be positive, for patients with other histological types the prognosis is dire. More than half of patients with adenosquamous and nearly two-thirds of those with clear cell cancers will be dead within 5 years. In addition, these results are not achieved without toxicity which is, perhaps in 6% of patients severe and in 2% debilitating.[1]

SCREENING

A disease which has the potential for screening should, according to the World Health Organization, fulfil a number of criteria. Amongst others, these include

Frank Lawton MD FRCOG
Consultant Gynaecological Cancer Surgeon, Guy's, King's and St Thomas' Gynaecological Cancer Centre, King's College Hospital, Denmark Hill, London SE5 9RS, UK

Table 1 Purported prognostic factors in endometrial carcinoma

Age
Tumour grade
Histology
Invasion into cervical stroma
Cervical glandular involvement
Lymphovascular space involvement
Pelvic/para-aortic nodal metastases
Depth of myometrial invasion ± positive peritoneal cytology
Extra-uterine disease
Mitotic activity of the tumour
Progestogen and oestrogen receptor status
Oncogene mutation
DNA ploidy
Post-surgical residual tumour mass
Use of post-surgical radiotherapy
Chromosomal abnormalities

that the natural history of the disease should be well understood, that it should have a recognisable early (premalignant?) stage, that treatment of the disease at an early stage should be of greater benefit than treatment started at a later stage, and that there should be a suitable test acceptable to the target population.

It is known that endometrial hyperplasias do have a malignant potential, the most important factor being the presence or absence of cytological atypia. A patient with endometrial hyperplasia without cytological atypia will have a less than 2% chance of progression to cancer compared with a 23% risk for one with atypia.[2] In addition, there are data to show that the hyperplasia can be modulated with progestogen therapy. More than 80% of patients with hyperplasia without atypia will revert to normal with medoxyprogesterone acetate therapy compared with only 50% of those with cytological atypia.[3] In addition, in the latter group, 25% will develop recurrent or resistant hyperplasia and 25% will develop cancer.

If we were able to distinguish reliably between hyperplasia with atypia and frank carcinoma would this be a step forward? On the grounds that until data on the therapeutic role of lymphadenecetomy become available, simple hysterectomy is the surgical management of choice for about 75% of patients with endometrial cancer (*i.e.* the proportion of patients who present with clinical stage I disease) and also would be recommended for patients with cytological atypia, then a screening programme that encouraged exactly the same surgical endeavour whether or not the patient had malignant or premalignant disease cannot be supported.

However, some patients at very high genetic risk of developing endometrial cancer should be considered for screening programmes. Hereditary non-polyposis colorectal cancer (HNPCC) is a relatively common syndrome which causes an individual to be at increased risk of developing malignancies of the colon, endometrium, ovary, stomach and small bowel as well as renal, hepatobiliary and brain tumours.[4] The syndrome is caused by autosomal dominant inheritance of a mutation in one of a group of DNA mismatch repair genes. Endometrial cancer is the second most common cancer in families with

HNPCC after colorectal cancer with the life-time risk estimated as up to 60%,[5] but some authors claim that the risk of developing endometrial cancer is even greater than that of colorectal cancer.[6] At this degree of risk and because the age at onset of endometrial cancer in HNPCC families is younger than the age of sporadic endometrial tumours, it has been recommended that endometrial sampling should begin at 30 years of age with annual screening, and that prophylactic hysterectomy should be carried out after the patient's family is complete.

The majority of women with endometrial cancer will present with postmenopausal bleeding (PMB) but in only about 15% of women is endometrial cancer the cause of PMB.[7] Traditionally, the investigation of all women with more than one episode of PMB included endometrial biopsy, either as an out-patient procedure using one of a number of patented aspiration devices or at dilatation and curettage under general anaesthesia. The former are uncomfortable for many patients and it may not be possible to get a satisfactory endometrial sample in nearly 20% of women over the age of 70 years.[8]

Vaginal ultrasonography to measure endometrial thickness may be used as a triaging technique in these patients with those with endometrial thickness of 5 mm or less being unlikely to have significant uterine pathology. In addition, vaginal ultrasound may be able to distinguish between cases of endometrial hyperplasia and those of cancer. In postmenopausal women with hyperplasia, the endometrium is thickened and hyperechogenic and the deeper endometrium becomes compacted but remains intact producing a subendometrial 'halo'. This disappears once invasion occurs.

A meta-analysis regarding endometrial thickness as a test for endometrial cancer in women with PMB has been published recently.[9] The authors reviewed nine studies identified from the Medline database using the key words 'vaginal ultrasonography' and 'endometrial thickness measurements' and in which they received supplementary information from the original authors regarding median endometrial thickness in the patients studied. In this meta-analysis, there were 3483 women without endometrial cancer and 330 with cancer. Whilst the median endometrial thickness for cancer cases was nearly 4 times that for unaffected women, 4% of the endometrial cancers would have been missed with a false positive rate as high as 50%. They concluded that endometrial thickness in symptomatic women does not reduce the need for formal endometrial sampling.[9]

In 2000, a meeting took place in the US to produce a consensus document regarding the evaluation of women with PMB. It concluded that either vaginal ultrasonography or endometrial sampling were equally safe and effective as first stage diagnostic steps.[10] However, the expertise of the ultrasonographer must be emphasised and a clinician should not be re-assured by a negative test (either by ultrasound or endometrial sample) in a woman who continues to be symptomatic.

The diagnostic superiority of endometrial sampling at hysteroscopy rather than blind sampling at traditional D and C is not doubted, but anxiety about possible dissemination of malignant cells into the peritoneal cavity at hysteroscopy has been expressed. A recent retrospective study compared the incidence of positive peritoneal cytology at laparotomy for endometrial cancer carried out immediately after hysteroscopy to determine possible endocervical disease.[11] In the study, 70 patients underwent hysteroscopy with carbon dioxide insufflation and 50 with normal saline. Of 8 patients with positive peritoneal cytology (6.7% of the total), 7 were in the normal saline group. The authors concluded that the risk of dissemination is real and may be more likely after saline hysteroscopy. It should be emphasised, of course, that formal D and C also carries such a risk.[12]

TAMOXIFEN AND THE ENDOMETRIUM

There is a consensus that the use of tamoxifen in a postmenopausal woman with breast cancer doubles or triples her risk of subsequently developing endometrial cancer. Tamoxifen is also associated with the development of a number of benign uterine pathologies such as polyps and hyperplasia; if these produce symptoms (*i.e.* vaginal bleeding), referral to a gynaecologist will in all likelihood be made. The future may see more referrals due to the increasing incidence of breast cancer and the use of tamoxifen for prevention of breast cancer. There is no standard protocol to manage such women. The American College of Obstetricians and Gynecologists recommends a yearly gynaecological examination for women taking tamoxifen but it uses terms such as 'close monitoring' and 'screening at the discretion of the individual clinician' which are not further defined and open to interpretation. The Royal College of Obstetricians and Gynaecologists recommends that women on tamoxifen with abnormal vaginal bleeding should undergo a Pipelle biopsy in the first instance with a negative result leading to hysteroscopy and pelvic ultrasound. Out-patient endometrial sampling may be an accurate diagnostic tool in cases of endometrial cancer but its ability to sample polyps is less good. Direct visualisation of the endometrial cavity is probably more accurate in these cases, but hysteroscopy is a more time-consuming procedure and has a greater cost to health-care budgets. Ultrasound examination is an accurate way of measuring endometrial thickness but some authors have shown that around 50% of women with an endometrial thickness of 5 mm or more will have no endometrial pathology.[13,14]

There are numerous management conundrums in monitoring women who have been prescribed tamoxifen. Should all women on tamoxifen whether symptomatic or not be screened? If so, how often and by what method? Could screening cease once the course of tamoxifen is completed or might there be longer term effects caused by the drug?

SURGERY

Since 1998, endometrial cancer has been staged surgically. Prior to this, the disease was staged clinically, the reason being that since almost all patients were treated with pre-operative radiotherapy only the information gained at initial D and C could be reliably used for prognostic purposes, all information obtained by examining the uterine specimen having been affected to some degree by the radiotherapy. With the increase in surgery followed by radiotherapy, it became apparent that factors such as depth of myometrial penetration, cervical glandular or stromal involvement, the presence of positive peritoneal cytology and nodal disease were important prognostic factors. The essential differences between clinical and surgical staging are shown in Table 2.

Table 2 Endometrial carcinoma: FIGO staging 1971 -v- 1988

FIGO staging	1971	1988
Stage 1	Confined to uterine corpus	Limited to endometrium
Stage II	Uterine corpus and cervix involvement	Endocervical or cervical stromal invasion
Stage III	Extra-uterine disease but not outside the true pelvis	Serosal/adnexal invasion or positive cytology, vaginal or nodal (pelvic/para-aortic) metastases
Stage IV	Extrapelvic/bladder or rectal mucosal invasion: spread to distant organs	Bladder/bowel mucosal invasion, intra-abdominal disease, inguinal node metastases

Although intercurrent disease, bodily habitus, *etc.* may make it impossible or inadvisable, surgery should be considered the primary modality in all cases of endometrial cancer. Surgery for stage III disease should be performed with the aim of carrying out hysterectomy and bilateral salpingo-oophorectomy and removal of parametrial, sidewall and abdominal disease using techniques similar to those for surgical management of advanced ovarian cancer. Even in stage IV disease, 'debulking' surgery may improve local control and assist in the palliation of discharge, bleeding, pain and bowel or urinary tract complications.

Traditionally, surgery for clinical stage I disease consisted of simple hysterectomy and removal of the uterine adnexa. A study published in 1970 showed that, in clinical stage I disease, pelvic node metastases would be found in nearly 6% of well-differentiated tumours and over a quarter of cases with poorly differentiated tumours.[15] A larger, later study conducted by The Gynecologic Oncology Group in the US revealed a similar proportion of patients with extra-uterine disease.[16] Yet compared with cervical cancer where a similar risk of nodal disease meant that radical hysterectomy was mandatory, most clinicians failed to address the question of lymphadenectomy in early endometrial cancer.

A retrospective study from the US has suggested that lymphadenectomy may be of some therapeutic benefit.[17] In this study, all patients underwent hysterectomy and bilateral salpingo-oophorectomy with peritoneal cytology; in addition, 212 patients had multiple-site pelvic node sampling, which the authors defined as nodes taken from at least four different sites, whilst 205 had 'limited sampling' (nodes taken from less than four sites) and 208 had no node sampling at all. Clearly, in a retrospective study, the reasons for the degree, or absence, of lymphadenectomy are many – patient general health, obesity, surgeons' skill or knowledge of the possibility of nodal disease, institutional practices, *etc.* and the results of the study must be viewed in that context. However, the overall survival for those patients who underwent multiple node sampling was significantly better than those who had hysterectomy only and the advantage was also seen in those patients who received neither pre- nor postoperative radiotherapy. When patients were categorised into high- and low-risk groups based on tumour grade, myometrial penetration and extra-uterine disease, this trend persisted. Although recurrence rates were higher in the non-node sampled group, of particular interest was the fact that neither the pattern of recurrence (pelvic, distant or both) nor the interval thereto was affected by lymphadenectomy, the median time to recurrence for all groups being 1 year.

The question of the therapeutic role of lymphadenectomy was also partially addressed in a large multicentre study of adjuvant hormonal therapy in patients with endometrial cancer.[18] All cases were high risk which the authors defined as either grade 1 endometrioid, adenosquamous, clear cell or serous papillary histological subtypes, with more than one-third myometrial penetration or cervical or adnexal involvement. The positive pelvic node rate was 13% (22% for patients with cervical involvement, 7% when disease was confined to the corpus). Following adjuvant radiotherapy plus or minus progestogen treatment, the authors reported that the recurrence rate was 14% in the node-negative group compared with 45% in those patients who were node positive (but the recurrence rate in those patients who did not undergo nodal dissection was 16.4%). Node-positive patients had a 2.5 times higher risk of recurrence or death compared with node-negative patients. The morbidity of lymphadenectomy, particularly in a group of women with a high chance of intercurrent medical/anaesthetic problems has been used to criticise those practitioners who have advocated more radical surgery in this disease; in the COSA study, 43% of patients who had lymphadenectomy and radiotherapy had some degree of morbidity compared with 35% who had radiotherapy without lymphadectomy. Other studies have shown that the added morbidity of lymphadenectomy is low.[19]

Is it possible, therefore, to select either pre-operatively or during hysterectomy those patients who would benefit from extended surgical staging comprising pelvic and possibly para-aortic lymph node dissection? The Gynecologic Oncology Group study examined the relationship between intra-operatively acquired pathological criteria and the incidence of nodal metastases.[16] Patients with well-differentiated tumours, with no myometrial penetration and no evidence of extra-uterine peritoneal disease (defined as 'low-risk) had a 0% chance of either pelvic or para-aortic disease. Those at moderate risk (grade 2 or 3 disease, inner or middle myometrial invasion and no peritoneal disease) had a 3% chance of pelvic nodes and a 2% chance of para-aortic disease if only one of the risk factors (grade or myopenetration) was present with the risk of pelvic disease doubling, but para-aortic risk unchanged, if both risk factors were present. The high-risk group (deep myometrial penetration, peritoneal disease) had an 18–61% chance of pelvic nodes depending on which, or both, factors were present and a 15–30% chance of para-aortic disease.

It would be difficult to support a treatment programme of TAHBSO only in the latter group: but, with a less than 5% chance of finding nodal disease in the other two groups, is the morbidity of extended surgical staging acceptable?

Pre-operative selection of patients for extended surgery

Serum tumour markers and the use of pelvic imaging to assess depth of myometrial penetration have been investigated in this setting. Serum CA125 levels are elevated in more than two-thirds of patients with extra-uterine disease compared with normal levels in more than 90% of patients with disease confined to the uterus.[20–22]

Vaginal ultrasound or MRI can predict accurately the depth of myometrial, penetration in 70% of patients or more.[23,24] However, can depth of myometrial penetration even combined with tumour grade predict the incidence of nodal disease and hence a referral to a gynaecological cancer surgeon?

This question was addressed in the management of 40 consecutive patients at King's College Hospital with clinical stage I disease all of whom underwent hysterectomy and surgical staging.[25] Of patients with greater than 50% myometrial penetration, 53% were node negative as were 45% of patients who would be included in the Gynecologic Oncology Group 'high risk group'. These patients would have in all probability been scheduled for postoperative pelvic teletherapy, but it seems illogical to treat the pelvic sidewall and add to the morbidity of treatment in node-negative women.

Intra-operative selection

Numerous strategies to limit, or extend, the intended surgical endeavour during laparotomy have been proposed. These include gross assessment of tumour size, depth of invasion or cervical involvement (either by frozen section or naked eye estimation), and the identification of lymphovascular space invasion at frozen section.

Tumour size was shown to be predictive of nodal metastases by the report of Schink et al.[26] who showed that, when tumour size was less than 2 cm, the incidence of positive nodes was around 6% compared with a rate of 21% for larger lesions and 40% when tumour occupied the whole uterine cavity.

Naked-eye estimation of depth of myometrial invasion has been reported by numerous investigators. Sensitivity in detecting a greater than 50% myometrial invasion has been achieved in over 70% of patients in recent series.[27,28] Using frozen section to estimate myometrial penetration and cervical spread has a similar detection rate.[29]

Since the idea of nodal sampling is to reduce the morbidity (and expense) of a 'radiotherapy for all' protocol, a number of studies have suggested that routine lymphadectomy for all patients with moderate-to-high risk disease (grade 2–3 tumours or macroscopic depth of myometrial invasion of > 50%) is a more cost-effective procedure than awaiting a frozen section report of the depth of myometrial penetration because a negative nodal biopsy would avoid the expense and morbidity of subsequent radiotherapy for a large number of patients.[17,30] The financial impact of treatment regimens will become under increasing scrutiny in health-care systems throughout the world.

Laparoscopic surgery

Data abound as to the feasibility and outcome of performing laparoscopically assisted vaginal hysterectomy for patients with benign uterine disease. There can be little doubt that the procedure has many benefits in terms of patient recovery, early mobilisation and discharge, pain relief requirements, etc. Laparoscopic pelvic lymphadectomy was first described by Reich in 1990.

Initial reports concerned laparoscopic lymphadectomy in patients with cervical cancer but, since the study by Childers and Surwit[31] of two cases of a combined laparoscopic and vaginal surgery for endometrial cancer, several reports have shown that lymph node harvest is similar whether or not lymphadenectomy is carried out by open laparotomy of laparoscopically.[32] The time has probably come to state that laparoscopically assisted vaginal surgery is the procedure of choice for women with endometrial cancer.

RADIOTHERAPY

Radiation therapy has always been integrated into management protocols for patients with endometrial cancer; despite being unproven, it was felt that the benefits of radiotherapy outweighed the side effects. However, in an extremely thorough review of 23 reports in the mid-1970s, Jones showed that for patients with clinical stage I disease 5-year survival was 75% for patients treated by surgery alone compared with 78% for those who received combined surgery and radiotherapy.[33]

The first (of only a very few) prospective randomised study to evaluate the role of postoperative radiotherapy was published in 1980 by Aalders and co-workers.[34] In this study, all 540 patients with clinical stage I disease underwent hysterectomy followed by a radiation dose of 6000 rad to the vaginal vault. The patients were then randomised to either no further treatment or to external field radiotherapy at a dose of 4000 rad to the pelvis. Over a follow-up interval of 3–10 years, there was a significant decrease in vaginal and pelvic recurrences in those patients receiving further treatment group compared with the control group (1.9% compared with 6.9%; $P < 0.01$), but the incidence of distant metastases was 9.9% compared with 5.4% and overall survival almost identical (89% versus 91%). It was concluded that only patients with poorly differentiated tumours with greater than 50% myopenetration might benefit, in gaining a 10% increase in survival, from additional external beam radiotherapy. This subgroup of patients would form less than 20% of a population of women with endometrial cancer.[16]

Despite these observations, most patients were still referred by gynaecologists for consideration of postoperative radiotherapy. This was based on the knowledge that radiation therapy alone could cure patients unfit for or unwilling to undergo hysterectomy and that radiotherapy could salvage a high proportion of patients who subsequently relapsed at the vaginal vault after surgery. It seemed appropriate, therefore, to try to prevent such recurrences with adjuvant radiotherapy. Piver et al.[35] reported a 7.5% vault recurrence rate in patients treated with surgery alone compared with a 4.5% rate for patients who also received pre-operative intracavitary brachytherapy and 0% for patients who received postoperative vault irradiation. In general, only patients with well-differentiated tumours, penetrating less than one-third of the myometrium and confined to the upper two-thirds of the uterine body, were spared adjuvant radiotherapy.[36] This practice continues and some centres treat all grades of endometrial cancer with postoperative radiotherapy even in cases of minimal myometrial invasion.[37,38]

With a vault relapse rate of 5% for patients with stage IB disease treated by surgery alone and a 100% salvage rate with subsequent radiotherapy,[39] a 'vault radiotherapy for all' approach cannot be justified. Indeed, some studies have shown that even for patients with stage IC disease there appears to be no benefit in their receiving postoperative radiotherapy.[40]

Therefore, the majority of patients with endometrial cancer will be cured by surgery alone because they are in a 'good prognosis' group. The majority of patients with poor prognosis disease will die of distant metastases with or without local recurrence as well. Radiotherapy clearly has no role in the prevention of distant disease but might lead to salvage of local recurrences. Should all such patients receive radiotherapy with its associated toxicity, or should radiotherapy be reserved to treat pelvic relapse? Is it justifiable to treat all patients with medium-risk disease as defined by the Gynecologic Oncology Group with radiotherapy when there is only a 3% chance of positive pelvic nodes?

If a blanket 'radiotherapy for all (or nearly all)' is to be avoided, can the group of patients who would really benefit from treatment over and above surgery alone be identified? Kadar et al.[41] queried whether the known prognostic variables of tumour grade, depth of myometrial penetration, tumour invasion of the cervix and lymphovascular space invasion were merely indicators of extra-uterine disease or were of prognostic significance even in patients with disease confined to the uterus. They used the above prognostic variables plus age and looked at their effect on survival. Analysis showed that the greatest negative effect on survival was seen comparing grade 1 versus grades 1 and 2 disease, more than inner one-third myoinvasion compared with less than one-third, the presence or absence of cervical stromal invasion and the presence or absence of lymphovascular space invasion. The combined effect of these variables was best shown by constructing three risk groups which consisted of patients with none or only one of these risk factors or those with two, or three or four. For patients with none or only one risk factor, the 5-year survival was 97% compared with 66% for those in the medium-risk group (two risk factors) and only 17% in those patients with three or four risk factors. They also reported a trend toward improved survival in the medium-risk group for those patients who received pelvic radiotherapy compared with those that did not (70% versus 50% at 5 years).

In another report, four statistically significant prognostic factors for patients with stage I disease were identified – myometrial invasion, vascular invasion, eight or more mitoses per 10 high-power fields and a negative progesterone receptor status.[42] All patients who died within 4 years of diagnosis had two or more of these prognostic factors.

A recent randomised study in medium-risk patients, defined as those with grade 1 tumours with > 50% myometrial invasion, grade 2 tumours with any degree of invasion and grade 1 tumours with superficial invasion, randomised them to either TAHBSO alone or surgery plus postoperative radiotherapy.[43] The 5-year locoregional recurrence rate was 14% in the surgery-only group compared with 4% in the irradiated group. This suggests that about 30% (4/14) of locoregional relapses are not controlled by radiotherapy: 5-year overall survival rates were 85% and 81%, respectively. In the surgery-only group, 40 patients developed a locoregional recurrence but only four died from it. It has been suggested that postoperative radiotherapy should not be given to medium-risk patients with stage I disease when so many can be salvaged at relapse with radiotherapy.[44] It should be noted, however, that radiation doses used to salvage locoregional recurrences are significantly higher than those used in a postoperative setting (70 Gray compared with 40 Gray). Considerably more toxicity is to be expected in a salvage setting but this has to be offset by the fact that radiation toxicity will be considerably less overall since many medium-risk patients will be cured by surgery alone.

HORMONAL THERAPY

Rather like radiation, hormonal therapy historically was given to patients after the diagnosis of endometrial cancer (*i.e.* before hysterectomy) and to almost all patients after surgery either in an immediate adjuvant setting or at relapse. Once again, prospective data are few but one study showed that adjuvant hormonal therapy does not improve cure rates.[45] In this study, after surgery patients with stage IB grade 1 or 2 disease were randomised to either no further treatment or 100 mg medoxyprogesterone acetate (MPA) twice daily for a year. Patients with stage IC disease and positive pelvic nodes were treated with radiotherapy with or without MPA. Relapse-free survival was high and almost identical for all groups.

In the large multicentre COSA-NZ-UK study, 1112 patients with high-risk disease (defined as grade 3 endometrioid, adenosquamous, clear cell or serous papillary cancer, any tumour invading more than one-third of the myometrium or involving the cervix or adnexa) were randomised, after surgery and radiotherapy, to receive either adjuvant MPA (200 mg bd) or no hormonal therapy for at least 3 years. Analysis of all patients showed significantly more relapses in the no treatment arm but no differences in survival.[46] Of 96 patients in the no treatment group, 49 received MPA at relapse. Median survival was 10 months compared with 4 months for those who were not treated. The group concluded that 'the use of adjuvant MPA at this dose and for this length of time has little place in the management of patients with high-risk endometrial cancer'. A meta-analysis of six randomised trials in endometrial cancer has not show any advantage to patients receiving adjuvant progesterone therapy.[47]

CHEMOTHERAPY

High cure rates by surgery/radiotherapy have precluded much interest in adjuvant chemotherapy in the majority of patients. Such trials that have been reported lack sufficient patient numbers or an agreed definition of 'risk'. The exception may be in the management of uterine papillary serous carcinoma, a rare (2–10% of all endometrial cancers) and aggressive histological variant which resembles ovarian serous papillary tumours and has a high propensity for extra-uterine spread at the time of presentation.[48] Standard chemotherapy regimens have not been defined but active regimens include combination cyclophosphamide, doxorubicin and cisplatin, achieving a 27% response rate, but with a median overall survival of only 7 months.[49] Toxicity is significant.

Many cytotoxics have been shown to have activity in advanced or recurrent disease (doxorubicin, cis- and carboplatin, ifosphomide, paclitaxel) with response rates of up to about 40% as single agents. However, most of these responses are only partial and of limited duration (8 months or less). Phase II studies of combination regimens seem to suggest higher response rates. Once again, there is a dearth of randomised prospective studies comparing cytotoxic regimens which reflects the difficulties in recruiting sufficient numbers of patients.

The relative lack of toxicity and different mode of action of progestational agents from cytotoxics makes it an attractive proposition to combine the two. Response rates vary from around 16% to over 80% (which suggests that different patient populations have been treated) but the studies are of small numbers and interpretation and comparison of the results are difficult. It would appear that the addition of progestogens adds little to the efficacy of cytotoxics.

HOW MIGHT THE MANAGEMENT OF ENDOMETRIAL CANCER BE IMPROVED?

The subtle alteration to this article's title is deliberate. Improvements in the prognosis for the majority of patients with endometrial cancer will not be apparent even with data from randomised studies because their prognosis is so good. Management will be improved for them, however, as we confirm that so few of them need adjuvant radiotherapy and those who do relapse can be salvaged successfully with radiotherapy. These data should allow us to be in a position to refine rather than define treatment protocols.

A greater ability to predict risk of recurrence within this 'good prognosis' group will allow a more rational use of adjunctive therapies. Pelvic nodal areas do not need to be irradiated in node-negative patients, but the upper abdomen ought to be considered at risk in patients with positive peritoneal cytology or biopsy proven upper abdominal disease.

More aggressive treatment strategies will be developed for high-risk groups and there is a very strong argument for entering these patients into randomised trials, comparing, for instance, whole abdominal radiotherapy with cytotoxics. For the more distant future, disease prevention is clearly the aim, but in the shorter term we are likely to encourage more (extended) surgery and less radiotherapy. Our patients should benefit from this.

References

1 Corn BW, Lanciano RM, Greven KM et al. Impact of improved radiation technique, age and lymph node sampling on the severe complication rate of surgically staged endometrial cancer patients: a multivariate analysis. J Clin Oncol 1994; 12: 510–515

2 Kurman RJ, Kaminski PF, Norris HJ. The behaviour of endometrial hyperplasia: a long term study of 'untreated' hyperplasia in 170 patients. Cancer 1985; 56: 403–407

3 Ferenczy A, Gelfland M. The biologic significance of cytologic atypia in progestogen-treated endometrial hyperplasia. Am J Obstet Gynecol 1989; 160: 126–130

4 Lynch HT, Smyrk TC, Watson P et al. Genetics, natural history, tumor spectrum and pathology of hereditary non-polyposis colorectal cancer: an updated review. Gastroenterology 1993; 104: 1535–1549

5 Aarnio M, Sankila R, Pukkala E et al. Cancer risk in mutation carriers of DNA-mismatch repair genes. Int J Cancer 1999; 81: 214–218

6 Dunlop MG, Farrington SM, Carothers AD et al. Cancer risk associated with germline DNA mismatch repair gene mutations. Hum Mol Genet 1997; 6: 105–110

7 Hacker NF, Moore JG. (eds) Essentials of Obstetrics and Gynecology. Philadelphia: WB Saunders, 1986; 467

8 Koss LG, Schreiber K, Oberlander SG et al. Screening of asymptomatic women for endometrial cancer. Obstet Gynecol 1981; 57: 681–685

9 Tabor A, Watt HC, Wald NJ. Endometrial thickness as a test for endometrial cancer in women with postmenopausal vaginal bleeding. Obstet Gynecol 2002; 99: 663–670

10 Goldstein RB, Bree RL, Benson CB et al. Evaluation of the woman with post-menopausal bleeding: Society of Radiologists in Ultrasound Consensus Conference statement. J Ultrasound Med 2001; 10: 1025–1036

11 Lo KWK, Cheung TH, Yim SF, Chung TKH. Hysteroscopic dissemination of endometrial carcinoma using carbon dioxide and normal saline: a retrospective study. Gynecol Oncol 2002; 84: 394–398

12 Kudela M, Pilka R. Is there a real risk in patients with endometrial carcinoma undergoing diagnostic hysteroscopy? Eur J Gynaecol Oncol 2001; 22: 342–345

13 Love CD, Muir BB, Scrimgeour JB, Leonard RC, Dillon P, Dixon JM. Investigation of endometrial abnormalities in asymptomatic women treated with tamoxifen and an evaluation of the role of endometrial screening. J Clin Oncol 1999; 17: 2050-2054

14 Lahti E, Blanco G, Kauppila A, Apaja-Sarkkinen M, Taskinen PJ, Laatikainen T. Endometrial changes in postmenopausal breast cancer patients receiving tamoxifen. Obstet Gynecol 1993; 81: 660–664

15 Lewis BV, Stallworthy JA, Cowdell R. Adenocarcinoma of the body of the uterus. J Obstet Gynaecol Br Cwlth 1970; 77: 343–348

16 Creasman WT, Morrow CP, Bundy BN, Homesley HD, Graham JE, Weller PB. Surgical pathologic spread patterns of endometrial cancer. A Gynecologic Oncology Group study. Cancer 1987; 60: 2035–2041

17 Kilgore LC, Partridge EE, Alvarez RD et al. Adenocarcinoma of the endometrium: survival comparisons with and without pelvic node sampling. Gynecol Oncol 1995; 56: 29–33

18 COSA-NZ-UK Endometrial Cancer Study Groups. Pelvic lymphadenectomy in high risk endometrial cancer. Int J Gynecol Cancer 1996; 6: 102–107

19 Homesley HD, Kadar N, Barrett RJ, Lentz SS. Selective pelvic and para-aortic lymphadenectomy does not increase morbidity in surgical staging of endometrial carcinoma. Am J Obstet Gynecol 1992; 167: 1225–1230

20 Niloff JM, Klug TL, Schaetzl E, Zurawski Jr VR, Knapp RC, Bast Jr RC. Elevation of serum CA125 in carcinomas of the fallopian tube, endometrium and endocervix. Am J Obstet Gynecol 1984; 148: 1057–1058

21 Patsner B, Mann WJ, Cohen C, Loesch M. Predictive value of preoperative serum CA125 levels in clinically localised and advanced endometrial carcinoma. Am J Obstet Gynecol 1988; 158: 399–402

22 Sood AK, Buller RE, Burger RA, Dawson JD, Sorosky JI, Berman M. Value of preoperative CA125 levels in the management of uterine cancer and prediction of clinical outcome. Obstet Gynecol 1997; 90: 411–417

23 Gordon AN, Fleischer AC, Reed GW. Depth of myometrial invasion in endometrial cancer: preoperative assessment by transvaginal ultrasonography. Gynecol Oncol 1990; 39: 321–327

24 Chen SS, Rumancik WM, Spiegel G. Magnetic resonance imaging in stage I endometrial carcinoma. Obstet Gynecol 1990; 75: 274–277

25 Lawton FG. The management of endometrial cancer. Br J Obstet Gynaecol 1997; 104: 127–134

26 Schink JC, Lurain JR, Wallemark CB, Chmiel JS. Tumor size in endometrial cancer: a prognostic factor for lymph node metastases. Obstet Gynecol 1987; 70: 216–219

27 Doering DL, Barnhill DR, Weiser EB, Burke TW, Woodward JE, Park RC. Intraoperative evaluation of depth of myometrial invasion in stage I endometrial adenocarcinoma. Obstet Gynecol 1989; 74: 930–933

28 Larson DM, Connor GP, Broste SK, Krawisz BR, Johnson KK. Prognostic significance of gross myometrial invasion in patients with endometrial cancer. Obstet Gynecol 1996; 88: 394–398

29 Shim JU, Rose PG, Reale FR, Soto H, Tak WK, Hunter RE. Accuracy of frozen section diagnosis at surgery in clinical stage I and II endometrial carcinoma. Am J Obstet

Gynecol 1992; 166: 1335–1338

30 Orr Jr JW, Holiman JL, Orr PF. Stage I corpus cancer: is teletherapy necessary? Am J Obstet Gynecol 1997; 176: 777–788

31 Childers J, Surwit E. Combined laparoscopic and vaginal surgery for the management of two cases of stage I endometrial cancer. Gynecol Oncol 1992; 45: 46–51

32 Fram KK. Laparoscopically assisted vaginal hysterectomy versus abdominal hysterectomy in stage I endometrial cancer. Int J Gynecol Cancer 2002; 12: 57–61

33 Jones III HJ. Treatment of adenocarcinoma of the endometrium. Obstet Gynecol Survey 1975; 30: 147–169

34 Aalders JG, Abeler V, Kolstad P, Onsrud M. Postoperative external irradiation and prognostic parameters in stage I endometrial carcinoma. Obstet Gynecol 1980; 56: 419–426

35 Piver MS, Yazigi R, Blumenson LE. A prospective trial comparing hysterectomy, hysterectomy plus vaginal radium and uterine radium plus hysterectomy in stage I endometrial carcinoma. Obstet Gynecol 1979; 54: 85–89

36 Aalders J. Treatment of endometrial cancer of the uterus. In: Blackledge GRP, Jordan JA, Shingleton HM. (eds) Textbook of Gynecologic Oncology. London: WB Saunders, 1991; 243–249

37 Maggino T, Romagnolo C, Landoni F, Sartori E, Zola P, Gadducci A. An analysis of approaches to the management of endometrial cancer in North America: a CTF study. Gynecol Oncol 1998; 68: 274–279

38 Lybeert MLM, van Putten WJL, Ribot JG et al. Endometrial carcinoma: high dose rate brachytherapy in combination with external irradiation; a multivariate analysis. Radiother Oncol 1989; 16: 245–252

39 Straughn JM, Huh WK, Kelly FJ et al. Conservative management of stage I endometrial carcinoma after surgical staging. Gynecol Oncol 2002; 84: 194–200

40 Chen SS. Operative treatment in stage I endometrial carcinoma with deep myometrial invasion and/or grade 3 tumor surgically limited to the corpus uteri: recurrence with only primary surgery. Cancer 1989; 63: 1843–1845

41 Kadar N, Malfetano JH, Homesley HD. Determinants of survival of surgically staged patients with endometrial carcinoma histologically confined to the uterus: implications for therapy. Obstet Gynecol 1992; 80: 655–659

42 Tormos C, Silva EG, El-Naggar A, Burke TW. Aggressive stage I grade 1 endometrial carcinoma. Cancer 1992; 70: 790–798

43 Creutzberg CL, van Putten WLJ, Koper PCM et al. Surgery and postoperative radiotherapy versus surgery alone for patients with stage I endometrial carcinoma. multicentre randomised trial. PORTEC Study Group Postoperative Radiation Therapy in Endometrial Carcinoma. Lancet 2000; 355: 1404–1411

44 Burger MPM. Management of stage I endometrial carcinoma. BMJ 2001; 322: 568–569

45 De Palo G, Mangioni C, Periti P, Del Vecchio M, Marubini E. Treatment of FIGO (1971) stage I endometrial cancer with intensive surgery, radiotherapy and hormonal therapy according to pathological prognostic groups. Long term results of a randomised multicentre study. Eur J Cancer 1993; 29A: 1133–1140

46 COSA-NZ-UK Endometrial Cancer Study Group. Adjuvant medoxyprogesterone acetate in high risk endometrial cancer. Int J Gynecol Cancer 1998; 8: 387–391

47 Martin-Hirsch PL, Lilford RJ, Jarvis GJ. Adjuvant progestogen therapy for the treatment of endometrial cancer. Review and meta-analysis of published, randomised controlled trials. Eur J Obstet Gynecol Reprod Biol 1996; 65: 201–207

48 Christopherson WM, Albertasky RC, Connelly PJ. Carcinoma of the endometrium. II: Papillary adenocarcinoma: a clinical pathological study of 46 cases. Am J Clin Pathol 1982; 77: 534–540

49 Price FV, Chambers SK, Carcanglu KE et al. Intravenous cisplatin, doxorubicin and cyclophosphamide in the treatment of uterine papillary serous carcinoma (UPSC). Gynecol Oncol 1993; 51: 583–589

Joseph Hanoch Angus McIndoe

22

Improving the prognosis of ovarian cancer

Ovarian cancer is the fourth most common cancer among women in the UK, and is a major source of morbidity and mortality. Each year, there are over 6820 new cases. Its high case-fatality rate reflects a delay in diagnosis: since patients often present with non-specific symptoms, diagnosis is generally made when disease has spread to the peritoneal cavity. The majority (65%) of patients are diagnosed with advanced cancer,[1] when 5-year survival is only 28%.[2] It presents an increasing challenge to the gynaecological oncologist, who is frustrated by the paucity of knowledge of the aetiological factors in ovarian cancer and by the failure to achieve any dramatic reduction in mortality due to these neoplasms during the past 6 decades.[3] It is the cause of more deaths than any other female genital tract cancer.

In the 1950s and 1960s, ovarian cancer was diagnosed by bimanual gynaecological exploration and laparotomy only, as sonography, computed tomography, and magnetic resonance imaging were unknown. The means of treatment was surgery: in cases of an 'operable tumour', total abdominal hysterectomy and bilateral salpingo-oophorectomy was mandatory. In case of peritoneal metastases a debulking of the tumour and omentectomy, as well as postoperative radiotherapy, were recommended.[4] In the more recent era, a multimodality therapy is established as the standard approach to treatment. Surgery remains a cornerstone of therapy for diagnosis, staging and treatment. Once the patients have had their primary debulking surgery, that by definition includes full surgical staging, the adjuvant therapy of choice for stages higher than Ia is usually Paclitaxel and platinum chemotherapy.[5]

Joseph Hanoch MD
Gynaecological Oncology Fellow. Department of Gynaecological Oncology, Hammersmith Hospital, Imperial College Medical School, Du Cane Road, London W12 0HS, UK
(for correspondence, E-mail: daniel5198@yahoo.com)

Angus McIndoe PhD FRCS MRCOG
Consultant Gynaecological Oncologist, Hammersmith Hospital, Imperial College Medical School, Du Cane Road, London W12 0HS, UK

The treatment of ovarian cancer has rapidly evolved in the past decade. Starting with the initial observation that alkylating agents were active in the treatment of this disease, new classes of agents have been rapidly incorporated in the therapeutic armamentarium. This has included the platinum compounds, taxanes and most recently, camptothecin derivatives, inhibitors of topoisomerase I. An intense search has been made for novel approaches to treatment of ovarian cancer, and several new treatments show promise.

This overall intense effort to improve survival in ovarian cancer patients is starting to show results, at least in the short-term survival assessment. Here, we describe and review these methods, old, new or combinations of both, that are aimed at improving the prognosis in this type of cancer, which has always been considered as the worst of all the gynaecological neoplasms.

SCREENING

The lower the stage, the better the prognosis. This general assumption is true for most cancers, if not all. Therefore, early detection should be a reasonable method of improving survival. The optimal analogy would be the cervical smear as screening for cervical cancer, that has had a major impact on the incidence of and death rate from cervical cancer.[3] Nevertheless, screening for ovarian cancer is still experimental, and early detection is currently more a matter of chance than a consequence of a scientific strategy, partly because of the fact that there is no single identifiable cause or marker for this disease.

The most commonly studied methods of early detection and screening are CA-125 and ultrasound. At the present time, they offer the best opportunity to detect ovarian cancers early; however, they are far from optimal. Laframboise et al.[6] reported a retrospective study on ovarian cancer screening in a high-risk female population using both CA-125 and ultrasound scan. This dual screening method was performed every 6 months. Overall, 33 of 1209 (2.7%) CA-125 results were abnormal, and 226 of 1342 (17%) ultrasounds were abnormal. In 7 years of screening, only one patient (0.3%) has been diagnosed with ovarian cancer.

Ultrasound is a very sensitive tool for identifying advanced stage ovarian cancer, but the identification of Stage I ovarian cancer with ultrasound screening is more problematic since only 25–50% of ovarian cancers are identified in low-risk and high-risk patients, respectively, using this technique.[7] Routine screening of premenopausal women or low-risk women after the menopause is unlikely to be cost-effective. At this time, ovarian cancer screening should probably be done in high-risk groups under careful investigational scrutiny. Transvaginal ultrasound is sensitive but not ideally specific for discriminating benign from malignant disease. The judicious use of colour Doppler evaluation may improve specificity.

A novel and promising technique described very recently by Petricoin et al.[8] is based on the concept that pathological changes within an organ might be reflected in proteomic patterns in serum. Generated by mass spectroscopy, proteomic patterns were identified in the serum, which could distinguish neoplastic from non-neoplastic disease within the ovary. The discriminatory pattern correctly identified all 50 ovarian cancer cases in a masked set, including all 18 stage I cases. This result yielded a sensitivity of 100%, specificity of 95%, and positive predictive value of 94%. These important findings need to be assessed in a prospective population-based study as a screening tool.

Recent advances in molecular technology are leading to the discovery of new tumour biomarkers that may be useful for cancer screening and early diagnosis. Mok et al.,[9] using transcriptional profiling of ovarian cancer cell lines, found that the levels of prostasin, a serine protease, are higher in cancerous ovarian epithelial cells and stroma than in normal ovarian tissue. Fourteen other candidate tumour markers have been found through these technological methods.[10] Novel markers like prostasin and others, that are, and will in the future be discovered from the emerging technologies of transcriptional profiling and proteomics should be investigated further as a screening or tumour marker, alone and in combination with CA-125, preferably following the guidelines of the National Cancer Institute's Early Detection Research Network (EDRN).[11]

There are currently at least three prospective, randomised clinical trials ongoing; however, unless results from these show differently, there are no reliable data that screening for ovarian cancer is effective in improving the length and quality of life in women with ovarian cancer.

PROPHYLACTIC SURGERY

Genetic testing for susceptibility to ovarian cancer is rapidly becoming integrated into the clinical practice of oncology. The identification of the BRCA genes and the availability of genetic testing for BRCA mutations have underscored the need for improvements in early detection and prevention of breast and ovarian cancer. Genetic testing for BRCA1 and BRCA2 is now recommended to most women with invasive ovarian cancer. Carriers of a mutation in BRCA1 are thought to have a 20–40% life-time risk of ovarian cancer. Women with a mutation in BRCA2 appear to have a 10–20% risk of ovarian cancer.[12] Alternatively, approximately 10% of women with ovarian cancer will have a positive test, including 4% of women without a family history of cancer. It also appears that women with ovarian cancer and a BRCA mutation experience better survival than women without a mutation.[12]

The indications for prophylactic oophorectomy, particularly in patients carrying the BRCA mutations, are well defined. Two very recent articles have validated this approach and supported a role for oophorectomy not only in the prevention of ovarian cancer, but also in reducing the risk of breast cancer.[14,15]

Prophylactic oophorectomy should be offered to all women with BRCA1–2 mutations, especially those beyond the years of childbearing.[16] From the surgical point of view, it seems prudent to perform adnexectomy rather than just oophorectomy, thus preventing the occurrence of fallopian tube carcinoma,[17] and reducing the risk of leaving ovary remnants in the mesovarium.[18] This surgery could easily use a laparoscopic approach.[18,19] Despite a sole report describing a higher risk of endometrial cancer in first-degree relatives of Jewish women with ovarian cancer who are BRCA1 mutation carriers,[20] performing a prophylactic oophorectomy does not seem to be an indication for a concomitant hysterectomy.

PRIMARY SURGICAL DEBULKING

Surgery is still the cornerstone in the management of advanced epithelial ovarian cancer patients. It has been a basic principle among many gynaecological oncologists that it is judicious to excise as much tumour as possible when disseminated disease is encountered at the time of primary operation for ovarian cancer. Substantial evidence exists to demonstrate that if surgery is performed by gynaecologists with a special training in gynaecological oncology, a survival advantage can be achieved.[21] Primary surgery with diagnostic and cytoreductive intent should be performed in accordance with the European Guidelines of Staging in Ovarian Cancer. Whether or not cytoreduction should systematically include lymphadenectomy is still a controversial issue. Different definitions exist for optimal cytoreduction. Griffiths[22] initially proposed that all metastatic nodules should be reduced to no greater than 1.5 cm in maximum diameter and showed that survival was significantly longer in such patients. Optimal debulking has been later re-defined to less than 2 cm, 1 cm or 5 mm tumour deposits, but it should be now recognised as the complete absence of disease at the end of the surgical procedure. Subsequently, it has been shown that the smaller the residual disease, the longer the patient's median survival.[23,24] Clearly, those patients whose disease has been completely resected have the best prognosis.[23] The extent of residual disease after primary surgery is an independent prognostic variable, and optimal cytoreduction is associated with improved survival even when there is a need for an en-bloc resection of rectosigmoid to achieve that,[25–27] and, although still controversial, probably also in stage IV disease.[28]

A very recent meta-analysis set to evaluate the effect of maximal cytoreductive surgery on survival among patients with advanced-stage ovarian carcinoma treated with platinum-based chemotherapy confirmed a statistically significant positive correlation between percentage maximal cytoreduction and log median survival time.[29]

INTERVAL DEBULKING

Retrospective analyses suggest that a subgroup of patients with Stage III and IV ovarian carcinoma can be treated with neo-adjuvant chemotherapy followed by interval debulking surgery, thus obtaining higher optimal resection rates, and consequently, a survival benefit.[30–32]

For those patients in whom optimal debulking would be clinically assessed to be possible, timely operation is mandatory. For the inoperable advanced cases, where optimal cytoreduction might not be achieved, usually because of metastases at sites where resection is impossible or due to uncountable peritoneal metastases, the chemotherapy-surgery-chemotherapy regimen could be recommended. Some authors consider also a large volume ascites to be a risk factor that would mandate a neo-adjuvant chemotherapy followed by interval debulking surgery.[33]

Kuhn et al.[34] have recently published a prospective study of patients with stage IIIc ovarian carcinoma. The study arm received 3 cycles of platinum/taxane-based chemotherapy, followed by surgical cytoreduction and 3 additional cycles of chemotherapy. They showed higher tumour resection rates and longer median survival in those patients who were treated by neoadjuvant chemotherapy compared to the patients in the control group, who were treated by the conventional therapy (tumour debulking surgery followed by 6 cycles of chemotherapy).

Neoadjuvant chemotherapy for primary unresectable ovarian carcinoma leads to the selection of a subset of patients sensitive to chemotherapy in whom optimal cytoreduction can be achieved after chemotherapy by standard surgery in a high proportion of cases. Conversely, aggressive surgery can be avoided in patients with initial chemoresistance, in whom the prognosis is known to be poor regardless of treatment.

The strategy of neoadjuvant chemotherapy, followed by interval debulking surgery, should be confirmed in a prospective randomised trial. The EORTC 55971 trial is currently addressing this issue.

SECONDARY DEBULKING

In recurrent ovarian cancer, secondary surgery may be an important opportunity to improve survival and quality of life. The median survival after secondary surgery has been reported ranging from 16 to 29 months, and seems to be longer in subjects with optimal debulked disease. Any benefit of treatment must be compared with potential morbidity. Postoperative complications are reported in a relatively high (25–30%) proportion of cases.[35]

In a recent prospective study by Scarabelli et al.,[36] 149 patients underwent secondary cytoreductive surgery following primary treatment. They found that residual tumour after secondary surgery was by far the most strongly predictive factor for patient survival, and concluded that patients who have documented gross disease pre-operatively should be selected for a secondary debulking operation.

Cormio et al.[37] published a retrospective review on 21 patients submitted to secondary cytoreductive surgery for apparently isolated and resectable recurrence of ovarian cancer; 71% had complete surgical debulking with no macroscopic tumour at the completion of the surgical procedure. Eleven complications were recorded in nine patients. The absence of residual disease after salvage surgery was the only factor associated with prolonged survival.

However, as with primary cytoreduction, it is difficult to establish whether the secondary debulking itself has a therapeutic, or even a lasting palliative effect, or whether the patients in whom the procedure is successful are those who have more indolent disease.

CHEMOTHERAPY

Since a relatively high response rate has been traditional with alkylating agent chemotherapy, there have been few trials with other single agents in patients who have not previously received chemotherapy

In 1976, Wiltshaw and Kroner[38] published their landmark report regarding the efficacy of cisplatin in ovarian cancer, which established the modern era of combination chemotherapy. They reported the treatment of 34 patients with advanced adenocarcinoma of the ovary that was resistant to the conventional chemotherapy of that time. A therapeutic response was shown in 26.5% of patients, with a median duration of 6 months. Several cisplatin-containing regimens soon became available, resulting in response rates as high as 90% and complete responses of 40–50%.[3]

In one carefully performed meta-analysis published by Hunter et al.,[39] 58 suitable studies that encompassed 6962 patients were studied to determine whether maximum cytoreductive surgery could benefit the survival of women with advanced ovarian cancer. The results showed that the cytoreductive surgery was associated with only a small improvement in median survival time, but platinum-containing chemotherapy improved median survival time substantially. Increased dose intensity also conferred a useful survival benefit. They concluded that cytoreductive surgery probably had only a small effect on the survival of women with advanced ovarian cancer, and that the type of chemotherapy used was more important.

In the early 1990s, the drug PTX (Paclitaxel) was first tested in ovarian cancer. It acts by promoting microtubular assembly and stabilises tubulin polymer formation. Although used primarily for salvage therapy, it has moved into trials of first-line therapy in combination with platinum, and since the GOG111 report in 1996 by McGuire et al.[40] has become the 'gold standard' in advanced disease. They randomly assigned 410 women with advanced ovarian cancer and residual masses larger than 1 cm after initial surgery to receive cisplatin with either cyclophosphamide or Paclitaxel. Among 216 women with measurable disease, 73% in the cisplatin-Paclitaxel group responded to therapy, as compared with 60% in the cisplatin-cyclophosphamide group ($P = 0.01$). Progression-free survival was significantly longer ($P < 0.001$) in the cisplatin-Paclitaxel group than in the cisplatin-cyclophosphamide group (median, 18 versus 13 months). Survival was also significantly longer ($P < 0.001$) in the cisplatin-Paclitaxel group (median, 38 versus 24 months). These favourable data were confirmed[41] by a European-Canadian Intergroup trial (OV10).

This choice of standard therapy might, however, be questioned based on the results of the hitherto largest randomised study in advanced ovarian cancer, ICON3. It compared Paclitaxel/Carboplatin with Carboplatin only or a platinum combination (cyclophosphamide/doxorubicin/cisplatin). There were no statistically significant differences in progression-free or overall survival. The results of ICON3, in accordance with GOG132 study[42] (that found similar overall survival rates for Paclitaxel combined with cisplatin, compared to Paclitaxel or cisplatin monotherapy), appear to contradict the earlier positive results seen for PTX and CP in the GOG-111 and OV10 trials.

Intraperitoneal therapy has been a controversial issue for a long time. Improved survival compared with intravenous therapy has yet to be confirmed.

High response rates are achieved with high-dose chemotherapy with stem cell support in the salvage situation but response duration is short.[43] Controlled data supporting survival benefit from high dose chemotherapy with haematological stem cell support are lacking. Phase III studies evaluating high-dose chemotherapy are ongoing.

Patients with recurrent disease frequently respond to second-line treatments, but the impact on survival remains uncertain. Topotecan, a drug with topoisomerase I-inhibitory activity, induces reversible single-stranded breaks. Toxicity of Topotecan can be significant, particularly bone marrow suppression. Several phase-II studies have shown a response rate of 13–14% in patients with platinum refractory ovarian cancer.[3] It is currently approved for use in the US as second-line therapy. Significant trials results to show survival benefit are still awaited for.

Radiation therapy techniques include intraperitoneal instillation of radioactive chromium phosphate and external-beam radiation to the abdomen and pelvis.

The use of salvage whole abdominopelvic radiation therapy (WAPRT) after cis-platinum failure or in women who have received more than one salvage chemotherapy regimen has been shown to be minimally effective and too toxic in this situation.[44–47]

However, more recent reports from radiation oncology investigators have questioned the above information, and proved that radiation therapy can be effective after chemotherapy.[48–50]

A recent retrospective review of radiation therapy for advanced ovarian carcinoma has shown that the response, survival, and tolerance rates compare favourably to those reported for current second- and third-line chemotherapy regimens.[51] Co-operative groups should consider evaluating prospectively the use of radiation therapy before non-platinum and/or non-Paclitaxel chemotherapy in these patients.

Another recent study,[52] looking into the survival effects of consolidation radiation therapy following cytoreductive surgery, chemotherapy and second-look laparotomy, showed that despite the initial survival advantage observed in irradiated patients, owing to late recurrences there was no significant difference in their long-term survival probability.

Low-dose radiation therapy with or without chemotherapy appears to be a promising area of investigation.

IMMUNOTHERAPY

In the last decades, realising that human tumours are immunogenic, there has been considerable interest in combining chemotherapy with immunotherapy for better results.

A prospective randomised study conducted by the GOG[53] compared treatment with Melphalan alone (63 patients) to treatment with Melphalan plus *Corynebacterium parvum* (45 patients). The effectiveness of chemoimmuno-therapy was evaluated in those previously untreated Stage III ovarian cancer patients. Response rate, progression-free interval, and survival were considerably better in the second (chemoimmunotherapy) group.

Advances in molecular biology and immunology now make it possible to explore immunotherapeutic approaches targeting proteins that play a role in the malignant transformation of a cell. The HER2/neu oncogenic protein is a particularly attractive therapeutic target, as it has been found that its overexpression is associated with a poor prognosis, and is correlated with more aggressive disease and potential resistance to standard doses of chemotherapy.[54] Passive immunotherapy strategies, such as the infusion of monoclonal antibodies specific for HER2/neu, have been shown to be of clinical benefit in patients with HER2/neu-overexpressing malignancies.[55] Inducing an active immune response by generating endogenous HER2/neu-specific antibodies and T cells may result in long-lived immunity and, hopefully, therapeutic benefit. Human clinical trials of active immunisation with HER2/neu-specific vaccines are just starting.

Table 1 Principal targets for gene therapy

Goal	Means
Repairing defects in tumour suppresser genes	p53 pathway Phosphatidyl-3-kinase (PI-3)/Akt pathway
Specific antitumour cell immunity	Inducing and promoting
Tumour cell cytotoxicity	Oncolytic adenoviruses Suicide gene delivery

GENE THERAPY

Gene therapy-based approaches have gained significant attention as more has been learned about the molecular basis of cancer, allowing for potential interventions at the molecular level for therapeutic purposes Table 1).

Since drug resistance to conventional chemotherapy can often occur within months, it is not surprising that other strategies are sought, and a number of groups have used virus gene therapy as one possible route to supplement conventional chemotherapy.

Adenovirus vectors have been used extensively for gene therapy because of their high infection efficiency in dividing and non-dividing cells and the wide prevalence of the coxsackie-adenovirus receptors (CARs) in a variety of cells and tissues.[56]

In a recent phase I clinical trial,[57] 10 patients with recurrent ovarian cancer were treated intraperitoneally with a replication-deficient recombinant adenovirus containing the herpes simplex virus thymidine kinase gene. Vector delivery was followed by intravenous administration of an antiherpetic prodrug and a topoisomerase I inhibitor. The results showed that median overall survival was about one-third longer than in previously reported second-and third-line trials.

On the whole, the use of viral vectors does offer a variety of routes to improved therapy, but progress has been disappointing. The future results of the new clinical trials will hopefully show enhanced survival.

VIRAL THERAPY

In the search for novel cancer therapies that can be used in conjunction with existing treatments, one promising area of research is the use of viral vectors and whole viruses. Viruses have evolved to infect, replicate in and kill human cells through diverse mechanisms. In the first half of the 20th century, many cancer patients had been treated with a variety of wild-type viruses, but that strategy was abandoned because of unacceptable toxicity.[58] However, following the first description by Martuza et al.[59] in 1991 of a virus engineered to replicate selectively in dividing cells, the field of viral therapy for cancer has been reborn and significantly expanded.

Targeting ovarian cancer, the first and most extensively studied and used in clinical trials is the Onyx-015, engineered from adenovirus. Another virus in clinical trials is a non-engineered agent, whose parental strain is the Newcastle disease virus.

Table 2 Major on-going clinical trials

Code name	Description	Projected accrual
GOG-175	Phase III randomised study of Carboplatin and Paclitaxel with or without low dose Paclitaxel in patients with early stage ovarian carcinoma	345 patients
EORTC-55005	Phase III randomised study of Carboplatin with or without Gemcitabine in patients with advanced ovarian epithelial carcinoma who failed prior first-line platinum-based therapy	250 patients
EORTC-55963	Phase III randomised study of chemotherapy with or without secondary cytoreductive surgery in patients with recurrent ovarian epithelial cancer	700 patients
EORTC-55012	Phase III randomised study of cisplatin and Topotecan followed by Paclitaxel and Carboplatin versus Paclitaxel and Carboplatin alone in patients with newly diagnosed Stage IIB–IV ovarian epithelial, primary peritoneal, or fallopian tube cancer	800 patients
EORTC-55971	Phase III randomised study of neoadjuvant chemotherapy followed by interval debulking surgery versus upfront cytoreductive surgery followed by chemotherapy with or without interval debulking surgery in patients with Stage IIIC or IV ovarian epithelial, peritoneal, or fallopian tube cancer	704 patients
EORTC-55981	Phase III randomised study of Paclitaxel and Carboplatin with or without Epirubicin as initial treatment in patients with Stage IIB, III, or IV invasive ovarian epithelial, fallopian tube, or peritoneal cancer	800 patients
GOG-0182	Phase III randomised study of Paclitaxel and Carboplatin with or without Gemcitabine, Doxorubicin-HCl liposome, or Topotecan in patients with Stage III or IV ovarian epithelial or primary peritoneal carcinoma	2000 patients
MRC-ICON4	Phase III randomised study of Paclitaxel with either Carboplatin or Cisplatin versus conventional platinum-based chemotherapy in patients with relapsed ovarian epithelial or peritoneal cancer	800 patients
EORTC-55955	Phase III randomised study of the benefit of early chemotherapy based on CA-125 level only versus delayed chemotherapy based on conventional clinical indicators in patients with relapsed ovarian cancer	800 patients
EBMT-OVCAT	Phase III randomised study of high-dose sequential chemotherapy versus standard chemotherapy in patients with optimally debulked Stage III or IV ovarian epithelial cancer	300 patients

Although phase 1 studies in patients with recurrent ovarian carcinoma[60] failed to show an objective response, the safety of its administration was demonstrated.

One of the advantages of viral therapy is the lack of cross-resistance with the standard therapies used for adjuvant treatments for ovarian cancer, such as chemo- or radiotherapy.

Virotherapy holds great promise as a treatment platform to improve prognosis in patients with advanced or recurrent ovarian cancer.

CLINICAL TRIALS

The most imminent and implementable answers in terms of new treatment strategies that might improve the prognosis of patients with ovarian cancer will probably emerge from the large-scale multicentred randomised on-going clinical trials. Numerous clinical trials are in progress to refine existing therapy and test the value of different approaches to postoperative drug and radiation therapy. Patients with any stage of ovarian cancer are appropriate candidates for clinical trials. The phase III on-going main studies are summarised in Table 2.

CONCLUSIONS

Despite improvements seen in median and overall survival, long-term survival rates for patients with advanced epithelial ovarian carcinoma remain disappointing. Lack of early warning signals and effective early detection techniques makes ovarian cancer a leading pelvic reproductive organ cancer health hazard, with poorer prognosis than other gynaecological cancers. Figures for England indicate that the 5-year survival rate is only about 26%.[61] The strong correlation between chemosensitivity, successful debulking surgery and survival, supports the concept that it is the biological characteristic of the disease rather than the aggressiveness of the surgeon that allows an optimal cytoreduction to achieve a significant survival benefit.

Consequences from the last decades of treatment of ovarian cancer include a much better diagnosis, a more correct staging, and improved peri- and postoperative care, with less mortality within the 28 days following the first laparotomy. Survival in all stages except Stage I have increased, partly by better differentiation.[62]

Biases and ethical issues have and will continue to hamper our ability to fully elaborate the benefits of surgery with respect to survival and quality of life regarding patients with advanced stage ovarian cancer.[63] Although questions persist regarding the relative effect of aggressive surgical cytoreduction on survival, surgery is still the cornerstone of treatment for this type of cancer. Women with advanced ovarian carcinoma should continue to be encouraged to participate in well-designed clinical trials.

Thanks to aggressive surgery and chemotherapy many patients should be able to reach a complete remission of their disease; nevertheless, most will die of recurrent disease.

Paclitaxel and platinum chemotherapy are still the treatment of choice after primary debulking surgery. Salvage chemotherapy with several single agents has only modest activity and does not prolong survival of patients with relapsed ovarian carcinoma. An intense search has been made for novel approaches to treatment of ovarian cancer, and several new treatments, such as immunotherapy and gene therapy, show promise; consequently, new treatment approaches are in need of large clinical trials.

Based on the results of phase II trials which demonstrated activity in previously treated patients with ovarian cancer, new combination regimens are being tested in which drugs such as gemcitabine, topotecan, or encapsulated doxorubicin are added to or sequenced with carboplatin plus Paclitaxel. In addition, new platinum and taxane analogues are also under clinical development.

Biological approaches to the treatment of patients with ovarian cancer are also in clinical development and include drugs that interfere with angiogenesis, matrix metalloproteinases, and signal transduction pathways. These drugs are currently being tested in previously treated patients with recurrent ovarian cancer.

Ovarian cancer remains a disease in search of highly sensitive screening test(s) and improved therapy. However, it is likely that the achieved improvement in short-term survival will be followed in the foreseeable future by a significant improvement in the long-term survival as well.

References

1 Ries LAG, Kosary CL, Hankey BF, Miller BA, Harras A, Edwards BK. SEER Cancer Statistics Review, 1973–1998, Bethesda, MD, National Cancer Institute, 2001

2 Greenlee RT, Hill-Harmon MB, Murray T, Thun M. Cancer statistics, 2001. Cancer J Clin 2001; 51: 15–36

3 DiSaia PJ, Creasman WT. (eds) Clinical Gynecologic Oncology, 6th edn. St Louis, MO: Mosby, 2002; 289–350

4 Berek JS, Hacker NF. (eds) Practical Gynecologic Oncology, 3rd edn. Philadelphia, PA: Lippincott Williams & Wilkins, 2000; 457–522

5 Peethambaram PP, Long HJ. Second-line and subsequent therapy for ovarian carcinoma. Curr Oncol Report 2002; 4: 159–164

6 Laframboise S, Nedelcu R, Murphy J, Cole DE, Rosen B. Use of CA-125 and ultrasound in high-risk women. Int J Gynecol Cancer 2002; 12: 86–91

7 Cohen L, Fishman DA. Ultrasound and ovarian cancer. Cancer Treat Res 2002; 107: 119–132

8 Petricoin EF, Ardekani AM, Hitt BA et al. Use of proteomic patterns in serum to identify ovarian cancer. Lancet 2002; 359: 572–577

9 Mok SC, Chao J, Skates S et al. Prostasin, a potential serum marker for ovarian cancer: identification through microarray technology. J Natl Cancer Inst 2001; 93: 1458–1464

10 Mills GB, Bast RC, Srivastava S. Future for ovarian cancer screening: novel markers from emerging technologies of transcriptional profiling and proteomics. Natl Cancer Inst 2001: 93(19); 1437–1439

11 Sullivan Pepe M, Etzioni R, Feng Z, Potter JD, Thompson ML, Thornquist M, Winget M, Yasui Y J. Phases of biomarker development for early detection of cancer. Natl Cancer Inst 2001: 93: 1054-1061

12 Haber D. Prophylactic oophorectomy to reduce the risk of ovarian and breast cancer in carriers of BRCA mutations. N Engl J Med 2002; 346: 1660–1662

13 Narod SA, Boyd J. Current understanding of the epidemiology and clinical implications of BRCA1 and BRCA2 mutations for ovarian cancer. Curr Opin Obstet Gynecol 2002; 14: 19-26

14 Kauff ND, Satagopan JM, Robson ME, Scheuer L, Hensley M, Offit K. Risk-reducing salpingo-oophorectomy in women with a BRCA1 or BRCA2 mutation. N Engl J Med 2002; 346: 1609–1615

15 . Rebbeck TR, Lynch HT, Neuhausen SL, Narod SA, Van't Veer L, Weber BL. Prophylactic

oophorectomy in carriers of BRCA1 or BRCA2 mutations. N Engl J Med 2002; 346(21): 1616–22

16 Cody III HS. Current surgical management of breast cancer. Curr Opin Obstet Gynecol 2002; 14: 45–52

17 Paley PJ, Swisher EM, Garcia RL et al. Occult cancer of the fallopian tube in BRCA-1 germline mutation carriers at prophylactic oophorectomy: a case for recommending hysterectomy at surgical prophylaxis. Gynecol Oncol 2001; 80: 176–180

18 Morice P, Pautier P, Mercier S, Spatz A et al. Laparoscopic prophylactic oophorectomy in women with inherited risk of ovarian cancer. Eur J Gynaecol Oncol 1999; 20: 202–204

19 Morice P, Pautier P, Delaloge S. Prophylactic surgery in patients with inherited risk of ovarian cancer. Gynecol Oncol 2001; 83: 445-447.

20 Narod SA, Brunet JS, Ghadirian P et al. Hereditary Breast Cancer Clinical Study Group. Tamoxifen and risk of contralateral breast cancer in BRCA1 and BRCA2 mutation carriers: a case-control study. Lancet 2000; 356: 1876–1881

21 Favalli G, Odicino F, Pecorelli S. Surgery of advanced malignant epithelial tumours of the ovary. Forum (Genova) 2000; 10: 312–320

22 Griffiths CT. Surgical resection of tumor bulk in the primary treatment of ovarian carcinoma. Natl Cancer Inst Monogr 1975; 42: 101–104

23 Hacker NF, Berek JS, Lagasse LD, Nieberg RK, Elashoff RM. Primary cytoreductive surgery for epithelial ovarian cancer. Obstet Gynecol 1983; 61: 413–420

24 Piver MS, Lele SB, Marchetti DL, Baker TR, Tsukada Y, Emrich LJ. The impact of aggressive debulking surgery and cisplatin-based chemotherapy on progression-free survival in stage III and IV ovarian carcinoma. J Clin Oncol 1988; 6: 983–989

25 Gillette-Cloven N, Burger RA, Monk BJ et al. Bowel resection at the time of primary cytoreduction for epithelial ovarian cancer. J Am Coll Surg 2001; 193: 626–632

26 Clayton RD, Obermair A, Hammond IG, Leung YC, McCartney AJ. The Western Australian experience of the use of en bloc resection of ovarian cancer with concomitant rectosigmoid colectomy. Gynecol Oncol 2002; 84: 53–57

27 Scarabelli C, Gallo A, Franceschi S, Campagnutta E, De G, Carbone A. Primary cytoreductive surgery with rectosigmoid colon resection for patients with advanced epithelial ovarian carcinoma. Cancer 2000; 88: 389–397

28 Naik R, Nordin A, Cross PA, Hemming D, de Barros Lopes A, Monaghan JM. Optimal cytoreductive surgery is an independent prognostic indicator in stage IV epithelial ovarian cancer with hepatic metastases. Gynecol Oncol 2000; 78: 171–175

29 Bristow RE, Tomacruz RS, Armstrong DK, Trimble EL, Montz FJ. Survival effect of maximal cytoreductive surgery for advanced ovarian carcinoma during the platinum era: a meta-analysis. J Clin Oncol 2002; 20: 1248–1259

30 Sun T, Feng Y, Zhu Y, Zheng Y. Therapeutic strategy in the management of stage II-IV epithelial ovarian carcinoma. Chin Med J (Engl) 2000; 113: 625–627

31 Zylberberg B, Dormont D, Janklewicz S, Darai E, Bretel JJ, Madelenat P. Response to neo-adjuvant intraperitoneal and intravenous immunochemotherapy followed by interval secondary cytoreduction in stage IIIc ovarian cancer. Eur J Gynaecol Oncol 2001; 22: 40–45

32 Kayikcioglu F, Kose MF, Boran N, Caliskan E, Tulunay G. Neoadjuvant chemotherapy or primary surgery in advanced epithelial ovarian carcinoma. Int J Gynecol Cancer 2001; 11: 466–470

33 Vergote I, de Wever I, Tjalma W, Van Gramberen M, Decloedt J, Van Dam P. Interval debulking surgery: an alternative for primary surgical debulking? Semin Surg Oncol 2000; 19: 49–53

34 Kuhn W, Rutke S, Spathe K, Schmalfeldt B, Florack G, Graeff H. Neoadjuvant chemotherapy followed by tumor debulking prolongs survival for patients with poor prognosis in International Federation of Gynecology and Obstetrics Stage IIIC ovarian carcinoma. Cancer 2001; 92: 2585–2591

35 Parazzini F, Raspagliesi F, Guarnerio P, Bolis G. Role of secondary surgery in relapsed ovarian cancer. Crit Rev Oncol Hematol 2001; 37: 121–125

36 Scarabelli C, Gallo A, Carbone A. Secondary cytoreductive surgery for patients with recurrent epithelial ovarian carcinoma. Gynecol Oncol 2001; 83: 504–512

37 Cormio G, di Vagno G, Cazzolla A, Bettocchi S, di Gesu G, Selvaggi L. Surgical

treatment of recurrent ovarian cancer: report of 21 cases and a review of the literature. Eur J Obstet Gynecol Reprod Biol 1999; 86: 185–188

38 Wiltshaw E, Kroner T. Phase II study of cis-dichlorodiamineplatinum(II) (NSC-119875) in advanced adenocarcinoma of the ovary. Cancer Treat Report 1976; 60: 55–60

39 Hunter RW, Alexander ND, Soutter WP. Meta-analysis of surgery in advanced ovarian carcinoma: is maximum cytoreductive surgery an independent determinant of prognosis? Am J Obstet Gynecol 1992; 166: 504–511

40 McGuire WP, Hoskins WJ, Brady MF, Kucera PR, Partridge EE, Davidson M. Cyclophosphamide and cisplatin compared with paclitaxel and cisplatin in patients with stage III and stage IV ovarian cancer. N Engl J Med 1996; 334: 1–6

41 Piccart MJ, Bertelsen K, James K, Cassidy J, Mangioni C, Pecorelli S. Randomized intergroup trial of cisplatin-paclitaxel versus cisplatin-cyclophosphamide in women with advanced epithelial ovarian cancer: three-year results. J Natl Cancer Inst 2000; 92: 699–708

42 Muggia FM, Braly PS, Brady MF, Sutton G, Niemann TH, Small JM. Phase III randomized study of cisplatin versus paclitaxel versus cisplatin and paclitaxel in patients with suboptimal stage III or IV ovarian cancer: a gynecologic oncology group study. J Clin Oncol 2000; 18:106–115

43 Hogberg T, Glimelius B, Nygren P. A systematic overview of chemotherapy effects in ovarian cancer. Acta Oncol 2001; 40: 340–360

44 Homesley HD, Scarantino CW, Muss HB, Welander CE. Concurrent chemotherapy and single high-dose plus whole abdominopelvic radiation for persistent ovarian carcinoma. Gynecol Oncol 1989; 34: 170–174

45 Linstadt DE, Stern JL, Quivey JM, Leibel SA, Lacey CG. Salvage whole-abdominal irradiation following chemotherapy failure in epithelial ovarian carcinoma. Gynecol Oncol 1990; 36: 327–330

46 Schray MF, Martinez A, Howes AE, Ballon SC, Podratz KC, Malkasian GD. Advanced epithelial ovarian cancer: toxicity of whole abdominal irradiation after operation, combination chemotherapy, and reoperation. Gynecol Oncol 1986; 24: 68–80

47 Shelley WE, Starreveld AA, Carmichael JA, O'Connell G, Roy M, Swenerton K. Toxicity of abdominopelvic radiation in advanced ovarian carcinoma patients after cisplatin/cyclophosphamide therapy and second-look laparotomy. Obstet Gynecol 1988; 71: 327–332

48 Cmelak AJ, Kapp DS. Long-term survival with whole abdominopelvic irradiation in platinum-refractory persistent or recurrent ovarian cancer. Gynecol Oncol 1997; 65: 453–460

49 Corn BW, Lanciano RM, Boente M, Hunter WM, Ladazack J, Ozols RF. Recurrent ovarian cancer. Effective radiotherapeutic palliation after chemotherapy failure. Cancer 1994; 74: 2979–2983.

50 Gelblum D, Mychalczak B, Almadrones L, Spriggs D, Barakat R. Palliative benefit of external-beam radiation in the management of platinum refractory epithelial ovarian carcinoma. Gynecol Oncol 1998; 69: 36–41

51 Tinger A, Waldron T, Peluso N, Katin MJ, Dosoretz DE, Orr Jr JW. Effective palliative radiation therapy in advanced and recurrent ovarian carcinoma. Int J Radiat Oncol Biol Phys 2001; 51: 1256–1263

52 Goldberg H, Stein ME, Steiner M, Sprecher E, Beck D, Kuten A. Consolidation radiation therapy following cytoreductive surgery, chemotherapy and second-look laparotomy for epithelial ovarian carcinoma: long-term follow-up. Tumori 2001; 87: 248–251

53 Creasman WT, Gall SA, Blessing JA, Schmidt HJ, Abu-Ghazaleh S, DiSaia PJ. Chemoimmunotherapy in the management of primary stage III ovarian cancer: a Gynecologic Oncology Group study. Cancer Treat Report 1979; 63: 319–323

54 Slamon DJ, Godolphin W, Jones LA, Holt JA, Wong SG, Ullrich A. Studies of the HER-2/neu proto-oncogene in human breast and ovarian cancer. Science 1989; 244: 707–712

55 Disis ML, Schiffman K. Cancer vaccines targeting the HER2/neu oncogenic protein. Semin Oncol 2001; 28 (Suppl 18): 12–20

56 Russell WC. Update on adenovirus and its vectors. J Gen Virol 2000; 81: 2573–25604

57 Hasenburg A, Tong XW, Fischer DC, Rojas-Martinez A, Nyberg-Hoffman C, Kieback DG. Adenovirus-mediated thymidine kinase gene therapy in combination with

topotecan for patients with recurrent ovarian cancer: 2.5-year follow-up. Gynecol Oncol 2001; 83: 549–554

58 Kirn D, Martuza RL, Zwiebel J. Replication-selective virotherapy for cancer: biological principles, risk management and future directions. Nat Med 2001; 7: 781–787

59 Martuza RL, Malick A, Markert JM, Ruffner KL, Coen DM. Experimental therapy of human glioma by means of a genetically engineered virus mutant. Science 1991; 252: 854–856

60 Vasey P, Shulman L, Gore M, Kirn D, Kaye S. Phase I trial of intraperitoneal Onyx-015 adenovirus in patients with recurrent ovarian carcinoma. Proc Am Soc Clin Oncol 2000; 19, 1512

61 Berrino F, Sant M, Verdecchia A et al. (eds) Survival of cancer patients in Europe: the EUROCARE study. Lyon: International Agency for Research on Cancer, 1995

62 Pfleiderer A. Is there any progress in the outcome of patients suffering from ovarian cancer? Treatment strategies since 1957. Gynecol Oncol 2001; 83: 451–456

63 Covens AL. A critique of surgical cytoreduction in advanced ovarian cancer. Gynecol Oncol 2000; 78: 269–274

Dudley Robinson Linda Cardozo

Oestrogens and urogenital atrophy

Urogenital atrophy is a manifestation of oestrogen withdrawal following the menopause and symptoms may appear for the first time more than 10 years after the last menstrual period.[1] The female genital and lower urinary tract share a common embryological origin from the urogenital sinus and both are sensitive to the effects of female sex steroid hormones. Oestrogen is known to have an important role in the function of the lower urinary tract throughout adult life and oestrogen and progesterone receptors have been demonstrated in the vagina, urethra, bladder and pelvic floor musculature.[1-4] Oestrogen deficiency occurring following the menopause is known to cause atrophic changes within the urogenital tract[5] and is associated with urinary symptoms such as frequency, urgency, nocturia, incontinence and recurrent infection. These may co-exist with symptoms of vaginal atrophy such as dyspareunia, itching, burning and dryness.

The role of oestrogen replacement in the treatment of these symptoms of urogenital atrophy has still not been clearly defined despite several randomised trials and wide-spread clinical use. This review presents an overview of the pathogenesis and management of urogenital symptoms and the role of oestrogen replacement therapy.

EPIDEMIOLOGY

Increasing life expectancy has led to an increasingly elderly population and it is now common for women to spend a third of their lives in the oestrogen-

Dudley Robinson MRCOG
Sub-specialty Trainee in Urogynaecology, Department of Obstetrics and Gynaecology, King's College Hospital, Denmark Hill, London SE5 9RS, UK (for correspondence, E-mail: dud@ukgateway.net)

Linda Cardozo MD FRCOG
Professor of Urogynaecology, Department of Obstetrics and Gynaecology, King's College Hospital, Denmark Hill, London SE5 9RS, UK

deficient postmenopausal state.[7] The average age of the menopause is 50 years although there is some cultural and geographical variation.[8] World-wide in 1990 there were approximately 467 million women aged 50 years or over and this is expected to increase to 1200 million over the next 30 years.[9] Furthermore, postmenopausal women comprise 15% of the population in industrialised countries with a predicted growth rate of 1.5% over the next 20 years. Overall, in the industrialised world, 8% of the total population have been estimated to have urogenital symptoms,[10] this representing 200 million women in the US alone.

UROGENITAL ATROPHY

The prevalence of symptomatic urogenital atrophy is difficult to estimate since many women accept the changes as being an inevitable consequence of the ageing process and thus do not seek help. It has been estimated that 10–40% of all postmenopausal women are symptomatic[11] although only 25% are thought to seek medical help. In addition, vaginal symptoms associated with urogenital atrophy are reported by two out of three women by the age of 75 years.[12]

More recently, a study assessing the prevalence of urogenital symptoms in 2157 Dutch women has been reported.[13] Overall, 27% of women complained of vaginal dryness, soreness and dyspareunia whilst the prevalence of urinary symptoms such as leakage and recurrent infections was 36%. When considering severity, almost 50% reported moderate-to-severe discomfort although only a third had received medical intervention. Interestingly, women who had previously had a hysterectomy reported moderate-to-severe complaints more often than those who had not.

The prevalence of urogenital atrophy and urogenital prolapse has also been examined in a population of 285 women attending a menopause clinic.[14] Overall, 51% of women were found to have anterior vaginal wall prolapse, 27% posterior vaginal prolapse and 20% apical prolapse. In addition, 34% of women were noted to have urogenital atrophy, 40% complaining of dyspareunia. Whilst urogenital atrophy and symptoms of dyspareunia were related to menopausal age, the prevalence of prolapse showed no association.

Whilst urogenital atrophy is an inevitable consequence of the menopause, women may not always be symptomatic. A recent study of 69 women attending a gynaecology clinic were asked to fill out a symptom questionnaire prior to examination and undergoing vaginal cytology.[15] Urogenital symptoms were found to be relatively low and were poorly correlated with age and physical examination findings although not with vaginal cytological maturation index. Women who were taking oestrogen-replacement therapy had higher symptom scores and physical examination scores. In conclusion, it would appear that urogenital atrophy is a universal consequence of the menopause although often women may be minimally symptomatic and hence treatment should not be the only indication for replacement therapy.

URINARY INCONTINENCE

The prevalence of urinary incontinence is known to increase with age, affecting 15–35% of community dwelling women over the age of 60 years[16] with other studies reporting a prevalence of 49% in women over 65 years.[17] In addition, rates of 50% have been reported in elderly nursing home residents.[18] A recent cross-sectional population prevalence survey of 146 women aged 15–97 years found that 46% experienced symptoms of pelvic floor dysfunction defined as stress or urge incontinence, flatus or faecal incontinence, symptomatic prolapse or previous pelvic floor surgery.[19]

Little work has been done to examine the incidence of urinary incontinence although a study in New Zealand of women over the age of 65 years found 10% of the originally continent developed urinary incontinence in the 3-year study period.[20]

ECONOMIC CONSIDERATIONS

The economic cost of urogenital atrophy is difficult to estimate due to under-reporting and also since some of the cost is borne by the patients themselves without involving the health services. The price of incontinence is slightly easier to estimate although is still affected by under-reporting. It is comprised of the 'direct' costs of treatment, supplies and provision of medical staff whilst 'indirect' costs relate to loss of earnings and productivity. A study performed in 1994 in Scotland estimated that the cost of pad supplies alone in the UK may be in the region of £57.3 million/year whilst the cost of incontinence has been estimated at $16 billion/year in the US. More recent data from the UK have shown the annual expenditure on incontinence to be £163 million with appliances and containment accounting for £59 million and £69 million, respectively, and the cost of drugs and surgery being £23 million and £12 million.[21]

OESTROGEN RECEPTORS AND HORMONAL FACTORS

The effects of the steroid hormone 17β-oestradiol are mediated by ligand-activated transcription factors known as oestrogen receptors which are glycoproteins sharing common features with androgen and progesterone receptors. The classic oestrogen receptor (ER-α) was first discovered by Elwood Jensen in 1958 and cloned from uterine tissue in 1986,[22] although it was not until 1996 that the second oestrogen receptor (ER-β) was identified.[23]

Oestrogen receptors have been demonstrated throughout the lower urinary tract and are expressed in the squamous epithelium of the proximal and distal urethra, vagina and trigone of the bladder,[24] although not in the dome of the bladder, reflecting its different embryological origin. Pubococcygeous and the musculature of the pelvic floor have also been shown to be oestrogen sensitive,[25,26] although oestrogen receptors have not yet been identified in the levator ani muscles.[27]

More recently, the distribution of oestrogen receptors throughout the urogenital tract has been studied with both α- and β-receptors being found in the vaginal walls and uterosacral ligaments of premenopausal women, although the latter was absent in the vaginal walls of postmenopausal women.[28] In addition, α-receptors are localised in the urethral sphincter and when sensitised by oestrogens are thought to help maintain muscular tone.[29] Interestingly, oestrogen receptors have also been identified in mast cells in women with interstitial cystitis[30] and in the male lower urinary tract.

PROGESTERONE AND ANDROGEN RECEPTORS

In addition to oestrogen receptors, both androgen and progesterone receptors are expressed in the lower urinary tract although their role is less clear. Progesterone receptors are expressed inconsistently, having been reported in the bladder, trigone and vagina. Their presence may be dependent on oestrogen status. In addition, whilst androgen receptors are present in both the bladder and urethra, their role has not yet been defined.[31]

More recently, the incidence of both oestrogen and progesterone expression has been examined throughout the lower urinary tract in 90 women undergoing gynaecological surgery; 33 were premenopausal, 26 postmenopausal without hormone replacement therapy and 31 postmenopausal and taking hormone replacement therapy.[32] Biopsies were taken from the bladder dome, trigone, proximal urethra, distal urethra, vagina and vesicovaginal fascia adjacent to the bladder neck. Oestrogen receptors were found to be consistently expressed in the squamous epithelia although were absent in the urothelial tissues of the lower urinary tract of all women, irrespective of oestrogen status. Progesterone receptor expression, however, showed more variability being mostly subepithelial, and was significantly lower in postmenopausal women not taking oestrogen replacement therapy.

LOWER URINARY TRACT FUNCTION

In order to maintain continence, the urethral pressure must remain higher than the intravesical pressure at all times except during micturition.[33] Oestrogens play an important role in the continence mechanism with bladder and urethral function becoming less efficient with age.[34] Elderly women have been found to have a reduced flow rate, increased urinary residuals, higher filling pressures, reduced bladder capacity and lower maximum voiding pressures.[35] Oestrogens may affect continence by increasing urethral resistance, raising the sensory threshold of the bladder or by increasing α-adrenoreceptor sensitivity in the urethral smooth muscle.[36,37] In addition, exogenous oestrogens have been shown to increase the number of intermediate and superficial cells in the vagina of postmenopausal women[38] and these changes have also been demonstrated in the bladder and urethra.[39]

More recently, a prospective observational study has been performed to assess cell proliferation rates throughout the tissues of the lower urinary tract.[40] Of 59 women studied, 23 were premenopausal, 20 were postmenopausal and not taking hormone replacement therapy, and 20 were post menopausal and taking hormone replacement therapy. Biopsies were taken from the bladder dome, trigone, proximal urethra, distal urethra, vagina and vesicovaginal fascia adjacent to the bladder neck. The squamous epithelium of oestrogen replete women was shown to exhibit greater levels of cellular proliferation than in those women who were oestrogen deficient.

BLADDER FUNCTION

Oestrogen receptors, although absent in the transitional epithelium of the bladder, are present in the areas of the trigone which have undergone squamous metaplasia.[24] Oestrogen is known to have a direct effect on detrusor function through modifications in muscarinic receptors[41,42] and by inhibition of movement of extracellular calcium ions into muscle cells.[43] Consequently, oestradiol has been shown to reduce the amplitude and frequency of spontaneous rhythmic detrusor contractions[44] and there is also evidence that it may increase the sensory threshold of the bladder in some women.[45]

NEUROLOGICAL CONTROL

Sex hormones are known to influence the central neurological control of micturition although their exact role in the micturition pathway has yet to be elucidated. Oestrogen receptors have been demonstrated in the cerebral cortex, limbic system, hippocampus and cerebellum,[46,47] whilst androgen receptors have been demonstrated in the pontine micturition centre and the pre-optic area of the hypothalamus.[48]

URETHRA

Oestrogen receptors have been demonstrated in the squamous epithelium of both the proximal and distal urethra[24] and oestrogen has been shown to improve the maturation index of urethral squamous epithelium.[49] It has been suggested that oestrogen increases urethral closure pressure and improves pressure transmission to the proximal urethra, both promoting continence.[50–53] Oestrogens have been shown to cause vasodilatation in the systemic and cerebral circulation and these changes are also seen in the urethra.[54–56] The vascular pulsations seen on urethral pressure profilometry secondary to blood flow in the urethral submucosa and urethral sphincter have been shown to increase in size following oestrogen administration[57] whilst the effect is lost following oestrogen withdrawal at the menopause.

COLLAGEN

Oestrogens are known to have an effect on collagen synthesis and they have been shown to have a direct effect on collagen metabolism in the lower genital tract.[58] Changes found in women with urogenital atrophy may represent an alteration in systemic collagenase activity[59] and urodynamic stress incontinence and urogenital prolapse has been associated with a reduction in both vaginal and periurethral collagen.[60–62] There is a reduction in skin collagen content following the menopause[63] and rectus muscle fascia has been shown to become less elastic with increasing age resulting in a lower energy requirement to cause irreversible damage.[64] Changes in collagen content have also been identified, the hydroxyproline content in connective tissue from women with stress incontinence being 40% lower than in continent controls.[65]

UROGENITAL ATROPHY

Withdrawal of endogenous oestrogen at the menopause results in well-documented climacteric symptoms such as hot flushes and night sweats in addition to the less commonly reported symptoms of urogenital atrophy.

Symptoms do not usually develop until several years following the menopause when levels of endogenous oestrogens fall below the level required to promote endometrial growth.[66] This temporal relationship would suggest oestrogen withdrawal as the cause.

Vaginal dryness is commonly the first reported symptom and is caused by a reduction in mucus production within the vaginal glands. Atrophy within the vaginal epithelium leads to thinning and an increased susceptibility to infection and mechanical trauma. Glycogen depletion within the vaginal mucosa following the menopause leads to a decrease in lactic acid formation by Doderlein's lactobacillus and a consequent rise in vaginal pH from around 4 to between 6 and 7. This allows bacterial overgrowth and colonisation with Gram-negative bacilli compounding the effects of vaginal atrophy and leading to symptoms of vaginitis such as pruritis, dyspareunia and discharge.

LOWER URINARY TRACT SYMPTOMS

Epidemiological studies have implicated oestrogen deficiency in the aetiology of lower urinary tract symptoms with 70% of women relating the onset of urinary incontinence to their final menstrual period.[6] Lower urinary tract symptoms have been shown to be common in postmenopausal women attending a menopause clinic with 20% complaining of severe urgency and almost 50% complaining of stress incontinence.[67] Urge incontinence in particular is more prevalent following the menopause and the prevalence would appear to rise with increasing years of oestrogen deficiency.[68] There is, however, conflicting evidence regarding the role of oestrogen withdrawal at the time of the menopause. Some studies have shown a peak incidence in perimenopausal women[69,70] whilst other evidence suggests that many women develop incontinence at least 10 years prior to the cessation of menstruation with significantly more premenopausal women than postmenopausal women being affected.[66,71]

Cyclical variations in the levels of both oestrogen and progesterone during the menstrual cycle have also been shown to lead to changes in urodynamic variables and lower urinary tract symptoms with 37% of women noticing a deterioration in symptoms prior to menstruation.[72] Measurement of the urethral pressure profile in nulliparous premenopausal women shows there is an increase in functional urethral length mid-cycle and early in the luteal phase corresponding to an increase in plasma oestradiol.[73] Furthermore, progestogens have been associated with an increase in irritative bladder symptoms[74,75] and urinary incontinence in those women taking combined hormone replacement therapy.[76] The incidence of detrusor overactivity in the luteal phase of the menstrual cycle may be associated with raised plasma progesterone following ovulation and progesterone has been shown to antagonise the inhibitory effect of oestradiol on rat detrusor contractions.[77] This may help to explain the increased prevalence of detrusor overactivity found in pregnancy.[78]

Urinary tract infection is also a common cause of urinary symptoms in women of all ages. This is a particular problem in the elderly with a reported incidence of 20% in the community and over 50% in institutionalised patients.[79,80] Pathophysiological changes such as impairment of bladder emptying, poor perineal hygiene and both faecal and urinary incontinence may partly account for the high prevalence observed. In addition, as previously described, changes in the vaginal flora due to oestrogen depletion lead to colonisation with Gram-negative bacilli which in addition to causing local irritive symptoms also act as uropathogens. These microbiological changes may be reversed with oestrogen replacement following the menopause which offer a rationale for treatment and prophylaxis.

OESTROGENS IN MANAGEMENT

Management of incontinence

Oestrogen preparations have been used for many years in the treatment of urinary incontinence[81,82] although their precise role remains controversial. Many of the studies performed have been uncontrolled observational series examining the use of a wide range of different preparations, doses and routes of administration. The inconsistent use of progestogens to provide endometrial protection is a further confounding factor making interpretation of the results difficult.

In order to clarify the situation, a meta-analysis from the Hormones and Urogenital Therapy (HUT) Committee has been reported.[83] Of 166 articles identified which were published in English between 1969 and 1992, only 6 were controlled trials and 17 were uncontrolled series. Meta-analysis found an overall significant effect of oestrogen therapy on subjective improvement in all subjects and for subjects with urodynamic stress incontinence alone. Subjective improvement rates with oestrogen therapy in randomised controlled trials ranged from 64% to 75% although placebo groups also reported an improvement of 10–56%. In uncontrolled series, subjective improvement rates were 8–89% with subjects with urodynamic stress incontinence showing improvement of 34–73%. However, when assessing objective fluid loss there was no significant effect. Maximum urethral closure pressure was found to increase significantly with oestrogen therapy although this outcome was influenced by a single study showing a large effect.[84]

A further meta-analysis performed in Italy has analysed the results of randomised controlled clinical trials on the efficacy of oestrogen treatment in postmenopausal women with urinary incontinence.[85] A search of the literature (1965–1996) revealed 72 articles of which only four were considered to meet the meta-analysis criteria. There was a statistically significant difference in subjective outcome between oestrogen and placebo although there was no such difference in objective or urodynamic outcome. The authors concluded that this difference could be relevant although the studies may have lacked objective sensitivity to detect this.

The role of oestrogen replacement therapy in the prevention of ischaemic heart disease has recently been assessed in a 4-year randomised trial, the Heart and Estrogen/progestin Replacement Study (HERS),[86] involving 2763 postmenopausal women younger than 80 years with intact uteri and ischaemic heart disease. In the study, 55% of women reported at least one episode of urinary incontinence each week, and were randomly assigned to oral conjugated oestrogen plus medroxyprogesterone acetate or placebo daily.

Incontinence improved in 26% of women assigned to placebo as compared to 21% receiving HRT while 27% of the placebo group complained of worsening symptoms compared with 39% in the HRT group ($P = 0.001$). The incidence of incontinent episodes per week increased an average of 0.7 in the HRT group and decreased by 0.1 in the placebo group ($P < 0.001$). Overall combined hormone replacement therapy was associated with worsening stress and urge urinary incontinence although there was no significant difference in daytime frequency, nocturia or number of urinary tract infections.

More recently, the effects of oral oestrogens and progestogens on the lower urinary tract have been assessed in 32 female nursing home residents[87] with an average age of 88 years. Subjects were randomised to oral oestrogen and progesterone or placebo for 6 months. At follow-up, there was no difference between severity of incontinence, prevalence of bacteriuria or the results of vaginal cultures although there was an improvement in atrophic vaginitis in the placebo group.

Management of stress incontinence

In addition to the studies included in the HUT meta-analysis, several authors have also investigated the role of oestrogen therapy in the management of urodynamic stress incontinence only. Oral oestrogens have been reported to increase the maximum urethral pressures and lead to symptomatic improvement in 65–70% of women[88,89] although other work has not confirmed this.[90,91] More recently, two placebo-controlled studies have been performed examining the use of oral oestrogens in the treatment of urodynamic stress incontinence in postmenopausal women. Neither conjugated equine oestrogens and medroxyprogesterone[92] or unopposed oestradiol valerate[93] showed a significant difference in either subjective or objective outcomes. Furthermore, a review of 8 controlled and 14 uncontrolled prospective trials concluded that oestrogen therapy was not an efficacious treatment for stress incontinence but may be useful for symptoms of urgency and frequency.[94]

From the available evidence, oestrogen does not appear to be an effective treatment for stress incontinence although it may have a synergistic role in combination therapy. Two placebo-controlled studies have examined the use of oral and vaginal oestrogens with the α-adrenergic agonist, phenylpropanolamine, used separately and in combination. Both studies found that combination therapy was superior to either drug given alone although whilst there was subjective improvement in all groups,[95] there was only objective improvement in the combination therapy group.[96] This may offer an alternative conservative treatment for women who have mild urodynamic stress incontinence.

Management of urge incontinence

Oestrogens have been used in the treatment of urinary urgency and urge incontinence for many years although there have been few controlled trials to confirm their efficacy. A double-blind, placebo controlled, crossover study using oral oestriol in 34 postmenopausal women produced subjective improvement in 8 women with mixed incontinence and 12 with urge incontinence.[97] However, a double-blind multicentre study of the use of oestriol (3 mg/day) in postmenopausal women complaining of urgency has failed to confirm these findings[98] showing both subjective and objective improvement but not significantly better than placebo. Oestriol is a naturally occurring weak oestrogen which has little effect on the endometrium and does not prevent osteoporosis although has been used in the treatment of urogenital atrophy. Consequently it is possible that the dosage or route of administration in this study was not appropriate in the treatment of urinary symptoms and higher systemic levels may be required.

The use of sustained release 17β-oestradiol vaginal tablets (Vagifem; Novo Nordisk) has also been examined in postmenopausal women with urgency and urge incontinence or a urodynamic diagnosis of sensory urgency or detrusor overactivity. These vaginal tablets have been shown to be well absorbed from the vagina and to induce maturation of the vaginal epithelium within 14 days.[99] However, following a 6-month course of treatment, the only significant difference between active and placebo groups was an improvement in the symptom of urgency in those women with a urodynamic diagnosis of sensory urgency.[100] A further double-blind, randomised, placebo-controlled trial of vaginal 17β-oestradiol vaginal tablets has shown lower urinary tract symptoms of frequency, urgency, urge and stress incontinence to be significantly improved although there was no objective urodynamic assessment performed.[101] In both of these studies, the subjective improvement in symptoms may simply represent local oestrogenic effects reversing urogenital atrophy rather than a direct effect on bladder function.

To try and clarify the role of oestrogen therapy in the management of women with urge incontinence, a meta-analysis of the use of oestrogen in women with symptoms of 'overactive bladder' has been reported by the HUT Committee.[102] In a review of 10 randomised placebo controlled trials, oestrogen was found to be superior to placebo when considering symptoms of urge incontinence, frequency and nocturia although vaginal oestrogen administration was found to be superior for symptoms of urgency. In those taking oestrogens there was also a significant increase in first sensation and bladder capacity as compared to placebo.

Management of recurrent urinary tract infection

Oestrogen therapy has been shown to increase vaginal pH and reverse the microbiological changes that occur in the vagina following the menopause.[103] Initial small uncontrolled studies using oral or vaginal oestrogens in the treatment of recurrent urinary tract infection appeared to give promising results[104,105] although unfortunately this has not been supported by larger randomised trials. Several studies have been performed examining the use of oral and vaginal oestrogens although these have had mixed results.

Kjaergaard and colleagues[106] compared vaginal oestriol tablets with placebo in 21 postmenopausal women over a 5-month period and found no significant difference between the two groups. However, a subsequent randomised, double-blind, placebo controlled study assessing the use of oestriol vaginal cream in 93 postmenopausal women during an 8-month period did reveal a significant effect.[107]

Kirkengen[108] randomised 40 postmenopausal women to receive either placebo or oral oestriol and found that although initially both groups had a significantly decreased incidence of recurrent infections, after 12 weeks oestriol was shown to be significantly more effective. These findings, however, were not confirmed subsequently in a trial of 72 women postmenopausal women with recurrent urinary tract infections randomised to oral oestriol or placebo. Following a 6-month treatment period and a further 6-month follow-up, oestriol was found to be no more effective than placebo.[109]

More recently, a randomised, open, parallel-group study assessing the use of an oestradiol-releasing silicone vaginal ring (Estring; Pharmacia and Upjohn, Sweden) in postmenopausal women with recurrent infections has been performed which showed the cumulative likelihood of remaining infection-free was 45% in the active group and 20% in the placebo group.[110] Estring was also shown to decrease the number of recurrences per year and to prolong the interval between infection episodes.

Management of urogenital atrophy

Symptoms of urogenital atrophy do not occur until the levels of endogenous oestrogen are lower than that required to promote endometrial proliferation.[66] Consequently, it is possible to use a low dose of oestrogen replacement therapy in order to alleviate urogenital symptoms whilst avoiding the risk of endometrial proliferation and removing the necessity of providing endometrial protection with progestogens.[111] The dose of oestradiol commonly used in systemic oestrogen replacement is usually 25–100 μg although studies investigating the use of oestrogens in the management of urogenital symptoms have shown that 8–10 μg of vaginal oestradiol is effective.[112] Thus only 10–30% of the dose used to treat vasomotor symptoms may be effective in the management of urogenital symptoms. Since 10–25% of women receiving systemic hormone replacement therapy still experience the symptoms of urogenital atrophy,[113] low-dose local preparations may have an additional beneficial effect.

A recent review of oestrogen therapy in the management of urogenital atrophy has been performed by the Hormones and Urogenital Therapy Committee.[114] Ten randomised trials and 54 uncontrolled series were examined from 1969 to 1995 assessing 24 different treatment regimens. Meta-analysis of 10 placebo-controlled trials confirmed the significant effect of oestrogens in the management of urogenital atrophy.

The route of administration was assessed and oral, vaginal and parental (transcutaneous patches and subcutaneous implants) were compared. Overall, the vaginal route of administration was found to correlate with better symptom relief, greater improvement in cytological findings, and higher serum oestradiol levels.

With regard to the type of oestrogen preparation, oestradiol was found to be most effective in reducing patient symptoms although conjugated oestrogens produced the most cytological change and the greatest increase in serum levels of oestradiol and oestrone.

Finally, the effect of different dosages was examined. Low dose vaginal oestradiol was found to be the most efficacious according to symptom relief although oral oestriol was also effective. Oestriol had no effect on the serum levels of oestradiol or oestrone whilst vaginal oestriol had minimal effect. Vaginal oestradiol was found to have a small effect on serum oestrogen although not as great as systemic preparations. In conclusion, it would appear that oestrogen is efficacious in the treatment of urogenital atrophy and low dose vaginal preparations are as effective as systemic therapy.

More recently, the use of a continuous low dose oestradiol-releasing silicone vaginal ring (Estring; Pharmacia and Upjohn, Sweden) releasing oestradiol 5–10 μg/day has been investigated in postmenopausal women with symptomatic urogenital atrophy.[110] There was a significant effect on symptoms of vaginal dryness, pruritis vulvae, dyspareunia and urinary urgency with improvement being reported in over 90% of women in an uncontrolled study. The patient acceptability was high and, whilst the maturation of vaginal epithelium was significantly improved, there was no effect on endometrial proliferation.

These findings were supported by a 1-year multicentre study of Estring in postmenopausal women with urogenital atrophy which found subjective and objective improvement in 90% of patients up to 1 year. However, there was a 20% withdrawal rate with 7% of women reporting vaginal irritation, two having vaginal ulceration, and three complaining of vaginal bleeding although there were no cases of endometrial proliferation.[115] Long-term safety has been confirmed by a 10-year review of the use of the oestradiol ring delivery system which has found its safety, efficacy and acceptability to be comparable to other forms of vaginal administration.[116] A comparative study of safety and efficacy of Estring with conjugated equine oestrogen vaginal cream in 194 postmenopausal women complaining of urogenital atrophy found no significant difference in vaginal dryness, dyspareunia and resolution of atrophic signs between the two treatment groups. Furthermore, there was a similar improvement in the vaginal mucosal maturation index and a reduction in pH in both groups with the vaginal ring being found to be preferable to the cream.[117]

SELECTIVE OESTROGEN RECEPTOR MODULATORS

A recent development in hormonal therapy has been the development of selective oestrogen receptor modulators (SERMS). These drugs have oestrogen-like actions in maintaining bone density and in lowering serum cholesterol but have anti-oestrogenic effects on the breast[118] and do not cause endometrial stimulation.[119] In theory, partial oestrogen antagonists may lead to a down-regulation of oestrogen receptors in the urogenital tract and consequently cause an increase in lower urinary tract symptoms and symptomatic urogenital atrophy. Early work would suggest that some SERMS in development, levormeloxifene and idoxifene, may increase the risk of urogenital prolapse[120] although there were some methodological problems noted in the study. However, in an analysis of three randomised, double-blind, placebo controlled trials investigating raloxifene in 6926 postmenopausal women there appeared to be a protective effect, with fewer treated women having surgery for urogenital prolapse; 1.5% versus 0.75% ($P < 0.005$).[121] At present, the long-term effect of SERMS on the urogenital tract remains to be determined and there is little data regarding effects on urinary incontinence and urogenital atrophy.

CONCLUSIONS

Oestrogens are known to have an important physiological effect on the female lower genital tract throughout adult life leading to symptomatic, histological and functional changes. Urogenital atrophy is the manifestation of oestrogen withdrawal following the menopause, presenting with vaginal and/or urinary symptoms. The use of oestrogen-replacement therapy has been examined in the management of lower urinary tract symptoms as well as in the treatment of urogenital atrophy although only recently has it been subjected to randomised placebo-controlled trials and meta-analysis.

Oestrogen therapy alone has been shown to have little effect in the management of urodynamic stress incontinence although when used in combination with an α-adrenergic agonists may lead to an improvement in urinary leakage. When considering the irritive symptoms of urinary urgency, frequency and urge incontinence oestrogen therapy may be of benefit although this may simply represent reversal of urogenital atrophy rather than a direct effect on the lower urinary tract. The role of oestrogen replacement therapy in the management of women with recurrent lower urinary tract infection remains to be determined although there is now some evidence that vaginal administration may be efficacious. Finally, low-dose vaginal oestrogens have been shown to be have a role in the treatment of urogenital atrophy in postmenopausal women and would appear to be as effective as systemic preparations.

References

1 Iosif CS. Effects of protracted administration of oestriol on the lower genitourinary tract in postmenopausal women. Acta Obstet Gynecol Scand 1992; 251: 115–120
2 Cardozo LD. Role of oestrogens in the treatment of female urinary incontinence. J Am Geriatr Soc 1990; 38: 326–328
3 Iosif S, Batra S, Ek A, Astedt B. Oestrogens receptors in the human female lower urinary tract. Am J Obstet Gynecol 1981; 141: 817–820
4 Batra SC, Fossil CS. Female urethra, a target for oestrogen action. J Urol 1983; 129: 418–420
5 Batra SC, Iosif LS. Progesterone receptors in the female urinary tract. J Urol 1987; 138: 130–134
6 Iosif C, Bekassy Z. Prevalence of genitourinary symptoms in the late menopause. Acta Obstet Gynecol Scand 1984; 63: 257–260
7 American National Institute of Health Population Figures. US Treasury Department, NIH, 1991
8 World Health Organization. Research on the Menopause in the 1990s. Report of a WHO Scientific Group. WHO Technical Report Series 866. Geneva: WHO, 1994
9 Hill K. The demography of the menopause. Maturitas 1996; 23: 113–127
10 Barlow D, Samsioe G, van Geelan H. Prevalence of urinary problems in European countries. Maturitas 1997; 27: 239–248
11 Greendale GA, Judd JL. The menopause: health implications and clinical management. J Am Geriatr Soc 1993; 41: 426–436
12 Samsioe G, Jansson I, Mellstrom D, Svanborg A. The occurrence, nature and treatment of urinary incontinence in a 70 year old population. Maturitas 1985; 7: 335–343
13 Van Geelen JM, Van de Weijer PH, Arnolds HT. Urogenital symptoms and resulting discomfort in non-institutionalised Dutch women aged 50–75 years. Int Urogynecol J Pelvic Floor Dysfunct 2000; 11: 9–14
14 Versi E, Harvey MA, Cardozo L, Brincat M, Studd JW. Urogenital prolapse and atrophy at menopause: a prevalence study. Int Urogynaecol J Pelvic Dysfunct 2001; 12: 107–110

15 Davila GW, Karapanagiotou I, Woodhouse S *et al*. Are women with urogenital atrophy symptomatic? Obstet Gynecol 2001; 97 (Suppl 1): S48

16 Diokno AC, Brook BM, Brown MB. Prevalence of urinary incontinence and other urological symptoms in the non-institutionalised elderly. J Urol 1986; 136: 1022

17 Yarnell J, Voyle G, Richards C, Stephenson T. The prevalence and severity of urinary incontinence in women. J Epidemiol Community Health 1981; 35: 71–74

18 Ouslander JG. Urinary incontinence in nursing homes. J Am Geriatr Soc 1990; 38: 289–291

19 MacLennan AH, Taylor AW, Wilson AW, Wilson D. The prevalence of pelvic floor disorders and their relationship to gender, age, parity, and mode of delivery. Br J Obstet Gynaecol 2000; 107: 1460–1470

20 Kok AL, Voorhorst FJ, Burger CW, Van Houten P, Kenemans P, Jannsens J. Urinary and faecal incontinence in community residing elderly women. Age Ageing 1992; 21: 211

21 Department of Health, 2001

22 Green S, Walter P, Kumar V *et al*. Human oestrogen receptor cDNA: sequence, expression and homology to v-erbA. Nature 1986; 320: 134–139

23 Kuiper G, Enmark E, Pelto-Huikko M, Nilsson S, Gustafsson J-A. Cloning of a novel oestrogen receptor expressed in rat prostate and ovary. Proc Natl Acad Sci USA 1996; 93: 5925–5930

24 Blakeman PJ, Hilton P, Bulmer JN. Mapping oestrogen and progesterone receptors throughout the female lower urinary tract. Neurourol Urodyn 1996; 15: 324–325

25 Ingelman-Sundberg A, Rosen J, Gustafsson SA. Cytosol oestrogen receptors in urogenital tissues in stress incontinent women. Acta Obstet Gynecol Scand 1981; 60: 585–586

26 Smith P. Oestrogens and the urogenital tract. Acta Obstet Gynecol Scand 1993; 72: 1–26

27 Bernstein IT. The pelvic floor muscles: muscle thickness in healthy and urinary-incontinent women measured by perineal ultasonography with reference to the effect of pelvic floor training. Oestrogen receptor studies. Neurourol Urodyn 1997: 16: 237–275

28 Chen GD, Oliver RH, Leung BS, Lin LY, Yeh J. Oestrogen receptor α and β expression in the vaginal walls and uterosacral ligaments of premenopausal and postmenopausal women. Fertil Steril 1999; 71: 1099–1102

29 Screiter F, Fuchs P, Stockamp K. Oestrogenic sensitivity of α receptors in the urethral musculature. Urol Int 1976; 31: 13–19

30 Pang X, Cotreau-Bibbo MM, Sant GR, Theoharides TC. Bladder mast cell expression of high affinity oestrogen receptors in receptors in patients with interstitial cystitis. Br J Urol 1995; 75: 154–161

31 Blakeman PJ, Hilton P, Bulmer JN. Androgen receptors in the female lower urinary tract. Int Urogynaecol J 1997; 8: S54

32 Blakeman PJ, Hilton P, Bulmer JN. Oestrogen and progesterone receptor expression in the female lower urinary tract, with reference to oestrogen status. Br J Urol Int 2000; 86: 32–38

33 Abrams P, Blaivas JG, Stanton SL *et al*. The standardisation of terminology of lower urinary tract dysfunction. Br J Obstet Gynaecol 1990; 97: 1–16

34 Rud T, Anderson KE, Asmussen M *et al*. Factors maintaining the urethral pressure in women. Invest Urol 1980; 17: 343–347

35 Malone-Lee J. Urodynamic measurement and urinary incontinence in the elderly. In: Brocklehurst JC. (ed) Managing and Measuring Incontinence. Proceedings of the Geriatric Workshop on Incontinence, July 1988

36 Versi E, Cardozo LD. Oestrogens and lower urinary tract function. In: Studd JWW, Whitehead MI. (eds) The Menopause. Oxford: Blackwell, 1988; 76–84

37 Kinn AC, Lindskog M. Oestrogens and phenylpropanolamine in combination for stress incontinence. Urology 1988; 32: 273–280

38 Smith PJB. The effect of oestrogens on bladder function in the female. In: Campbell S. (ed) The Management of the Menopause and Postmenopausal Years. Carnforth: MTP, 1976; 291–298

39 Samsioe G, Jansson I, Mellstrom, D, Svandborg A. Occurrence, nature and treatment of urinary incontinence in a 70 year old female population. Maturitas 1985; 7: 335–342

40 Blakeman PJ, Hilton P, Bulmer JN. Cellular proliferation in the female lower urinary tract with reference to oestrogen status. Br J Obstet Gynaecol 2001; 8: 813–816

41 Shapiro E. Effect of oestrogens on the weight and muscarinic receptor density of the rabbit bladder and urethra. J Urol 1986; 135: 1084–1087

42 Batra S, Anderson KE. Oestrogen induced changes in muscarinic receptor density and contractile responses in the female rat urinary bladder. Acta Physiol Scand 1989; 137: 135–141

43 Elliott RA, Castleden CM, Miodrag A, Kirwan P. The direct effects of diethylstilboestrol and nifedipine on the contractile responses of isolated human and rat detrusor muscles. Eur J Clin Pharmacol 1992; 43: 149–155

44 Shenfield OZ, Blackmore PF, Morgan CW, Schlossberg SM, Jordan GH, Ratz PH. Rapid effects of oestriol and progesterone on tone and spontaneous rhythmic contractions of the rabbit bladder. Neurourol Urodyn 1998; 17: 408–409

45 Fantl JA, Wyman JF, Anderson RL et al. Post menopausal urinary incontinence: comparison between non-oestrogen and oestrogen supplemented women. Obstet Gynecol 1988; 71: 823–828

46 Maggi A, Perez J. Role of female gonadal hormones in the CNS. Life Sci 1985; 37: 893–906

47 Smith SS, Berg G, Hammar M. (eds) The Modern Management of the Menopause. Hormones, Mood and Neurobiology – A Summary. Carnforth: Parthenon, 1993; 204

48 Blok EFM, Holstege G. Androgen receptor immunoreactive neurones in the hypothalamic preoptic area project to the pontine micturition centre in the male cat. Neurourol Urodyn 1998; 17: 404–405

49 Bergman A, Karram MM, Bhatia NN. Changes in urethral cytology following oestrogen administration. Gynaecol Obstet Invest 1990; 29: 211–213

50 Rud T. The effects of oestrogens and gestogens on the urethral pressure profile in urinary continent and stress incontinent women. Acta Obstet Gynecol Scand 1980; 59: 365–270

51 Hilton P, Stanton SL. The use of intravaginal oestrogen cream in genuine stress incontinence. Br J Obstet Gynaecol 1983; 90: 940–944

52 Bhatia NN, Bergman A, Karram MM et al. Effects of oestrogen on urethral function in women with urinary incontinence. Am J Obstet Gynecol 1989; 160: 176–180

53 Karram MM, Yeko TR, Sauer MV et al. Urodynamic changes following hormone replacement therapy in women with premature ovarian failure. Obstet Gynecol 1989; 74: 208–211

54 Ganger KF, Vyas S, Whitehead RW et al. Pulsatility index in the internal carotid artery in relation to transdermal oestradiol and time since the menopause. Lancet 1991; 338: 839–842

55 Jackson S, Vyas S. A double blind, placebo controlled study of postmenopausal oestrogen replacement therapy and carotid artery pulsatility index. Br J Obstet Gynaecol 1998; 105: 408–412

56 Penotti M, Farina M, Sironi L et al. Long term effects of postmenopausal hormone replacement therapy on pulsatility index of the internal carotid and middle cerebral arteries. Menopause 1997; 4: 101–104

57 Versi E, Cardozo LD. Urethral instability: diagnosis based on variations in the maximum urethral pressure in normal climacteric women. Neurourol Urodyn 1986; 5: 535–541

58 Falconer C, Ekman-Ordeberg G, Ulmsten U et al. Changes in paraurethral connective tissue at menopause are counteracted by oestrogen. Maturitas 1996; 24: 197–204

59 Kushner L, Chen Y, Desautel M, Moak S, Greenwald R, Badlani G. Collagenase activity is elevated in conditioned media from fibroblasts of women with pelvic floor weakening. Int Urogynaecol 1999; 10 (Suppl 1): 34

60 Jackson S, Avery N, Shepherd A et al. The effect of oestradiol on vaginal collagen in postmenopausal women with stress urinary incontinence. Neurourol Urodyn 1996; 15: 327–328

61 James M, Avery N, Jackson S, Bailey A, Abrams P. The pathophysiological changes of vaginal skin tissue in women with stress urinary incontinence: a controlled trial. Int Urogynaecol 1999; 10 (Suppl 1): 35

62 James M, Avery N, Jackson S, Bailey A, Abrams P. The biochemical profile of vaginal tissue in women with genitourinary prolapse: a controlled trial. Neurourol Urodyn 1999; 18: 284–285

63 Brincat M, Moniz CF, Studd JWW. Long term effects of the menopause and sex hormones on skin thickness. Br J Obstet Gynaecol 1985; 92: 256–259

64 Landon CR, Smith ARB, Crofts CE, Trowbridge EA. Biochemical properties of connective tissue in women with stress incontinence of urine. Neurourol Urodyn 1989; 8: 369–370

65 Ulmsten U, Ekman G, Giertz G. Different biochemical composition of connective tissue in continent and stress incontinent women. Acta Obstet Gynecol Scand 1987; 66: 455

66 Samicoe G. Urogenital ageing – a hidden problem. Am J Obstet Gynecol 1998; 178: S245–S249

67 Cardozo LD, Tapp A, Versi E, Samsioe G, Bonne Erickson P. (eds) The lower urinary tract in peri- and postmenopausal women. In: The Urogenital Deficiency Syndrome. Bagsverd, Denmark: Novo Industri, 1987; 10–17

68 Kondo A, Kato K, Saito M et al. Prevalence of hand washing incontinence in females in comparison with stress and urge incontinence. Neurourol Urodyn 1990; 9: 330–331

69 Thomas TM, Plymat KR, Blannin J et al. Prevalence of urinary incontinence. BMJ 1980; 281: 1243–1245

70 Jolleys JV. Reported prevalence of urinary incontinence in a general practice. BMJ 1988; 296: 1300–1302

71 Burgio KL, Matthews KA, Engel B. Prevalence, incidence and correlates of urinary incontinence in healthy, middle aged women. J Urol 1991; 146: 1255–1259

72 Hextall A, Bidmead J, Cardozo L, Hooper R. Hormonal influences on the human female lower urinary tract: a prospective evaluation of the effects of the menstrual cycle on symptomatology and the results of urodynamic investigation. Neurourol Urodyn 1999; 18: 282–283

73 Van Geelen JM, Doesburg WH, Thomas CMG. Urodynamic studies in the normal menstrual cycle: the relationship between hormonal changes during the menstrual cycle and the urethral pressure profile. Am J Obstet Gynecol 1981; 141: 384–392

74 Burton G, Cardozo LD, Abdalla H, Kirkland A, Studd JWW. The hormonal effects on the lower urinary tract in 282 women with premature ovarian failure. Neurourol Urodyn 1992; 10: 318–319

75 Cutner A, Burton G, Cardozo LD, Wise BG, Abbot D, Studd JWW. Does progesterone cause an irritable bladder? Int Urogynaecol J 1993; 4: 259–261

76 Benness C, Gangar K, Cardozo LD, Cutner A. Do progestogens exacerbate urinary incontinence in women on HRT? Neurourol Urodyn 1991; 10: 316–318

77 Elliot RA, Castleden CM. Effect of progestogens and oestrogens on the contractile response of rat detrusor muscle to electrical field stimulation. Clin Sci 1994; 87: 342

78 Cutner A. The urinary tract in pregnancy. MD Thesis, University of London, 1993

79 Sandford JP. Urinary tract symptoms and infection. Annu Rev Med 1975; 26: 485–505

80 Boscia JA, Kaye D. Asymptomatic bacteria in the elderly. Infect Dis Clin North Am 1987; 1: 893–903

81 Salmon UL, Walter RI, Gast SH. The use of oestrogen in the treatment of dysuria and incontinence in postmenopausal women. Am J Obstet Gynecol 1941; 14: 23–31

82 Youngblood VH, Tomlin EM, Davis JB. Senile urethritis in women. J Urol 1957; 78: 150–152

83 Fantl JA, Cardozo LD, McClish DK and the Hormones and Urogenital Therapy Committee. Oestrogen therapy in the management of incontinence in postmenopausal women: a meta-analysis. First report of the Hormones and Urogenital Therapy Committee. Obstet Gynecol 1994; 83: 12–18

84 Henalla SM, Hutchins CJ, Robinson P, Macivar J. Non–operative methods in the treatment of female genuine stress incontinence of urine. Br J Obstet Gynaecol 1989; 96: 222–225

85 Zullo MA, Oliva C, Falconi G, Paparella P, Mancuso S. Efficacy of oestrogen therapy in urinary incontinence. A meta-analytic study. Minerva Ginecol 1998; 50: 199–205

86 Grady D, Brown JS, Vittinghoff E, Applegate W, Varner E, Synder T. Postmenopausal hormones and incontinence: the Heart and Estrogen/progestin Replacement Study. Obstet Gynaecol 2001; 97: 116–120

87 Ouslander JG, Greendale GA, Uman G, Lee C, Paul W, Schnelle J. Effects of oral oestrogen and progestin on the lower urinary tract among female nursing home residents. Am Geriatr Soc 2001; 49: 803–807

88 Caine M, Raz S. The role of female hormones in stress incontinence. In: Proceedings of the 16th Congress of the International Society of Urology, 1993, Amsterdam, The Netherlands

89 Rud T. The effects of oestrogens and gestagens on the urethral pressure profile in urinary continent and stress incontinent women. Acta Obstet Gynecol Scand 1980; 59: 265–270

90 Wilson PD, Faragher B, Butler B, Bullock D, Robinson EL, Brown ADG. Treatment with oral piperazine oestrone sulphate for genuine stress incontinence in postmenopausal women. Br J Obstet Gynaecol 1987; 94: 568–574

91 Walter S, Wolf H, Barlebo H, Jansen H. Urinary incontinence in postmenopausal women treated with oestrogens: a double-blind clinical trial. Urol Int 1978; 33: 135–143.

92 Fantl JA, Bump RC, Robinson D et al. Efficacy of oestrogen supplementation in the treatment of urinary incontinence. Obstet Gynecol 1996; 88: 745–749

93 Jackson S, Shepherd A, Brookes S, Abrams P. The effect of oestrogen supplementation on post-menopausal urinary stress incontinence: a double-blind, placebo controlled trial. Br J Obstet Gynaecol 1999; 106: 711–718

94 Sultana CJ, Walters MD. Oestrogen and urinary incontinence in women. Maturitas 1995; 20: 129–138

95 Beisland HO, Fossberg E, Moer A et al. Urethral insufficiency in post-menopausal females: treatment with phenylpropanolamine and oestriol separately and in combination. Urol Int 1984; 39: 211–216

96 Hilton P, Tweddel AL, Mayne C. Oral and intravaginal oestrogens alone and in combination with alpha adrenergic stimulation in genuine stress incontinence. Int Urogynecol J 1990; 12: 80–86

97 Samsicoe G, Jansson I, Mellstrom D, Svanberg A. Urinary incontinence in 75 year old women. Effects of oestriol. Acta Obstet Gynecol Scand 1985; 93: 57

98 Cardozo LD, Rekers H, Tapp A et al. Oestriol in the treatment of postmenopausal urgency: a multicentre study. Maturitas 1993; 18: 47–53

99 Nilsson K, Heimer G. Low dose oestradiol in the treatment of urogenital oestrogen deficiency – a pharmacokinetic and pharmacodynamic study. Maturitas 1992; 15: 121–127

100 Benness C, Wise BG, Cutner A, Cardozo LD. Does low dose vaginal oestradiol improve frequency and urgency in postmenopausal women. Int Urogynaecol J 1992; 3: 281

101 Eriksen PS, Rasmussen H. Low dose 17β-oestradiol vaginal tablets in the treatment of atrophic vaginitis: a double-blind placebo controlled study. Eur J Obstet Gynecol Reprod Biol 1992; 44: 137–144

102 Cardozo L, Versi E, McClish D, Lose G. 4th Report of the Hut Committee. Acta Scand 2004, In press

103 Brandberg A, Mellstrom D, Samsioe G. Low dose oral oestriol treatment in elderly women with urogenital infections. Acta Obstet Gynecol Scand 1987; 140: 33–38

104 Parsons CL, Schmidt JD. Control of recurrent urinary tract infections in postmenopausal women. J Urol 1982; 128: 1224–1226

105 Privette M, Cade R, Peterson J et al. Prevention of recurrent urinary tract infections in postmenopausal women. Nephron 1988; 50: 24–27

106 Kjaergaard B, Walter S, Knudsen A et al. Treatment with low dose vaginal oestradiol in postmenopausal women. A double blind controlled trial. Ugeskr Laeger 1990; 152: 658–659

107 Raz R, Stamm WE. A controlled trial of intravaginal oestriol in postmenopausal women with recurrent urinary tract infections. N Engl J Med 1993; 329: 753–756

108 Kirkengen AL, Anderson P, Gjersoe E et al. Oestriol in the prophylactic treatment of recurrent urinary tract infections in postmenopausal women. Scand J Prim Health Care 1992; 10: 142

109 Cardozo LD, Benness C, Abbott D. Low dose oestrogen prophylaxis for recurrent urinary tract infections in elderly women. Br J Obstet Gynaecol 1998; 105: 403–407

110 Eriksen B. A randomised, open, parallel-group study on the preventative effect of an oestradiol-releasing vaginal ring (Estring) on recurrent urinary tract infections in postmenopausal women. Am J Obstet Gynecol 1999; 180: 1072–1079

111 Mettler L, Olsen PG. Long term treatment of atrophic vaginitis with low dose oestradiol

vaginal tablets. Maturitas 1991; 14: 23–31

112 Smith P, Heimer G, Lindskog, Ulmsten U. Oestradiol releasing vaginal ring for treatment of postmenopausal urogenital atrophy. Maturitas 1993; 16: 145–154

113 Smith RJN, Studd JWW. Recent advances in hormone replacement therapy. Br J Hosp Med 1993; 49: 799–809

114 Cardozo LD, Bachmann G, McClish D, Fonda D, Birgerson L. Meta-analysis of oestrogen therapy in the management of urogenital atrophy in postmenopausal women: Second report of the Hormones and Urogenital Therapy Committee. Obstet Gynecol 1998; 92: 722–727

115 Henriksson L, Stjernquist M, Boquist L, Cedergren I, Selinus I. A one-year multicentre study of efficacy and safety of a continuous, low dose, oestradiol-releasing vaginal ring (Estring) in postmenopausal women with symptoms and signs of urogenital aging. Am J Obstet Gynecol 1996; 174: 85–92

116 Bachmann G. Oestradiol-releasing vaginal ring delivery system for urogenital atrophy. Experience over the last decade. J Reprod Med 1998; 43: 991–998

117 Ayton RA, Darling GM, Murkies AL et al. A comparative study of safety and efficacy of low dose oestradiol released from a vaginal ring compared with conjugated equine oestrogen vaginal cream in the treatment of postmenopausal vaginal atrophy. Br J Obstet Gynaecol 1996; 103: 351–358

118 Park WC, Jordan VC. Selective oestrogen receptor modulators (SERMS) and their roles in cancer prevention. Trends Mol Med 2002; 8: 82–88

119 Silfen SL, Ciaccia AV, Bryant HU. Selective oestrogen receptor modulators: tissue selectivity and differential uterine effects. Climacteric 1999; 2: 268–283

120 Hendrix SL, McNeeley SG. Effect of selective oestrogen receptor modulators on reproductive tissues other than endometrium. Ann NY Acad Sci 2001; 949: 243–250

121 Goldstein SR, Neven P, Zhou L, Taylor YL, Ciacca AV, Plouffe L. Raloxifene effect on frequency of surgery for pelvic floor relaxation. Obstet Gynecol 2001; 98: 91–9

Jo Hockey Vineeta Verma Nicholas Panay

24

The wider role of intra-uterine progestogens

The concept of the intra-uterine administration of progesterone for contraception was introduced in the US in the 1970s. Following this work, the levonorgestrel-releasing intra-uterine system was devised in Finland gaining a licence there for contraception in 1990 and soon after in the UK. Its excellent contraceptive benefits have led to its wide-spread use. Since that time, the non-contraceptive health benefits of these systems secondary to the effect of the local action of the progestogen on the endometrium have been observed and researched. This evidence has supported the granting of a licence for the use of the levonorgestrel-releasing system for the non-contraceptive indication of menorrhagia and for the development of different types of intra-uterine system designed for the treatment of other non-contraceptive indications.

Here, we explore the evidence obtained from the use of these intra-uterine hormone delivery systems to provide a review of their current and proposed wider clinical applications, advantages and disadvantages of such devices.

STRUCTURE

The aim of any intra-uterine hormone delivery system is to deliver a small, predictable, daily dose of hormone into the uterine cavity. This predictable release should be sustained for a number of years[1] and can be achieved by mixing the steroid with a polymer to form a steroid reservoir. If this is contained within a polymeric sleeve or membrane, a controlled, daily release

Jo Hockey MD MRCOG
Speciaist Registrar, Queen Charlotte's and Chelsea Hospital, London, UK
(for correspondence, E-mail: johockey@doctors.org.uk)

Vineeta Verma MBBS MD MRCOG
Speciaist Registrar, Queen Charlotte's and Chelsea Hospital, London, UK

Nicholas Panay BSc MRCOG MFFP
Consultant Obstetrician and Gynaecologist, Queen Charlotte's and Chelsea Hospital, London, UK

of steroid can be achieved. The polymer polymethylsiloxane, developed in the 1970s, has been shown to provide a predictable sustained release of progesterone and the much more potent progestogen, levonorgestrel and is used widely in intra-uterine systems as well as subdermal contraceptive hormone implants.[1-4] The steroid reservoir is then attached to a frame (rendered radio-opaque by the impregnation of barium sulphate) which nestles within the uterine cavity or a fibrous frameless device anchored to the uterine fundus with a radio-opaque fastening clip.

There are four types of intra-uterine hormone releasing system – Progestasert, Mirena, Mirena MLS and Fibroplant. The latter two are still undergoing clinical trials.

Progestasert (PIPS) was the first progestogen-releasing system on the market. This has a drug reservoir of 38 mg of progesterone within its polymer of polydimethyl siloxane incorporated onto a T-shaped polymeric platform. The covering membrane allows a release of 65 µg of progesterone daily into the uterine cavity for 18–24 months. It was manufactured in the US and received FDA approval in 1976 for use as a contraceptive in parous women for 1 year with a 2-year bio-availability.[5] It was available briefly in the UK until marketing for this product ceased in the summer of 2001.[6]

The Mirena Intrauterine System (LNG-IUS) has a T-shaped frame (based on the Nova T IUCD) 32 mm by 32mm made of polyethylene surrounded by an elastomer sleeve in its vertical part. This sleeve is a 1:1 mixture of 52 mg of levonorgestrel and polymethylsiloxane. The membrane (also made of polymethylsiloxane) allows a controlled release of 20 mcg of levonorgestrel daily at a constant rate over 5 years. At the end of 5 years, the rate slowly decreases to 15 mcg a day and decreases further to 12 mcg at 7 years.[6] The LNG-IUS was first introduced in Finland in 1990 and is currently marketed in most European countries and in the US since 2000.[1]

A new low dose LNG IUS the Mirena MLS delivering 10 mcg daily to the uterine cavity is currently undergoing clinical trials to evaluate its effectiveness as the progestogenic opposition in HRT to suppress the endometrium in menopausal women.

A frameless delivery system, Fibroplant, is also undergoing clinical trials. This system has its 3 or 4 cm long 1.2 mm wide steroid reservoir and sustained release mechanism (delivering 10 or 14 mcg levonorgestrel, respectively) bound onto a fibrous flexible stem. This stem is attached to the fundus of the uterus by a metal clip and anchoring thread. The anchoring knot is implanted into the fundal myometrium using the Gynae-Fix insertion instrument. This system, due to its flexibility, can thus adapt to fit both uniform and non-uniform uterine cavities.[7] The duration of predictable release is at least 3 years.

PHARMACOKINETICS

The LNG-IUS releases levonorgestrel into the uterine cavity from which it is quickly absorbed into the capillaries of the endometrium and then into the systemic circulation. Levonorgestrel can be detected in the plasma within 15 min of insertion.[8] This plasma levonorgestrel is mainly bound to SHBG which may protect it from metabolism which rapidly occurs if free in the serum to a less potent steroid metabolite.[9,10] Maximum levels are achieved within a few hours and plateau after the first few weeks. The levels at the plateau are much lower than those achieved with the subcutaneous depot levonorgestrel implant, Norplant, the combined oral contraceptive pill and the progesterone only pill, without the serum levels exhibiting peaks and troughs as in the latter 2 modes of administration.[11-14] In the LNG-IUS, both the serum and intra-uterine levels remain constant over the life-time of the device in one individual. There is a wide variation of serum levels between individuals (0.3–0.6 nmol/l).[9]

EFFECTS ON OVARIAN FUNCTION

The effect of the LNG-IUS on ovarian function is minimal as suppression of ovarian function depends on the systemic absorption of 50 mcg levonorgestrel/24 h. As the Mirena LNG-IUS releases only 20 mcg and Fibroplant only 14 mcg, these suppressive levels are not achieved. Over 85% of women have ovulatory cycles using the LNG-IUS.[15] In general, those who have anovulatory cycles exhibit higher plasma levonorgestrel levels than those with ovulatory cycles. This is generally in the first year of use, the levels often declining and ovulation returning after this year. The endometrial levels remain constant.[15-17]

The observed bleeding pattern reflects neither the serum levonorgestrel concentration nor the presence or absence of ovarian activity. It is purely the effect of the device on the endometrium.[16,18] Oestrodiol levels are maintained at the normal pre-menopausal levels in women with both ovulatory and anovulatory cycles, in women with amenorrhea or those normally menstruating. Premenopausal women can be re-assured that the LNG-IUS only weakly affects ovarian function, particularly after the first year of use. Any change is reversible following removal of the device.[9]

Plasma levels of exogenous progesterone are not detectable in women using the Progestasert system and thus ovarian function is unaffected.

ENDOMETRIAL EFFECTS

The endometrium is constantly changing due to the effect of cyclical ovarian hormones. The development of the endometrial layers is regulated by a complex mechanism involving these steroid hormones, their receptors and local molecular systems which mediate their action.

The presence of the LNG-IUS causes profound changes within the endometrium down to the hormonally non-responsive basalis. The concentration of levonorgestrel is 200–800 times higher in the endometrium than in the adjacent myometrium or fallopian tubes.[19] An understanding of the endometrial effects of the LNG IUS underpins the mechanism of most of the significant non-contraceptive therapeutic effects of this system.

The endometrium undergoes structural, histological changes in response to the intra-uterine levonorgestrel system. These changes are uniform throughout the endometrial mucosa as far as the basal layer irrespective of the proximity of the device.[20] Histopathological studies have shown a thinning of the endometrium, atrophy of the endometrial glands, decidualisation of the endometrial stroma, capillary thrombosis and inflammatory cell infiltrate.[21,23]

These features are consistent with a progestogenic effect and the presence of a mechanical device.[21] The thinning of the endometrium, as a result of endometrial atrophy, occurs in the first 3 months following insertion.[22,23] Cyclical changes in the endometrium in relation to the menstrual cycle are abolished.[24] Local blood flow is also altered. The presence of the LNG IUS has been associated with the development of thin-walled blood vessels in the superficial myometrium.[25] Comparative Doppler blood flow studies have demonstrated a decrease in subendometrial flow in the spiral arteries in women with a LNG IUS *in situ*.[26] This is not shown in women with a copper-containing IUCD. In both groups, there was no change in the blood flow in the cervical branch of the uterine artery.

Local biochemical factors are important in the process of cellular atrophy within the endometrium. These include an alteration in the dynamics of growth factor mechanisms, an increase in apoptosis (or programmed cell death) within the endometrial glands and the suppression of a gene coding for a receptor for thrombin. These may all have a role although their relationship remains unclear.

The insulin-like growth factor system modulates the effects of oestrogen. There are two main types of factor, IGF 1 which when stimulated by oestrogen stimulates the endometrium to proliferate, and IGF 2 which causes and maintains differentiation within the endometrium. Endometrial stromal cells produce IGF 1 and IGF 2 and their binding proteins, IGFBP 1 and IGFBP 2.

Women using LNG IUS have been shown to have an increase in IGFBP 1 and a subsequent decrease in IGF 1 activity. There is also a rise in the concentration of IGF 2.[27,28] This will result in a weak proliferation of the endometrium, which is well differentiated and maintained.

Another marker of endometrial proliferation is ki-67 which is abundant in the endometrial cells of menorrhagic women. This has been shown to be reduced in women using the LNG IUS.[29] Endometrial plasminogen activator inhibitor has been shown to be induced by the presence of the LNG IUS[30] and this is thought to have a role in reducing menstrual blood flow.

Apoptosis or programmed cell death in endometrial glands and stroma has been reported as rare in normal, ectopic or adenomyotic endometrial tissue. At 3 months post-insertion of LNG IUS, it has been shown to be much more common.[31]

The LNG IUS has been shown to down-regulate the gene that codes for a receptor for thrombin (protease activated receptor–1). An alteration in the expression of this receptor affects both growth and haemostatic activity in the endometrium.[32]

In summary, the thinning of the endometrium occurs in the early weeks following insertion with changes in local endometrial blood flow only. Biochemical modulators may mediate this as a reduction of cell proliferation and an increase in programmed cell death. When taken together, this results in a reduction in the endometrial thickness. These changes are reversible even after long-term use; normal menstruation is restored 1 month after the removal of the system.[33]

The non-contraceptive therapeutic indications for the LNG IUS are generally based on this principle of endometrial suppression and these include beneficial effects on menorrhagia, use of the system as the progestogenic component of combined HRT, use of the system in the treatment of hyperplastic and endometriotic endometrium and for the treatment of fibroids and their symptoms. Other health benefits include a reduction in pelvic inflammatory disease and ectopic pregnancy and a possible application in the treatment of premenstrual syndrome.

ROLE IN THE MANAGEMENT OF MENORRHAGIA

Menorrhagia is experienced by up to 30% of women of reproductive age;[34] it accounts for 60% of general practice consultations for menstrual dysfunction,[14] 12% of gynaecology referrals[35] and is the commonest cause of iron-deficiency anaemia affecting 20–25% of healthy fertile women in the UK.[13,14]

One in 20 women aged 30–49 years consult their general practitioner each year with menorrhagia.[36] Of women referred to secondary care, 60% are likely to have a hysterectomy within 5 years of referral as shown by Coulter *et al.*[37] and in most of these women there is no demonstrable pelvic pathology.[14]

In 1993–1994, 73,517 hysterectomies were carried out in England, there was a decline in 1997–1998 when 63,345 operations were carried out.[38] Endometrial ablations had risen markedly from 9945 to 36,440 in the same period.[39]

This trend towards endometrial destructive procedures, away from hysterectomy, is not surprising. These procedures are associated with lower complication rates and mortality. They also have higher patient satisfaction.[40] However, these procedures may not always be successful; re-operation rates range from 11–40%[41] and about a third of women will eventually require a hysterectomy.[42]

Although patient satisfaction with hysterectomy remains high as the definitive cure for menorrhagia,[43,44] considerable morbidity and occasional mortality may occur. Complication rates up to 42% have been shown to be associated with abdominal hysterectomy, the commonest route used in UK, compared from 24% for vaginal hysterectomy.[45] Substantial costs are incurred due to a long convalescence in both hospital and at home.[38,44]

MEDICAL THERAPIES

Women warrant a trial of effective medical therapies before proceeding to definitive surgical treatment.[46] Many drug therapies, however, are ineffective and suffer from poor patient compliance.

A meta-analysis and survey of general practice prescription patterns showed that norethisterone was most widely used by 40.9% of general practitioners. Low-dose luteal phase regimens are often ineffective and may even increase the blood flow in some cases.[47]

Reduction of menstrual blood loss by different forms of medical treatment reported in various studies[48–51] ranges from 25% (mefenamic acid), 40% (oral contraceptive pill), 50% (tranexamic acid), 75% (gonadotrophin releasing hormone analogues) and 80% (danazol)

Andersson and Rybo[52] used the LNG IUS in 20 women with confirmed menorrhagia and observed significant reduction in menstrual loss of 85% at 3 months' usage and a further reduction of up to 97% at 12 months of LNG IUS usage. There was also significant increase in mean serum ferritin by 47% in the first year of use. Spotting was commonly reported in the first 3 months and 35% of women were amenorrhoeic at 1 year.

In an observational study, involving 10 Chinese women who were anaemic and had objectively measured blood loss of > 80 ml, the LNG IUS resulted in significant reduction of menstrual blood loss of 54%, 87% and 95% in the first, third and sixth month of treatment, respectively, and an increase in mean haemoglobin by 19.2 % at 6 months compared with pre-treatment cycles.[53]

The progesterone-releasing system (Progestasert) has also been shown to reduce menstrual blood loss (65% reduction 12 months post-insertion),[54] but this is not to the same extent as the LNG-IUS.

In a study by Wildermeersch and Schacht,[55] the lower dose levonorgestrel releasing Fibro plant IUS was inserted in 32 women with a normal uterus. A reduction of menstrual blood loss of at least 80% occurred in the 1–23 month follow-up with reduction seen as early as 1 month.

Stewart et al.[56] conducted a systematic review to address the effectiveness of levonorgestrel releasing systems in menorrhagia. They identified 34 studies using the LNG IUS releasing 20 mcg levonorgestrel and reporting menstrual loss. Only 10 studies fulfilled inclusion criteria because they had objective evidence of menorrhagia. Five studies were randomised controlled trials[57-61] and reported the use of the LNG IUS in 110 women with menorrhagia, and five case series[52,53,62-64] reported on use in a further 101 women. The main outcome measures were reduction in menstrual blood loss (MBL), serum ferritin/Hb level, side effects, satisfaction with treatment at 3 months and decision to cancel hysterectomy.

The results of the meta-analysis showed the use of the LNG IUS could significantly reduce menstrual blood loss (range, 74–97%) in women with confirmed menorrhagia. However, to establish the effectiveness and cost effectiveness relative to other treatments and effect on surgical waiting lists, larger, more powerful, randomised, controlled trials with longer follow-up are required.

LNG-IUS APPLICATIONS

LNG-IUS versus other medical therapies

Only two of the randomised trials have directly compared LNG IUS to other forms of medical treatments.[57,58] In the study by Irvine et al.,[57] the efficacy and acceptability of the LNG IUS was compared with higher doses of norethisterone 5 mg three times daily, from days 5 to 26 of cycle for three cycles. Reduction of menstrual blood loss by the LNG IUS was 94% and oral norethisterone 87%, after three cycles. Of the women in the LNG IUS group, 76% wished to continue with the treatment compared with 22% of the norethisterone group, even though 52% (10/19) in the LNG IUS group were still experiencing intermenstrual bleeding. Women in the norethisterone group objected to taking 64 tablets a month.[57]

The LNG-IUS compares well to other medical therapies. The mean menstrual blood loss reduction at 12 months was much higher with the LNG IUS reducing blood loss by 96% compared to 21% with flurbiprofen and 44% with tranexamic acid.[58]

In the Cochrane Database Review,[65] no studies were found comparing progesterone/levonorgestrel IUS to placebo or no treatments. Progestasert had been compared to other medical therapies in one small study but no conclusions could be made on its effectiveness.

LNG IUS compared to surgical management

The reduction in menstrual loss by the LNG IUS has reduced the demand for hysterectomy or transcervical resection of the endometrium. Reports suggest that the treatment was so effective that 64–82% of women who had previously failed medical therapy, and who were awaiting surgery, came off the waiting list. This compared to around 14% of women continuing with existing medical therapies.[59,62]

Recent results of Nagrani and Bowen-Simpkins[66] of 4–5-year long-term follow-up of the patients recruited in their original study[62] demonstrated a continuation rate of 50% after a mean 54 months' follow-up. The more important observation from this study was that only 26.4% eventually had surgical treatment despite 50% not continuing with the LNG IUS and an overall 67.4% avoided surgery.[66]

Comparing the LNG IUS with endometrial resection demonstrates a mean menstrual blood loss reduction of 79–90% with the LNG IUS at 12 months. This is less than that achieved with endometrial resection with mean menstrual blood loss rates of 89–98% but these findings between the two groups are not always found to be significant.[60,61,67] Satisfaction was high in both groups, 85% in the LNG-IUS group and 94% in the resection group.[60] Health-related quality of life perception was not significantly different in the two treatment groups.

If menstrual loss is measured using a pictorial assessment chart,[68] treatment success, defined as a Pictorial Blood Assessment Chart (PBAC) score of ≤ 75 at 12 months, has been shown in similar comparisons.[69] Treatment success was achieved in 67% (20/30) of the LNG-IUS group and 90% (26/29) of the resection group. In the Visual Analogue Scale (VAS) assessment of the subjective symptoms, sleeping problems were slightly increased in the TCRE group, general feeling of genital health was increased and menstrual pain decreased over time in both the groups.

The SMART study (Satisfaction with Mirena and Ablation: a Randomised Trial) aimed to determine women's satisfaction and assessment of heaviness by pictorial charts at 12 months' post-treatment. This study was terminated due to a poor recruitment rate owing to high reluctance to be randomised to the LNG-IUS arm.[70]

Johnson et al.[71] are more optimistic about a similar randomised trial, TALIS (Thermo-Ablation versus the Levonorgestrel Intrauterine System), in Auckland where recruitment has been more successful. This is possibly due to women being more favourable towards research and the LNG-IUS, and due to a better study design allowing more decision time and use of one/two–stop menstrual disorder clinics in the research trial.[71]

Hurskainen et al.[72] conducted a trial on quality of life and cost effectiveness of the LNG IUS versus hysterectomy for treatment of menorrhagia in 236 women. After 12 months, 20% of the women in the LNG IUS group underwent hysterectomy and 68% continued to use the system, with 69% experiencing amenorrhea or minimal bleeding. Amongst those randomised for hysterectomy, 91% went to have the operation. Health-related quality of life (HRQoL) and indices of psychosocial well-being improved significantly in both groups .There was no significant difference between the two groups except that women with the hysterectomy had less pain. Overall costs were 3 times higher for the hysterectomy group than for the IUS group.[72]

The LNG-IUS provides an effective, efficient, well-tolerated, cost-effective alternative to other medical and surgical management of menorrhagia.

LNG-IUS as the progestogenic component of HRT

Hormone replacement therapy is currently used by 33% of British women.[73] Unfortunately, studies have shown that about 50% of women who start hormone replacement therapy discontinue within a year.[74] It has been reported that patients are more likely to discontinue therapy if they experience side effects related to treatment and are more likely to continue if side effects are less common.[75] Women with an intact uterus need progestogen administration whenever oestrogen replacement therapy is used. This avoids endometrial hyperplasia and neoplasia,[76,77] the risk of developing hyperplasia at 1 year is 20% and the relative risk of developing endometrial cancer in women taking unopposed oestrogen is 2–3.[78] Cyclical administration of progestogen causes withdrawal bleeding which has been shown to decrease compliance.[79,80] Other factors cited as reducing compliance include mastalgia, weight gain, fear of cancer and symptoms of pre-menstrual tension.[81]

Continuous combined hormone replacement therapy or 'period-free' hormone replacement therapy was first used 20 years ago in Scandinavia to overcome some of these problems and improve patient satisfaction and compliance.[82] Continuous combined regimens have proved to be at least as effective as cyclical regimens in preventing endometrial hyperplasia, reducing the risk to virtually nil,[76,78] and may even be more protective against endometrial cancer than cyclical regimens.[83] In addition, women on a continuous combined regimen have a lower rate of abnormal vaginal bleeding than those on cyclical schemes and consequently undergo fewer gynae-cological investigations.[84] The use of continuous combined regimens is, however, reserved for those women who report more than 12 months' amenorrhoea and are thought to be menopausal. If the continuous, combined, hormone replacement therapy is administered to perimenopausal women, erratic vaginal breakthrough bleeding may be experienced due to inconsistent endogenous hormone levels being produced from the ovaries.[81]

Progesterone and its derivatives in the systemic circulation have an essentially anti-oestrogenic effect and could potentially counteract the beneficial effects of oestrogens depending on the type and dosage used.[85] The intra-uterine administration of progestogen minimises the problems associated with systemic progestogenic side effects and may increase the suitability of continuous combined therapy in the perimenopausal woman.

The levonorgestrel intra-uterine system has been shown in studies to be effective in providing progestogenic opposition in perimenopausal and post-menopausal women using oral,[86] transdermal[7] and implanted oestrogen.[87,88]

Transvaginal ultrasonography and endometrial biopsies were used in the studies to confirm atrophy. There were no cases of endometrial hyperplasia in any of the levonorgestrel intra-uterine system users. The proportion of women with amenorrhoea using the intra-uterine system after 1 year was up to 80% in one study.[87]

Endometrial suppression is also achieved by using an intra-uterine system delivering only 5 mcg of levonorgestrel to the uterus. Both a 5 mcg and 10 mcg system produced histologically non-proliferative endometrium after 12 months with similar bleeding patterns in both groups of women.[89]

The only intra-uterine system currently available in the UK is the Mirena. The Mirena is currently licensed for contraception and the treatment of menorrhagia. Clinical trials are currently on-going in the development of intra-uterine systems specifically for the purpose of endometrial suppression in women using oestrogen replacement therapy. Lower doses of levonorgestrel intra-uterine system Mirena MLS 10 mcg and Fibroplant, delivering either 10 mcg or 14 mcg, have been shown to be a safe and effective method for suppressing the endometrium during oestrogen replacement therapy in perimenopausal and postmenopausal women. It induces atrophy of the endometrium and amenorrhoea in the majority of women.[7,90] No difference in the endometrial effect between the two Fibroplant dosage forms was reported following ultrasound examination. Slight, scanty, bloody discharge can occur mainly in perimenopausal women but is found to be infrequent and of little significance.

Effects on lipid and lipoprotein metabolism

Postmenopausal women have a different lipid profile when compared with women of fertile age. The levels of serum cholesterol and low-density lipoprotein cholesterol (LDL-cholesterol) as well as triglycerides increase and levels of high-density lipoprotein cholesterol (HDL-cholesterol) may decrease after the menopause.[91] High serum cholesterol and LDL-cholesterol levels are associated with a high risk of cardiovascular disease.

Oestrogen replacement therapy reduces cholesterol and LDL-cholesterol levels in serum and increases the HDL-cholesterol fraction.[92] When a progestogen is added to the oestrogen replacement therapy, either as sequential or as a continuous combined therapy, the lipid and lipoprotein profile may be adversely altered in a dose- and duration-dependent manner.[93]

A recent study by Raudaskoski et al.[90] using 2 mg oestradiol valerate and the Mirena intra-uterine system showed HDL-cholesterol remaining at baseline level after 12 months of treatment. This result is similar in the group of patients using 2 mg oestradiol valerate and oral medroxyprogesterone acetate. However, an increase in mean concentration of HDL-cholesterol was shown in the group using the lower 10 mcg menopausal levonorgestrel intra-uterine system. Similar results were shown in the study by Wollter-Svensson et al.,[94] where 5 mcg and 10 mcg levonorgestrel intra-uterine systems were used. The increase in HDL-cholesterol levels must be considered as an oestrogenic effect that was not opposed by the low doses of levonorgestrel, which strongly indicates that the influence of levonorgestrel on HDL-cholesterol is dose dependent.

The LDL-cholesterol levels were reduced by all the levonorgestrel intra-uterine system doses.[90,94] These results showed that the continuous combined hormone replacement therapy with an intra-uterine administration of levonorgestrel in low doses did not abolish the beneficial lipid metabolic effects usually seen after oestrogen administration. These changes might be favourable in cardioprotection.

LNG IUS and endometriosis

Women with endometriosis have a higher baseline mean menstrual score than normal according to the visual chart devised by Higham *et al.*[68] It has been speculated that this may account for some of the dysmenorrhoea suffered by such women.[95] A pilot study[96] investigating the tolerability and efficacy of the LNG IUS in the long-term treatment of recurrent dysmenorrhoea associated with endometriosis demonstrated a greatly reduced visual analogue scale for menstrual pain which was associated with a 76% mean reduction in PBLA chart score. The system was tolerated at 1 year. Further studies are needed to show if this improvement is sustained in the long term.

The LNG IUS has been shown to be effective as a therapy for endometriosis of the rectovaginal septum.[97] This small study in women with deep endometriosis showed that dysmenorrhoea, pelvic pain and deep dyspareunia greatly improved when assessed after 12 months. The size of the endometrial deposits, measured by transrectal and transvaginal ultrasound, were significantly reduced by treatment. This finding supports earlier work which showed endometriosis to be arrested by the treatment of LNG IUS.[98] Adenomyosis-related menorrhagia has been successfully treated by the LNG IUS[63] in women with regular intra-uterine cavities and also in those with irregular , enlarged cavities due to severe adenoyosis.[99]

Fibroids

There is conflicting evidence regarding the use of the LNG IUS in the treatment of the symptoms of fibroids and for the treatment for the fibroids themselves.

When compared to copper IUD users, women with the LNG IUS are less likely to develop fibroids or have fibroid-related surgery in the long term (after 7 years).[100] Another study showed 13% of women had fewer fibroids at 12 months using the LNG IUS than controls.[101] One report has demonstrated a measurable reduction in the size of fibroids in 5 menorrhagic women with fibroids after 6–18 months of treatment with LNG IUS.[102] Other studies suggest no change in the size of existing fibroids with the LNG IUS[103] or the use of the new frameless levonorgestrel IUS, Fibroplant (releasing 14 mcg per day),[104] although there was significant improvement in symptoms due to a marked reduction in menstrual blood loss.

The exact biological mechanism underlying cessation of growth or reduction in the size of fibroids is not clearly established. Fibroids all show evidence of decreased apoptosis in keeping with other tumours, together with an increase in insulin-like growth factors. The modulation of these factors may play a part,[105] although intra-uterine levonorgestrel will reduce proliferation and increase apoptosis in normal myometrium. Its effects on leiomyoma cells is less clear and may even stimulate leiomyoma cell growth *in vitro*.[106]

Patients do, however, receive good symptomatic relief from fibroid-related menorrhagia.[104,107] The development of the frameless device, Fibroplant, may assist in treating women with uterine cavities distorted by fibroids as the fibrous structure is firmly anchored. This device appears less likely to be dislodged and expelled than the framed devices in these women.[104,108,109]

The intra-uterine levonorgestrel systems provide an improvement in fibroid-related menorrhagia with a reduction in dysmenorrhoea. It may protect against the development of fibroids although its role in the direct treatment of the fibroids themselves seems less clear.

Endometrial hyperplasia

The antiproliferative and suppressive effects on the endometrium when either the progesterone or levonorgestrel IUS are used can treat endometrial hyperplasia. This was first demonstrated with the Progestasert[110] which was found to be successful in 81% of cases but with a high recurrence rate after removal. The LNG IUS can achieve a faster regression of endometrial hyperplasia than the Progestasert probably due to the greater efficacy of androgenic progestogens over progesterone in achieving secretory transformation.[111,112] These changes involve the whole thickness of the endometrium and occur irrespective of the pattern of the initial hyperplasia.[111–113]

Tamoxifen-induced endometrial hyperplasia

Tamoxifen is currently one of the most commonly used hormonal treatments for breast cancer. Tamoxifen is not a pure anti-oestrogen, as it has oestrogenic effects in the skeletal system, in lipid metabolism[114] and in the uterus.[115] This unopposed oestrogenic effect promotes occult uterine lesions to develop into polyps, fibroids and endometrial hyperplasia and is responsible for a 2–3-fold increase in endometrial cancer. The use of systemic progestogens may blunt the efficacy of tamoxifen to prevent recurrence of breast cancer. Levonorgestrel-releasing intra-uterine systems have shown a protective action against the uterine effects of tamoxifen with uniform decidualisation of the endometrium.[116]

Treatment of early endometrial cancer

Intra-uterine progesterone has been studied in the treatment of early endometrial cancer.[117] This could be particularly useful as patients associated with a high risk of endometrial cancer (*e.g.* obesity, diabetes mellitus and hypertension) are also associated with a high operative risk. Severe or fatal peri-operative morbidity has been reported in as many as half of these patients.[118] Systemic progestogen compounds have reversed the neoplastic process, but are not always well tolerated.[120] Montz *et al.*[117] showed that intra-uterine progesterone appears to eradicate some cases of presumed stage 1a grade 1 endometrial cancer in women with a high risk of peri-operative morbidity.

Pelvic inflammatory disease

The most important factor regarding acquisition of pelvic inflammatory disease (PID) is a predisposition to sexually transmitted infection.[6] Many studies showed an increase in infection in the first month following insertion but this increased rate was linked to pre-existing infection. Diagnosis and treatment prior to insertion eliminated this increase rise of infection.[121] The LNG IUS, unlike the copper IUD, seems to prevent PID. A large randomised study in 5 European countries[122] concluded that women using the LNG IUS had a significantly lower rate of PID than IUCD users. There is also a protective effect in the long term, preventing sexually transmitted infection developing into PID,[123] although it confers no protection against sexually transmitted infection.[6]

Premenstrual syndrome

Effective treatment of premenstrual symptoms includes the suppression of ovulation by continuous exogenous oestrogen thereby reducing symptoms of natural cyclical oestrogen. Such treatment also demands protection of the endometrium by progestogens. When taken systemically, these progestogens are a major cause of troublesome side effects in over 40% of patients.[124] Intra-uterine levonorgestrel with its minimal systemic effects should prove to be useful in minimising side effects in these patients. In one study, 56% of users who had premenstrual symptoms claimed to have been cured of their symptoms by the LNG IUS.[62] The improvement in the menorrhagia and dysmenorrhoea may, in itself, relieve the fear associated with the premenstrual expectancy of these symptoms.

Prevention of ectopic pregnancy

The failure rates in prevention of pregnancy are low in every age group of women using LNG IUS.[125] This, in turn, makes the ectopic pregnancy rate very low. Luukkainen[6] reported from a collection of trials representing 12,000 women-years of LNG IUS use without a single ectopic pregnancy. The multicentre study in Europe[121] reported one case in 5000 women-years giving a rate of 0.02 per 100 women. This compares well to IUCD use (0.25 per 100 women years) and women not using contraception (1.2–1.6 per 100 women-years).

The risk of ectopic pregnancy in women using Progestasert was less re-assuring. Ectopic pregnancy rates were as high as 0.5 per 100 women-years. The risk of ectopic pregnancy during its use may even be increased.[126] This increased risk together with the short contraceptive life-time of the device (1 year) have limited the use of Progestasert.[6] It would still have a use as progestogenic opposition for oestrogen therapy in post-menopausal women, and for premenopausal women using oestrogen patches for the treatment of premenstrual syndrome.

DISADVANTAGES

Ovarian cyst formation

Functional ovarian cysts have been shown to be commoner in LNG IUS users compared to IUCD users 1.2 versus 0.4 per 100 women-years[100] and in other studies when compared to controls.[127,128] A more recent study has described the natural evolution of these cysts.[129] These cysts were symptomless, relatively small and showed a high rate (94%) of spontaneous resolution. Occurrence was not related to age or FSH levels.

Fitting the system

The intra-uterine system should only be fitted by doctors trained in the fitting and the insertion technique. As a consequence of the steroid reservoir, the intra-uterine system has a slightly wider diameter vertical stem compared to the copper intra-uterine contraceptive device. This has necessitated a wider insertion tube in the case of the Mirena. The insertion diameter is greater with Progestasert due to the arms initially folded down against the stem. These wider diameters may lead to difficulty in fitting of the systems and may require some gentle cervical dilatation prior to insertion.

The smaller, lower-dose menopausal levonorgestrel intra-uterine system (MLS) and the frameless Fibroplant try to address this issue. The initial trial result showed that the insertion of the smaller menopausal levonorgestrel intra-uterine system was often easier than Mirena. The diameter of menopausal levonorgestrel intra-uterine system is 2.3 mm whereas the diameter of Mirena is 3.2 mm. A smaller intra-uterine system did not result in an increased expulsion rate.[90] In another study by Wollter-Svensson et al.,[89] a much smaller intra-uterine system (delivering 5 mcg/day or 10 mcg/day of levonorgestrel) with horizontal arms of only 14 mm length, combined with oral oestradiol valerate, was expelled in 5 of 108 perimenopausal women during 1 year of study. It seems that the length of 28 mm of the horizontal arms in the smaller menopausal intra-uterine system maybe the ideal size to eliminate the risk of expulsion.

Fibroplant has a diameter of 1.2 mm and seems to be fitted without discomfort and resulting abdominal pains. However, until the smaller intra-uterine system becomes available, the prospect of cervical dilatation has to be considered for insertion of Mirena. Adequate analgesia required prior to dilatation can usually be achieved either by the administration of a non-steroidal anti-inflammatory drug, given 1 h before insertion or by the use of paracervical block using a fine dental syringe or a 1% lignocaine or xylocaine cervical spray.

Adequate attention and care to achieve asepsis must be observed when inserting the intra-uterine system as complications such as perforation, embedment, expulsion and infection can occur.

Unscheduled vaginal bleeding

A universal problem with all the intra-uterine systems is the occurrence of irregular vaginal bleeding and spotting in the first few months after insertion. This usually settles within 3–6 months,[130] as it takes 3 months for full endometrial transformation to occur. In premenopausal women, after this time, the breakthrough bleeding has not been shown to be related to either ovarian function or plasma levonorgestrel levels.[16,17]

Women in the perimenopause experience more episodes of spotting and bleeding than postmenopause.[131,132] The majority of these episodes settle after

6–12 months.[86,133] The occurrence of spotting is in combination with all types of continuous oestrogen therapy oral or transdermal. Raudaskoski et al.[90] noted that the bleeding was described as mainly spotting and did not reduce haemoglobin values.

Amenorrhoea is seen in as many as 35% of premenopausal women at the end of the first year of use. This can be worrying for women unless they are adequately counselled prior to insertion that amenorrhoea is common, not due to ovarian failure, confers health benefits and improved quality of life, and normal menstruation will return once the device is removed.

There have been several case reports where a patient presented with a recurrence of heavy vaginal bleeding after a period of oligomenorrhoea. These were investigated and endometrial pathology detected. In one case, a polyp was found and in the other two, adenocarcinoma of the endometrium was discovered.[134,135] These cases serve as a reminder that prior to insertion, intra-uterine pathology should be excluded by taking a careful history and investigating any abnormal bleeding. Abnormal symptoms, which persist after insertion, should also be investigated.

Progestogenic side effects

Despite very low serum levonorgestrel levels in the use of LNG IUS, some women do complain of hormonal side effects. These include oedema, weight gain, headache, breast tenderness, acne and hirsutism[136] and metabolic side effects such as a decrease in LDL level.[137] One case of hypersensitivity has been reported.[138] The multicentre contraceptive study in Europe[121] noticed no difference in the weight gain between LNG IUS users and copper IUD users at any time over the 5-year period. However, more women attributed their weight gain over this time to the LNG IUS. Over a 5-year period, the discontinuation rate was higher in the LNG IUS group than the copper IUD group attributed to a higher degree of vaginal spotting. However, when the LNG IUS is used for therapeutic reasons in women with menorrhagia, these discontinuation rates fall.

CONCLUSIONS

The levonorgestrel releasing intra-uterine systems provide a wide spectrum of benefit beyond their contraceptive capabilities. Side effects, or nuisance symptoms, can be reduced by careful pre-insertion counselling; and insertion difficulties minimised by practitioners who are trained fitters.

The systems have proved to be a useful tool in the treatment of menorrhagia and seem set to achieve a place in the hormone replacement armoury. The beneficial effects are mainly related to the effect of local levonorgestrel in the endometrium and these effects could lead to the development of the system in the treatment of endometrial disease.

KEY POINTS FOR CLINICAL PRACTICE

- Intra-uterine systems deliver high doses of hormone to the endometrium with minimal serum concentrations.

- Endometrial effects are uniform throughout the endometrium and achieved by 3 months' post-insertion. These include thinning of the endometrium, decidualisation of the endometrial stroma and atrophy of the endometrial glands.

- Reduction of menstrual blood loss compares favourably to both medical and surgical management.

- The LNG-IUS may be useful in providing progestogenic endometrial protection in women using oestrogen replacement therapy.

- The LNG-IUS is an effective treatment of endometrial hyperplasia and may have a place in the treatment of early endometrial cancer in some women.

- There is some evidence of the LNG IUS having a beneficial effect in endometriosis. There are conflicting reports of its usefulness in the treatment of fibroids, but it is useful in the management of fibroid-related menorrhagia.

- A reduction in pelvic inflammatory disease as compared to IUCD users has been shown. A lower rate of ectopic pregnancy is also demonstrated with the Mirena IUS versus IUCD.

- Ovarian cyst formation may occur but this is short lived and rarely causes problems.

- Unscheduled vaginal bleeding in the first few months is the most commonly reported side effect, which causes fewer complaints if the patient is properly counselled.

References

1 Lahteenmaki P, Rauramo I, Backman T. The levonorgestrel intra-uterine system in contraception. Steroids 2000; 65: 693–697

2 Nilsson CG, Johansson ED, Jackanizz TM, Lukkainen T. Biodegradable polyactate as a steroid releasing polymer: intra-uterine administration of d–norgestrel. Am J Obstet Gynecol 1975; 122: 90–95

3 El-Margoub S. d-Norgestrel slow releasing T device as an intra-uterine contraceptive. Am J Obstet Gynecol 1975; 123: 133–138

4 Segal SI, Croxatto HB. Single administration hormones for long term control of reproductive function. Presented at XXII Meeting of the American Fertility Society, Washington DC, 1967

5 Soderstrom RM. Progestasert intra-uterine progesterone contraceptive system. In: Bardin CW, Mishell Jr DR (eds) Proceedings from the Fourth International Conference on IUDs. Newton, MA: Butterworth Heinemann 1994; 314–327

6 Luukainen T, Pakarinen P, Toivonen J. Progestin-releasing intra-uterine systems. Semin Reprod Med 2001; 19: 355–363

7 Wildemeersch D, Schacht E. Endometrial suppression with a new 'frameless' levonorgestrel releasing intra-uterine system in perimenopausal and postmenopausal women. Maturitas 2000; 36: 63–68

8 Luukainen T. Levonorgestrel-releasing intra-uterine device. Ann NY Acad Sci 1991; 626: 43–49

9 Sturridge F, Guillebaud J. A risk benefit assessment of the levonorgestrel-releasing intra-uterine system. Drug Safety 1996; 15: 430–440

10 Victor A, Weiner E, Johansson EDB. Sex hormone binding globulin the carrier protein for d-norgestrel. J Clin Endocrinol Metab 1976; 43: 244–247

11 Weiner E, Victor A, Johansson EDB. Plasma levels of d-norgestrel after oral administration. Contraception 1976; 14: 563–570

12 Nilsson CG, Lahteenmaki PLA, Luukkainen T et al. Sustained intra-uterine release of levonorgestrel over five years. Fertil Steril 1986; 45: 805–807

13. Reid B, Gangar K. The medical management of menorrhagia in general practice. Diplomate 1994; 1: 92–98

14 McPherson A, Anderson ABM. (eds) Women's Problems in General Practice. Oxford: Oxford University Press, 1983; 21–41

15 Scholten PC. The Levonorgestrel IUD. Clinical performance and impact on menstruation. Thesis, University of Utrecht, 1989; 94

16 Nilsson C. Pertti L, Lahteenmaki A. Ovarian function in amenorrhoeic and menstruating users of a levonorgestrel device. Fertil Steril 1984; 41: 52–55

17 Xaio B, Zeng T, Shangchun W et al. Pharmacokinetic and pharmacodynamic studies of levonorgestrel-releasing intra-uterine devices. Contraception 1990; 41: 353–361

18 Barbosa I, Bakos O, Olsson SE. Ovarian function during use of a levonorgestrel-releasing IUD. Contraception 1990; 42: 51–56

19 Nilsson CG, Haukkamaa M, Vierola H, Luukainen T. Tissue concentrations of levonorgestrel in women using a levonorgestrel releasing IUD. Clin Endocrinol 1982; 17: 529–536

20 Perino A, Quartararo P, Castinella E, Genova G, Cittadini E. Treatment of endometrial hyperplasia with levonorgestrel releasing intra-uterine devices. Acta Eur Fertil 1987; 18: 137–140

21 Phillips V, Graham CT, Manek S, McCluggage WG. The effect of levonorgestrel intra-uterine system on endometrial morphology. J Clin Pathol 2003; 56: 305–307

22 Rutanen EM, Salmi A et al. mRNA expression of insulin like growth factors (IGF-1) is suppressed and those of IGF-11 and IGF-binding protein-1 are constantly expressed in endometrium during the use of an intra-uterine levonorgestrel system. Mol Hum Reprod 1997; 3: 749–754

23 Luukkainen T, Allonen H, Haukkamaa M et al. Five years' experience with levonorgestrel releasing IUDs. Contraception 1986; 33: 139–148

24 Parkarinen P, Luukainen T, Laine H et al. The effect of local intra-uterine levonorgestrel administration in endometrial thickness and uterine blood circulation. Hum Reprod 1995; 10: 2390–2394

25 McGavigan CJ, Dockery P, Metax-Mariaton V et al. Hormonally mediated disturbance of angiogenesis in the human endometrium after exposure to intra-uterine levonorgestrel. Hum Reprod 2003; 18: 77–84

26 Zalel Y, Shulman A, Lidor A, Achinon R, Mashiach S, Gamzu R. The local progestational effect of the levonorgestrel-releasing intra-uterine system: a sonographic and Doppler flow study. Hum Reprod 2002; 17: 2878–2880

27 Erickson RE, Mitchell C, Pharriss BB, Place VA. The intra-uterine progesterone contraceptive system. In: Advances in Planned Parenthood. Princeton; Exerpta Medica, 1976; 167–174

28 Rutanen E-M. Insulin-like growth factors and insulin-like growth factor binding proteins in the endometrium: effect of intra-uterine levonorgestrel delivery. Hum Reprod 2000; 15 (Suppl 3): 173–181

29 Hurskainen R et al. Expression of sex steroid receptors and Ki-67 in the endometria of menorrhagic women: effects of intra-uterine levonorgestrel. Mol Hum Reprod 2000; 6: 1013–1018

30 Rutanen E, Hurskainen R, Finne P et al. Induction of endometrial plasminogen activator-inhibitor. A possible mechanism contributing to the effect of intra-uterine levonorgestrel in the treatment of menorrhagia. Fertil Steril 2000; 73: 1020–1024

31 Maruo T et al. Effects of the levonorgestrel-releasing intra-uterine system on proliferation and apoptosis in the endometrium. Hum Reprod 2001; 16: 2103–2108

32 Hague S, Oehler MK, Mackenzie IZ, Bicknell R, Rees MC. Protease activated receptor-1 is down-regulated by levonorgestrel in endometrial stromal cells. Angiogenesis 2002; 5: 93–98

33 Silverberg SG, Haukkamaa M, Arko H *et al.* Endometrial morphology during long-term use of levonorgestrel-releasing intra-uterine devices. Int J Gynaecol Pathol 1986; 5: 235–241

34 Luukkainen T. Levonorgestrel-releasing intra-uterine device. Ann NY Acad Sci 1991; 626: 43–49

35 Bradlow J, Coulter A, Brooks P. Patterns of Referral. Oxford: Oxford Health Service Research Unit, 1992; 20–21

36 Vessey MP *et al.* The epidemiology of hysterectomy: findings in a large cohort study. Br J Obstet Gynaecol 1992; 99: 402–407

37 Coulter A *et al.* Outcomes of referrals to gynaecology outpatient clinics for menstrual problems: an audit of general practice records. Br J Obstet Gynaecol 1991; 98: 789–796

38 Anon. Hospital Episode Statistics vol 1. Finished consultant episodes by diagnosis operation and speciality. London: HMSO, 1995

39 Natural Health Service Executive. National Schedule of Reference Costs. May 1999: Appendix 1A. London: Department of Health, 1999

40 Dwyer N, Hutton J, Stirrat GM. Randomised controlled trial comparing endometrial resection with abdominal hysterectomy for the surgical treatment of menorrhagia. Br J Obstet Gynaecol 1993; 100: 237–243

41 Anon. Guidelines for Management of Heavy Menstrual Bleeding. Auckland, New Zealand: National Advisory Committee on Health and Disability, 1998

42 Lilford RJ. Hysterectomy: will it pay the bills in 2007? BMJ 1997; 314: 160–161

43 Coulter A, Peto V, Jenkinson C. Quality of life and patient satisfaction following treatment for menorrhagia. Fam Pract 1994; 11: 394–401

44 Coulter A, Kelland J, Long A *et al.* The management of menorrhagia. Effective Health Care Bulletin 1995; No. 9

45 Dicker RC *et al.* Complications of abdominal and vaginal hysterectomy among women of reproductive age in the United States. The collaborative review of sterilization. Am J Obstet Gynecol 1982; 144: 841–848

46 Duckitt K, Shaw RW. Is medical management of menorrhagia obsolete? Br J Obstet Gynaecol 1998; 105: 569–572

47 Coulter A *et al.* Treating menorrhagia in primary care. An overview of drug trials and a survey of prescribing practice. Int J Technol Assess Health Care 1995; 11: 456–471

48 Bonnar J, Sheppard BL. Treatment of menorrhagia during menstruation: randomised controlled trial of ethamsylate, mefenamic acid, and tranexamic acid. BMJ 1996; 313: 579–582

49 Fraser IS, McCarron G. Randomized trial of 2 hormonal and 2 prostaglandin-inhibiting agents in women with a complaint of menorrhagia. Aust NZ J Obstet Gynaecol 1991; 31: 66–70

50 Chimbira TH *et al.* The effect of danazol on menorrhagia, coagulation mechanisms, haematological indices and body weight. Br J Obstet Gynaecol 1979; 86: 46–50

51 Thomas EJ, Okuda KJ, Thomas NM. The combination of a depot gonadotrophin releasing hormone agonist and cyclical hormone replacement therapy for dysfunctional uterine bleeding. Br J Obstet Gynaecol 1991; 98: 1155–1159

52 Andersson JK, Rybo G. Levonorgestrel-releasing intra-uterine device in the treatment of menorrhagia. Br J Obstet Gynaecol 1990; 97: 690–694

53 Tang GW, Lo SS. Levonorgestrel intra-uterine device in the treatment of menorrhagia in Chinese women: efficacy versus acceptability. Contraception 1995; 51: 231–235

54 Bergqvist A, Rybo G. Treatment of menorrhagia with intra-uterine release of progesterone. Br J Obstet Gynaecol 1983; 90: 255–258

55 Wildemeersch D, Schacht E. Treatment of menorrhagia with a novel 'frameless' intra-uterine levonorgestrel-releasing drug delivery system: a pilot study. Eur J Contracept Reprod Health Care 2001; 6: 93–101

56 Stewart A *et al.* The effectiveness of the levonorgestrel-releasing intra-uterine system in menorrhagia: a systematic review. Br J Obstet Gynaecol 2001; 108: 74–86

57 Irvine GA *et al.* Randomised comparative trial of the levonorgestrel intra-uterine system and norethisterone for treatment of idiopathic menorrhagia. Br J Obstet Gynaecol 1998; 105: 592–598

58 Milsom I *et al.* A comparison of flurbiprofen, tranexamic acid, and a levonorgestrel-

releasing intra-uterine contraceptive device in the treatment of idiopathic menorrhagia. Am J Obstet Gynecol 1991; 164: 879–883

59 Lahteenmaki P et al. Open randomised study of use of levonorgestrel releasing intra-uterine system as alternative to hysterectomy. BMJ 1998; 316: 1122–1126

60 Crosignani PG et al. Levonorgestrel-releasing intra-uterine device versus hysteroscopic endometrial resection in the treatment of dysfunctional uterine bleeding. Obstet Gynecol 1997; 90: 257–263

61 Kittelsen N, Istre O. A randomized study comparing levonorgestrel intra-uterine system and the transcervical resection of the endometrium in the treatment of menorrhagia: preliminary results. Gynecol Endosc 1998; 7: 61–65

62 Barrington JW, Bowen-Simpkins P. The levonorgestrel intra-uterine system in the management of menorrhagia. Br J Obstet Gynaecol 1997; 104: 614–616

63 Fedele L et al. Treatment of adenomyosis-associated menorrhagia with a levonorgestrel-releasing intra-uterine device. Fertil Steril 1997; 68: 426–429

64 Scholten PC, Christiaens GCML, Haspels AA. Treatment of menorrhagia by intra-uterine administration of levonorgestrel. In: Scholten PC. (ed) The Levonorgestrel IUD: clinical performance and impact on menstruation (thesis). Utrecht; The Netherlands: Utrecht University Hospital, 1989; 47–55

65 Lethaby AE, Cooke I, Rees M. Progesterone/progestogen releasing intra-uterine systems versus either placebo or any other medication for heavy menstrual bleeding. *Cochrane Database System Rev* 2000(2)

66 Nagrani R, Bowen-Simpkins P, Barrington JW. Can the levonorgestrel intra-uterine system replace surgical treatment for the management of menorrhagia? Br J Obstet Gynaecol 2002; 109: 345–347

67 Zhu P, Hongzhi L, Wenliang S et al. Observation of the activity of factor VIII in the endometrium of women pre- and post-insertion of three types of IUDs. Contraception 1991; 44: 367–387

68 Higham JM, O'Brien PM, Shaw RW. Assessment of menstrual blood loss using a pictorial chart. Br J Obstet Gynaecol 1990; 97: 734–739

69 Istre O. Trolle B. Treatment of menorrhagia with the levonorgestrel intra-uterine system versus endometrial resection. Fertil Steril 2001; 76: 304–309

70 Rogerson L et al. Management of menorrhagia – SMART study (Satisfaction with Mirena and Ablation: a Randomised Trial). Br J Obstet Gynaecol 2000; 107: 1325–1326

71 Johnson N et al. The management of menorrhagia – SMART study (Satisfaction with Mirena and Ablation: a Randomised Trial). Br J Obstet Gynaecol 2001; 108: 773–774

72 Hurskainen R et al. Quality of life and cost-effectiveness of levonorgestrel-releasing intra-uterine system versus hysterectomy for treatment of menorrhagia: a randomised trial. Lancet 2001; 357: 273–277

73 Million Women Study Collaborators. Patterns of use in hormone replacement therapy in 1 million women in Britain 1996–2000. Br J Obstet Gynaecol 2002; 109: 1319

74 Ryan P, Harrison R, Blake G, Fogelman I. Compliance with hormone replacement therapy after screening for postmenopausal osteoporosis. Br J Obstet Gynaecol 1992; 99: 325–328

75 Schneider H, Gallagher J. Moderation of the daily dose of HRT: benefits for patients. Maturitas 1999; 33 S25–S29

76 Grady D, Gebretsadik I, Kerlikowske K, Ernster V, Petitte D. Hormone replacement therapy and endometrial cancer risk: a meta analysis. Obstet Gynaecol 1995; 85: 304–312

77 Rogiero A and The Editorial Board of the North American Menopause Society. Role of progestogen in hormone therapy for post menopausal women: position statement of the North American Menopause Society. Menopause 2003; 10: 113–132

78 Feely M, Wells M. HRT and the endometrium. J Clin Pathol 2001; 54: 435–440

79 Smith RN, Holland EF, Studd JW. The symptomology of progestogen intolerance. Maturitas 1994; 18: 87–91

80 Hope S, Rees MCP. Why do British women start and stop hormone replacement therapy? J Br Menopause Soc 1995; 1: 26–27

81 Ng C, Cloke B, Panay N. Low dose hormone replacement therapy and phyto-oestrogens. In: Barter J, Hampton N. (eds) The Year in Gynaecology 2001. Clinical Publishing Services, 2001; 193–214

82 Staland B. Continuous treatment with natural oestrogens and progestogens: a method to avoid endometrial stimulation. Maturitas 1981; 3: 145–156

83 Weiderpass E, Adami HD, Baron JA. Risk of endometrial cancer following oestrogen replacement with and without progestins. J Natl Cancer Inst 1999; 91: 1131–1137

84 Ettinger B, Li DK, Klein R. Unexpected vaginal Bleeding and associated gynecologic care in post menopausal women using hormone replacement therapy: a comparison of cyclic versus continuous combined schedules. Fertil Steril 1998; 69: 865–859

85 Panay N, Studd J. Progestogen intolerance and compliance with hormone replacement therapy in menopausal women. Hum Reprod Update 1997; 3: 159–171

86 Andersson K, Mattsson LA, Rybo G, Stadberg E. Intrauterine release of levonorgestrel – a new way of adding progestogen in hormone replacement therapy. Obstet Gynecol 1992; 79: 963–967

87 Raudaskoski T, Tytti H, Lahti *et al*. Transdermal estrogen with a levonorgestrel-releasing intra-uterine device for climacteric complaints: clinical and endometrial responses. Am J Obstet Gynecol 1995; 172: 114–119

88 Suhonen S, Holmstrom T, Lahteenmaki P. Three year follow up of the use of a levonorgestrel-releasing intra-uterine system in hormone replacement therapy. Acta Obstet Gynecol Scand 1997; 76: 145–150

89 Wollter-Svensson LO, Stadberg E, Andersson K, Mattisson LA, Odling V, Persson I. Intrauterine administration of levonorgestrel 5 and 10 mcg/24 hours in perimenopausal hormone replacement therapy. Acta Obstet Gynecol Scand 1997; 76: 449–454

90 Raudaskoski T, Tapanainen E, Tomas E *et al*. Intrauterine 10 mcg and 20 mcg levonorgestrel systems in postmenopausal women receiving oral oestrogen replacement therapy: clinical, endometrial and metabolic response. Br J Obstet Gynaecol 2002; 109: 136–144

91 Matthews KA, Meilahn E, Kuller LH, Kelsey SF, Caggiula AW, Wing RR. Menopause and risk factors for coronary heart disease. N Engl J Med 1989; 321: 641–646

92 Barnes RB, Roy S, Lobo RA. Comparison of lipid and androgen levels after conjugated estrogen or depo medroxyprogesterone acetate treatment in postmenopausal women. Obstet Gynecol 1985; 66: 216–219

93 Jensen J, Nilas L, Christiansen C. Cyclic changes in serum cholesterol and lipoproteins following different doses of combined postmenopausal hormone replacement therapy. Br J Obstet Gynaecol 1986; 93: 613–618

94 Wollter-Svensson H *et al*. Intrauterine administration of levonorgestrel in two low doses in HRT. A randomised clinical trial during one year: effects on lipid and lipoprotein metabolism. Maturitas 1995; 22: 199–205

95 Vercellini P, De Giorgi O, Aimi G, Panazza S, Uglietti A, Crosignani PG. Menstrual characteristics with and without endometriosis. Obstet Gynecol 1997; 90: 264–268

96 Vercellini P, Aimi G, Panazza S, De Giorgi O, Pesole A, Crosignani PG. A levonorgestrel-releasing intra-uterine system for the treatment of dysmenorrhea associated with endometriosis. A pilot study. Fertil Steril 1999; 72: 505–508

97 Fedele L, Branchi S, Zanconato G, Portuese A, Raffaelli R. Use of a levonorgestrel-releasing IUD in the treatment of rectovaginal endometriosis. Fertil Steril 2001; 75: 485–488

98 Xiao B, Zeng T, Wu S, Sun H, Xiao N. Effect of levonorgestrel-releasing intra-uterine device on hormonal profile and menstrual pattern after long term use. Contraception 1995; 51: 359–365

99 Fong YF, Singh K. Medical treatment of a grossly enlarged adenomyotic uterus with the levonorgestrel-releasing IUS. Contraception 1999; 60: 173–175

100 Sivin I, Stern J. Health during prolonged use of levonorgestrel 20 mg/d and the Copper T Cu 380 Ag intra-uterine contraceptive devices: a multicentre study. Fertil Steril 1994; 61: 70–77

101 Gerdner FJ, Konje JC, Abrams KR *et al*. Endometrial protection from tamoxifen-stimulated changes by a levonorgestrel-releasing IUS; a randomised controlled trial. Lancet 2000; 356: 1711–1717

102 Singer A, Ikomi A. Successful treatment of fibroids using an intra-uterine progesterone device. Int J Gynecol Obstet 1994: 46: 55

103 Hagenfeldt K, Landgren BM, Edstrom K, Johanisson E. Biochemical and morphological

changes in the human endometrium induced by the Progestasert device. Contraception 1977; 16: 183–197

104 Wildemeersch D, Schacht E et al. The effect on menstrual blood loss in women with uterine fibroids of new 'frameless' intra-uterine levonorgestrel-releasing system; a pilot study. Eur J Obstet Gynecol Reprod Biol 2002; 102: 74–79

105 Pekonen F, Nyman T, Lahteenmaki P. Intrauterine progestin induces continuous insulin like growth factor binding protein 1 production in the human endometrium. J Clin Endocrine Metab 1992; 75: 660–664

106 Marao T, Matsuo H, Samoto T et al. Effects of progesterone on uterine leiomyoma growth and apoptosis. Steroids 2000; 65: 585–592

107 Ikome A, Pepia E. Effect of the levonorgestrel intra-uterine system in treating menorrhagia, actualities and ambiguities. J Fam Plan Reprod Health Care 2002; 28: 99–100

108 Wildemeersch D, Schacht E, Wildemeersch P, Janssens D, Thiery M. Development of a miniature low dose frameless intra-uterine levonorgestrel-releasing system for contraception and treatment; a review of initial clinical experience. Reprod Biomed Online 2002; 4: 71–82

109 Wildemeersch D, Schacht E, Wildemeersch P. Treatment of primary and secondary dysmenorrhea with a novel frameless intra-uterine levonorgestrel-releasing drug delivery system. A pilot study. Eur J Contracept Reprod Health Care 2001; 6: 192–198

110 Volpe A, Botticelli A, Abrate M et al. An intra-uterine progesterone contraceptive system (52 mg) used in pre- and peri-menopausal patient with endometrial hyperplasia. Maturitas 1982; 4: 73–79

111 Perino A, Quartararo P, Catinella E et al. Treatment of endometrial hyperplasia with levonorgestrel-releasing intra-uterine devices. Acta Eur Fertil 1987; 18: 137–140

112 Scarselli G, Tantini C, Colofrancesch M et al. Levonorgestrel nova T and precancerous lesions of the endometrium. Eur J Gynaecol Oncol 1988; 9: 284–286

113 Wildemeersch D, Dhont M. Treatment of nonatypical and atypical endometrial hyperplasia with levonorgestrel-releasing intra-uterine system. Am J Obstet Gynecol 2003; 188: 1297–1298

114 Love RR, Wieve DA, Newcomb PA et al. Effects of tamoxifen on cardiovascular risk factors in postmenopausal women. Ann Intern Med 1991; 115: 860–864

115 Kedar RP, Bourne TH, Powles TJ et al. Effects of tamoxifen on uterus and ovaries of postmenopausal women in a randomised breast cancer prevention trial. Lancet 1994; 343: 1318–1321

116 Gardner FJ, Konje JC et al. Endometrial protection from tamoxifen stimulated changes by a levonorgestrel releasing intra-uterine system: a randomised controlled trial. Lancet 2000; 356: 1711–1717

117 Montz F, Bristow R, Bovicelli A, Tomacruz R, Kuiman R. Intrauterine progesterone treatment of early endometrial cancer. Am J Obstet Gynecol 2002; 186: 651–657

118 Harris WJ. Complications of hysterectomy. Clin Obstet Gynecol 1997; 40: 928–938

119 Kim YB, Holschneider CH, Ghosh K, Nieberg RK, Montz FJ. Progestin alone as a primary treatment endometrial carcinoma in premenopausal women. Cancer 1997; 79: 320–327

120 Thigpen JY, Brady MF, Alvarez RD, Adelson MD, Homesley HD. Oral medroxyprogesterone acetate in the treatment of advanced or recurrent endometrial carcinoma, a dose response study of the Gynecologic Oncology Group. J Clin Oncol 1999; 17: 1736–1744

121 Andersson K, Odling V, Rybo G. Levonorgestrel-releasing and copper releasing (Nova T) IUDs during 5 years of use. A randomised comparative trial. Contraception 1994; 49: 56–72

122 Luukainen T, Allonen H, Haukkamaa M et al. Effective contraception with levonorgestrel-releasing intra-uterine device. 12 Month report of a European multicentre study. Contraception 1987; 36: 169–179

123 Toivonen J, Luukainen T, Allonen H. Protective effect of intra-uterine release of levonorgestrel in pelvic infection. 3 years comparative experience of levonorgestrel and copper releasing IUD. Obstet Gynecol 1991; 77: 261–264

124 Smith RNJ, Studd JW, Zamblera D. A randomised comparison over 8 months of 100 and

200 micrograms twice weekly doses of transdermal oestradiol in the treatment of severe premenstrual syndrome. Br J Obstet Gynaecol 1995; 102: 475–484

125 Toivonen J, Luukainen T. Progestin-releasing intra-uterine devices. In: Bardin CW. (ed) Current Therapy in Endocrinology and Metabolism. St Louis, MO: Mosby, 1997; 281–285

126 Rantakyla P, Ylostalo P, Jarvinen PA, Vierjke A. Ectopic pregnancies and the use of intrauterine device and low progestogen contraception. Acta Obstet Gynecol Scand 1977; 56: 61–62

127 Barbosa I, Bakos O, Olsson SE, Odlind V, Johansson ED. Ovarian function during use of a levonorgestrel releasing IUD. Contraception 1990; 42: 51–66

128 Borgfedt C, Andolf E. Transvaginal scan ovarian findings in a random sample of women 25–40 years old. Ultrasound Obstet Gynecol 1999; 13: 345–350

129 Inki P, Hurskainen R, Palo P et al. Comparison of ovarian cyst formation in women using the levonorgestrel-releasing IUS vs hysterectomy. Ultrasound Obstet Gynecol 2002; 20: 381–385

130 Nilsson CG, Lahteenmaki P, Luukkainen T. Levonorgestrel plasma concentrations and hormone profiles after insertion and after one year of treatment with a levonorgestrel-IUD. Contraception 1980; 21: 225–233

131 Panay N, Studd J. Non-contraceptive uses of the hormone releasing intra-uterine systems. Prog Obstet Gynaecol 1998; 13: 379–395

132 Wildemeersch D, Schacht E, Wildemeersch P. Performance and acceptability of intra-uterine release of levonorgestrel with a miniature delivery system for hormonal substitution therapy, contraception and treatment in peri and post menopausal women. Maturitas 2003; 44: 237–245

133 Suhonen S, Holmstrom T, Allonen M et al. Intrauterine and subdermal progestin administration in postmenopausal hormone replacement therapy. Fertil Steril 1995; 63: 336–342

134 Jones K, Georgiou M, Hyatt D, Spencer T, Thomas H. Endometrial carcinoma following insertion of Mirena IUCD. Gynecol Oncol 2002; 87: 216–218

135 Brechin S, Cameron ST, Paterson AM, Williams AR Critchley HO. Intrauterine polyps. A cause of unscheduled bleeding in women using the levonorgestrel intra-uterine system: a case report. Hum Reprod 2000; 15 :650–652

136 Wan LS, Ying-Chih H, Manik G, Bigelow B. Effects of the Progestasert® on the menstrual pattern, ovarian steroids and endometrium. Contraception 1977; 16: 417–434

137 Raudaskoski TH, Tomas EI, Paakkari IA, Kauppila AJ, Laatikainen TJ. Serum lipids and lipoproteins in postmenopausal women receiving transdermal oestrogen in combination with a levonorgestrel intra-uterine device. Maturitas 1995; 22: 47–53

138 Piereira A, Coker A. Hypersensitivity to Mirena – a rare complication. J Obstet Gynaecol 2003; 23: 81–92

John W.W. Studd

Benefits and side effects of HRT after the Women's Health Initiative (WHI) and Million Women's Study (MWS) reports

Until recently, hormone replacement therapy (HRT) was quite straightforward. Oestrogen prevented the symptoms of the climacteric, particularly flushes, sweats, vaginal dryness, depression, loss of energy and loss of libido. Cyclical or continuous progestogen although possibly producing PMS-type side-effects in women who were progestogen-intolerant, protected the endometrium. There were also long-term benefits of protection from osteoporosis, reduction in colon cancer and both primary and secondary prevention of heart attacks. It was always possible that this 50% reduction of coronary artery disease was due to selection of patients with the healthier, non-smoking normotensive patients receiving HRT but most laboratory studies in women and primates supported the hypothesis of this protective role.

There was a possible slight increase in breast cancer but as virtually all studies showed an increased survival in these women, it was easy to believe that this apparent increase was an artefact due to increased surveillance in women receiving HRT or a problem of precise pathological diagnosis in the grey area between ductal *in situ* or invasive cancer.

RECENT ADVERSE PUBLICITY

The HERS study[1] first challenged the optimism that oestrogens exerted a protective effect in women with established coronary artery disease and more recently the paper from the Women's Health Initiative (WHI)[2] study and the Million Women Study (MWS)[3] have caused enormous alarm by reporting that heart attacks, strokes, venous thrombo-embolism and breast cancer are more common in women who are receiving treatment. In December 2003, the UK CSM following the lead of EMAS advised that HRT should no longer be the

John W. W. Studd DSc MD FRCOG
Professor of Gynaecology and Consultant Gynaecologist, Academic Department of Obstetrics and Gynaecology, Chelsea and Westminster Hospital, 369 Fulham Road, London SW10 9NH, UK (E-mail: harley@studd.co.uk)

first choice for the prevention and treatment of osteoporosis. We strongly disagree with this opinion as did one of the two gynaecologists on the committee who resigned in protest. The MWS was attended by a hostile and superficial editorial[4] which read like a political polemic rather than a scientific comment.

Although the latter two studies are now recognised to be greatly flawed at many levels, they were both the subject of press conferences before publication with the front pages of the newspapers reporting the bad news before the studies were in any way discussed by the scientific community.[5] The fault lay not with the press who reported the facts as presented to them but with the authors making the best of their data. It is certain that bad-news epidemiology obtains more press coverage and more research funds for departments. Similarly, medical charities wish to be seen making a contribution to women's health. All this encourages the denial of critical discussion by experts before publication. Although the design and conclusions of these two studies have been roundly criticised by epidemiologists and clinicians, the damage has been done. The errors in the studies were so manifest that they would have been improved with prior discussion but we are left with the fact that the putative side-effects of HRT are now fixed in the public memory regardless of any final scientific revision of the conclusions from these papers.

If that were not enough, a subsequent paper from the WHI study indicated that the quality of life was not improved with treatment after all.[6] Not surprisingly, there has been a 50% reduction of HRT taking in the US and a significant, but rather less, reduction in Europe.

To add further to the confusion, we now know (from 2 March 2004) that the oestrogen-only arm of the WHI study has been stopped because the increase in stroke has been confirmed after 7 years with an extra 8 more strokes per year for every 10,000 women than on placebo. But there is no increase in breast cancer or heart attacks. The definitive paper has yet to be published but no wonder both patients and doctors are confused.

THE HERS STUDY

The anxiety about HRT started with the HERS study which evaluated the effect of oestrogens on women with established coronary artery disease. There had been many clinical papers and studies of lipids and coronary blood flow and physiology which indicated that oestrogens had a profound protective effect on the normal coronary arteries and there was also persuasive clinical evidence that this treatment could be used in women who had had coronary artery disease with advantage. Although a primary prevention study (the future WHI study) was being considered, it was considered that a secondary protection study would give the answer with fewer patients over a shorter period of time.

This HERS study consisted of a randomised, placebo-controlled trial of 2763 women with a mean age of 66.7 years with established coronary artery disease. They were given either 0.625 mg of conjugated equine oestrogen with 2.5 mg of MPA or placebo. The follow-up was for 6.8 years. Although this therapy produced the expected beneficial biochemical effects on lipids, such as lowering the LDL by 11% and increasing HDL by 10%, there was an increased rate of venous thrombo-embolic events and no change in the overall rate of CHT events either non-fatal MI or CHD death in either group. There was, in fact, a small increase in heart attacks in the first year but this had ceased and there was even a non-significant decrease by the end of the fourth year. The concept of oestrogens producing 'early harm' even if they might ultimately produce benefit was born.

The study was discontinued prematurely and hence an important opportunity was missed. The conclusion from this study was that HRT in this form was not recommended for the secondary prevention of CHD. There now seems to be much agreement on this point.

THE WOMEN'S HEALTH INITIATIVE (WHI) STUDY

The WHI study, which so adversely affected patients' confidence, was a large trial using the wrong hormone combination on the wrong patients which bears no relationship to the treatment that is given to patients of the appropriate age with the appropriate symptoms.

A total of 16,809 women aged 50–79 years were recruited from 40 centres in the US and randomised to active HRT and placebo. The mean age was 63 years with 21% of the patients being between 70–79 years. In the study group, 7.7% had prior cardiovascular disease and 1.1% (HRT) and 1.5% (placebo) had had a previous coronary artery bypass operation; 36% were hypertensive and 7% were taking statins at commencement of the study. They were asymptomatic but a further report from this group informs us that 10% had vasomotor symptoms. They were overweight.

They were treated with continuous-combined oestrogen and progestogen therapy (CCEP) in the form of conjugated equine oestrogens 0.625 mg daily and MPA 2.5 mg daily or premarin 0.625 mg in hysterectomised women.

In spite of this, 42% of the treatment group dropped out compared with 38% of the placebo group. Thus, this is one of the rare studies when the drop-out is more common in the active preparation than the placebo. The CCEP arm was discontinued after 5.2 years because of an excess of complications but the oestrogen-only study continues. We do not know the change in the incidence of statin therapy when the study was discontinued but it is very likely that these high-risk American patients chose to take statins when they soon realised in this barely-blinded study that they were having placebo.

The results of CCEP therapy in this population make depressing reading. There was an increase in coronary artery disease with a Risk Ratio of 1.29 (95% CI, 1.02–1.63). Stroke was increased RR 1.41 (95% CI, 0.7–1.85). There was double the incidence of VTE with a RR of 2.11 (95% CI, 1.58–2.82) and an increase in breast cancer RR 1.26 (95% CI, 1.0–1.94).

In spite of this negative information, it was the first randomised study that showed a decrease in the hip fracture of 34% (95% CI, 0.45–0.98) and a similar decrease in vertebral fracture (95% CI, 0.44–0.98). There was also a demonstrable decrease in colon cancer of 37% (95% CI, 0.43–0.92). No doubt this improvement was seen in the study because the age group was appropriate for prevention of osteoporotic fractures and occurrence of colon cancer regardless of the type of oestrogen and progestogen preparation used.

The increase in coronary heart disease and VTE began from year one and the increase in stroke appeared from year two supporting the view of early harm. The increase in breast cancer was only apparent after 4 years.

There is a great difference between the re-assuring observational studies compared with the interventional (RCT) studies in HRT users. There are now more than 30 observational case-controlled studies showing protection. The most important of these is the Nurses' Health Study of 70,533 post-menopausal women followed up from 1976 to 1996 with 1258 major coronary events.[8] The Risk Ratio in current users of HRT was reduced to 0.61 (95% CI, 0.52–0.71).

Regardless of the other recent large studies showing an unchanged or a decrease in breast cancer[9] or cardiac deaths,[10] the large, greatly flawed WHI study has been used unwisely to erase the entire clinical laboratory and animal studies supporting its use in the primary prevention of CHD. These publications of inappropriate optimistic therapy seemed to impress NAMS and other American medical bodies.

NAMS RESPONSE

The NAMS Advisory Panel report (3 October 2002) on the HERS and WHI studies made the following recommendations:
1. Treatment of menopausal and vasomotor symptoms and pelvic atrophy remain the major indications for HRT.
2. Progestogens are to be used in women with a uterus to no HRT for primary or secondary prevention of coronary vascular disease.
3. Physicians should try alternatives to HRT for osteoporosis.
4. Use shortest duration.
5. Lower than standard dosage should be considered.
6. Try alternative medications.

Two weeks later (23/24 October 2002) at a meeting with NAMS/ACOG and AHA confirmed that:
1. HRT was not to be used for prevention of coronary vascular disease.
2.) It had no place for the prevention of chronic conditions.
3. It is indicated for treatment of vasomotor symptoms 'if severe enough'.
4. Lowest possible dose should be used for as short a time as possible.
5. Oestrogen/progestogen HRT is not the first choice for prevention or treatment of osteoporosis but can be used if other treatments are not tolerated and if there are vasomotor symptoms.
6. The CE/MPA formulation in WHI cannot be extrapolated to other E/P HTs but the safety of other formations cannot be assumed until proven.

These recommendations continue to produce outrage from experienced workers in the menopause. The advice concerning cardiovascular disease, particularly primary prevention, and osteoporosis was too negative.

OBJECTIONS TO WHI STUDY

It is important to consider some of the details of this study. In years 2, 3, 4, and 6 there was no significant increase in coronary heart disease. There was, as in the HERS study of secondary protection, a slight increase in the first year. The number of CHD events remained stationary over the next 6 years although the trend was decreasing. The statistically significant Risk Ratio in year 5 is because of unexplained large fall in the placebo cases. It was this as much as breast cancer data which triggered the alarm bells to stop the study. There was in fact no increase in incidence of coronary heart disease in the treatment group in spite of the high cardiovascular risk of the study group.

As these older 60- and 70-year-old hypertensive women are not the patients who would normally commence treatment with HRT, we must ask what the information specifically about the younger patients is. Naftolin has deduced the following. This study had 287 patients aged 50–54 years. As the age-corrected number of expected events found in the Nurses' Health Study is 0.7 events per 475 women per 5 years, it would require greater than 4000 women in each arm to show a statistically significant difference between the groups or so with a 42% drop-out rate the number of subjects needed per group becomes 9000. Thus the WHI randomised control trial is 10-fold underpowered to test the cardioprotective effect of HRT in women entering the menopause. Although the authors claim to show the same increase in risk at each decile of age, there clearly is inadequate or virtually no information about the 45–55-year-old typically menopausal patients that we treat. However looking at the data related to 'years from menopause' does show a benefit in the women with a recent menopause.

The misguided advice based on the WHI study is so persuasive that a recent guidelines on HRT from The Royal College of Physicians of Edinburgh begin by stating that 'the administration of oestrogens may produce heart attacks'. It is worth pointing out again that the cardioprotective benefits of starting hormone treatment at the time of the menopause cannot be ruled out by the WHI study. Similarly, the cardiovascular consequences of stopping long-term hormone therapy that began at the time of the menopause cannot be evaluated by these data.

This study is the wrong population, the wrong drug, and clearly came to the wrong conclusions as it is treatment that is rarely used (in Europe) in women who we do not treat. It will take time to erase the unjustified conclusions from the WHI study but many smaller studies including the WISP study of Stevenson using the correct hormone – oestradiol – in well-supervised patients of the correct age for the appropriate pathology or symptoms are likely to produce a message, one way or another, which we can believe.

The interpretation of this study is the same as concluding that appendicectomy is not the appropriate treatment for women with gallbladder disease. We know this but it tells us nothing about the value of appendicectomy nor how to treat gallbladder disease. The WHI study is similarly ill conceived.

BREAST CANCER

The data on the extra risk of breast cancer are mixed and confused with almost as many publications reporting a decrease as showing an increase. However the conclusion from Beral's meta-analysis[11] which reports a duration-dependent increase in incidence seems now to be increasingly accepted .It is reported that after 5, 10 and 15 years of HRT use, there are 2, 6 and 12 extra cases/1000 HRT users, respectively.

The majority of papers looking at mortality from breast cancer in women taking HRT have found this to be greatly reduced by as much as 30%. An exception is Chlebowski et al.[12] from the WHI group reporting a higher mortality in these tumours which were more commonly metastatic at the time of diagnosis. These authors are alone with this finding.

THE MILLION WOMEN STUDY

The Million Women Study (MWS) is a very influential publication of a large group of patients. A total of 1,084,110 UK women aged 50–64 years attending for mammography were studied by questionnaire. There were 9364 cases of invasive breast cancers at 2.6 years of follow-up but only 7140 were analysed. These exclusions are important as they have biased the conclusions by turning the control group into low risk while the active group remains the same.

There were 637 breast cancer deaths at 4.1 years of follow-up of current users. This gave an overall RR of 1.66 with a 1.22 Risk Ratio of death from breast cancer. The results were shown to be worse in the oestrogen plus progestogen group RR 2.0 (95% CI, 1.88–2.12). Oestradiol only was 1.30 RR with 95% CI, 1.21–1.40. Being a large study, it was able to study different oestrogens and different routes of administration. There was no significant difference whether oestrogens were taken by the oral route, by patch or by implant. Tibolone also showed an increase of breast cancer RR 1.44 (95% CI, 1.25–1.68).

The breast cancers were diagnosed on average 1.2 years after recruitment with the mean time of death from diagnosis of only 1.7 years. These are extraordinary results as it takes 5–8 or more years for a few malignant cells to become a 1 cm tumour. Many of these must have been interval tumours missed at mammography not related to oestrogen therapy. Although such tumours have a poor prognosis, the short survival of 1.7 years from diagnosis in this study is hardly believable being less than the 3-year survival of women from diagnosis who have metastatic breast cancer. Can these MWS data really be correct?

The study should have excluded all cancers mostly interval cancers, found in the first and perhaps even the second year of oestrogen taking as our knowledge of the biology of breast cancer makes the therapeutic association unlikely. Any real excess of cancer would have shown up after 5 or more years if there was a causal link. But the cancers which were excluded made a difference in the direction of risk. Of the fatal cases, 48% (485 out 1002) were excluded creating an imbalance which can not be calculated from the information given. The authors also excluded 60,606 50–52-year-old HRT takers with a low mortality (18 deaths) because they considered that the menopausal status would be confused by treatment.

In current users of each type of HRT, the risk of breast cancer increased with increasing total duration of use. The authors estimate that 10 years use of HRT results in five additional breast cancers per thousand users of oestrogen-only preparations and 19 additional cancers per 1000 users of oestrogen and progestogen combinations.

Furthermore, the authors extrapolate the data by claiming that HRT used by women aged 50–64 years in the UK within the past decade has resulted in an estimated 20,000 extra breast cancers. This claim is not supported by UK (or US) cancer statistics where breast cancer numbers have plateaued since 1993.

Another oddity is the finding of no increase in breast cancer incidence or breast cancer deaths in past users. If oestrogens really are carcinogenic this is different to other promoters of malignancy such as tobacco, asbestos or even nulliparity or a late menopause where the excess risk does not reach zero 2 years after the exposure.

There are many critiques of this study,[13–15] but my own views are that the following points need to be addressed:

1. Is the percentage of women taking HRT in the UK correct? Of the women recruited for MWS, 50% were ever-users and 33% were current users. These very high percentages contradict publications concerning the frequency of HRT use in the UK. This is an atypical population as at least two-thirds of ERT/HRT users stop hormonal intake within 1 year and according to the study of European countries including the UK only 10% of all women use ERT long-term.

2. Unfortunately, after the initial questionnaire and categorisation, it was not possible for the authors to have information about continuation of HRT or changes in treatment as there was no follow-up questionnaire. This inadequacy of information is not corrected by the large numbers involved in the study as claimed by Beral and colleagues as it may re-inforce errors rather than cancel them out. Not only are the results of the MWS based on one time data collection by questionnaire with no follow-up, but not all centres have reported back. No clinical statement concerning the conditions of treatment can be made on the basis of these data as indications for treatment, dosage route, consideration of contra-indications and compliance is not recognisable from the paper. This is an important point since the rate of side-effects is directly related to the quality of treatment such as individualisation, and choice of preparation and dose according to the symptoms or pathology to be treated.

3. Are women attending for mammography in some way selective regarding risk and anxiety? It is likely that a high-grade selection has occurred in that women registered voluntarily for screening on long-term HRT considered they were risk cases for on-going breast cancer. Also women taking ERT are more willing to register for safety screening.

4. Why is the excess of breast cancers during the first year of HRT not excluded as it is a biological impossibility for such tumours if caused by oestrogen to be apparent as an invasive tumour within the first year of treatment?

5. If oestrogens are carcinogenic why are recent past-users clear of risk? This sudden return to normality does not occur with other carcinogens.

6. The pathology was not checked by a second independent pathologist. This has been the fault of all of the previous papers showing an excess of breast cancer of a better prognosis in women taking HRT. A Swedish study[15] re-evaluated the histology of endometrial cancer associated with oestrogen use and downgraded more than 33% to a lesser diagnosis of atypical or adenomatous hyperplasia. This should be done with the MWS data which show an increase in the first 2 years and no excess on stopping HRT as

this sounds more like ductal *in situ* carcinoma stimulated with oestrogens than invasive cancer. This diagnostic grey area occurs in about 4% of cases and should be investigated and, if appropriate, excluded.

7. The increased risk from Tibolone is surprising. There has been a belief that Tibolone acting like a SERM may have a protective effect upon the breast – a view supported by considerable laboratory and clinical work. It has, therefore, been common-place for Tibolone to be prescribed for higher risk women with a family history or in the presence of benign breast disease. There must have been a degree of selective prescribing.

8. A table refers to ethinyloestradiol at 10 times the correct dose even if this oestrogen was never used in HRT. It is not. This is clearly a mistake missed by the authors, the reviewers and the editors. It would have been picked up if there had been the most rudimentary clinical input into the study which would also have revealed the more eccentric claims and conclusions of the study. There are also at least 15 other errors of data presentation in the text and tables including multiple discrepant estimates given in the abstract, the text and the figures together with incorrect arithmetic in both text and tables. As things stand, we have an influential and hastily written paper of such carelessness above the surface that it brings into question the validity of the mathematics and statistics below the surface and indeed any of the conclusions made.

CURRENT ADVICE FOR HRT PRESCRIBING

1. Oestrogen treatment should be used for the treatment of specific symptoms and low bone density. Although licensing authorities have stated that oestrogens should not be first choice therapy for the prevention or treatment of osteoporosis, most gynaecological endocrinologists would strongly disagree.

2. Although oestrogens appear to have no place for the secondary prevention of cardiovascular disease, we believe it is still indicated in the early menopausal women for protection against CHD and perhaps strokes and Alzheimer's disease. There is a window of opportunity in 45–60-year-old symptomatic women who may show long-term cardiovascular and neurological benefits from early oestrogen therapy.

3. Oestrogens commenced in older women of 60–79 years may do 'early harm' in the form of heart attacks, strokes and vascular dementia before any benefit is achieved.

4. The dose and route will depend upon the symptoms, and the age of the patient. Peri-menopausal and post-menopausal patients with vasomotor symptoms should be given either oral or transdermal oestradiol with cyclical progestogen for endometrial protection.

5. Proven benefits of HRT confirmed in randomised trials are an improvement of symptoms such as hot flushes, night sweats, insomnia, vaginal dryness, and peri-menopausal depression and also a decrease in colon cancer, vertebral and hip fractures.

6. Major side effects of HRT are VTE, breast cancer (perhaps only with oestrogen/progestogen preparations) and strokes and heart attacks in older high-risk women receiving premarin.

7. The usual duration of progestogen is 14 days: however, if the extra risk to the breasts from progestogen is confirmed, it would be sensible to reduce the duration to 7 days. This shortened course is useful in women with progestogen intolerance.

8. Patients may wish to avoid bleeding by using low- dose oestrogen and progestogen or have insertion of a Mirena IUS or use Tibolone.

9. Patients with hormone-responsive mood disorders should have a higher dose of transdermal oestrogens either by patch, gel or implant. As these are often progestogen-intolerant, 7-day cycles of progestogen are permissible.

10. If loss of libido and loss of energy remain a problem, the addition of testosterone should be considered.

11 The lowest effective dose should be used remembering that the dose for the elimination of vasomotor symptoms will be less than the dose required for mood disorders or low bone density.

12. The indication and the need for HRT should be reviewed each year with discussion of the current views on risk.

13. A 5-year duration has been recommended but, in reality, women remain on HRT if they are feeling well with relief of symptoms. It is difficult to persuade these women to stop even after 10 or more years.

14. A mammogram should be performed each year and breast examination every 6 months.

Note added in proof

- The recently published WHI oestrogen only arm is most interesting.[16] Although the editorial and the press coverage reported that the study had been discontinued because of an increased risk of strokes without any increase in breast cancer or heart attacks, the stratified results by age are very different.

- If the patients aged 50–59 are examined there is: a 42% decrease in heart attacks (16v29); a 28% decrease in breast cancer (25v35); a 41% decrease in colorectal cancer (8v14); a 27% decrease in mortality (34v47); and a 20% decrease in 'global index' of complications (104v132). There was a 22% increase in VTE (18v15), and allegedly an 8% increase in strokes (19v19).

- It does appear that HRT, particularly oestrogen only is not only safe but beneficial in the age group which in this country is normal for commencing treatment.

References

1 Hulley, Grady, Bush T et al. Randomized trial of estrogen plus progestin for secondary prevention of coronary heart disease in post-menopausal women.

2 Writing Group for Women's Health Initiative Investigators. Risks and benefits of estrogen plus progestin in healthy postmenopausal women; principal results from the Women's Health Initiative randomized controlled trial. JAMA 2002; 288: 321–333

3 Beral V. and Million Women Study Collaborators (Breast cancer and hormone-replacement therapy in the Million Women Study. Lancet 2003; 362: 419–427

4 Lagro-Jannsen T, Rosser WW, van Weel C. Breast cancer and hormone-replacement therapy; up to general practice to pick up the pieces. Lancet 2003; 362: 414–415

5 Studd J. Up to general practice to pick up the pieces – what pieces? – a response to WHI and MWS. Maturitas 2003; 46: 95–97

6 Hays J, Ockene JK, Brunner RL et al. and Women's Health Initiative Investigators. Effects of estrogen plus progestin on health-related quality of life. N Engl J Med 2003; 348: 1839–1856

7 Stampfer MJ, Colditz GA, Willett WC et al. Post menopausal estrogen therapy and cardio-vascular disease; ten year follow-up from the Nurses' Health Study. N Engl J Med 1991; 325: 756–762

8 De Lignieres B, de Vathaire F, Fournier S, Urbinelli R, Allaert F, Le MG et al. Combined hormone replacement therapy and risk of breast cancer in a French cohort study of 3175 women. Climacteric 2002; 5: 332–340

9 Sourander L, Rajala T, Raiha I, Makinen J, Erkkola R, Helenius H. Cardiovascular and cancer morbidity and mortality and sudden cardiac deaths in postmenopausal women on oestrogen replacement therapy (ERT). Lancet 1998; 352: 1965–1969

10 Collaborative Group on Hormonal Factors in Breast Cancer. Breast cancer and hormone replacement therapy; collaborative reanalysis of data from 51 epidemiological studies of 52,705 women with breast cancer. Lancet 1997; 350: 1047–1059

11 Chlebowski RT, Hendrix SL, Langer RD et al. and WHI Investigators. Influence of estrogen plus progestin on breast cancer and mammography in healthy postmenopausal women: the Women's Health Initiative Randomised Trial. JAMA 2003; 289: 3243–3253

12 Speroff L. The Million Women Study and breast cancer. Maturitas 2003; 46: 1–6

13 Genazzani AR, Gambacciani M. The sound of an international anti-HRT herald. Maturitas 2003; 46: 105–106

14 Sturdee DW, MacLennan AH. Is combined estrogen/progestogen hormone therapy worth the risk? Climacteric 2003; 6: 177–179

15 Persson I, Adami HO, Lindgren A, Norlinder H, Pettersson B, Silver S. Reliability of endometrial cancer diagnoses in a Swedish Cancer Registry – with special reference to classification bias related to exogenous estrogens. Acta Pathol Microbiol Immunol Scand 1986; 94: 187–194

16. Studd JWW. Second thoughts on the WHI and MWS –The importance of age for HRT safety. 2004 (In press)

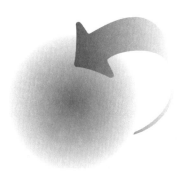

Index